ROBERT D. DRIPPS, M.D.
Late Vice-President for Health Affairs and
Professor, Department of Anesthesia,
The University of Pennsylvania School of Medicine,
Philadelphia

JAMES E. ECKENHOFF, M.D.
Dean and Professor of Anesthesia,
Northwestern University Medical School,
Chicago

LEROY D. VANDAM, M.D.
Professor of Anaesthesia, Harvard Medical School;
Anesthesiologist-in-Chief, Peter Bent Brigham Hospital,
Boston

Introduction to
ANESTHESIA

THE PRINCIPLES OF SAFE PRACTICE

Fifth Edition

Line Drawings by Dr. Vandam

W. B. SAUNDERS COMPANY
Philadelphia • London • Toronto

W. B. Saunders Company: West Washington Square
Philadelphia, PA 19105

1 St. Anne's Road
Eastbourne, East Sussex BN21 3UN, England

1 Goldthorne Avenue
Toronto, Ontario M8Z 5T9, Canada

Introduction to Anesthesia: The Principles of Safe Practice   ISBN 0-7216-3193-2

© 1977 by W. B. Saunders Company. Copyright 1957, 1961, 1967 and 1972 by W. B. Saunders Company. Copyright under the International Copyright Union. All rights reserved. This book is protected by copyright. No part of it may be reproduced, stored in a retrieval system, or transmitted in any form or by any means, electronic, mechanical, photocopying, recording, or otherwise, without written permission from the publisher. Made in the United States of America. Press of W. B. Saunders Company. Library of Congress catalog card number 76-51011.

Last digit is the print number: 9   8   7   6   5   4   3

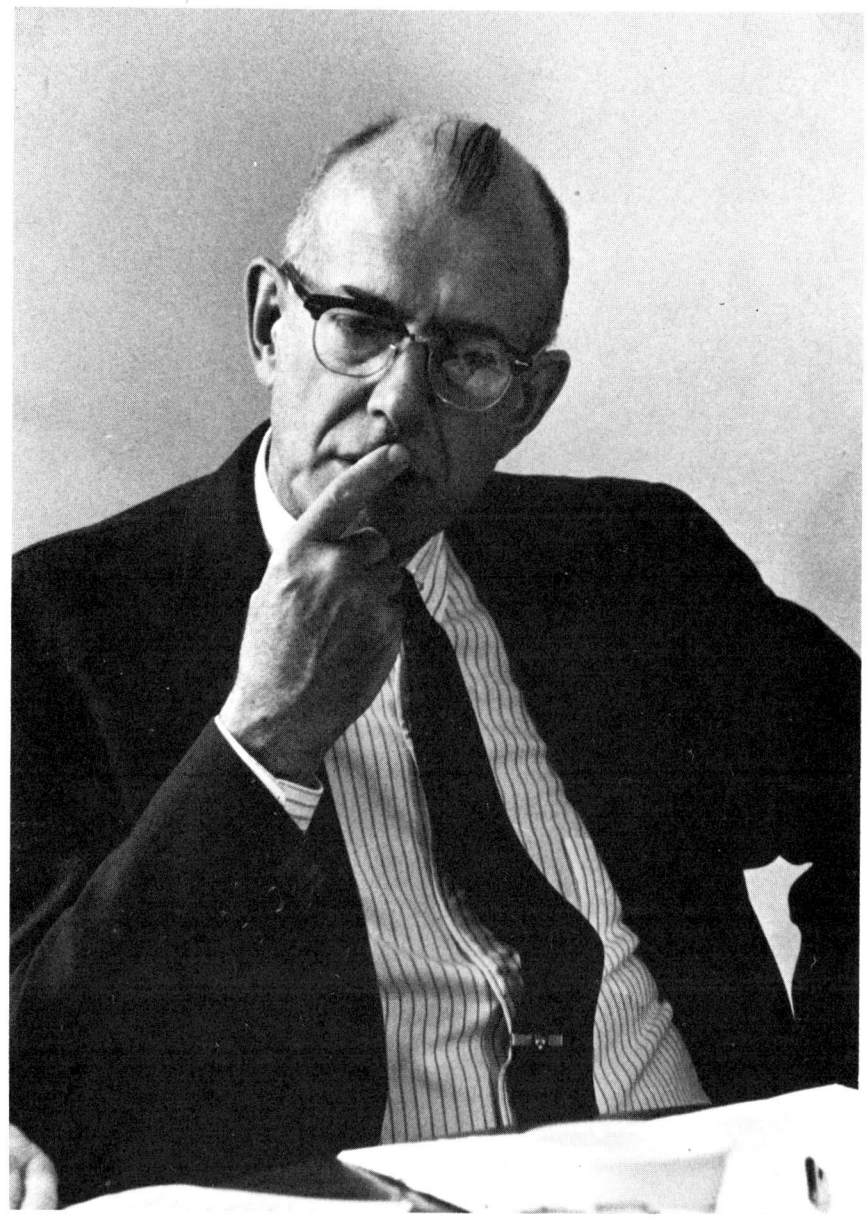

This book is dedicated to the memory of
ROBERT D. DRIPPS,
our tutor, colleague, and cherished comrade.
He remains very much alive in these pages.

PREFACE TO THE FIFTH EDITION

Approximately 20 years ago, three anesthesiologists at the University of Pennsylvania resolved to publish a text on anesthesia in the belief that the need was great. The idea was conceived in October of 1956, a first draft was completed at Barnegat Light, New Jersey, one cold week in January, the final manuscript was sent to W. B. Saunders Company in March, and the book was published in September of 1957 at a price of $4.75. Our purpose was fourfold: to offer an introductory text, to write the material as succinctly as possible, to base the message strictly on fact, and to keep the price of the book at a minimum.

In each subsequent edition we have striven to abide by the original intentions. But as the field of anesthesia broadened and the available information expanded, the book inevitably grew larger. We have resisted the pressure to prepare a more comprehensive work. As our respective professional burdens increased, it became increasingly difficult to prepare the material by ourselves; in this, as in the last edition, our associates have helped us beyond measure. However, the text remains our sole responsibility. As will be apparent, there have been both deletions and additions in this latest effort, more than a few chapters have been entirely rewritten, the references have been brought up to date, and the material has been made consistent with current practice.

No one of us has been solely responsible for the original edition or any of the revisions, always a product of all three. If an impasse was reached, R. D. Dripps, by agreement as senior, had the last word. But seldom was he prompted to take a stance. We edited each others' chapters with vigor—even at times tore them apart! Little passed unchallenged. As a result, a rare synthesis of ideas was achieved.

Upon Bob Dripps' untimely and lamentable death in October of 1973, we were unsure of the wisdom of approaching a fifth edition. However, we were persuaded to do so by many friends, who thought that neglect of the task might constitute a disservice to anesthesiology. Hence we present a fifth edition, still under the authorship and style of Dripps, Eckenhoff, and Vandam. The first edition was dedicated to a dear surgeon friend, I. S. Ravdin. Dedications are usually not altered in subsequent editions, but we dare to break with tradition and dedicate the fifth to the memory of Robert Dunning Dripps, to whom both of us and all of medicine owe so much.

James Eckenhoff and Leroy Vandam are uncertain if there will be another edition to appear under their coauthorship. If still active in practice, we may well try again. Otherwise, if the hope is not realized, we trust that those whom we have taught and counseled will continue to work at the goal where we have left off—that of an introductory text, succinctly written, based on fact, and modestly priced.

JAMES E. ECKENHOFF
LEROY D. VANDAM

ACKNOWLEDGMENTS

DAVID L. BRUCE, M.D.
  Professor of Anesthesia, Northwestern University Medical School.
Pharmacologic Principles and Drug Interactions.

EDWARD A. BRUNNER, M.D., Ph.D.
  Professor and Chairman, Department of Anesthesia, Northwestern University Medical School.
Fundamentals of Inhalation Anesthesia; Inhalation Anesthetics; Evaluation of the Response to Anesthetics; Ambulatory Anesthesia Services.

JAY S. DEVORE, M.D.
  Assistant Professor of Anesthesia and of Obstetrics, Northwestern University Medical School.
Obstetric Anesthesia and Perinatology.

VLADIMIR FENCL, M.D.
  Associate Professor of Physiology (Anaesthesia), Harvard Medical School.
Respiration and Respiratory Care.

RONALD A. GABEL, M.D.
  Assistant Professor of Anaesthesia, Harvard Medical School.
Monitoring; Cardiopulmonary Resuscitation.

RONALD A. HARRISON, M.D.
  Assistant Professor of Clinical Anesthesia, Northwestern University Medical School.
Intravenous Fluids and Acid-Base Balance; Blood Component Therapy.

STANLEY LEE SON, M.D.
  Instructor in Anaesthesia, Harvard Medical School.
Anesthesia for Extracorporeal Circulation.

RICHARD M. LEVIN, M.D.
  Associate Professor of Clinical Anesthesia and Pediatrics, Northwestern University Medical School.
Pediatric Anesthesia.

HARRY W. LINDE, Ph.D.
Professor of Anesthesia, Northwestern University Medical School.

Anesthesia Equipment; Electric Hazards, Fires, and Explosions.

STEPHEN J. PREVOZNIK, M.D.
Associate Professor of Anesthesia, University of Pennsylvania Medical School.

Intravenous Anesthesia.

BARRY A. SHAPIRO, M.D.
Associate Professor of Clinical Anesthesia, Northwestern University Medical School.

Inhalation and Chest Physiotherapy.

BARBARA E. WAUD, M.D.
Professor of Anesthesia, University of Massachusetts Medical Center.

Neuromuscular Blocking Agents.

PREFACE TO THE FIRST EDITION

This book is a descendant of a smaller work privately printed in 1949 and circulated in the Department of Anesthesiology of the Hospital of the University of Pennsylvania. It was called "Organization and Procedures." A second and larger edition appeared in 1953. The third lineal descendant is now being made available to others.

Much of the teaching of anesthesia is by word of mouth. Beginners seek to learn countless details that cannot be found in general texts. This is the lore of anesthesia that must be passed on from individual to individual. A good bit of the material gathered in this volume might be classified as being in this rather shadowy area, including such topics as the philosophy of records, surgeon-anesthetist relations, the value of death reports, hazards of the immediate postoperative period, the treatment of immediate postoperative pain and excitement, and the determination of the depth of general anesthesia.

The subjects and the manner of their presentation represent the thinking and ultimate distillation into teaching practice of the senior staff at Pennsylvania, augmented and refined by all who came within teaching range. One who contributed much to the early editions and whose influence may be discerned in the present volume is Austin Lamont. We mention him with respect and give thanks to others who will find bits of their practice and philosophy in print.

Chapters dealing with fundamental aspects of certain techniques and with basic considerations of the drugs used in anesthesia have been included in the hope that such material can contribute to the safer practice of anesthesia. These are guides; they contain what we believe to be established precepts, but they are not covered in detail nor can they be regarded as complete.

We have intentionally omitted discussion of most of the specialized aspects of anesthesia such as hypothermia, deliberate hypotension, hypnosis, the technical considerations of regional anesthesia, and problems of the treatment of pain. These constitute advanced study in the field. We believe that the students for whom this book is intended should not be confronted by them until later in their training.

We trust that this book will be instructive for all students of anesthesia and those in other fields who would learn a little something of this specialty. We hope that it may be a useful introductory volume of interest before one proceeds to wider reading. Although we have listed only a few references as guides for further study, it has not been our intention to slight individuals who have made important contributions. Doubtless, omissions and reasons for disagreement will be found.

Dr. Henry L. Price, Dr. Ronald Woolmer and others of our associates have contributed valuable suggestions. Miss Sally Van de Water has performed yeoman service as our secretarial assistant. We acknowledge these contributions with gratitude.

ROBERT D. DRIPPS
JAMES E. ECKENHOFF
LEROY D. VANDAM

CONTENTS

Chapter 1
THE BROAD REALM OF ANESTHESIOLOGY 1

Section 1
PRELIMINARY CONSIDERATIONS

Chapter 2
PREANESTHETIC CONSULTATION AND CHOICE OF
ANESTHESIA 11

Chapter 3
PHARMACOLOGIC PRINCIPLES AND DRUG
INTERACTIONS 22

Chapter 4
PREMEDICATION, TRANSPORT TO THE OPERATING
ROOM, AND PREPARATION FOR ANESTHESIA 36

Section 2
ESSENTIAL PREANESTHETIC CONSIDERATIONS

Chapter 5
MEDICOLEGAL CONSIDERATIONS 51

Chapter 6
ANESTHESIA EQUIPMENT 59

Chapter 7
AN APPROACH TO ASEPSIS IN ANESTHESIA 78

Chapter 8
MONITORING 87

Chapter 9
THE ANESTHESIA RECORD 101

Section 3
ANESTHESIA AND OPERATION

Part A Inhalation Anesthesia

Chapter 10
FUNDAMENTALS OF INHALATION ANESTHESIA 115

Chapter 11
INHALATION ANESTHETICS 133

Chapter 12
TECHNIQUES OF INHALATION ANESTHESIA 162

Part B Intravenous Anesthesia and Tracheal Intubation

Chapter 13
INTRAVENOUS ANESTHESIA 174

Chapter 14
NEUROMUSCULAR BLOCKING AGENTS 195

Chapter 15
INTUBATION OF THE TRACHEA 216

Chapter 16
EVALUATION OF THE RESPONSE TO ANESTHETICS:
THE SIGNS AND STAGES 231

Part C Regional Anesthesia

Chapter 17
LOCAL ANESTHETICS 242

Chapter 18
SPINAL ANESTHESIA 260

Contents xv

Chapter 19
PERIDURAL AND CAUDAL ANESTHESIA 278

Chapter 20
REGIONAL NERVE BLOCKS.. 288

Part D   Intravenous Supportive Therapy

Chapter 21
INTRAVENOUS FLUIDS AND ACID-BASE BALANCE 309

Chapter 22
BLOOD COMPONENT THERAPY 330

Part E   The Specialties

Chapter 23
OBSTETRIC ANESTHESIA AND PERINATOLOGY 346

Chapter 24
PEDIATRIC ANESTHESIA 364

Chapter 25
AMBULATORY ANESTHESIA SERVICES... 388

Chapter 26
SPECIAL TECHNIQUES 396

Part F   Untoward Sequelae of Anesthesia

Chapter 27
ARTERIAL HYPOTENSION DURING ANESTHESIA 409

Chapter 28
COMPLICATIONS OF ANESTHESIA 427

Chapter 29
ELECTRIC HAZARDS, FIRES, AND EXPLOSIONS.......................... 436

Section 4
ANCILLARY ANESTHESIA CARE

Chapter 30
CARDIOPULMONARY RESUSCITATION 447

Chapter 31
THE IMMEDIATE POSTOPERATIVE PERIOD: RECOVERY AND INTENSIVE CARE 460

Chapter 32
INHALATION AND CHEST PHYSIOTHERAPY 471

Chapter 33
RESPIRATION AND RESPIRATORY CARE 485

Appendix: I. *Common Abbreviations* 522
II. *Numerical Equivalents* 523

Index 525

Chapter 1

THE BROAD REALM OF ANESTHESIOLOGY

Anesthesia is recognized as a major American contribution to medicine. News of the first successful demonstration of ether in Boston, in 1846, spread rapidly to Europe where leading surgeons were quick to try this remarkable substance. Within a year another general anesthetic, chloroform, was used in England, and the introduction of the two agents set the stage for the development of the specialty of anesthesia in the two countries. Chloroform was introduced by an eminent obstetrician, James Y. Simpson. It was both a respiratory and circulatory depressant, requiring great skill in administration and lethal in unskilled hands. A large number of deaths attested to the potency of chloroform; therefore only physicians were judged competent to administer it.

In the United States, dentist William T. G. Morton, who had publicly introduced ether, was challenged for the priority by his collaborator, scientist Charles Jackson, by dentist Horace Wells who earlier introduced nitrous oxide, and finally by physician Crawford W. Long, who had first given ether in 1842 but without audience or publication. The attempts at establishing patents and the controversy over who should receive recognition for its discovery placed anesthesia under a cloud. In contrast to chloroform, ether stimulated both respiration and circulation, which was thought to be a built-in protection for the patient and the reason why a skilled person did not have to administer it. Students, nurses, newly graduated physicians, specialists in other fields, and even custodians were called upon to be "etherizers." When toward the end of the century nurses were encouraged to become full-time anesthetists, patients received better care because someone with continuing experience was anesthetizing them.

Some 60 years elapsed before the first American physician began to devote full time to anesthesia. While the strides made by surgery around the turn of the century were great, little change occurred in anesthesia, even though some surgeons pleaded for anesthesia specialists. Two separate series of events sparked the development of anesthesia as a discipline. The first comprised two world wars, which created a need for large numbers of anesthetists to care for battle casualties. The second was the increasingly complex nature of operations, which produced a demand for

1

more skilled help. In 1931 there were enough specialists on hand to form the American Society of Anesthetists, and in 1937 the American Board of Anesthesiologists began to certify specialists. New agents and equipment appeared, and the older agents were studied anew in the laboratory and clinic. Training programs arose throughout the country, the better ones attracting many trainees at the conclusion of World War II. The introduction of curare, with the accompanying need for control of pulmonary ventilation during and after operations, and the organization of postanesthesia recovery rooms provided further breadth for the fledgling specialty. By 1950 anesthesiologists' activities began to spread beyond the confines of the operating room.

For more than 100 years after the introduction of ether surgeons had dominated the operating room, everyone bowing to their authority. This dominance now began to wane. Operating teams evolved consisting of several surgeons, anesthetists, and highly competent nurses. The development of new agents, adjuvants, equipment, and techniques had changed anesthesia into a discipline now beyond the training of surgeons who had formerly supervised technicians or had given the anesthetics themselves. Therefore most surgeons readily welcomed physician anesthetists as full partners in the surgical team.

Over the past two decades, anesthesiology has emerged as a clearly defined specialty recognized and respected throughout the country. In every medical school anesthesiology functions mostly as an autonomous academic department, in some as a division of surgery. There are approximately 2300 physicians in training in 164 anesthesiology residency programs in the United States. The American Board of Anesthesiologists to date has certified over 8000 specialists, and the Board has been recognized as a leader among specialty boards in setting standards and improving techniques of examination. Approximately 4.5 per cent of all physicians practicing in the United States are anesthesiologists. There are more than a few national societies and an impressive number of journals and texts is published each year on the subject.

NURSE ANESTHETISTS AND ANESTHESIOLOGISTS

About one half of the 20 million anesthetics given annually in the United States are administered by nonphysicians. Thus the public is confused as to the difference between a nurse anesthetist and an anesthesiologist. To become certified as a registered nurse anesthetist (CRNA) the nurse must have a high school education, an average of three years of nursing training, plus two additional years of anesthesia training followed by an examination. To become an anesthesiologist, after college and award of the medical degree a physician must have four years of postgraduate training in an approved residency program, with one year devoted to medicine, surgery, or other clinical discipline. Two years are spent in clinical anesthesia and the optional fourth in a specialized area of choice. Some engage in practice for two years in lieu of the optional fourth year. Those qualified take an examination to become diplomates of the American Board of Anesthesiology. In the United States, neither a nurse nor a physician has to pass certification to practice anesthesiology, nor indeed, any other specialty. It is possible to administer anesthesia without formal training if a hospital will accept the lack of credentials!

It is apparent that the physician anesthesiologist offers greater depth of training than the nurse anesthetist, but this does not necessarily qualify the physician as a better anesthetist. By achieving the technical skills and the appropriate experience and knowledge, a conscientious nurse can easily surmount the gap in training. An anesthesiologist, acting as a technician, who fails to keep abreast of advances in medicine soon loses the advantage.

In general, the CRNA is an employee of a hospital; a few practice on a fee-for-service basis, as do most anesthesiologists. Their malpractice liability is less than that of physicians (see Chapter 5). For the most part their activities are confined to the operating room; they often do not participate in pre- or postoperative care and are not in a position by virtue of their background to exercise medical judgment. In the eyes of the law they function under the medical direction of physicians, either the surgeon or an anesthesiologist.

In most large hospital departments nurse and physician anesthetists and technicians work in harmony. Cases are assigned by physicians who evaluate the patients preoperatively, write preoperative notes and preanesthetic orders, assist as necessary during anesthesia, remain available for consultation, and care for patients postoperatively in the event of complications. Considering the extensive national demands for anesthesia care it is unlikely that all anesthetics will ever be given solely by physicians. As paralleled by the trend toward midwifery in obstetrics, there is and always will be a need for nurse anesthetists.

FUNCTIONS OF THE ANESTHESIOLOGIST

The principal tasks of the anesthesiologist are to provide relief from pain for patients during operation and optimal operative conditions for surgeons, both in the safest possible manner. To do this the anesthesiologist must be a competent physician and a clinical pharmacologist, with a broad knowledge of surgery and the ability to utilize and interpret correctly a variety of monitoring devices.

In addition to anesthetics, drugs employed by anesthesiologists include: opioids and antagonists, antisialagogues, barbiturates, tranquilizers, vasopressors, vasodilators, antiarrhythmics, cardiotonics, antihypertensives, neuromuscular blockers and antagonists, analeptics and steroids – to cite just a few. In recent years the interaction of drugs and their pathways of elimination have assumed increasing importance, not only from the viewpoint of widespread drug usage by patients but also because inhalation anesthetics, once thought inert, are now known to undergo metabolic transformation, interacting with other drugs and body components.

Anesthetists must combine a knowledge of the patient's disease, the drugs taken, the demands of the operation, and the patient's concerns in order to arrive at a proper choice of agent and technique. Most monitoring devices in use in intensive care units today are modifications and extensions of equipment first used by anesthetists in operating suites. Recovery rooms arose out of the need for continued individual patient care, and today both surgical and medical intensive care units extend such attention to all critically ill patients. Blood pressure via direct or indirect recording, heart and breath sounds, blood gas analysis, central venous pressure, body temperature, and pulmonary wedge pressure commonly are measured during anesthesia and an electrocardiogram and an electroencephalogram taken.

Fluid replacement during operation is supervised by the anesthetist, who establishes the routes of administration and the kinds of fluids given while keeping track of blood loss and therefore determining blood or blood component therapy needed. In this sphere, consultation between surgeon and anesthetist is essential.

Anesthetists spend more time in the operating room than any other group of physicians. It is logical, therefore, that many institutions have appointed an anesthesiologist chief of the operating room, responsible for day to day scheduling and overall supervision of activities.

In the United States, prior to the introduction of curare, the principal anesthetic used was ether. Because of its stimulant effect on respiration, control of ventilation was of little importance. Cyclopropane depressed respiration in light planes of anesthesia, allowing for easier control of respiration, but failed to provide good abdominal relaxation. Curare altered all of this; with muscle relaxation came respiratory paralysis. Not only was the patient unconscious but unable to breathe as well. By necessity, anesthetists became respiratory physiologists and experts at managing ventilatory inadequacy. New ventilators were devised, monitoring equipment was introduced to ensure ventilatory exchange, and blood gas analysis was perfected. Again, such expertise could not be restricted to the operating room. Anesthetists began to be consulted in intensive care and respiratory care units, in the care of traumatized patients and those with neurologic deficits. In many hospitals today, anesthesiologists manage respiratory and inhalation therapy services; an appreciable number are solely involved in these endeavors (see Chapters 32 and 33).

SPECIALIZED ANESTHESIA SERVICES

Some anesthetists allied with general surgical services have found the field too broad and have preferred to specialize. While a few have elected neurosurgical or cardiothoracic operations, even more have opted for pediatric and obstetric anesthesia. Management of the critically ill child, the infant, or the neonate is quite a challenge, as is made evident in Chapter 24; techniques used, responses to agents, monitoring, and the rapidity with which physiologic changes take place differ from what occurs in the adult. Only recently have anesthetists chosen to care for obstetric patients. Anesthesia remains a leading cause of maternal mortality, and fetal monitoring is a developing field (see Chapter 23). Nevertheless, the problems of pain relief during labor; opportunities for the selection of regional or general anesthesia; the anesthetic care of two lives simultaneously; neonatal resuscitation; and the not uncommon emergencies that arise all add up to a challenging and rewarding activity.

Anesthetists have been in the vanguard in establishing ambulatory or day care surgical services. Operations performed on an ambulatory basis minimize costs and reserve available hospital beds for the critically ill and those requiring major procedures. Anesthetists arrange the schedule, interview and instruct patients before the day of operation, admit and examine them, anesthetize, supervise recovery, and discharge them (see Chapter 25). Anesthesia for the outpatient is quite different from in-hospital care; only reasonable risks for anesthesia can be accepted, and only agents that dissipate rapidly are administered.

Relief of pain during operations can be provided by means other than general anesthesia. Regional anesthesia, without loss of the patient's consciousness, is afforded by injection of local anesthetics into either the subarachnoid or the epidural space, in proximity to nerve trunks, or infiltrated into areas in which the incision will be made. Skill with the needle need not be confined to operation. Various neurosurgical and circulatory illnesses are amenable to nerve blocks, which are of value therapeutically, diagnostically, and prognostically. Anesthesiologists have established pain clinics, evaluated the newer local anesthetics, and published detailed observations on pain and its relief. Others have been concerned with major investigations into the actions and effectiveness of opioids and their antagonists as well as analgesics, sedatives, and tranquilizers.

Every day, anesthetists face cardiorespiratory emergencies in and out of the operating room. It is only natural that they should have organized cardiopulmonary resuscitation teams throughout hospitals, evolved rescue and transport systems for cases of cardiac arrest and drowning, and instructed firemen, the police, and civilians in emergency procedures.

RESEARCH

The opportunities for research in anesthesia are boundless. After all, the mechanism by which general anesthetics act is still unknown, 130 years after their discovery. Curare was a laboratory curiosity for nearly 90 years until anesthetists put it to use in clinical anesthesia. Every patient to whom anesthesia is administered presents the opportunity to record clinical observations and accumulate data, provided that the ethics of research are observed. Standard monitoring equipment is of better quality than that used in most laboratories several decades ago.

Nearly all academic departments of anesthesia support laboratories for fundamental investigations. In the two decades following World War II most basic studies on anesthesia largely involved the respiratory or circulatory systems. Now we have moved in the direction of biochemical and metabolic research, with emphasis on the pharmacokinetics of anesthetics, enzyme induction, toxicology, and cellular and immunologic effects. There is opportunity for full-time research in anesthesia, and most departments have one or more people so engaged. Many residency programs offer one or two years of training in research techniques during the years required for board certification. Moreover, more than a few anesthesiologists spend part of their time engaged in clinical activities and the remainder in either laboratory or clinical investigation.

TEACHING

Anesthesiology bridges the gap between basic and clinical science. Of all the disciplines, it is most suited to reinforcement of information learned in biochemistry, physiology, and pharmacology in the context of a patient's disease. Anesthesia practice is the ideal setting in which to teach ventilatory control and adequacy of respiratory exchange, circulatory monitoring, care of the comatose, assessment of levels of consciousness, and fluid replacement. Tracheal intubation, insertion of venous cannulas, and spinal tap are also logically taught on an anesthesia service. Postgraduate training in anesthesia differs from that in other fields because it must be individualized. Considering the breadth of the surgical and obstetric fields, the specialty has wide exposure to many disciplines and has the advantage of receiving information from all. Practically all university departments of anesthesia still seek qualified anesthesiologists interested in teaching and research as well as in clinical practice.

SURGEON-ANESTHETIST RELATIONS

Surgeons and anesthetists constitute a team of physicians dedicated to the welfare of the surgical patient whose interest is best served if each member of the team recognizes his or her responsibilities, yet remains aware of the problems faced by colleagues. The anesthetist's position on the team is clearly defined: he or she must have a thorough knowledge of the patient's medical history, the operation proposed, and the risks involved. The stresses placed upon the bodily systems by the contemplated anesthesia and surgical procedure must be understood. There must be discussion with the surgeon and other consultants concerning unfamiliar aspects of the patient's disease. The surgeon should be informed of the patient's progress, not by routine recitation of vital signs but by instant transmission of important information. A multitude of details must be constantly monitored that would distract the surgeon's attention from the technical problems of operation. Care of the patient in the crucial immediate postoperative period must be closely supervised while the surgeon is engaged elsewhere.

A surgeon should consult with the anesthetist before operation and discuss the details of surgical management. It is unwise to insist upon unnecessary speed in induction of anesthesia, since this can be detrimental to the patient. A particular anesthetic or technique rarely should be demanded, as the surgeon may not know the limits of an anesthetist's capabilities or the potential for harm of certain anesthetics and techniques. Cadaveric relaxation never is needed and cannot be produced with genuine safety under any circumstance. Problems peculiar to anesthesia must be realized and time allowed for their solution. On occasion the surgeon must agree to rapid conclusion of the operation if the anesthetist believes that the patient's condition is deteriorating; development of malignant hyperthermia is a good example (see Chapter 28).

A team is at its best when its members have worked together repeatedly. It takes time for individuals to learn where they fit into the scheme of things and how associates perform their particular tasks. Good teamwork arises from mutual respect. A new member of the team must be proved worthy before acceptance on the same basis as the others.

Surgical teams work under a variety of circumstances. In most operations there should be little tension, but in difficult operations or those in which complications arise, tempers may flare and harsh words may be exchanged. The care of the patient may suffer as a result. Surgeon and anesthetist must visualize each other's predicament. Technically simple operations may be performed under trying anesthetic conditions, while an intricate, difficult operation may be performed without anesthetic incident. If irritability is displayed by any member of the team, the others must assess the situation and minimize friction if possible. The operating room is no place for verbal battle. Words spoken in anger can be withdrawn later on, but if the patient has suffered, irreparable damage may ensue.

The inexperienced observer sometimes believes that the anesthetist occupies a position subordinate to that of the surgeon. This feeling often arises from lack of experience with the team performance of complex operations, although the anesthetist may contribute to his or her subordinate status by failing to participate fully in medical care. Evidence that an anesthetist is first a physician and then a competent specialist will assure acceptance as an equal in the overall care of patients.

Confusion often exists in the minds of both surgeons and anesthetists as to medicolegal responsibility in anesthesia. A study of court rulings confirms that surgeons are responsible for the anesthetic only if administered by a nurse or technician under their medical direction. Anesthetics given by anesthesiologists constitute their legal responsibility.

One might summarize the essentials of successful surgeon-anesthetist relations as comprising mutual professional confidence, understanding, frankness, honesty, courtesy, and fair-mindedness.

APPRAISAL

Anesthesiology is now a mature specialty, but its limits have not yet been clearly defined. We are unable to fill all the academic and clinical positions available, some in eminent institutions. Because of the intimate association with so many other specialty areas, a discerning anesthetist is more likely than not to stay abreast of the advances in medicine. The relationship with the basic sciences is close, perhaps more so than in other specialties. Some have charged that the practice of anesthesiology is too routine and lacks intellectual challenge. This is a matter of individual opinion, for certainly the authors of this text have not lacked for challenge. Every branch of medicine has its share of routine. How much of a pediatrician's day is spent in examining normal infants and children, in giving prophylactic injections, or in treating respiratory infections? Obstetricians deal mostly with normal women who will deliver without incident, and a day in an internist's office has more than its share of routine work. So with anesthesia! Most patients will be healthy, undergo elective, uncomplicated operations, and recover from anesthesia without incident. Few specialists, however, encounter such a high ratio of stressful moments in which a wrong or a tardy decision may spell disaster.

REFERENCES

Bunker JP: The Anesthesiologist and the Surgeon. Partners in the Operating Room. Boston, Little, Brown Co, 1972.
Eckenhoff JE: Anesthesia from Colonial Times. Philadelphia, J B Lippincott Co, 1966.
Greene NM: Anesthesiology and the University. Philadelphia, J B Lippincott Co, 1975.
Vandam LD: Early American anesthetists: The origins of professionalism in anesthesia. Anesthesiology 38:264, 1963.

Section 1

PRELIMINARY CONSIDERATIONS

Chapter 2

PREANESTHETIC CONSULTATION AND CHOICE OF ANESTHESIA

At one time the crucial phase of a surgical illness was thought to be the operation—the chance of survival depending upon the patient's response to anesthesia. A question often posed was whether a patient in poor physical condition could tolerate the anesthetic; this concern has now undergone modification. Anesthesia is still of major importance, to be given with skill and good judgment, but it is the quality of pre- and postanesthetic care that largely determines whether the outcome will be satisfactory. This overall approach to anesthesia has led to a decrease in the number of intraoperative complications and to a reduction in postoperative morbidity and mortality despite the extremes of age and the greater severity of disease in patients coming to operation.

Participation by the anesthetist in preparation of the patient for operation improves the outcome because the anesthetist is knowledgeable in the pathophysiology of disease as it pertains to the action of anesthetics. Anesthetists must establish their reputations with the expectation that they will be asked to consult on operability and to help prepare the patient for the procedure. The attitude that this is "their" patient goes a long way toward dispelling the notion that anesthetists lack responsibility in patient care. Surgeons and referring physicians should avail themselves of anesthetists' advice and acquaint them with specific aspects of the illness as well as the procedure planned.

GUIDELINES FOR THE PREANESTHETIC VISIT

Every patient should be seen by an anesthetist before operation. For this reason it is necessary that patients be admitted to the hospital early enough to permit a complete examination. Past and present hospital records should be reviewed with attention focused on prior experiences and the physiologic alterations induced by disease. The ability to tolerate adverse effects of anesthesia and operation depends largely upon the normality of respiration and circulation and of the homeostatic functions of the liver, kidneys, endocrines, and central nervous system.

There is no substiture for talking to patients, listening to their problems, and acquainting them with the procedure planned. Thus the visit is a subtle educational process for both patient and anesthetist; the patient learns what anesthesia has to offer, and if misconceptions exist they can be dispelled. The interview should be unhurried and tactful; if the patient is eating or receiving special therapy it is better to return at another time. If visitors are present they should be asked to leave before the examination.

If a patient has not yet been informed of the decision to operate, anesthesia can be described as though it were to take place in the future. It is best to avoid discussion of matters in the surgeon's domain. Questioning should proceed along lines of past anesthetic experiences, familial problems with anesthetics, routine use of drugs, and unusual reactions to drugs and the concurrent illness (see Chapter 3).

While assessing the patient's emotional state, one should look for physical characteristics that may cause technical difficulties during anesthesia. The individual with a short, stout neck readily develops respiratory obstruction once unconscious; the athlete requires more medication than the asthenic. If there are loose or carious teeth or delicate dental work, the patient should be warned that dislodgement or damage may occur upon airway insertion, and a note to that effect should be written on the chart. Patients should be told to remove dentures and leave them in the room so that they will not be broken or misplaced.

An anesthetist should perform those elements of a physical examination deemed necessary. Simple tests of pulmonary function may be performed and reserves of the cardiopulmonary system ascertained by questioning the patient about tolerance to exercise. A patient may be asked to walk in the corridor or up a flight of stairs to detect shortness of breath or claudication. In a patient with a history of myocardial infarction, presence or absence of angina pectoris provides an essential but not always conclusive index of sufficiency of coronary blood flow. Adequacy of digitalization can be determined by counting the pulse after exercise; a rise in rate from 72 to 120 beats per minute as a result of walking 20 to 30 feet suggests the need for a higher dose. A history of palpitation, or appearance of premature atrial or ventricular beats or left bundle block on the electrocardiogram may be the only clues to myocardial disease. If regional anesthesia is planned it is essential to inspect and palpate the site selected for injection of spinal or caudal anesthesia. It helps to test the effect of the operative position on circulation and respiration; for example, the arthritic patient may not tolerate the lithotomy position.

Once the preliminaries are over, the patient is told of the plans for anesthesia. Reactions will vary; some patients will accede readily, while others who fear the face mask or needle puncture will wish to be unconscious before going to the operating room. Still others will be concerned about postoperative vomiting or pain. Many object to spinal anesthesia, having heard that headache or paralysis may follow. Explanation and reassurance usually settle most of these problems, but the anesthetist should not be unyielding in choice of agent or technique. Finally, a plan is elected in the patient's best interest, bearing in mind the surgeon's needs. Most patients accept a physician's advice when confidence is inspired.

Special examinations and laboratory work should be carried out when necessary. If the patient has been admitted to the hospital late in the afternoon it may be necessary to wait until the morning of operation for a complete record, but there should be no compromise in quality even at this late time.

Patients should have a good night's sleep. They should be told when medications will be given and warned not to eat or drink during the six to eight hours preceding anesthesia; the reasons for this should be made explicit. The time and manner of transport to the operating room should be discussed, as well as the plan for postoperative observation in the recovery or intensive care area.

When the anesthetist leaves the patient preliminary data are recorded on the anesthesia chart, a physical status category assigned, preanesthetic orders written, and a note made in the patient's record summarizing the results of the visit and the proposed anesthetic management. From a medicolegal point of view, this summary is more meaningful than a signed anesthesia permit, although an operation permit must be signed, particularly for minors and those incompetent to make judgments. Anesthetists in training should discuss their plans with the supervising anesthetist.

Anesthetists should develop enough judgment of their own to make a surgical diagnosis and to predict the effect of the surgical position and operation on physiologic processes. Occasionally an operation must be postponed, such as when the patient contracts a respiratory infection or digitalization is inadequate. Rarely should there be disagreement over proper preparation of a patient for operation. On the other hand, standard practice may have to be abandoned in an emergency. Operation may be necessary even though a full stomach or an exceptionally low hematocrit reading would otherwise dictate delay. Immediate operation is the primary resuscitative measure in uncontrolled hemorrhage, rapidly increasing intracranial pressure, or perforated viscus. We believe that an anesthetist can hardly ever refuse to give anesthesia if surgical opinion suggests that immediate operation offers a patient the best chance for survival.

PHYSICAL STATUS AND RISK

Questions are often raised concerning the chance of survival or the risk involved in undergoing anesthesia. In 1954 Beecher and Todd found that anesthesia played a primary or contributory role in the death of one patient in every 1500 operations. On the other hand, in a later study Dripps and his coworkers (1961) reported an incidence of anesthetic-related death as one in 780 for spinal and one in 259 for general anesthesia. The disparity in figures arises in part from the difficulty in defining death caused by anesthesia and in making a distinction between the effects of the patient's disease, the operation, and the anesthesia. From the standpoint of the individual, "risk" encompasses many variables. In addition to factors already mentioned, risk might involve the technical skills of an anesthetist or surgeon, socioeconomic factors in the home or hospital environment, extremes of atmospheric conditions, or duration of operation. Too often a patient is called a "poor risk" only after a catastrophe has taken place; this may represent a conscious or subconscious effort on the part of a physician to conceal errors in diagnosis or management. From a statistical or prognostic standpoint, therefore, the term "risk" is untenable and improvement in patient care does not lie in attempting to establish the degree of risk.

A solution to the problem is found by categorizing the relative physical conditions of all patients as representing constants among the many variables of the surgical experience. For example, when physical status is quantified, prognosis and evaluation of therapy for heart disease are aided immeasurably by a functional classification. Thus, the classification of the American Heart Association bears relevance to anesthetic problems. Such a classification is helpful in designating the resilience or reserves of the cardiac patient approaching operation, but it does not quite apply to other types of disease. For the purposes of anesthesia, therefore, the classification of physical status adopted by the American Society of Anesthesiologists is most useful.

Class 1. The patient has no organic, physiologic, biochemical or psychiatric disturbance. The pathologic process for which operation is to be performed is localized and does not entail a systemic disturbance. Examples: a fit patient with inguinal hernia; fibroid uterus in an otherwise healthy woman.

Class 2. Mild to moderate systemic disturbance caused either by the condition to be treated surgically or by other pathophysiologic processes. Examples: non- or only slightly limiting organic heart disease, mild diabetes, essential hypertension, or anemia. Some might choose to list the extremes of age here, either the neonate or the octogenarian, even though no discernible systemic disease is present. Extreme obesity and chronic bronchitis may be included in this category.

Class 3. Severe systemic disturbance or disease from whatever cause, even though it may not be possible to define the degree of disability with finality. Examples: severely limiting organic heart disease; severe diabetes with vascular complications; moderate to severe degrees of pulmonary insufficiency; angina pectoris or healed myocardial infarction.

Class 4. Indicative of the patient with severe systemic disorders that are already life-threatening, not always correctable by operation. Examples: patients with organic heart disease showing marked signs of cardiac insufficiency, persistent anginal syndrome, or active myocarditis; advanced degrees of pulmonary, hepatic, renal, or endocrine insufficiency.

Class 5. The moribund patient who has little chance of survival but is submitted to operation in desperation. Examples: the burst abdominal aneurysm with profound shock; major cerebral trauma with rapidly increasing intracranial pressure; massive pulmonary embolus. Most of these patients require operation as a resuscitative measure with little if any anesthesia.

Emergency Operation (E). Any patient in one of the classes listed previously who is operated upon as an emergency is considered to be in poorer physical condition. The letter E is placed beside the numerical classification. Thus, the patient with an hitherto uncomplicated hernia now incarcerated and associated with nausea and vomiting is classified 1E.

Although there may be problems in assigning the appropriate physical status, usually because of the implications of the operation to be performed, an estimate should be made in every instance. Other factors being equal, one might anticipate that the patient with poor physical status would not fare as well as the patient in good condition. Thus, Dripps and coworkers found no deaths caused by anesthetics in physical status Class 1, whether spinal or general anesthesia was given. However, Beecher and Todd noted that among patients in poor physical status (Classes 3 and 4), mortality was four to five times greater than that of patients in good condition, a finding confirmed by Dripps and coworkers. A similar experience has been reported by anesthesia commissions—groups formed on a voluntary basis to investigate the causes of anesthetic death. Almost as a rule, death in the better physical categories was deemed preventable from the standpoint of anesthetic management. Several reports also suggest that intraoperative cardiac arrest is more frequent in the poorer physical status categories.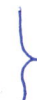

Physical status, therefore, provides us with a common language and a method of examining anesthetic morbidity and mortality. Here is a means of assessing the relative safety of new techniques of anesthetics upon an unchanging background of the patient's physical competence. A poor classification should alert the surgical team to employ greater safeguards. Lastly, physical status provides a means whereby one anesthetist's experience can be compared with others against a common background.

EXAMPLES OF PREANESTHETIC CONSULTATION NOTES

A well-written consultation note provides instruction for all involved, likewise serving to illustrate the anesthetist's concern about all phases of the patient's illness.

Physical Status 1E. First admission to hospital for this 16-year-old unmarried woman with complaint of profuse vaginal bleeding. Several episodes of pneumonia in infancy but no other major illnesses. She has not had anesthesia before, takes no drugs, and knows of no allergy to medications either familial or personal. She ate and drank last about ten hours prior to admission. On examination she is anxious, blood pressure 110/80, pulse 96, temperature 37°C. No airway problem. Teeth in good repair. Heart and lungs normal on percussion and auscultation. Urine shows many red blood cells. Hematocrit 29 per cent, BUN 11 mg per 100 ml, and blood glucose 122 mg per 100 ml. Physical status 1E. Immediate dilation of cervix and evacuation of uterus contemplated. Plan: induce anesthesia with thiopental followed by nitrous oxide by mask and meperidine intravenously as supplement. Patient accepts plan. Operation and anesthesia permits have been signed by mother. Please crossmatch two units of blood.

Physical Status 3. Fourth admission to hospital of this 73-year-old woman with massive hematemesis ten days before admission followed by weakness and lethargy. Prior admissions for saphenous vein ligation performed with spinal anesthesia, and for urinary tract infection and hematemesis. Other operations include tonsillectomy and adenoidectomy, appendectomy, and ovarian cystectomy many years ago; anesthesia tolerated well. On last admission diagnosis of Laennec's cirrhosis of liver made and esophageal varices demonstrated by barium swallow. Heavy alcohol intake for years, does not smoke, and knows of no drug allergy. Present medications include digitalis leaf daily, iron for anemia, and Maalox. Weight steady at 67 kg. She becomes short of breath after one flight of stairs. Prominent family history of arteriosclerotic heart disease. During the ten days in the hospital the following studies are of note: hematocrit, at first 31 per cent, has risen to 38 per cent with transfusion of whole blood and packed RBC; BUN 50 mg per 100 ml; urine loaded with RBC. Intravenous pyelogram showed slight bilateral decrease in dye density; total protein within normal limits; LDH 264 U per ml; SGOT 20 U per ml; bilirubin 1.5 to 2.0 mg per 100 ml; ECG normal sinus rhythm, left ventricular hypertrophy, no changes since prior tracing. Chest x-ray compatible with mild obstructive lung disease.

She is obese, somewhat anxious. Blood pressure 180/80, pulse 96, temperature 37.0°C. No airway problem. Mouth edentulous. Distant breath sounds, no rales. Heart not easily percussed. At apex and base, grade II to VI systolic murmurs, former transmitted to left sternal border. Liver 7 cm below costal margin, spleen just palpable. Neurologic examination normal.

Anesthesia problems in this woman for portacaval shunt: arteriosclerotic, cardiac and renal disease, probable aortic stenosis, well compensated on digitalis. Borderline liver failure with corrected anemia. Obesity and possible pulmonary emphysema. Physical status 3. She will do best with light general anesthesia with nitrous oxide-oxygen (at most 2:1) and thiopental supplemented by *d*-tubocurarine. Management: tracheal intubation, followed by controlled respiration; monitor blood pressure, pulse, respiration, central venous pressure, pulmonary artery wedge pressure, urine output, and body temperature. Give warm intravenous fluids and blood. Crossmatch about 10 units and have several units of fresh blood available. Very likely postoperative ventilatory assistance will be necessary. Continue to measure blood gases and to monitor progress as intraoperatively.

CHOICE OF ANESTHESIA

The evolution of anesthetic practice is mirrored in the present-day choice of agents and techniques. Originally the choice was among ether, nitrous oxide, and chloroform, given with simple devices. It is remarkable that ether lasted until modern times and that nitrous oxide is at present the most frequently used inhalation anesthetic. A second phase was marked by the introduction of cocaine, then procaine (Novocain) for regional anesthesia, most techniques in use today having been developed at the turn of the century. Synthesis of new inhalation agents, notably cyclopropane, and discovery of the short-acting barbiturates for intravenous use marked the 1930s. At this time the practice arose of giving combinations of agents in a balanced technique, each agent for a specific purpose — regional anesthesia for analgesia and muscle relaxation, thiopental intravenously for loss of consciousness, and an inhalant for maintenance of unconsciousness. Neuromuscular blocking agents added another dimension, providing pure muscle paralysis, while pain was relieved with nitrous oxide and opioids and unconsciousness was afforded by thiopental. Artificial hibernation and neuroleptanalgesia are modifications of balanced anesthesia. The provision of deliberate hypotension or hypothermia offers certain advantages in addition to the main anesthetic techniques. Over the last 15 years new halogenated hydrocarbons have come upon the scene — nonflammable halothane (Fluothane) and methoxyflurane (Penthrane), and slightly flammable fluroxene (Fluoromar). While halothane survives, methoxyflurane is used only sparingly, and fluroxene is no longer manufactured. The most recent addition is enflurane (Ethrane), while isoflurane (Forane) is still in the investigational stage.

An anesthetist skilled in a variety of techniques and well versed in the pharmacology of anesthesia can solve the problem of choice of anesthesia in many ways. But choice is dictated by several considerations: the patient as a human being (age, prior anesthetic experience, and complicating disease); the operation to be performed; the habits and skill of the surgeon; and the position required for the procedure. Thus it is illogical to state categorically that there is only one agent or technique for a specific situation. This does not imply that there are not definite contraindications to some methods of management (see chapters on agents and techniques). An ancillary concern is the avoidance of an agent or technique that could unjustifiably be implicated if a complication were to arise; for example, not using halothane for cholecystectomy because jaundice might develop postoperatively.

THE PATIENT

If a patient has had a bad experience with anesthesia in the past, this will be evident in the reaction to choice of anesthesia. Not infrequently relatives of the patient will have opinions on anesthetic choice contrary to those of the anesthetist, thus influencing the patient's response. In these situations analysis of the reasons for the choice presented in a confident manner usually saves the day. Nevertheless, a patient's preference ought to be considered. The law, under the doctrine of assault, dictates against imposing the anesthetist's will on a patient.

Emotional status must be taken into account in planning for anesthesia. Almost all patients have some degree of anxiety; the nature and extent of these feelings must be evaluated. A woman emerging from anesthesia following the performance of biopsy for possible cancer often shows agitation or delirium because of preoperative apprehension. In some, emotional instability or apprehension may require heavy premedication, which may predispose to circulatory and respiratory depression intra- and postoperatively. Under trying emotional conditions intravenous induction of anesthesia is preferred, as is avoidance of regional techniques. Even in the stolid person, a long operative procedure for which regional anesthesia has provided good pain relief may be quite trying.

Certain pathophysiologic changes justify exclusion of specific agents or techniques. For example, wishing to avoid the pharmacologic action of an anesthetic that could enhance an underlying abnormality, one might avoid halothane in the presence of increased intracranial pressure because of the cerebrovascular dilation produced. When coronary arteriosclerosis is present, addition of epinephrine to a local anesthetic solution can increase the work of the heart.

Body habitus must be considered. The asthenic, elderly, or chronically ill generally require minimal anesthesia. Conversely, the robust often need sustained higher concentrations of anesthetics. The obese patient presents special problems. Among other things, pulmonary ventilation will require careful attention because the short, thick-necked, obese individual readily develops soft tissue airway obstruction and may require tracheal intubation even for a minor operation.

Elsewhere we will touch upon other matters that influence choice of anesthesia, such as drug therapy and physical status. It is worthwhile at this point to delve deeper into the matter of complicating disease.

Circulatory Abnormalities

In general the goals during anesthesia are to avoid an increase in myocardial irritability that can result in tachyarrhythmias and to prevent serious degrees of circulatory depression, both leading to hypotension and even cardiac arrest. These aims entail a comprehension of circulatory abnormalities already present, knowledge of the drugs used in treatment of heart disease, and a thorough understanding of the circulatory effects of anesthetics. The rule has always been to ensure adequate oxygenation, elimination of carbon dioxide, and maintenance of a safe blood pressure. But a modest decrease in the mean arterial pressure will decrease the afterload and the work of the heart, thereby lessening oxygen consumption, while an increase in pulse rate and in myocardial inotropic action also increases heart work and the demand for oxygen. Therefore, during anesthesia, an appropriate balance must be struck between avoiding a low blood pressure and avoiding those factors that increase the myocardial need for oxygen. This matter is discussed in succeeding chapters.

Respiratory Insufficiency

Respiratory abnormalities either at the central or peripheral level raise the possibility of the development of respiratory failure when anesthetics are superimposed. Commonly encountered pulmonary problems are bronchitis, bronchospastic states, emphysema, and restrictive defects. Central depression of respiration owing to intracranial disease, carbon dioxide retention, or drugs may be encountered as well as neuromuscular disability secondary to poliomyelitis, muscular dystrophy, myasthenia gravis, arthritis, or kyphoscoliosis. With the resulting diminution in pulmonary function and the relative inefficiency of defense mechanisms, alveolar ventilation, and cough, patients with these problems are highly susceptible to development of postoperative atelectasis and bronchopneumonia. The approach to these problems is as follows: tests of pulmonary function and determination of blood gas values to define the extent of respiratory insufficiency; treatment of bronchospasm and infection by eliminating smoking and use of bronchodilating drugs with intermittent positive pressure breathing (IPPB); practice for the patient in pulmonary physiotherapy; and administration of antibiotics for known infection. IPPB serves to accustom the patient to the type of postoperative treatment to be received in order to encourage deep breathing and cough. Several days or more are required to arrive at full benefit when lung disease is severe. Opioids should be avoided because of diminution in the respiratory response to carbon dioxide and the depression of cough. During anesthesia, controlled ventilation is carried out to maintain gas exchange as indicated by repeated blood gas analyses. Postoperatively, a stir-up regimen of deep breathing and physiotherapy is used, particularly if opioids are required for relief of pain. If inadequate pulmonary exchange is found, tracheal intubation and assisted or controlled ventilation are continued until a patient can be weaned from this regimen.

Liver Disease

The many homeostatic functions of the liver are readily influenced by anesthetics through their effects on splanchnic blood flow, their potentially hepatotoxic properties, and the role of the liver in biotransformation of anesthetic compounds. Parenchymatous disease must be severe before biotransformation of drugs such as short-acting barbiturates, succinylcholine (Anectine), and opioids is influenced. Acute stages of serum or infectious hepatitis, terminal phases of portal or biliary cirrhosis, advanced hemochromatosis, and extensive replacement of the liver by primary or metastatic neoplasms are associated with a high surgical death rate.

Thus, maximal improvement in liver function should be sought preoperatively. In portal cirrhosis, for example, prothrombin and serum albumin should be at least at minimally acceptable levels, as should liver function tests—Bromsulphalein excretion, alkaline phosphatase, plasma cholinesterase, and serum glutamic oxalic transaminase (SGOT)—to mention just a few used as guidelines. Drugs used to treat the liver failure of cirrhosis (e.g., cortisone and neomycin), as noted elsewhere, may complicate anesthetic administration.

Kidney Disease

Excretion of anesthetic drugs and their metabolites by the kidney and its role in acid-base and water metabolism are essential considerations in anesthetic management. In a patient with minimal renal reserves, compounds excreted by the kidneys—the long-acting barbiturates, gallamine (Flaxedil), and succinylcholine given by constant infusion—are to be avoided. Recently problems have been encountered in the reversal of the actions of pancuronium (Pavulon). Before the era of hemodialysis, which maintains the renal failure patient in a reasonable state of biochemical balance, such patients presented a formidable array of problems: high serum potassium levels, low sodium and calcium, metabolic acidosis, and increased susceptibility to infection. Drugs used to treat these conditions added to the problems of anesthesia—antihypertensive medications, digitalis, antibiotics, and cortisone. In preparation for nephrectomy or renal transplantation, chronic dialysis returns physiologic and biochemical abnormalities toward normal values, and the risks of anesthesia and operation consequently are lessened. But optimal conditions must be attained before operation. Starting with a borderline high serum potassium level, from 5.5 to 6.0 mEq per liter, several events during anesthesia may elevate potassium levels to the point of cardiac standstill or ventricular fibrillation: use of succinylcholine with attendant release of potassium; transfusion of large volumes of cold bank blood of low pH and high serum potassium; and use of sympathomimetic drugs. Hypoxia, hypercarbia, and low flow states also add to K^+ load, and low flow states with concomitant blood transfusion or release of myoglobin from traumatized tissues and the use of sympathomimetic drugs that cause renal vasoconstriction predispose to postoperative acute tubular necrosis.

Endocrine Disease

Each endocrine abnormality calls for a specific anesthetic approach, problems becoming more complicated as new hormones are discovered (aldosterone, angiotensin, 5-hydroxytryptamine [serotonin], prostaglandins). Further, certain neoplasms may exhibit endocrine activity. Carcinoma of the lung or thyrotoxicosis may be accompanied by a myasthenic state; in a few instances new growths have been shown to secrete adrenocorticotropic hormone (ACTH). Diseases of the pituitary-adrenal axis may require correction of electrolyte imbalance, replacement therapy with steroids, and the use of nonstressful anesthetics like the halogenated compounds. Although thyrotoxicosis can now be controlled by specific therapy affecting the release of thyroxine at one of several levels, the possibility of thyroid storm calls for elimination of atropine as a preanesthetic medication and avoidance of ether or cyclopropane because of sympathetic stimulating properties. Resection of a pheochromocytoma is now approached with alpha- and beta-adrenergic blocking drugs on hand and the prior use of alpha blockers to correct the known plasma volume deficit. The choice of anesthesia in this disease entails use of nonautonomic stimulating agents.

APPRAISAL

In this chapter we have depicted the many facets of a preanesthetic visit to patients: how best to approach them, how to categorize physical status, and how to write a consultation note. Using the background of the information thus obtained, when determining choice of anesthesia the anesthetist must then take into account complicating ailments, particularly those involving the vital organs and homeostatic systems. As experience is gained the anesthetist will find that the preanesthetic visit, above all else, sets the stage for a safe course both during and after operation.

REFERENCES

American Society of Anesthesiologists: New classification of physical status. Anesthesiology 24:111, 1963.

Beecher HK, Todd DP: A study of the deaths associated with anesthesia and surgery based on a study of 599,548 anesthetics in ten institutions 1948–1952, inclusive. Ann Surg 140:2, 1954.

Bodlander FMS: Deaths associated with anaesthesia. Br J Anaesth 47:36, 1975.

Dripps RD, Lamont A, Eckenhoff JE: The role of anesthesia in surgical mortality. JAMA 178:261, 1961.

Marx GF, Mateo CV, Orkin LR: Computer analysis of postanesthetic deaths. Anesthesiology 39:54, 1973.

Saklad M: Grading of patients for surgical procedures. Anesthesiology 2:281, 1941.

Wylie WD: "There, but for the grace of God. . . ." Ann R Coll Surg Engl 56:171, 1975.

Chapter 3

PHARMACOLOGIC PRINCIPLES AND DRUG INTERACTIONS

Since the previous edition of this text, interest in drug interactions has increased. Recent research has been designed to detect the ways in which concurrent medical treatment influences anesthetic drug metabolism. This change in emphasis has been prompted by the growing proportion of patients requiring anesthesia while taking drugs for other conditions, and because anesthetics once thought to be inert are now known to be metabolized in varying degree. The pharmacokinetics and metabolism of drugs will be reviewed, followed by specific considerations of concurrent drug therapies of interest. Figure 3–1 provides an overview of the pharmacokinetic phases discussed here.

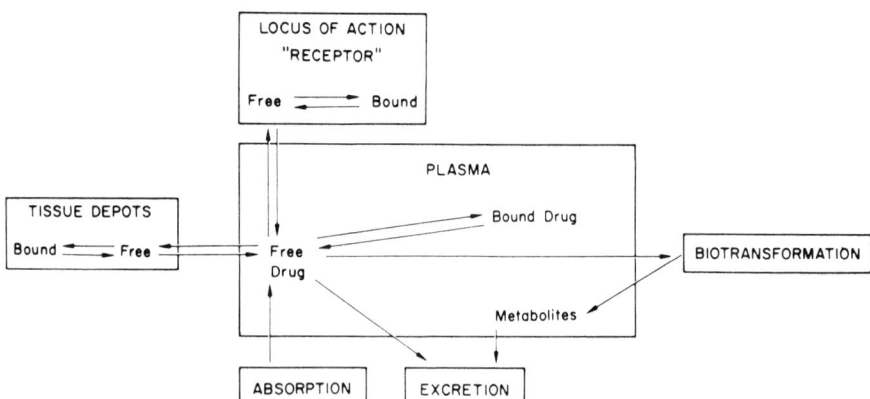

Figure 3–1. Schematic representation of the interrelationship of the absorption, distribution, binding, biotransformation, and excretion of a drug and its concentration at its locus of action. (From Goodman LS, Gilman A (eds): The Pharmacological Basis of Therapeutics. 5th ed, New York, Macmillan Publishing Co, 1975.)

BASIC PHARMACOLOGIC PRINCIPLES

DRUG UPTAKE

Uptake is influenced by route of administration, tissue blood flow, physical-chemical factors such as molecular size and ionization, binding by proteins in plasma and tissues, and availability of "receptors" at target cells. The uptake and distribution of inhaled and intravenous anesthetics are discussed in Chapters 10 and 13. Uptake entails delivery of an agent to the circulation, a process that occurs instantaneously when the drug is given intravenously and rapidly when an aqueous solution is injected intramuscularly.

The vehicle in which the drug is dissolved relates to its solubility, relevant in absorption from any site but of particular importance for drugs given orally. Volume and acidity of gastric juice may alter absorption. Some drugs are precipitated in acid solution and thereby absorbed slowly; others dissolve more easily at low pH. The presence of food slows absorption of most drugs but improves absorption of lipid-soluble drugs taken with fatty foods. Drugs are also absorbed from the intestine and bowel, with motility governing the rate of delivery to absorption sites and, in irritable states, limiting absorption. High concentrations favor absorption, but circulation to the site must be adequate for the process.

Once in the circulation, regardless of route of administration, the drug molecule behaves according to principles dictated by structure. The compound may exist in a free state, but most drugs are inactivated functionally to some extent by plasma protein binding. Once attached to a large protein molecule in the circulation, drugs are unable to reach extravascular target cells. Binding is influenced by pH; the higher pH is above the isoelectric point of the protein molecule, the more negative the net charge on that molecule. This is the principle underlying serum electrophoresis, in which proteins migrate in an electric field at pH 8.8. With an isoelectric point of 4.7 albumin travels farthest because its charge is most negative at this pH, while gamma globulin migrates little since its isoelectric point is near pH 7.0. At the pH of blood—7.4—albumin has a negative charge, greater than that of other proteins; drugs with a positive charge are thereby bound. Nonelectrostatic binding also may occur as a result of covalency or van der Waals' forces; this may account for binding of pancuronium to gamma globulins.

Ionization of a drug is likewise important, not only in protein binding but also in determining lipid solubility and rapidity in crossing cell membranes. Most drugs are weak electrolytes, present in aqueous solution in ionized and non-ionized forms, the proportions depending upon the pH of the solution, the pK_a of the drug, and whether the drug is an acid or base. The relationship is defined by the Henderson-Hasselbalch equation:

$$pH = pK_a + \log \frac{\text{Salt}}{\text{Acid}}$$

pK$_a$ is the negative logarithm of the dissociation constant of a weak acid, HA, which ionizes to H$^+$ and A$^-$. The equation may be rewritten:

$$pH = pK_a + \log \frac{A^-}{HA}$$

Many drugs, local anesthetics for example, contain a tertiary nitrogen to which a hydrogen atom attaches reversibly. By pharmacologic convention, their dissociation is also described by pK$_a$ and the equation becomes:

$$pH = pK_a + \log \frac{B}{BH^+}$$

Since an acid acts as an H$^+$ donor, dissociation of both acids and bases are described by the equation:

$$pH - pK_a = \log \frac{A^-}{HA} \text{ or } \log \frac{B}{BH^+}$$

Thus, for a given pK$_a$, as pH increases the ionized form of an acid increases whereas the ionized form of a base decreases. Which is the active form of the drug? Must the drug penetrate lipid cell membranes in order to act? Uncharged species of the molecule penetrate membranes more easily than the ionized form. Thus, acidic drugs are easily absorbed from gastric juice whose pH may be 1.4; an acid drug with pK$_a$ of 4.4 exists in a ratio of 1000 parts HA to 1 part A$^-$ and is readily absorbed. At the pH of blood, 7.4, the ratio is reversed. Concentration gradients for one drug form can be produced across cell membranes simply by changes in pH. In addition, carrier-mediated membrane transport occurs as an active process. Drugs eventually reach not only their sites of action via the circulation but sites of metabolic degradation and elimination as well.

The effects on regional blood flow produced by anesthetics will be described elsewhere, but a few general remarks are relevant. Of greatest concern are the cerebral, coronary, pulmonary, splanchnic, and renal circulations. Each depends upon cardiac output, although there is some autoregulation in the cerebral, coronary, and renal circulations that maintains perfusion in the face of changes in perfusion pressure. Of these, splanchnic blood flow is most directly related to drug metabolism since it is by this route that orally administered drugs eventually reach the liver. Splanchnic flow is compromised directly or indirectly by most general anesthetics.

BIOTRANSFORMATION

Once carried to the liver, a drug is subject to biotransformation both to inactivate the drug and to allow its elimination. Drugs that exist in a nonpolar, lipid-soluble form cross cell membranes easily and tend to remain in the body, since such molecules are easily reabsorbed by renal tubular cells. Modification of molecules by oxidation, reduction, or hydrolysis to polar compounds renders them less lipid soluble and thus they are more easily eliminated in urine.

Drug metabolism is mediated both by microsomal and nonmicrosomal enzymes. Hepatic drug-metabolizing microsomal enzyme systems have been the most thoroughly studied. First, it should be noted that "microsomes" are a laboratory product, not a biological reality. Liver cells contain a system of membranes or endoplasmic reticulum (ER), divisible into smooth and rough kinds. Upon differential ultracentrifugation, the smooth ER (Fig. 3–2) is fragmented into tiny structures that assume spherical forms called microsomes. These are rich in enzymes and contain cytochrome P-450, a primary component of the mixed function oxidase system. Cytochrome P-450 is a hemoprotein with iron in an oxidized (Fe^{3+}) or reduced (Fe^{2+}) form. Drugs combine with the oxidized form, and the drug complex is then reduced by a nicotinamide adenine dinucleotide phosphate (NADPH)–cytochrome c reductase reaction, with NADPH as the primary electron donor. The drug-Fe^{2+}-cytochrome complex then combines with molecular oxygen, the oxidized drug splits off, and the Fe^{3+} form of the cytochrome P-450 is regenerated. Two binding sites or two types of cytochrome P-450 exist, so that drugs are designated as type I or type II according to characteristic changes produced in P-450 absorbance spectra.

Enzyme induction describes the increased activity of microsomal enzymes brought about by many drugs, chemicals, or environmental agents (Fig. 3–2*B*). The prototype is phenobarbital, which causes proliferation of endoplasmic reticulum and increased synthesis of cytochrome P-450 and NADPH–cytochrome c reductase, reactions blocked by inhibitors of protein or nucleoprotein synthesis. Liver weight and blood flow increase, as does overall hepatic protein synthesis. There are also nonmicrosomal enzyme reactions in drug metabolism, examples being conjugation of salicylates with glycine, *N*-methylation of catecholamines, hydrolysis of procaine and lidocaine, and oxidation of ethanol. Nonmicrosomal enzymes are not inducible.

EXCRETION

The kidney is largely responsible for elimination of drugs and their metabolites. Nonpolar compounds are eliminated slowly owing to reabsorption by renal tubular cells. Water-soluble, polar drugs or metabolites are readily eliminated. Volatile anesthetics are for the most part exhaled via the lungs but significant quantities of polar metabolites are produced from several inhalation agents.

If drugs are not bound to plasma proteins, elimination is proportional to glomerular filtration rate. In the proximal renal tubules, certain organic cations and anions are added by active tubular secretion. Reabsorption of non-ionized substances occurs chiefly in the distal tubules in proportion to the rate of water and sodium reabsorption. The pH effect is important,

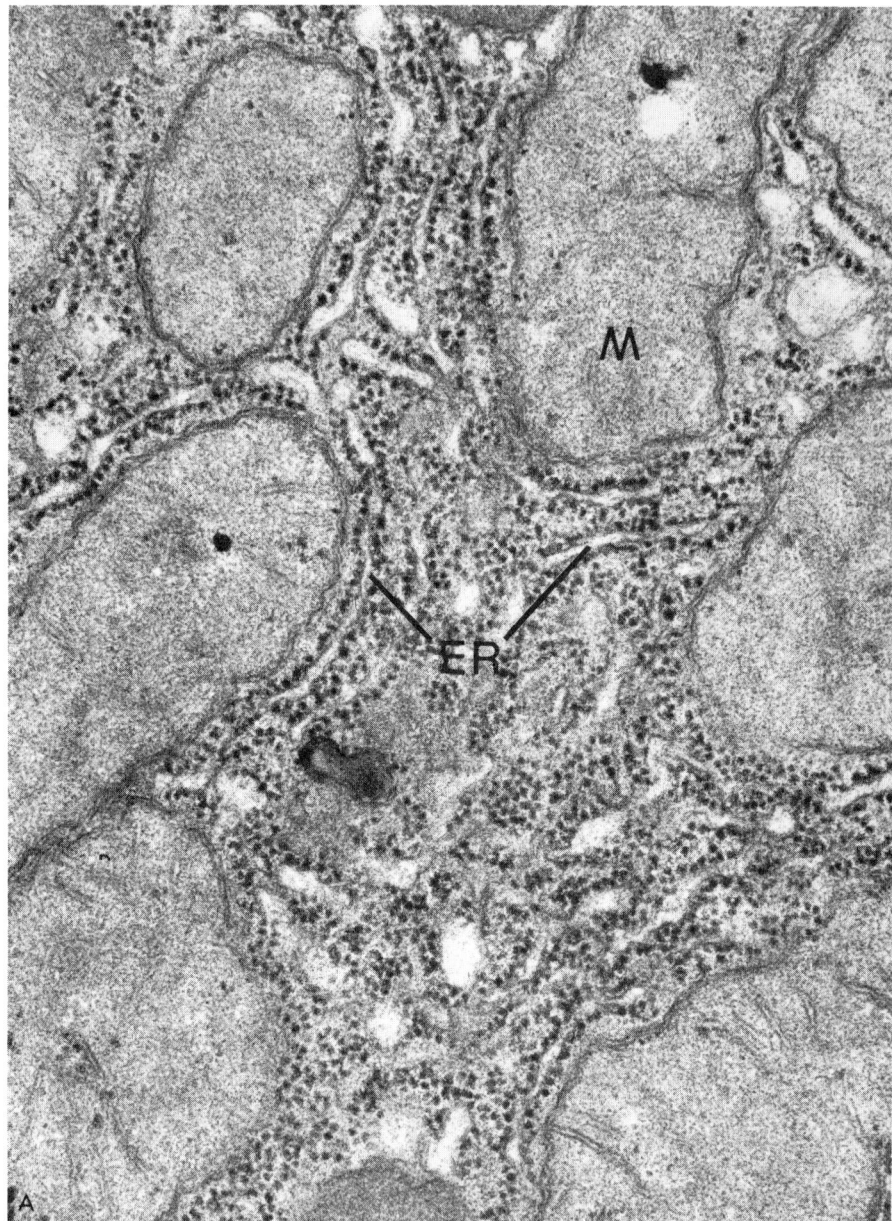

Figure 3-2. Electron micrographs (×42,500) of mouse liver. Control (A) animal given saline injections daily for five days; induced (B) animal given 40 mg/kg phenobarbital intraperitoneally daily for five days. Both animals fasted 24 hours prior to sacrifice. Livers fixed in 1 per cent OsO_4. Symbols: M — mitochondria; ER — rough endoplasmic reticulum with attached ribosomes appearing as black beads; SER — smooth endoplasmic reticulum, seen best in transverse views, where it circumscribes vacuolar (cisternal) spaces. (Micrographs courtesy of Dr. RM Hinkley.)

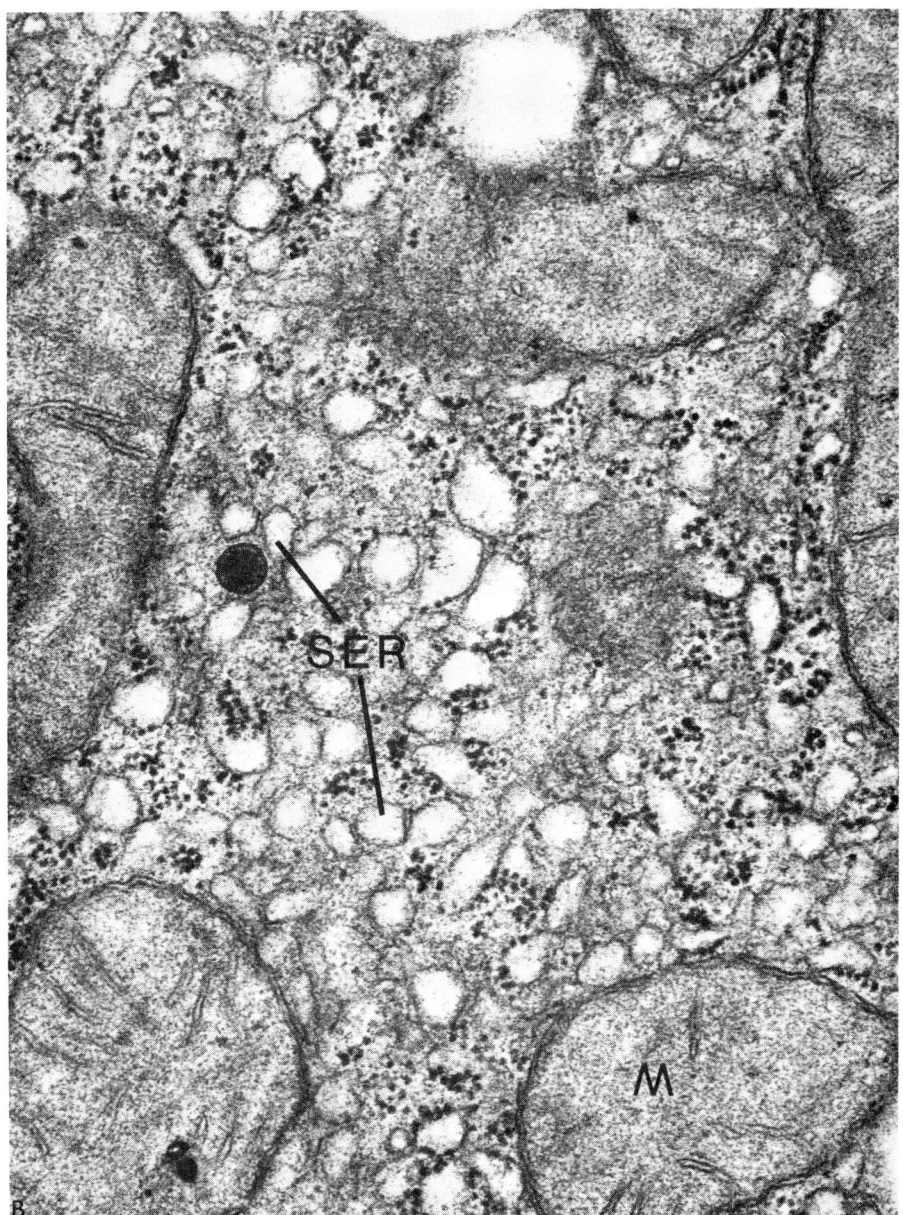

Figure 3-2 (*Continued*).

since in the presence of alkalinized urine weak acids are ionized and rapidly excreted. However, weak bases become less ionized as pH rises. Some drug metabolites are excreted in bile and either reabsorbed in the bowel for eventual renal clearance or excreted in feces, not an important mode of elimination

CONCURRENT DRUG THERAPY

CARDIOVASCULAR DRUGS

Cardiac Glycosides

Probably the best studied of all anesthetic–concurrent drug interactions are those involving the cardiac glycosides. Morrow showed that digitalis toxicity occurs at a low total dose when dogs are anesthetized with cyclopropane, and that a higher digitalis dose is required in the presence of halothane or methoxyflurane. Thus, digitalis toxicity may be unmasked by cyclopropane, while an inadequately digitalized patient may require more drug during halothane anesthesia. Recently, it was found that enflurane, isoflurane, and ether all raised the dose of ouabain necessary to produce ventricular tachycardia in the dog.

Antiarrhythmics

Many patients with cardiac arrhythmias are treated with the antiarrhythmic drugs quinidine or procainamide, which depress myocardial conduction velocity, contractility, and excitability. The combined depressant actions of these drugs and the inhalation anesthetics have not been extensively studied, but the reduction of cardiac contractility common to both groups suggests the need for caution in their use.

Since Ahlquist, in 1947, categorized catecholamine actions into alpha and beta types, the actions of a pure beta agonist, isoproterenol, have been studied extensively. This ultimately led to the synthesis and clinical use of beta-adrenergic blocking agents such as propranolol (Inderal). This drug, now widely used in the treatment of angina pectoris, cardiac arrhythmias, and hypertension, carries obvious implications for anesthetic practice. The drug is taken orally in widely varying dosage, is well absorbed, and about 90 per cent is bound to plasma proteins; the plasma half-life of an intravenous dose is about three to four hours. The liver binds propranolol and is responsible for nearly all of its metabolism, followed by urinary excretion of metabolites, at least one of which may have a biologic effect.

The beta-adrenergic responses of heart and smooth muscle to catecholamine stimulation are blocked by propranolol, resulting in a decreased heart rate and cardiac output, prolongation of mechanical systole, slight lowering of blood pressure, and increase in bronchomotor tone.

Older anesthetics, such as ether and cyclopropane, provide some safety against circulatory depression via catecholamine liberation during the course of anesthesia. In the presence of propranolol, this response may be compromised and the overall effect of the anesthetics becomes depressive. Newer volatile agents do not evoke such catecholamine responses, and directly depress the myocardium, while propranolol may render a patient more susceptible to anesthetic overdose. Some clinicians arbitrarily discontinue propranolol therapy 24 hours preoperatively; we believe that the possibility of exacerbation of the disease for which propranolol was given may outweigh possible advantages of discontinuance. We therefore continue with therapy, but cautiously, during and after anesthesia.

Antihypertensives

Similar reasoning applies to antihypertensive drugs as to the antiarrhythmics. At one time reserpine was discontinued two weeks preoperatively to allow reaccumulation of catecholamine stores depleted by the chronic treatment. Today, we believe that reappearance of hypertension with its accompanying myocardial stress is more of a danger than continuance of the drug. Mildly hypertensive patients are sometimes treated with phenobarbital, the prototypical enzyme-inducing agent, or more commonly with chlordiazepoxide or diazepam, which have not as yet been shown to be enzyme inducers. Seriously hypertensive patients are often treated with methyldopa, which interferes with biosynthesis of norepinephrine (NE) and was once thought to lower blood pressure by reducing tissue NE stores. Later studies failed to support this explanation. Methyldopa action is now ascribed to the action of a metabolic by-product—alpha-methylnorepinephrine—on the central nervous system, abetted by the sedation produced by the drug.

Diuretics

A major part of antihypertensive therapy entails the use of diuretics which are given to modify water and electrolyte balance. The most commonly used diuretics are the thiazides, which are rapidly absorbed from the gut, actively secreted into the proximal renal tubules, and excreted within three to four hours with minimal biotransformation. They inhibit renal tubular reabsorption of sodium, chloride, and, to a lesser extent, potassium while obligatory water excretion takes place. Water and electrolytes are lost, the plasma volume reduced, myocardial work decreased, and vascular reactivity improved, thus enhancing the response to other antihypertensive drugs. While the overall effect is beneficial, chronic potassium loss may result in hypokalemia which affects peripheral nerve conduction, conduction in the myocardium and hence the electrocardiogram, and the duration and extent of action of neuromuscular blockers; this also favors digitalis toxicity. Therefore a three-way interaction among diuretics, digitalis, and anesthetics makes for a confusing clinical assessment of a patient's condition.

Anticoagulants

Patients with thromboembolic disease may receive the anticoagulants heparin or bishydroxycoumarin (Dicumarol) when presenting for anesthesia. There is minimal effect of general anesthetics on coagulation, but anesthetic management may be dictated by concurrent anticoagulation in that regional anesthetic techniques are contraindicated unless the clotting and prothrombin times are near normal. Enzyme-inducing agents such as the barbiturates shorten the action of bishydroxycoumarin by stimulating enzyme systems responsible for its degradation.

DRUGS AFFECTING ENDOCRINE ORGANS

Thyroid

With modern drug therapy, rarely does a patient come to operation in a thyrotoxic state; the well-treated patient poses no special problems in premedication. Occasionally, however, the thyrotoxic patient may respond poorly or become sensitive to methimazole (Tapazole), or an operation other than thyroidectomy is necessary before thyrotoxicosis can be brought under control. In these circumstances the prophylactic use of reserpine or propranolol serves to diminish the excessive sympathetic nervous activity that accompanies hyperthyroidism, and these drugs must be taken into account in anesthetic management. The thyrotoxic patient is unduly anxious, has tachycardia, is intolerant of warm temperatures, and may have lost considerable body weight plus have developed muscle weakness. One worries about the development of thyroid storm, in which the hypermetabolic condition leads to hyperpyrexia with excessive demands on the circulation, tachyarrhythmias, heart failure, and progressive fever. Heavy sedation is required for prophylaxis; atropine is avoided because of the tendency toward tachycardia and heat retention. For anesthesia, agents and techniques that do not stimulate the sympathetic nervous system are chosen, with provision made for body cooling. The eyes are protected when exophthalmus is present.

The hypothyroid patient presents with an opposite picture, although usually is euthyroid following thyroid substitution therapy. The tendency is to use lesser amounts of sedatives in these patients.

Diabetes

Diabetics are of concern to the anesthetist not only because they require special metabolic management and often have other concurrent diseases, but also because of interactions between anesthetics and insulin. Insulin release is stimulated by beta-adrenergic agonists and inhibited by epinephrine and norepinephrine through their alpha-adrenergic actions.

Stresses such as hypoxia, burns, or operation increase circulating catecholamines, thus inhibiting insulin release and causing glycogenolysis; both of these conditions elevate blood sugar. During anesthesia a diabetic type of response follows an intravenous glucose tolerance test. Intravenous insulin has a half-life of nine minutes, metabolic degradation occurring rapidly with about 40 per cent of the dose destroyed in both the liver and the kidneys. This approaches the hepatic limit for catabolism of insulin; appreciable renal insufficiency may overload the liver's capacity and prolong the action of insulin. Since glucose is the main substrate for energy metabolism in the brain, a gross oversupply of insulin leads to disordered metabolism and irreversible cerebral damage may occur. During anesthesia, the usual symptoms of hypoglycemia are absent; sweating and tachycardia may be modified or masked. Hypoglycemia is more serious than hyperglycemia; if in doubt it is prudent to give glucose liberally to patients who have received insulin.

Adrenals

Corticosteroids are given for a variety of diseases, obligating the anesthetist to know why the drugs have been used and how they act. Cortisol, the prototypical glucocorticoid, secreted in normal humans at the rate of about 20 mg/24 hours, exerts a negative feedback influence on the hypothalamus and adrenocorticotropic hormone (ACTH) release. Prolonged treatment with steroids in excess of the normal 24-hour cortisol equivalent may result in functional impairment of the adenohypophysis, adrenal atrophy, and dependence upon exogenously supplied steroids. Because regulation of carbohydrate, fat, and protein metabolism, water and electrolyte balance, and cardiovascular, renal, and neuromuscular function all depend upon normally functioning adrenals, insufficiency of steroids renders the patient incapable of adjusting to the stress of anesthesia and operation. For a variety of reasons plasma cortisol levels double during operation, particularly with the use of cyclopropane and ether, but this is not evident if the pituitary-adrenal axis is depressed. If steroid therapy has been stopped two or more months previously steroid pretreatment may not be needed, but hydrocortisone should be available for intravenous use during operation if cardiovascular collapse develops. A patient receiving systemic steroids within two months of operation, at a level above the equivalent of 20 mg cortisol (5 mg prednisone) daily should probably be given a "cover" of intramuscular hydrocortisone with the premedication and about 300 mg intravenously daily, gradually tapering off the dose postoperatively.

ANTIBIOTICS

Neuromuscular blocking agents and antibiotics used to irrigate body cavities or given intravenously interact in a dangerous manner: all of the "mycin" drugs—neomycin, kanamycin, and to a lesser extent, streptomycin—prolong the muscle paralysis induced by nondepolarizing neuromuscular blockers. The paralysis is relatively resistant to reversal by anticholinesterases and may respond to intravenous calcium salts, although most anesthetists perfer mechanical ventilation until the respiratory paralysis disappears. This complication occurs most often in patients with peritonitis when irrigation is done at wound closure. A patient may develop respiratory insufficiency when no longer under observation by the surgical team; therefore recovery room nurses should be alerted to the possibility. The antibiotics of concern are excreted primarily by the kidney; patients with renal disease are more susceptible to the complication because the plasma level of antibiotic is higher for a given dose.

Antibiotics are metabolized and excreted by the liver and kidney or a combination of the two. Toxicity of any drug is usually directed toward the organ principally concerned in its elimination. In relation to postanesthetic organ dysfunction, the anesthetist should be aware that hepatitis or nephritis may relate to antibiotic treatment rather than to the general anesthetic given. Patients with high output renal failure following methoxyflurane anesthesia who are concurrently receiving tetracycline have demonstrated oxalate crystal deposition in renal parenchyma representative of breadown products of either the antibiotic or the anesthetic. Tetracycline also has caused fatal hepatitis in pregnant women given the drug to treat pyelonephritis. If these patients had been anesthetized with halothane the liver damage might have been ascribed to the anesthetic.

CNS ACTIVE AGENTS

Alcohol

Many patients routinely ingest drugs to alter mood or behavior, either socially or as medical prescription. In terms of numbers affected, alcohol heads the list. The problems presented to the anesthetist range from patients with the well-known functional effects and physical damage caused by alcohol to those injured while intoxicated who must then be anesthetized. Since alcohol is depressant to all excitable tissues, caution is advised in using additional depressant drugs. Many patients use alcohol in addition to other psychoactive drugs, such as diazepam or barbiturates; although they are seemingly alert, there may be a thin line between consciousness and coma. Some may require large doses of intravenous induction agents, but most require minimal general anesthesia once consciousness is lost.

Alcohol in modest doses affects the heart, increasing stroke volume, heart rate, and myocardial oxygen consumption; in larger amounts it decreases contractility and slows electrical conduction, with the appearance of atrial or ventricular premature beats. These effects resemble those produced by potent anesthetics; therefore the actions of alcohol and anesthetic may be additive.

A fasting person who drinks large quantities of alcohol evidences hypoglycemia with blood sugar levels approaching 30 mg per 100 ml. Glucose should be given to all acutely intoxicated patients. Alcohol taken acutely inhibits the release of antidiuretic hormone from the posterior pituitary, but chronic usage results in antidiuresis and overhydration; fluid overload occurs easily in such patients.

Hepatic function may be impaired, ranging from mild fatty infiltration to portal cirrhosis in advanced stages, interfering with metabolism of drugs and hepatic synthesis of albumin and other proteins. A low serum albumin decreases drug binding, thereby altering drug requirements. Finally peripheral neuropathy is common in chronic alcoholics, affecting application of regional anesthetic techniques.

Alcohol and its metabolites are highly water-soluble, do not accumulate in the endoplasmic reticulum, and probably are not enzyme inducers, despite reports to the contrary. More convincing is the evidence that alcohol interferes with microsomal enzymes responsible for barbiturate inactivation, potentiating barbiturate effects if taken concomitantly. An additive effect of many CNS depressants and alcohol occurs, and surprisingly, tricyclic antidepressants potentiate the depression of alcohol.

Sedatives and Tranquilizers

Two other groups of psychoactive agents widely used are the tranquilizers and barbiturates. The three most commonly prescribed kinds of tranquilizers are phenothiazines (chlorpromazine), propanediol carbamates (meprobamate), and benzodiazepines (diazepam), all generally of low toxicity. Phenothiazines, meprobamate, and the barbiturates induce microsomal enzymes. Cholestatic jaundice occurs in about 2 per cent of patients taking chlorpromazine and all the phenothiazines occasionally produce postural hypotension. The chief concern to the anesthetist is that other agents will add to the sedation produced by tranquilizers or barbiturates possibly resulting in untoward sensitivity to anesthetics or prolonged recovery from anesthesia. Convulsions may occur following abrupt withdrawal from long-term tranquilizer or barbiturate therapy. It is best to maintain such patients on the accustomed drug regimen throughout the operative experience.

Psychoactive Drugs

"Mood elevators" or antidepressants are prescribed to combat depression. The two general classes are the tricyclic antidepressants and the monoamine oxidase inhibitors (MAO). Tricyclics (imipramine and amitriptyline) are slightly sedative, act through modulation of the metabolism of brain amines, exert prominent anticholinergic effects, and cause tachycardia; they also may cause orthostatic hypotension, cardiac arrhythmias, blunting of normal cardiovascular reflexes, and T wave changes in the

ECG. For these reasons patients on high doses of tricyclic drugs requiring anesthesia for electroconvulsive therapy present serious risks.

The monoamine oxidase inhibitors (tranylcypromine, phenelzine) are not widely used today but result in vitally important drug interactions. Monoamine oxidase, an enzyme localized intracellularly in the mitochondria, is involved in the degradation of intracellular sympathomimetic amines and serotonin. MAO inhibition increases the tissue content of epinephrine, norepinephrine, dopamine, and serotonin, and exaggerates the effect of exogenously administered amines. In addition to mood elevation, the compounds can lower blood pressure and orthostatic hypotension is common. During anesthesia, hypotension must be treated with extreme caution because administration of sympathomimetics may result in sudden, severe hypertension. A similar reaction occurs after ingestion of foods and beverages containing tyramine. The use of meperidine is hazardous in these patients because hypertension also occurs.

ANTI-PARKINSON THERAPY

The treatment of Parkinson's disease has changed dramatically since the introduction of levodopa, the levo-isomer of dihydroxyphenylalanine. This agent enters the brain and there is converted to dopamine, a neurotransmitter normally present in pathways between the substantia nigra and corpus striatum but absent or diminished in patients with this disease. Upon ingestion most of the levodopa is converted to dopamine in the liver, but this metabolite does not cross the blood-brain barrier. At the onset of levodopa therapy, most patients develop orthostatic hypotension which disappears after a time. The cardiac effects are manifested by ectopic beats, tachycardia, palpitation, dyspnea, and angina pectoris. Anesthetics that sensitize the myocardium to catecholamines, notably cyclopropane and, to a lesser extent, the halogenated hydrocarbons, should be given cautiously to patients being treated with levodopa. Some prefer to discontinue levodopa for 24 hours prior to operation; however, this is unnecessary if proper precautions are taken.

OPIOIDS AND ADDICTION

Anesthetists often encounter patients receiving opioids preoperatively for pain. The hazard of opioids lies mostly in postoperative morbidity. During surgical stimulation, the respiratory depressant action of opioids is offset by painful stimuli, but these are absent after operation. Thus depression of respiration may last for many hours after therapeutic doses of morphine, particularly in the presence of hepatic or renal failure.

Additional problems are posed by the opioid addict. If in a treatment program, the addict is often unaware of the maintenance dose and tends to exaggerate drug needs; thus the unwary physician may inadvertently prescribe an overdose. Too small a dose of opioid is equally important, since withdrawal symptoms may occur. Hospitalization for operation is not the time to alter maintenance programs or otherwise to treat addiction. The maintenance plan should be continued and if treatment of pain is required, additional opioid should be given. Pentazocine (Talwin) should not be given because it is an opioid antagonist and may precipitate the withdrawal syndrome. Many opioid addicts are dependent on other drugs as well, notably the barbiturates and alcohol. Withdrawal symptoms may result from withholding any of these agents. Obtaining a preoperative history is important in the event that problems arise during the postoperative period when information cannot be obtained.

Other drugs used illegally for mood and behavior alteration are not as well studied in relation to anesthesia. Amphetamine, a sympathomimetic agent, exerts CNS excitatory actions; anesthetic requirements are higher when this drug is taken acutely as one dose, but lower when taken chronically. This probably relates to the increased turnover rates of norepinephrine and dopamine. Anesthetics sensitizing the myocardium would seem to be contraindicated. Even less clear are the additive effects of lysergic acid diethylamide (LSD), mescaline, and marijuana on the actions of anesthetics. All these drugs, in the acute stage, are sympathomimetics resulting in tachycardia and hypertension.

REFERENCES

Barbeau A, McDowell FH (eds): L-Dopa and Parkinsonism. Philadelphia, F. A. Davis Company, 1970.

Bigger JT Jr: Arrhythmias and antiarrhythmic drugs. Adv Intern Med 18:251, 1972.

Conney AH: Pharmacological implications of microsomal enzyme induction. Pharmacol Rev 19:317, 1967.

Freedman DX, Senay EC: Methadone treatment of heroin addiction. Annu Rev Med 24:153, 1973.

Liberti P, Stanbury JB: The pharmacology of substances affecting the thyroid gland. Annu Rev Pharmacol 11:113, 1971.

Merin RG, Samuelson PN, Schalch DS: Major inhalation anesthetics and carbohydrate metabolism. Anesth Analg 50:625, 1971.

Morrow DH, Townley NT: Anesthesia and digitalis toxicity: an experimental study. Anesth Analg 43:510, 1964.

Myerson RM: Effects of alcohol on cardiac and muscular function. *In* Israel Y, Mardones J (eds): Biological Basis of Alcoholism. New York: John Wiley & Sons Inc, 1971, pp 183–208.

Page LB, Sidd JJ: Medical management of primary hypertension. N Engl J Med 287:960; 1018; 1074, 1972.

Pittinger C, Adamson R: Antibiotic blockade of neuromuscular function. Annu Rev Pharmacol 12:169, 1972.

Schildkraut JJ: Neuropharmacology of the affective disorders. Annu Rev Pharmacol 13:427, 1973.

Sellers EM, Kalant H: Drug therapy: Alcohol intoxication and withdrawal. N Engl J Med 294:757, 1976.

Thorn GW (ed): Symposium on the adrenal cortex. Am J Med 53:529, 1972.

Chapter 4

PREMEDICATION, TRANSPORT TO THE OPERATING ROOM, AND PREPARATION FOR ANESTHESIA

During preanesthetic rounds the anesthetist observes the mental and physical condition of a patient, and, after due consideration of the patient's problems, the surgeon's requirements, and the anesthetist's own skills, a decision is made on the conduct of anesthesia. Premedication can be given rationally only after these considerations have been taken into account. Selection of preanesthetic drugs should be the prerogative of the anesthetist, since the anesthesia may be said to begin when these drugs are given. Wise choice of medication can pave the way for an uncomplicated anesthetic and postoperative course; improper choice can lead to an unsatisfactory experience for all concerned.

The kinds and amounts of preanesthetic drugs chosen depend upon the anesthetist's goals. As noted subsequently, some agents are meant to diminish salivary secretions and vagal effects on the heart; to eliminate the possibility of awareness during light planes of anesthesia; and to act as basal analgetics when intravenous barbiturates and nitrous oxide are administered. We prefer that patients come to the operating room awake though drowsy, free from apprehension, and fully cooperative. If confidence has been gained by the patient during the preanesthetic visit, apprehension will usually be less and the need for sedation reduced. This contention had long been based on clinical impression until Egbert and his coworkers (1963) evaluated the comparative calming effects of a placebo, pentobarbital (Nembutal), and an informative, reassuring preoperative visit. The interview involved frank discussion of the patient's fears, analysis of problems, statement of the time required for the operation, the nature of the anesthetic, and a description of immediate postoperative effects. Their findings, summarized in Table 4–1, clearly indicate that instruction, suggestion, and encouragement are useful nonpharmacologic antidotes to anxiety.

Table 4-1. PREMEDICATION VS. PREOPERATIVE VISIT
BY ANESTHETIST*

	No Visit No Drug	Visit Alone	Drug Alone	Drug and Visit
	Per Cent			
Feel nervous	58	40	61	38
Feel drowsy	18	26	30	38
Judged adequately sedated	35	65	48	71

*Comparison of effects of pentobarbital 2 mg per kg intramuscularly, one hour before induction of anesthesia, with those of a reassuring, informative preoperative visit by the anesthetist. (Modified from Egbert LD, Battit, GE, Turndorf, H, et al: JAMA 185:553, 1963.)

It should be emphasized that drowsiness or sleepiness does not guarantee freedom from apprehension. For many genuinely frightened patients, relief of anxiety comes only with considerable dulling of consciousness. One may be tempted, therefore, to agree to the frequent request that the patient be unconscious before leaving the floor. However, if unconsciousness is induced before the journey to the operating room additional hazards are created, resulting not only from central depressant effects of the drugs but also from complications such as respiratory obstruction and circulatory instability. A word to the patient that the practice is unsafe usually settles the issue.

The physical and mental condition of the patient determines the need for as well as the dosage of premedicants. The more ill, the more elderly, and the less robust and active the patient, the smaller is the requirement for sedatives and analgetics. A degree of physical depression difficult to define is already present in these individuals, and, in general, the greater the body mass, the larger is the distribution volume for the drugs given.

THE PREMEDICANTS

In general drugs used for premedication include the sedatives, opioids, tranquilizers, and anticholinergics.

SEDATIVES

The term sedative or hypnotic does not connote a specific kind of action, because the wide variety of drugs used for these purposes produces a spectrum of effects ranging from mere sedation through general anesthesia, deep coma, and terminating in death with gross overdose. The relationship between sleep-producing properties and chemical constitution is not well defined. Few of these drugs mimic the action of natural sleep in terms of rapid eye movement (REM) activity. To a large extent the efficacy of a drug depends upon the pharmacokinetics involved, that is, the rate and extent of absorption, distribution in the body fluid compartments, degree of protein-binding, and the rapidity and nature of metabolism and excretion. For passage across the blood-brain barrier, a matter of high lipoid solubility, a sedative should offer a low degree of ionization at body pH.

Barbiturates

Most patients scheduled for operation do better when given a hypnotic the night before operation, since apprehension, the newness of surroundings, and the disturbances in a hospital all cause insomnia. When used for this purpose, the barbiturates offer a long record of safety. There is no known teratogenic effect when they are given during pregnancy. Generally pentobarbital (Nembutal) or secobarbital (Seconal) in a dose from 100 to 200 mg is given orally at bedtime and repeated once if necessary. These drugs produce maximal sedation in one to one and one-half hours, the action largely dissipating after three to four hours. Although duration of action is an intrinsic property of the barbiturate chosen, classification of these drugs into short- and long-acting compounds has not been supported by controlled studies. Large doses of any of the barbiturates will result in a prolonged action. It is best to inquire whether a patient has been taking sedatives; if accustomed to a particular kind, this may be repeated remembering that tolerance may have developed and that a larger dose is required. Barbiturates can induce hepatic microsomal enzymes involved in the metabolism of other drugs as well as the barbiturates themselves (see Chapter 3).

We prefer to give a barbiturate as the principal drug for premedication and favor secobarbital or pentobarbital in doses from 75 to 200 mg for the adult. Doses for infants and children are discussed in Chapter 24. Barbiturates offer an advantage over opioids in that sedation is the principal action. In usual amounts they rarely depress respiration (Fig. 4-1) or circulation. Allergic responses are not uncommon and an occasional subject may become excited and confused rather than quieted. A barbiturate may be given orally two hours before operation with a sip of water, a convenient route of administration, with the duration of action as stated. When injected intramuscularly, an effect is usually noted within 30 minutes, disappearing in two to three hours. The intramuscular route is more certain and necessary when a gastric tube is in place. Barbiturates cause pain when injected because of the glycol solvent.

Depending upon the barbiturate chosen, metabolism and excretion may differ. The so-called short-acting drugs are metabolized and conjugated principally in the liver, and they therefore are useful in the patient with advanced renal disease in whom excretion of another kind of barbiturate would be delayed. In the presence of severe hepatic disease, however, the effects may be exaggerated and prolonged. Phenobarbital is excreted mostly by the kidney and hence is the barbiturate of choice in patients with liver failure. High doses of barbiturates cause respiratory depression, and

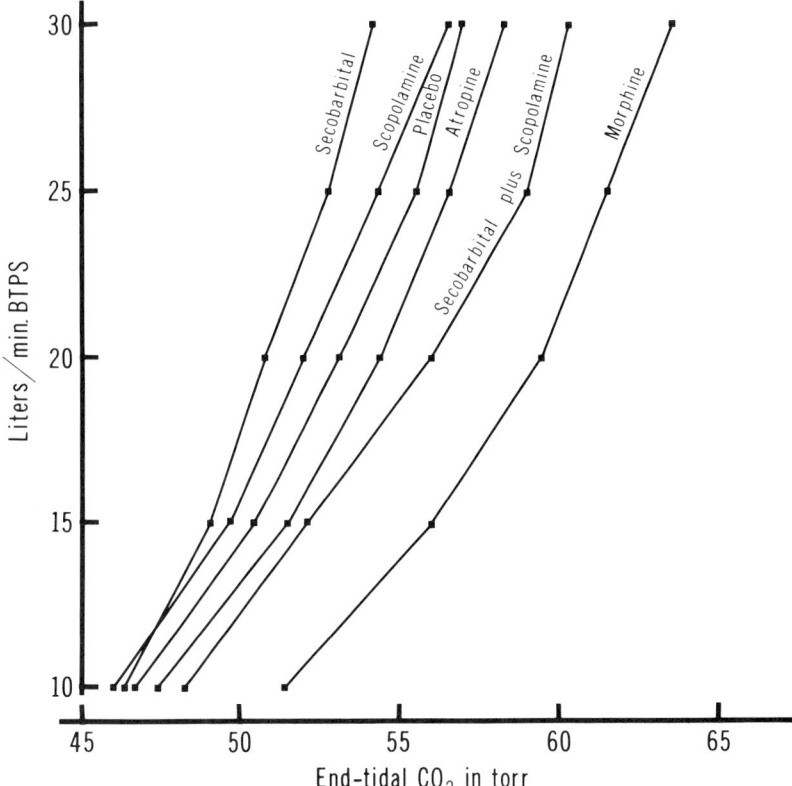

Figure 4–1. Effects of premedicant drugs upon respiratory response to carbon dioxide in man. Ten subjects rebreathed carbon dioxide in a closed system. Average end-tidal carbon dioxide tension required to produce minute ventilations of 10, 15, 20, 25, and 30 L/min are plotted. Secobarbital and scopolamine individually are mild respiratory stimulants (although clinically insignificant), while in combination they are depressant (although not so severely as 10 mg of morphine). (Reproduced with permission from Smith TC, Stephen GW, Zeiger L, et al: Anesthesiology 28:883, 1967.)

the drugs should not be given in the presence of acute intermittent porphyria because a crisis may be precipitated.

The central stimulating properties of local anesthetics such as muscle tremor, agitation, and convulsions can be treated with low doses of barbiturates, although diazepam (Valium) is the drug of choice. Either one is given intravenously, together with inhalation of oxygen (see Chapter 17). The belief has long been held that administration of a barbiturate before regional anesthesia would minimize toxic reactions. There are no data to support this contention, and some claim that a higher mortality may result from additive circulatory depression. Diazepam given prophylactically does increase the median lethal dose of local anesthetic in laboratory animals.

If barbiturates rather than opioids are given preoperatively, the anesthetist might anticipate that the patient will awaken more quickly from general anesthesia, experience pain earlier, and exhibit restlessness as consciousness is regained, which is believed to reflect an antianalgetic action of barbiturates. The incidence of postoperative nausea and vomiting can be expected to be lower when these drugs are given for premedication, as compared with opioids.

Nonbarbiturate Sedatives and Major Tranquilizers

Under a number of circumstances other sedatives are preferable to the barbiturates, such as when allergic reactions have been experienced or when hyperactivity rather than sedation is anticipated. It is believed that when barbiturates are given to the elderly a higher incidence of disorientation, agitation, and transient psychoses may result; hence chloral hydrate 0.5 to 1.0 gm in capsule form, by mouth, is sometimes used as a substitute. Probably chloral hydrate thus given merely represents a lower sedative dose.

In addition to promethazine (Phenergan), sometimes given with an opioid, other phenothiazine derivatives, tranquilizers such as hydroxyzine (Vistaril), and certain butyrophenones may be given for premedication. Hydroxyzine, in particular, has been shown to potentiate the analgetic effect of opioids without an increase in major side effects. The use of all these is predicated upon a number of pharmacologic effects: sedative action *per se*, potentiation of the effect of opioids and general anesthetics, alpha-adrenergic blockade, blockage of certain autonomic reflexes, and antiemetic and antihistaminic activity. The major differences between these drugs and the barbiturates is that they are not anticonvulsants and do not lead to respiratory depression or physical dependence, although a few produce extrapyramidal effects. Some of these substances offer considerable antiemetic activity, but we believe it unwise to prescribe drugs routinely preoperatively for this purpose. If there is a history of protracted postanesthetic vomiting, an antiemetic can be given intramuscularly 15 to 20 minutes before the end of the operation, or to treat nausea or vomiting already present. According to some, promazine (Sparine), triflupromazine (Vesprin), and propiomazine (Largon) also exert a mild analgetic action. Other phenothiazines such as promethazine appear to increase sensitivity to pain if used independently of the opioids.

The benzodiazepines are among the most widely prescribed drugs in clinical medicine. As a group these compounds are used as sedative-hypnotics, for the treatment of anxiety (chlordiazepoxide), behavioral disorders, neuromuscular disease, seizures, and the alcohol withdrawal syndrome. Diazepam, used in 5 to 10 mg doses either orally or intravenously (the intramuscular route results in poor absorption), is employed before cardioversion and for both prevention and treatment of the central stimulant properties of local anesthetics. Others use the drug as a sedative alone, for endoscopic procedures, to ease labor and delivery, and for intravenous induction of general anesthesia (see Chapter 13). The pain experienced upon intravenous injection probably results from precipitation of drug crystals from the glycol solvent. A localized sterile thrombophlebitis is, therefore, not an uncommon complication.

Excessive dosage of any of the benzodiazepines can, in addition to coma, result in respiratory and circulatory depression. However, in contrast to the barbiturates, the addiction liability is less, and hepatic enzyme induction does not seem to occur. For these reasons, in addition to the fact that REM sleep is more closely approximated, flurazepam (Dalmane) rather than a barbiturate is used as a sleep medicine, in doses of 15 to 30 mg orally.

OPIOIDS

This group of drugs comprises the potent analgetics and is classified as follows: (1) natural alkaloids of opium (morphine, codeine) and mixtures of the alkaloids (omnopon [Pantopon]), (2) semisynthetic modifications of these compounds (dihydromorphinone [Dilaudid]), and (3) synthetics (meperidine [Demerol]). Although pain is not common prior to operation, it has been customary to prescribe the analgetics in part for sedation but mostly to diminish the amount of general anesthetic subsequently required. The efficacy of the analgetics in reducing the concentration of general anesthetic needed to produce a given depth of anesthesia is evidenced by a lowering of the minimum alveolar concentrations (MAC) (see Chapter 10).

It is common practice to give an analgetic to patients who are to be anesthetized with less potent combinations of general anesthetics like nitrous oxide and thiopental and to combine an opioid with a barbiturate or diazepam for regional anesthesia. Under these circumstances, the action of the opioid is probably more like that of a basal anesthetic. The respiratory depressant action of analgetics may be useful, since most volatile anesthetics increase the respiratory rate in the light planes; tidal volumes may become inadequate and respiratory acidosis result. An analgetic may counter this tendency by maintaining a more satisfactory rate and depth of breathing. On the other hand, uptake of the anesthetic may be slowed by respiratory depression and respiratory assistance may be required.

Undesirable Effects of the Analgetics

All analgetics decrease alveolar ventilation, as shown by a diminished response to a carbon dioxide challenge. The degree and duration are dose-related, but with approximately the same effect in equianalgetic doses. The duration of effect is longer than is generally appreciated. Figure 4-2 illustrates this response, showing that fentanyl (Sublimaze), a potent opioid with relatively brief analgetic action, continues to exert an effect on breathing for a matter of hours. A single dose of morphine has been shown to be active for 12 hours or more after intramuscular injection. Respiratory depression is also evident in the newborn as a result of placental transfer of an opioid. For the same reasons, the use of analgetics is associated with a higher incidence of postoperative pulmonary complications: atelectasis

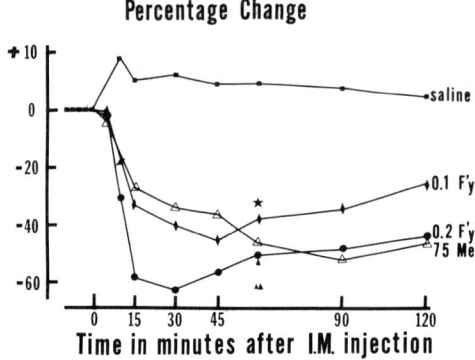

Figure 4-2. Prolonged respiratory action of narcotic analgetics. The end-tidal carbon dioxide was kept at 46 torr by addition of variable amounts of carbon dioxide to inspired gas. F'y'l = fentanyl; Mep = meperidine. Doses in mg.

may result because of elimination of spontaneous intermittent sighing and depression of the cough reflex.

A reduction in the ability of the circulation to react to stress is evidenced by an increased incidence of hypotension and fainting following head-up tilt; this is the result of a direct vasodilating action on peripheral vascular smooth muscle, possibly owing to release of histamine. When cyclopropane was a popular anesthetic, the addition of morphine caused a reduction in cardiac output over a normal or increased state resulting from endogenous output of catecholamines. However, morphine given intravenously in high doses, 0.5 to 3.0 mg per kg, usually has little adverse effect on circulatory dynamics in the supine individual, except for the occasional person who develops profound hypotension. In this way morphine has been used as the major analgetic supplemented by moderate concentrations of nitrous oxide and neuromuscular blockers for the performance of major cardiac operations during extracorporeal circulation. Respiratory depression is profound, requiring ventilatory assistance well into the postoperative period. Meperidine may cause tachycardia and in rare instances convert auricular fibrillation to flutter with a correspondingly higher ventricular rate.

So far as the bowel is concerned, after initial duodenal spasm and increased gastric emptying time, peristalsis and intestinal tone are decreased and constipation results. Analgetics can cause nausea and vomiting prior to induction of anesthesia and they contribute to postoperative nausea and vomiting in part through an effect on the vestibular apparatus leading to motion sickness, or through stimulation of the chemoreceptor trigger zone in the medulla. Sphincteric tone is increased and smooth muscle is constricted in other areas such as the biliary tract, ureter, and bronchioles. Release of antidiuretic hormone by opioids has been shown in the dog; in patients it may contribute to dilutional hyponatremia.

New opioids are introduced from time to time, each purporting to produce the same degree of analgesia provided by morphine but with fewer undesirable side effects. As a rule, these contentions are unfounded because the drugs in question have not been compared in controlled clinical studies with the analgesia produced by morphine in a standard dose of 10 mg per 70 kg body weight.

Attention has focused on the opioid antagonists as useful analgetics because they are nonaddictive and some produce analgesia in their own right. Nalorphine (Nalline) is a satisfactory analgetic, but accompanying hallucinatory effects preclude its use. Pentazocine (Talwin), a benzomorphan related to phenazocine (Prinadol), is both a weak opioid antagonist and an analgetic in humans, a dose of 30 to 60 mg corresponding to 10 mg of morphine. However, in equianalgetic dosage, respiratory and other adverse effects differ little from those of the other opioids. Likewise the belief that the drug is nonaddictive is incorrect, although the dependence potential is minimal; in certain individuals unpleasant hallucinatory phenomena occur. In order to avoid the possibility of addiction, a phenothiazine derivative, methotrimeprazine (Levoprome) was introduced, 15 to 20 mg given intramuscularly being the equivalent of 10 mg morphine. But methotrimeprazine causes marked postural hypotension and excessive sedation.

Analgetics are given before anesthesia by the subcutaneous or intramuscular route; in the former, the optimal effect is reached in approximately 45 to 60 minutes. Intramuscular injection provides a more rapid onset but shorter duration. Medication may also be given intravenously just before induction of anesthesia; under these conditions injection is made slowly and the dose reduced since respiratory depression may follow.

A schedule for preanesthetic use of opioids in children is provided in Chapter 24. The dose of morphine in the adult varies from 5 to 10 mg per 60 to 70 kg body weight, with corresponding doses of meperidine from 50 to 125 mg. When an analgetic is combined with a barbiturate, the dose of analgetic is reduced.

Combination of an opioid with an opioid antagonist has been suggested with the idea that analgesia could be preserved and respiratory or circulatory depression prevented. However, when a mixture of opioid and antagonist in appropriate ratio is given to a patient who has not had an opioid previously respiratory depression develops. There are no convincing data to show that the combination minimizes the postural hypotension sometimes observed. If enough antagonist is given, analgesia will be counteracted; thus it is more rational to give the opioid and antagonist separately.

During the preanesthetic visit, patients sometimes ask that a particular analgetic not be given because of allergy. Questioning usually reveals that the symptoms consisted of nausea, vomiting, or vertigo — common side effects rather than allergy. However, a history of protracted vomiting, excitement, urticaria, or wheezing suggests that the offending opioid should be omitted. If analgesia is required, an analgetic of different chemical configuration should be given. When time permits, a small test dose can be given several days beforehand.

Elderly patients, those in poor physical condition, or patients with circulatory instability should be given lower doses of the analgetics because of the higher incidence of side effects, particularly those relating to circulation and respiration. In the presence of liver failure, opioids should be used cautiously lest coma result. Patients with pulmonary emphysema, bronchial asthma, kyphoscoliosis, or cor pulmonale may react poorly to analgetics because diminished respiratory reserves and lack of compensation may result in respiratory failure. Therefore, a sharp reduction in dosage is indicated when pain relief is necessary. Preferably some other means of relieving pain should be tried, for example, intercostal or epidural nerve block for thoracic or abdominal incisional pain.

ANTICHOLINERGICS

The copious respiratory tract secretions seen during open drop administration of ether anesthesia suggested the prophylactic use of a parasympatholytic agent, and atropine came to be used routinely for this purpose. As new, less irritating inhalation anesthetics were introduced, the need for antisialogogues diminished. Routine use of atropine or scopolamine certainly causes uncomfortable dryness of the mouth. More than a few studies describe the apparently safe administration of general anesthesia without prior use of anticholinergics. Although atropine or scopolamine is still given preoperatively by many anesthetists, we believe that these drugs should be used only for specific indications.

There are other uses for these drugs, such as the prevention or treatment of severe reflex slowing of the heart during anesthesia. When this follows intrathoracic manipulation, traction on abdominal viscera, or stimulation of the carotid sinus, intravenous injection of atropine should restore heart rate and arterial pressure to normal. Prophylactically, in order to block reflex vagal effects on the heart, a dose of atropine of at least 1.0 mg per 60 kg body weight is required. Bradycardia may also be seen in association with increase in intraoccular pressure, with traction on extraocular muscles during operation for squint, or when a dose of succinylcholine is repeated within a short period of time. Bradycardia is also common in infants and children after injection of succinylcholine and inhalation of halothane. While the drying effect of scopolamine is superior to that of atropine, the former is not as effective in preventing reflex bradycardia during general anesthesia.

The sedative action of scopolamine is marked and useful for preanesthetic sedation and amnesia. However, many patients become restless and irritable—even disoriented—after its use and the incidence of agitation during emergence from general anesthesia is high, a reaction commonly seen in response to pain. These reactions can be controlled by the intravenous injection of physostigmine (Antilirium), which crosses the blood-brain barrier to counteract the central anticholinergic action of several kinds of drugs. Physostigmine should be given slowly in 1 mg doses, not exceeding 3 mg, to avoid dangerous degrees of cholinergic activity peripherally as seen with neostigmine (Prostigmine).

Atropine and scopolamine are usually ordered in doses of 0.4 to 0.6 mg per 60 kg body weight. However, if major vagal blockade is needed prior to use of neostigmine or to treat organophosphate poisoning, much higher doses are needed (1 to 3 mg). The effects of atropine or scopolamine on heart rate differ to some extent, of some importance when digitalis has produced slowing of the rate in auricular fibrillation or flutter, or neostigmine is given for reversal of neuromuscular blockade. Both atropine and scopolamine given intravenously in low doses may slow the heart rate for a matter of seconds. Atropine thereafter causes more prolonged tachycardia, whereas scopolamine is associated with bradycardia. Scopolamine, then, would seem to be the choice for the digitalized patient. In children who are febrile and dehydrated, or with tachycardia, or in thyrotoxicosis, the dose of anticholinergic drug should be reduced or eliminated. Some anesthetists avoid these drugs in the presence of bronchial asthma or bronchitis, fearing inspissation of secretions and inability to eliminate them through cough. Both drugs, however, are bronchodilators and increase the physiolgic dead space. Except for the narrow-angle variety, glaucoma does not contraindicate their use, since a rise in intraocular pressure does not occur unless the usual clinical doses are exceeded. Moreover, an effect on smooth muscle of the iris can be counteracted by pilocarpine instilled locally. The concept that an anticholinergic drug can prevent laryngospasm in light planes of general anesthesia is not tenable; the striated muscles of the larynx do not respond to drugs that in ordinary doses have no effect on neuromuscular transmission.

In spite of their universal acceptance the belladonna alkaloids, atropine and scopolamine, have shortcomings in their relatively short duration of action, their central nervous system stimulating properties, and their varying effects on pulse rate. For these reasons the quaternary ammonium compound, glycopyrrolate (Robinul), an anticholinergic drug long used in the treatment of gastrointestinal disorders, merits consideration as a premedicant. On a milligram for milligram basis, this drug is twice as potent an antisialogogue as atropine, in both adult and child, and the duration of action at least three times as long. Although the tachycardia produced is less, protection against vagal-induced bradycardia is greater than with atropine. Finally, because the blood-brain barrier is not crossed, the central stimulation and confusion are lacking with glycopyrrolate.

PREPARATION FOR ANESTHESIA

Anesthesia is given safely only if thoughtful preparations are made beforehand, beginning with the preanesthetic visit when the anesthetist envisions the problems that may be encountered and then orders premedication. Planning presupposes a thorough understanding of the surgical procedure contemplated and the anesthetic selected. If matters are complex, it is helpful to issue detailed descriptive protocols, as, for example, use of deliberate hypotension, or management for implantation of a cardiac pacemaker or for extracorporeal circulation. Sound practice calls for departments of anesthesia to convene on the afternoon before or at the start of the day's schedule to discuss problems and management of patients to be anesthetized. Larger training programs can make "block assignments," placing staff and resident anesthetists in the same specialty area of an operating suite for weeks or months. This facilitates preoperative discussion, preparation, demonstration, and supervision during anesthesia, as well as postoperative teaching rounds.

Transport of the Patient

A patient should be brought to the operating area in sufficient time so that anesthesia need not be hurried. Rapid induction is not in the best interests of the patient nor is it conducive to instruction of beginners. Careful transport to the operating room is essential, if possible under the supervision of a nurse or nurse's aide. Detailed instructions for transfer are written when needed; for example, one should specify that the orthopneic patient should be in the head-up position or the desperately ill patient accompanied by a physician. Upon arrival, the patient must be identified. Preparation may proceed either in a holding room or in the operating room proper. Use of anesthesia induction rooms is no longer recommended because some believe it unsafe to anesthetize patients in one area and then move them to another, although others believe better operating room utilization is achieved this way and that the practice is not a hazardous one. Regardless of opinion, patients should await anesthesia in a quiet area where an intravenous infusion can be started and a blood pressure cuff applied. They should not be subjected to the sights and sounds of the operating room as they lie strapped to a litter in a busy corridor. The purposes of premedication are defeated by this practice.

Immediate Preanesthetic Care

The patient should be assisted in the transfer from litter to operating table. Care in movement is important in the extremely ill, the patient in pain, the osteoporotic, and for those whose circulation is precarious. Intravenous infusions, drainage catheters, and traction apparatus must be protected. The patient should be covered with a clean bed sheet or cotton blanket for modesty and warmth. A lifting sheet should be present beneath the back, and a broad restraining strap above the knees. The arms and legs should be comfortably restrained to protect against peripheral nerve injury, and the legs not crossed. Some patients find that flexion of the operating table provides more comfort. When there is a potential explosion or electric hazard, the patient should be grounded to the table by means of a conductive strap. An operating room cap should be applied to protect the hair and promote asepsis. Whether every patient should wear a mask is a matter of opinion, although this should be the case when virulent pulmonary infections are present. Once placed on an operating table or litter, a patient should not be left alone.

The beginner tends to concentrate on technical matters, although obviously assessment of the patient's condition should be the first consideration. The patient is asked when he or she last ate or drank and whether medication was given. The nurse's record is consulted for preoperative vital signs and temperature, to be sure dentures have been removed, and for dosage and time of administration of medicines. The latest recordings of laboratory data are noted. Of particular interest here are serum electrolyte levels, coagulation defects, hematocrit reading, the electrocardiogram, and the chest x-ray. These are recorded on the anesthesia record with the assessment of the degree of sedation and other changes in physical or mental condition. Cancellation of the operation may be necessary if preparation has been inadequate.

Stethoscope and blood pressure cuff are applied to the arm and the stethoscope taped to the chest; these remain in place throughout the operation. The blood pressure cuff can be protected against contact at the side of the operating table by a tobogganlike device. Baseline blood pressure, pulse, and respiratory rate are recorded. Monitoring devices such as electrocardiograph leads may be applied or a central venous catheter inserted at this time, with care taken not to cause pain or alarm the patient (see Chapter 8). When there is a deviation from the expected in symptoms or signs, an explanation must be sought. The supervising anesthetist, surgeon, and consulting internist should determine whether to proceed.

Technical Procedures

An intravenous infusion is started except for brief procedures in which fluid is not needed or an intravenous anesthetic is not used. Intravenous techniques and fluid therapy are discussed in Chapter 21. Venipuncture and venous or arterial cutdowns may be less disturbing to the patient after consciousness has been lost and peripheral vasoconstriction abolished through the action of general anesthetics. Likewise, bladder catheterization or passage of a gastric tube or esophageal stethoscope is better completed after the patient is asleep. Present-day anesthesia practices may require several infusions: for giving drugs, and for fluid and blood replacement. For some operations, such as major vascular or radical cancer procedures, an important part of anesthetic management lies in the anticipation, measurement, and replacement of blood loss, for which large cannulas are inserted.

Artificial airways, endotracheal tubes, laryngoscope, and suction catheters and apparatus are arranged neatly on the anesthetist's work table. Each piece of apparatus should be clean and working properly. Dirty equipment is placed in a container kept separate from clean supplies. A source of suction is at hand. Drugs used for induction such as neuromuscular blockers are drawn into labeled syringes beforehand.

A second person can be of considerable help during induction to restrain the patient when there is excitement, aid in positioning for operation, observe the pulse at crucial times, prepare injections, start an intravenous infusion, or seek additional help when necessary. Anesthesia for complicated operations may require the continuous attention of two or more anesthetists.

The value of a prescribed routine in the preparation of the patient is appreciated only after the beginner has encountered difficulties during induction. Extra time set aside for preparation permits one to deal with the unexpected. Anesthetists should be prompt; if tardy, they take unnecessary chances and perform poorly under the scrutiny of an impatient operating team. Calm, unhurried activity, neatness, cleanliness, and punctuality mark the skilled clinician.

APPRAISAL

After reading the contents of this chapter, both anesthetists and other physicians will understand why the prescription of premedication is so much an essential part of anesthetic administration *per se*. Once routine practice, consisting for the most part of the administration of atropine and morphine, premedication today entails a knowledge not only of the pharmacology of dozens of compounds but of the patient, the complicating ailments, drugs concurrently given, and the anesthetic technique planned. Trite as the dictum may seem, preanesthetic medication may very well set the stage for all that follows, both good and bad.

REFERENCES

Egbert LD, Battit GE, Turndorf H, et al: The value of the preoperative visit by an anesthetist. JAMA 185:553, 1963.
Giuffrida JG, Bizzari DV, Saure AC, et al: Anesthetic management of drug abusers. Anesth Analg 49:272, 1970.
Gravenstein JS (ed): Pharmacology for the preoperative visit. Int Anesthesiology Clin 6 (1), 1968.
Greenblatt DJ, Shader RI: Drug therapy. Anticholinergics. N Engl J Med 288:1215, 1973.
Greenblatt DJ, Shader RI: Drug therapy. Benzodiazepines. N Engl J Med 291:1011, 1239, 1974.
Koch-Weser J, Greenblatt DJ: Editorial—The archaic barbiturate hypnotics. N Engl J Med 291:790, 1974.
Lasagna L: Drug therapy. Hypnotic drugs. N Engl J Med 287:1182, 1972.
Watt RH Jr, Keats AS: Prophylaxis and treatment of nausea and vomiting. Pharmacol Physicians 2 (12), 1968.

Section 2

ESSENTIAL PREANESTHETIC CONSIDERATIONS

Chapter 5

MEDICOLEGAL CONSIDERATIONS

Since publication of the last edition of this text, the incidence of malpractice actions against physicians and health care facilities and the problem of obtaining protection against such actions have reached the level of a national crisis. The number of suits filed has risen precipitously, while the costs of protection against suits has become so financially unrealistic that some physicians seek early retirement and others are on strike or threatening to strike in seeking relief from the high premium costs. Many in the high-risk specialties cannot afford to start private practice, and some practice without insurance protection (according to an AMA survey, 27 per cent, with an additional 30 per cent threatening to do so). The crisis was studied by a national commission which did not recommend attempt at solution by the national government but suggested action at the state level. Thus in 1976 nearly every state was debating or acting upon or had recently enacted new malpractice laws; some have been found unconstitutional within a year of enactment. Under these circumstances there is little reason to discuss solutions to the malpractice protection problem; the solutions will evolve at the state level, probably on a basis different from previous practice. This discussion will confine itself to definitions, exposures, causes, and prevention of litigation.

Lest the anesthetist in training become alarmed at the prospects of medicolegal suit, a conclusion of the national Commission on Medical Malpractice is appropriate. "Despite the publicity resulting from a few large malpractice cases, a medical malpractice incident is a relatively rare event, claims are even rarer, and jury trial rarer still." In 1970, the Commission found that 59.9 per cent of all awards were under $3000 and only 3 per cent were over $100,000.

THE CHARACTER OF LAW SUITS

What is malpractice? Conditions of law under which suits may be filed and the judgments awarded vary among the states. An excellent defense in one state may constitute no defense at all in another. Legal precedent may even be reversed and new principles of law established. Although generalizations can be made, the anesthetist should be familiar with procedures in his or her own area.

Malpractice may be criminal, a violation of law with prosecution by the state; or civil, not in violation of law, with prosecution in a civil court. Most malpractice suits fall into the latter category. Use of the term malpractice is unfortunate because it suggests criminal conduct; seldom is this the case.

Malpractice implies negligence in the care of a patient or failure to employ methods, agents, or skills ordinarily considered appropriate, but to characterize all malpractice cases as negligence is an injustice to the medical profession. One judge has observed that "persons undertaking to administer anesthetics in the course of medical or dental treatment . . . are not insurers against harm nor guarantors of a favorable result, but are required only to exercise ordinary or reasonable care or skill under the circumstances, that is, . . . the skill and diligence of the ordinary person engaged in similar practice at the time, and in the locality where the defendant undertook to act." That the hoped-for result does not follow or that complications occur does not imply liability unless the physician has promised a specific result or the complication arises from improper care. The usual professional liability policy excludes claims based upon a warranty of cure or guaranteed result. A physician is not responsible for an error in judgment unless it is so gross as to be inconsistent with the skill expected of every physician.

Proof of malpractice can be established in several ways. The most common requirement is that the plaintiff produce expert testimony establishing the standard of care applicable to the specialty involved. This is not easily done because the facts may not warrant such testimony. Physicians who once were reluctant to testify in a manner that would adversely affect a colleague are less reluctant today, especially in significant departures from standard modern patient care; thus the complaint of "conspiracy of silence" may no longer be applicable. The matter is complicated in that courts usually apply a liberal interpretation of what constitutes an "expert" witness, and the jury is left to decide upon the expert's qualifications. Many physicians harbor preconceived notions, frequently not well founded, concerning their obligation to testify.

Because physicians were once reluctant to participate, the law recognized the doctrine of *res ipsa loquitur,* which for practical purposes eliminates the need for expert testimony. Literally, the doctrine means "the act speaks for itself." This has usually been applied in situations in which harm could not have occurred except through negligence and the technique or treatment causing the harm was under the control of the physician. In cases in which the doctrine is invoked, the physician must prove that negligence was not involved. The doctrine is apt to be invoked when a malpractice case heard on actual facts might otherwise fail for lack of proof. If there is an indication that lack of expert testimony for the plaintiff results from inability of the patient to secure it, a court may rule *res ipsa loquitur*. With physicians now more ready to testify, in recent years seldom has a case of merit been wanting for expert testimony. Many county and state medical societies provide a plaintiff with expert witnesses in meritorious cases.

CAUSES OF MALPRACTICE ACTIONS

Failure of physicians to establish a rapport with their patients is the principal cause of suits against physicians. Anesthetists are frequently negligent in this regard. While having worked hard for recognition of the specialty as an independent discipline, they have failed to appreciate the responsibility of a closer identification with their patients. Unfortunately, custom and tradition have not required the usual patient-physician relationship. Opportunities for contact with patients outside the operating room are less than those afforded most other specialists, and too often visits are hastily completed. When a preoperative examination has been omitted and postoperative visits are not made, the only recollection the patient may have of the anesthetist is receipt of a bill for services. Obviously under these circumstances a bond of understanding between patient and physician has not been established. With the patient usually unconscious during the time when the anesthetist makes a major contribution, the stage is set for resentment against an unknown physician.

Other factors render anesthetists susceptible to suit. They work as a team, some members of which are even more liable to suit, and the present tendency in malpractice actions is to name all members of a team as well as the hospital.

Some patients are "suit conscious," believing that they should receive compensation for anything other than a perfect result and for inadvertent accidents, unexpectedly long periods of convalescence, and even hurt feelings. An attorney described this attitude as follows: "The present philosophy of the bulk of American people is that they are entitled to absolute protection from someone for every misfortune of human life, regardless of whether caused by divine providence, human frailty, or their own improvidence or misconduct." The emotional component of a medical malpractice case may be strong. In the ordinary personal injury action unrelated to medical practice, plaintiffs wish to be compensated for the injury and the damage caused, but they believe that the award will be paid by an insurance company and they may harbor no ill will or malice toward the person or organization thought to be responsible. However, in medical malpractice suits, although the source of payment again is thought to be an insurance company, bitterness is likely to arise if an illness or deformity is unsuccessfully treated. The patient may have regarded the doctor as a last hope and the treatment failed to measure up to expectations.

Finally, malpractice suits can provide substantial revenue for the plaintiff's attorney, who may urge clients to institute malpractice suits in the hope of obtaining, on a contingency basis, 30 per cent or more of whatever judgment is awarded, sometimes amounting to hundreds of thousands of dollars. In 1968, a successful plaintiff received only an average of 27 per cent of the sum awarded, the remainder going for costs and attorney's fees. In countries in which contingency fees are not permitted, the incidence of medicolegal suits is low.

Dornette has summarized the origin of malpractice problems, as shown in Figure 5–1.

RESPONSIBILITY OF MEDICAL STUDENTS, RESIDENTS, AND NURSE ANESTHETISTS

Medical students and resident physicians are not immune to court action and should be protected by malpractice insurance. Rarely are they named as sole defendants but more likely as one of several, including the supervising anesthetist, the surgeon, and the hospital administrator. Medical students pursuing courses for credit and registered with a university or college are usually protected against suit through the institution, sometimes by the hospital, and occasionally by both. However, students on preceptorships or in elective courses not approved by the medical school, or those

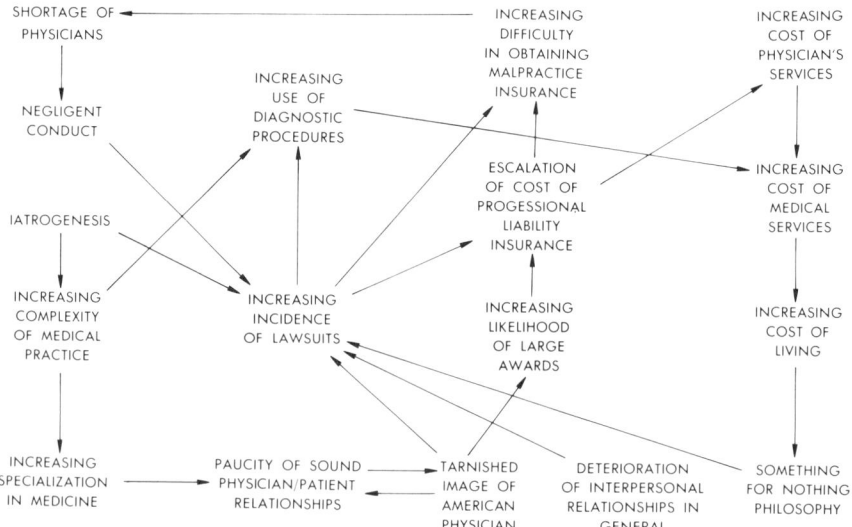

Figure 5–1. Pathogenesis of the malpractice insurance problem. (Reproduced with permission from Dornette WHL: Anesthesiology 33:535, 1970.)

taking training in hospitals or working with physicians unaffiliated with a medical school should inquire as to their protection rather than assume they are protected or carry no risk. House staff likewise are protected through the hospital or medical center in which they are training, but they should inquire as to insurance protection and, if need be, secure it for themselves. Dornette (1970) has suggested that the question is not whether a resident should be protected but by whom and to what policy limits. He points out that even residents in government-supported hospitals should purchase insurance and that, in general, protection should be held with the same carrier used by the majority of surgeons in the institution. A resident should also discover who carries protection for the anesthesia staff. Residents who indulge in "moonlighting" should notify the insurance carrier of their activities so that they are not unprotected outside the parent institution.

A nurse anesthetist can be held liable for negligence in the administration of an anesthetic. This person is assumed to be responsible for the technical administration of the anesthetic, for the observation and recording of vital signs, and for the well-being of the patient. Most certified registered nurse anesthetists avail themselves of malpractice protection. However, the likelihood is that responsibility for the actions of the nurse will be shared at least in part by others. If a surgeon of anesthetist supervises a nurse in the administration of an anesthetic, under the doctrine of *respondeat superior* the nurse is the assistant of the physician and the latter must assume responsibility. If a nurse's work is unsupervised while an employee of the hospital, the hospital is responsible under the same doctrine. If an anesthetist employs the nurse or advises the hospital as to the qualifications or conditions of employment, the anesthetist is responsible even though not directly concerned in supervision at the time of an alleged act of negligence.

HOW TO MINIMIZE LEGAL RISK

Preoperative Preparation for Anesthesia. Anesthetists' responsibilities commence before the patient arrives in the operating room; they should conduct themselves after the manner suggested in Chapter 2. Pertinent points of the history should be summarized on the patient's chart with the results of the physical examination and interview, including a statement of any unusual risk involved and the type of anesthesia planned. If such a procedure always were followed, many a law suit might have been avoided.

The problem of "informed consent" must be considered at the time of the interview with the patient and a notation made on the chart. Not only must patients sign a statement authorizing the operation and anesthesia, but they must thoroughly understand what is to be done. The surgeon explains the operative procedure, and the anesthetist that which he or she proposes to do. The patient should be given the opportunity to ask questions or to make a choice if any is to be made. Choice should not be interpreted to mean that the anesthetist presents the patient with a "shopping list" of agents and techniques; few patients have the competence to make such selections. The choice is more likely to involve regional versus general anesthesia, intravenous induction versus inhalation induction, and so on. Barring questions, the anesthetist need not go into detail about possible complications unless an unusual technique is to be used, a new drug employed, or the physical condition of the patient renders him particularly complication-prone, such as the possibility of dislodgment of loose or diseased teeth during laryngoscopy. One must inform but at the same time try to avoid arousing undue apprehension. The note on the record should include a statement that the anesthetist has described the proposed anesthesia and that the patient understands. When new drugs or techniques are to be used, it is best to have the patient sign for both approbation and consent.

In the Operating Room. Anesthetists are responsible for the immediate preoperative preparation and care (Chapters 4 and 6). While it is their duty to see that gas cylinders are properly attached to the anesthesia machine, adequately filled, and identified by color and label, they are not charged with the manufacturer's responsibility of providing correctly identified gases of acceptable purity. They must identify all drugs injected and assure themselves that the materials used for injection satisfy requirements for sterility. Protective devices such as suction, airways, and the like must be provided. Although there is no law requiring that all safety devices such as endotracheal equipment or a defibrillator be immediately at hand for every procedure, this equipment should be conveniently available in the operating theater.

Transport of patients is a shared responsibility, but the hospital provides the means for safe transportation. Once a patient has been delivered into the hands of the anesthetist, the anesthetist assumes control except when this is shared by the surgeon. If surgeons supervise positioning of the patient for operation, complications arising therefrom may be wholly their responsibility.

During anesthesia, the anesthetist exercises care in protection of the patient against injury as outlined in subsequent chapters. In the event that anesthetists employ a new technique, equipment, or agents, they should be able to substantiate familiarity with these methods and understanding of any complications that may arise from their use.

Electric and Combustion Hazards. Anesthetists are not ordinarily responsible for maintenance of equipment in operating rooms insofar as electric and combustion hazards are concerned. They should, however, point out to the hospital administration any inadequacies in conductive flooring, lack of explosion-proof electric connections, lack of approved storage facilities for flammable agents, improper control of humidity and ventilation, and explosion and electrocution hazards associated with the electrocautery, the electrocardiograph, and other devices. The surgeon should inform the anesthetist of any intended use of electric equipment. Prevention of electric accidents, fires, and explosions is discussed in Chapter 29. If anesthetists choose to administer flammable anesthetics, they should observe the necessary precautions and be able to defend the choice, showing that they were aware of the hazard and that steps to avoid an accident were taken.

Records. The best protection an anesthetist can have is an accurate and complete anesthesia record with written observations at regular intervals as operation and anesthesia progress. A record should never be altered *post facto.* If items of information are subsequently recorded, these must be clearly indicated as additions.

Blood Transfusion. The kinds and quantities of parenteral fluids given during operation are best determined by mutual consent between surgeon and anesthetist. The physician who starts a transfusion is responsible for identifying each unit of blood given and determining that the blood has been properly crossmatched. The anesthetist must be aware of the hazards of blood transfusion and be certain that the indications for transfusion are valid.

Postoperative Care. Responsibilities of the anesthetist do not cease when the patient has been taken from the operating room. Observation continues until care is assigned to another competent person. If dissatisfied with the patient's condition, the anesthetist should remain in attendance. In most institutions the recovery room is supervised by anesthetists. A detailed record of the patient's progress in the recovery room is essential.

During postoperative visits, discussion of the anesthesia experience should be encouraged by the anesthetist. If the patient is dissatisfied, this is usually apparent. It is the disgruntled patient not given the opportunity to express dissatisfaction who may ultimately sue.

WHAT SHOULD BE DONE IN THE EVENT OF AN ACCIDENT?

It is inconceivable that medicine can be practiced without accidents or complications. Most patients are understanding and are satisfied by frank discussion of the problems. If, however, the physician belittles or ignores a complication or fails to impart sympathetic understanding, the stage is set for the malpractice action.

In the event of an accident or complication definitely or possibly related to anesthesia, the anesthetist should document the facts on the patient's chart in chronological order during or immediately following the administration of anesthesia. Treatment should be noted and consultative opinions included. Subsequent notations should be made on the chart periodically during the remainder of the hospital stay and a record of treatment kept.

The physician should immediately provide the hospital and the insurance company with a complete account of the accident. Should a suit be threatened or legal inquiry made concerning a patient, the physician should immediately notify the carrier. Failure to do so within a reasonable period has resulted in loss of protection in more than a few instances.

APPRAISAL

The attitude of the courts toward malpractice suits undergoes continuous revision. The body of law lies between the tradition that liability must be predicated upon fault and one calling for reinbursement of those who suffer injury. When care may have been improper, malpractice or negligence can be accepted as descriptive of the defendant's action, and the traditional concepts of law apply. In such cases, physicians should be willing to testify on behalf of a plaintiff; most cases are settled out of court.

More perplexing problems involve those instances in which the physician's conduct has been blameless according to accepted standards, but the patient has had a poor result and seeks compensation. When the terms malpractice and negligence are used in this context, they are not applicable. There is increasing pressure to settle out of court, as a large judgment may be made when a jury views a poor result and is unable to understand the situation facing the physician at the time of treatment. At the present time, few courts seem willing to recognize that there is an irreducible risk in the practice of medicine. Nonetheless, when fault is not involved, settlement should not be made and the case should be brought to trial. Several countries are exploring no fault patient injury insurance as a solution to this dilemma.

Meanwhile the best protection against medicolegal action lies in a thorough and up-to-date practice of anesthesia, coupled with sympathetic interest in the patient and compilation of detailed records of the course of anesthesia.

REFERENCES

Curran WJ: Malpractice insurance. N Engl J Med 292:1223, 1975.
Dornette WHL: Professional liability insurance. Anesthesiology 33:535, 1970.
Dornette WHL: The medical malpractice problem, and some possible solutions. Anesthesiology 44:230, 1976.
Louisell DW, Williams H: Trial of Medical Malpractice Cases. Albany, New York, Matthew Bender & Co Inc, 1960.
Report of the Secretary's Commission on Medical Malpractice (DHEW Publication No OS 73-88) Washington DC, US Government Printing Office, January 16, 1976.
Shindell S: A survey of the law of medical practice. JAMA 194:281, 1965.
Waltz JR, Imbau, FE: Medical Jurisprudence. New York, The Macmillan Company, 1971.
Wasmuth CE: Liability of the anesthesiologist and the surgeon. JAMA 172:1473, 1960.
Wasmuth CE: The causes of malpractice action. Anesthesiology 26:659, 1965.

Chapter 6

ANESTHESIA EQUIPMENT

ANESTHESIA MACHINES

Every anesthetist should be conversant with the mechanism and physical principles governing use of an anesthesia machine. There are various makes of machine, all with the same basic elements. These include (Fig. 6-1): a source of oxygen and anesthetic gases; the means for measuring and controlling their delivery; a means to volatilize and deliver liquid anesthetics; and safety devices. The anesthetic-oxygen mixture delivered from the machine is administered to the patient through a breathing system. One system, the circle absorber, is shown in Figure 6-1. Others are described in Chapter 12.

COMPRESSED GASES

In the first few decades after the introduction of anesthesia, there was little need for compressed gases or anesthesia machines, for ether and chloroform were given as vapors in atmospheric air. When nitrous oxide was used, the gas was supplied from a generating apparatus. Though the vital importance of oxygen was known, it was not until 1868 that Andrews introduced mixtures of nitrous oxide and oxygen. This created an interest in apparatus for simultaneous administration of the gases. In 1872 the Johnston Brothers Concern began to supply liquid nitrous oxide in metal cylinders, requiring measurement of pressure and flow rate of gases; this, in turn, led to the development of anesthesia machines.

Gases used in anesthesia are available in cylinders mounted on the machine (Fig. 6-1) or, for oxygen and nitrous oxide, they may be piped in from a central container or bank of cylinders. There are precautions necessary for both systems, some specific for one or the other. Because a central supply may fail, it is essential to mount cylinders on machines for emergency use.

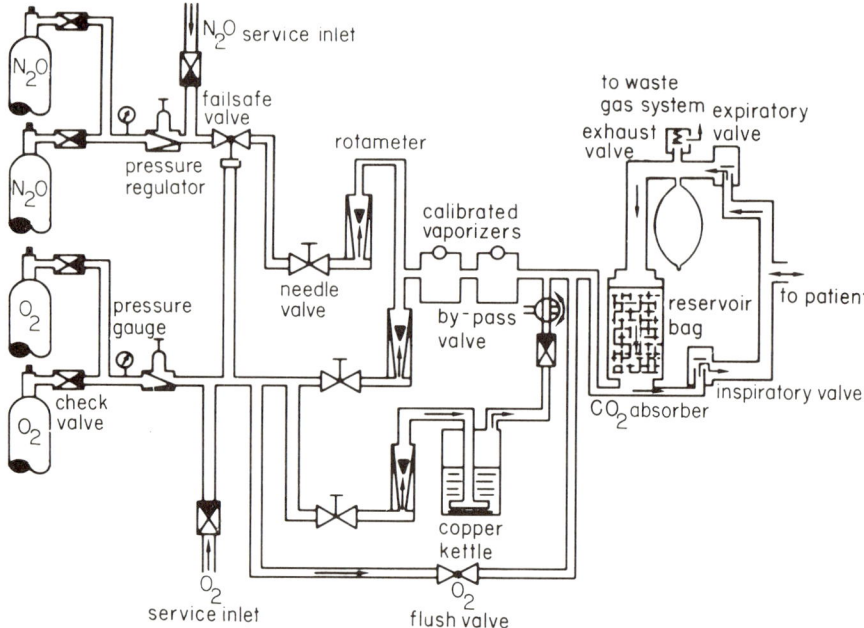

Figure 6-1. Anesthesia machine circuit. Oxygen and nitrous oxide enter the machine from cylinders, or from the hospital service supply. Pressure regulators reduce cylinder pressure to about 3 kg/cm^2. Check valves prevent transfilling of cylinders or gas flow from cylinders to service line. The fail-safe valve prevents flow of nitrous oxide if the oxygen supply fails. Needle valves control flows to rotameters. Calibrated vaporizers provide a preselected concentration of volatile anesthetics. The Copper Kettle delivers the saturated vapor of any agent; thus the effluent must be diluted. The bypass valve vents vapor from the Kettle when it is not in service. Gases are delivered to the circle absorber, where unidirectional valves assure flow from patient through carbon dioxide absorber. Excess gas is vented through the exhaust valve into a waste gas scavenger system. The reservoir bag compensates for variations in respiratory demand.

In the United States, specifications for identity and purity of medical gases are established by the United States Pharmacopeia and supervised by the Food and Drug Administration. Safe practice for manufacture, packaging, shipping, handling, and storing of gases is set by the Department of Transportation (DOT), the Compressed Gas Association (CGA), and the National Fire Protection Association (NFPA). Among other things, these organizations regulate safety devices and markings on cylinders, uniformity of valve threads on large cylinders, and the pin-indexing system (Fig. 6-2) for post-type valves on small medical cylinders. Manufacturing and testing data can be learned from the markings on a cylinder (Fig. 6-2). Manufacturers and distributors of medical gases are required to maintain cylinders and valves in good condition, to insure the purity and identity of gases, and to test periodically the effect of high pressures on the cylinder.

Anesthesia Equipment

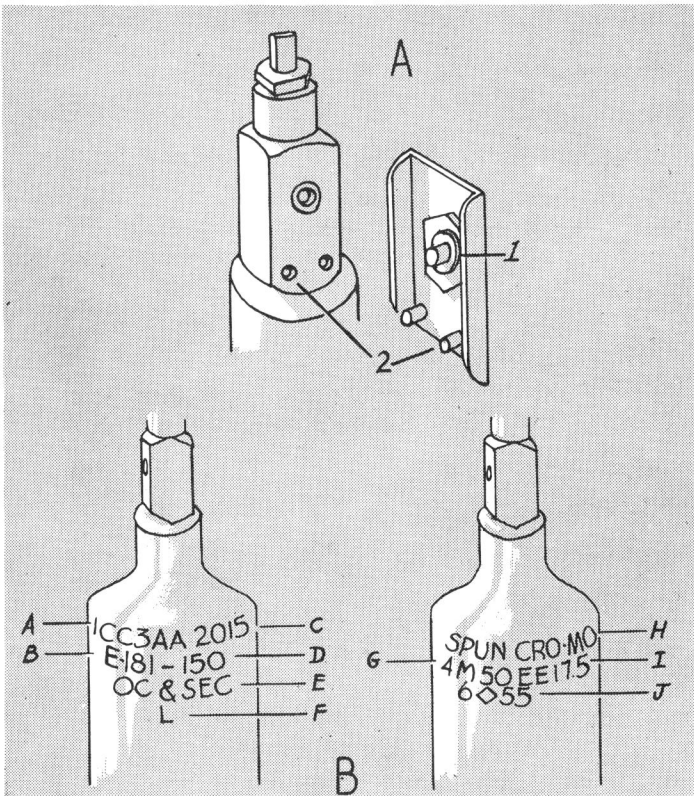

Figure 6-2. Features of gas cylinders. *A*, Cylinder valve and yoke connection: *1*, washer; *2*, pin-index system specific for each anesthetic gas. *B*, Cylinder markings: *A*, Interstate Commerce Commission (now Department of Transportation, DOT) specifications; *B*, cylinder size; *C*, maximum working pressure in pounds per square inch; *D*, manufacturer's serial number; *E*, ownership; *F*, inspector's mark; *G*, manufacturer's mark and date of original test; *H*, chrome-molybdenum (steel); *I*, elastic expansion in ml at 3360 psi; *J*, retest dates.

Compressed gases should be handled carefully to minimize the risk of fire or explosion. Oxidizing gases, oxygen and nitrous oxide, are stored apart from flammable gases. All gases must be stored at temperatures below 52° C. Detailed specifications are given in "Standard for the Use of Inhalation Anesthetics" and "Nonflammable Medical Gas Systems" published by the NFPA as well as in publications of the CGA.

The following recommended practices are based on those of the CGA:
1. Never permit oil, grease, or combustible material to come in contact with cylinders, valves, regulators, gauges, or fittings. Oil may react with oxygen or nitrous oxide with explosive violence.
2. Never lubricate regulators, fittings, or gauges.
3. Open the high pressure valve on the cylinder before connecting the apparatus to the patient.

4. Open cylinder valves slowly, with the face of the gauge on the regulator pointing away from personnel.
5. Never drape a cylinder with sheets, hospital gowns, masks, or caps.
6. Never use gas fittings, valves, regulators, or gauges for service other than for the purpose intended.
7. Never mix gases in cylinders. Never refill cylinders.
8. Always use oxygen from a cylinder through a pressure regulator.
9. Do not use regulators in need of repair or cylinders with valves not operating properly.
10. Defective equipment should be repaired or replaced by the manufacturer or an authorized agent.

Additional precautions are taken when cylinders are placed in service. Paper wrappings are removed so that identifying labels are clearly visible. Valves are opened completely when the cylinder is in use and closed tightly when idle, an economic as well as a safety measure. The flowmeter valve on the anesthesia machine is closed before a cylinder valve is opened; if the valve is open, a high gas flow may damage the flowmeter or cause the bobbin to stick at the top. Compressed gas cylinders are connected to the machine by means of yokes with hand screws and washers of nonflammable material. Pin-indexed cylinders and yokes prevent attachment of a cylinder to the wrong yoke (Fig. 6-2).

The gauges indicate cylinder pressures (Fig. 6-1). Before anesthesia is induced, the cylinder or supply system is tested to be sure that sufficient gas is available. Anesthesia machines usually have double yokes so that two cylinders of oxygen or nitrous oxide are at hand. Check valves prevent one cylinder from transfilling the other. Metal tubing conducts the gases from cylinders to pressure-reducing valves.

The physical properties of commonly used anesthetic gases are given in Table 6-1. Compression of gas to a liquid state offers the most economic supply and smallest volume, but the physical properties limit the conditions under which this may be accomplished. Compressed oxygen can only be supplied as a gas because its critical temperature, above which liquefaction cannot occur, is below ambient temperature. Liquid oxygen, however, is now in common use and is vaporized for supply throughout a hospital. It is stored in large, insulated containers under pressures of 5 to 10 atm, with corresponding temperatures from $-160°$ to $-150°$ C. Unlike oxygen, nitrous oxide is compressible to a liquid at temperatures up to $36°$ C. Compressed cyclopropane and carbon dioxide are also liquids at ordinary temperatures.

As compressed oxygen is used from a cylinder a gradual decrease in pressure occurs. Thus cylinder contents are judged by pressure levels on the gauge: at a given temperature when the original pressure is reduced by half, the cylinder will be half full. For example, an E cylinder containing 625 L of oxygen when full will have 312 L remaining when the pressure decreases to 77 kg/cm^2 (1100 psi). With nitrous oxide, as long as some liquid remains, that is until the cylinder is about 75 per cent exhausted, cylinder pressure is equal to the vapor pressure of nitrous oxide, about 52

Table 6-1. PROPERTIES OF MEDICAL GASES

		Oxygen	Nitrous Oxide	Cyclopropane	Carbon Dioxide
Symbol		O_2	N_2O	C_3H_6	CO_2
Molecular weight		32	44	42	44
Cylinder color		Green*	Blue	Orange	Gray
Physical state in cylinder (20°C)		Gas	Liquid	Liquid	Liquid
Specific gravity of gas (Air = 1)		1.11	1.53	1.48	1.53
Critical temperature (°C)		−118.8	36.5	124.6	31.3
Boiling point (°C)		−183.0	−89.5	−32.8	−78.4§
Cylinder contents (L)	E	625	1590	D = 870	1590
	G	5300	12,110		12,110
Gas weight (kg)†	E	0.8	3.0	D = 1.6	3.0
	G	7.0	22.7		22.7
Cylinder pressure (kg/cm²) (psi)‡		155	52	5.6	59
		2200	745	79	838

*The World Health Organization specifies that medical oxygen cylinders be painted white while U.S. standards require green.

†Empty E cylinder including valve weighs approximately 7 kg.
 Empty G cylinder including valve weighs approximately 45 kg.

‡Nominal filling pressures at 21°C. Values for nitrous oxide, cyclopropane, and carbon dioxide are their vapor pressures at 21°C. One kg/cm² = 14.22 psi.

§Sublimes.

kg/cm² (745 psi) at room temperature. The pressure, therefore, does not indicate the amount of gas remaining. Carbon dioxide and cyclopropane behave similarly. The vaporization of liquefied gases as well as the expansion of compressed gases absorb heat which is extracted from the metal cylinder and the surrounding air. For this reason atmospheric water vapor may condense or freeze on cylinders and valves during high gas flows; to prevent internal icing, liquefied and compressed gases must be free of water vapor.

PRESSURE-REDUCING VALVES

Pressure-reducing valves or regulators serve to lower cylinder pressure to a less hazardous and more easily controlled level (Fig. 6-1). Oxygen pressure in a full cylinder at 155 kg/cm² is reduced to about 3 kg/cm² before delivery to the needle valves on flowmeters. Reducing valves also maintain a constant outlet pressure, providing a constant pressure at needle valves and a stable flow for a given valve setting.

Fail-Safe Devices. To eliminate the possibility of administering an hypoxic gas mixture resulting from failure of the oxygen supply, systems have been developed to regulate the flow of other gases in proportion to the oxygen pressure. The essentials of one such system are shown in Figure 6-3. A master oxygen regulator supplies a reference pressure to slave regula-

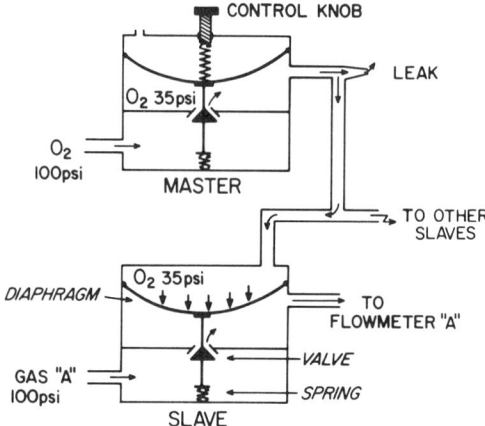

Figure 6-3. Master-slave fail-safe system. Master oxygen reference pressure on slave diaphragm permits gas "A" to flow.

tors controlling the pressure of other gases. If the reference oxygen pressure decreases, so will oxygen flow but the reference pressure in other slave regulators will also decline, thus resulting in a proportionate reduction of all gas flows. Incorporation of a fixed-ratio gas mixer for oxygen and nitrous oxide downstream from the master-slave regulators provides additional safety. The mixer delivers a constant 25 per cent oxygen at variable gas flows. Higher concentrations are provided by adding oxygen through a supplementary flowmeter.

FLOWMETERS

Rotameters measure the flow of a gas based on the principle that flow past a resistance is proportional to pressure. Proportionality between pressure and flow is determined by the shape of the resistance and the physical properties of gases. If the resistance is an orifice, density is the controlling factor; if the resistance is tubular, viscosity becomes dominant. At low flow rates a rotameter acts as tube; at high flow rates as an orifice. Since few gases have the same viscosity and density, rotameter calibrations are not interchangeable. In a rotameter (Fig. 6-1), gas flows from below through a tapered tube, raising a bobbin or float. The channel through which the gas flows varies in diameter according to the height of the bobbin: the higher the flow, the larger the channel. The bobbin comes to rest when the force of gravity is balanced by the fall in pressure caused by the bobbin.

RESERVOIR BAG

Flows having been adjusted, gases are then delivered to the patient. Most anesthetics are administered by means of a system that permits at least partial rebreathing of the gases, a matter of economy. A reservoir bag (Fig. 6-1) is needed to compensate for variations in respiratory demand. At peak inspiration, gas flows of 30 to 60 L per minute may be required, while during respiratory pause and exhalation, no gas flow is required. In the former instance, the larger quantity of gas needed is obtained from the reservoir bag, and in the latter, gas accumulates in the reservoir. In addition, the reservoir bag permits manual assistance or control of ventilation. Movement of the bag is unreliable as an index of adequacy of respiration. However, if the bag does not move, the cause must be sought immediately. The patient may be apneic, the airway obstructed, a faulty connection present, or there may be a poor mask fit.

VAPORIZERS

VAPORIZATION OF VOLATILE LIQUIDS

The first volatile anesthetics, ether and chloroform, were inhaled from masks or containers in which the anesthetic was vaporized by air drawn over the surface of the liquid. This simple method is still utilized in open drop techniques, in portable vaporizers utilizing trichloroethylene or methoxyflurane, and in vaporizers placed within the breathing circuit. With ether and chloroform the vapor concentrations obtained were erratic; sudden high concentrations led to overdosage, while at other times the concentrations were insufficient to attain anesthesia. An understanding of the physics of vaporization led pioneers like Snow and Clover to devise apparatus that provided predictable and nearly uniform concentrations. The surface area for vaporization was increased and the metal containers were surrounded by warm water to maintain constant temperature and vapor pressure. These lessons were largely forgotten when compressed gas came to be used as the carrying vehicle for anesthetic vapors. Although oxygen was used instead of atmospheric air, the high flow of gases over liquid surfaces or bubbling through the liquid produced vapor concentrations that were hardly predictable.

An ideal vaporizer should yield a constant concentration of anesthetic under varying conditions of gas flow, liquid volume, and ambient temperature. Vapor concentration should be controlled with an accuracy equal to that for gases metered by flowmeters. Three physical characteristics are fundamental to the design of vaporizers: dependence of vapor pressure on temperature; latent heat of vaporization; and intimacy of the gas-liquid contact. The maximum partial pressure (concentration) of a volatile liquid that can be obtained in the vapor phase is limited by the vapor pressure at the existing temperature. If the temperature of the liquid fluctuates, vapor concentration changes proportionately. The relation between vapor pressure and temperature for some of the volatile anesthetic agents is given in Figure 6-4. Heat is required for the change to a gaseous state. If heat is

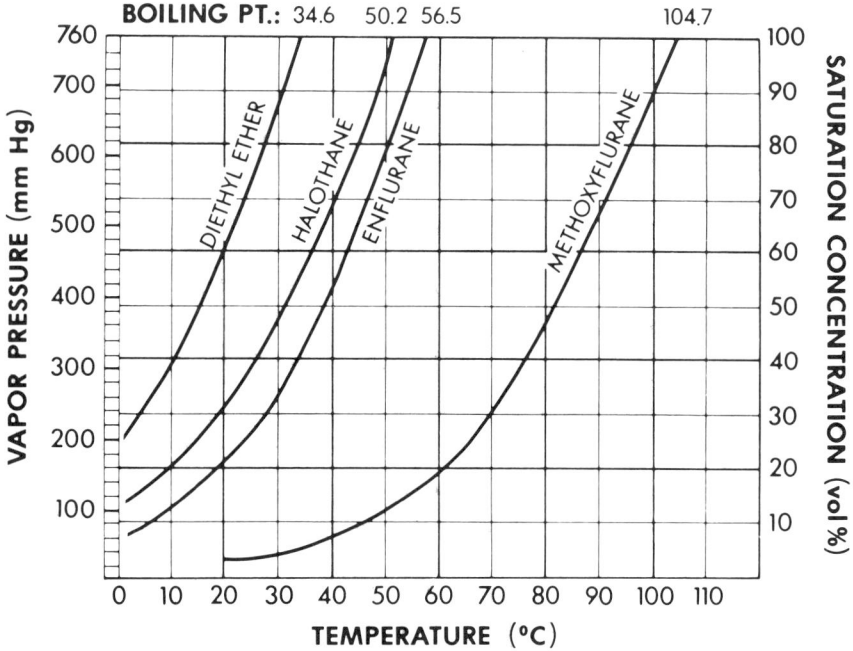

Figure 6–4. Vapor pressure curves of liquids commonly used for anesthesia. (Reproduced with permission from Macintosh R, Mushin WW, Epstein HG: Physics for the Anaesthetist. 3rd ed, Philadelphia, F. A. Davis Company, 1963.)

not provided by the surroundings, it is derived from the liquid itself, with cooling as a consequence. Finally, in order to vaporize a liquid by a stream of gas, the two must be brought into contact. Since contact time is limited, a large gas-liquid interface like that provided by many small bubbles, assures more efficient vaporization.

CURRENTLY USED VAPORIZERS

These physical concepts were incorporated by Morris in his design of the Copper Kettle vaporizer (Fig. 6–5). To provide a relatively constant temperature, a heavy copper container with its high heat capacity and good conductivity is employed. A separately metered flow of oxygen passes through the container while intimate gas-liquid contact is assured by dispersing the gas through a sintered bronze disc to form streams of fine bubbles. Gas exiting from the vaporizer is nearly saturated with anesthetic vapor, the concentration equal to its vapor pressure at that temperature divided by atmospheric pressure.

$$\text{per cent vapor} = \frac{\text{vapor pressure}}{\text{atmospheric pressure}} \times 100 = \frac{\text{ml vapor} \times 100}{\text{ml oxygen} + \text{ml vapor}}$$

Anesthesia Equipment

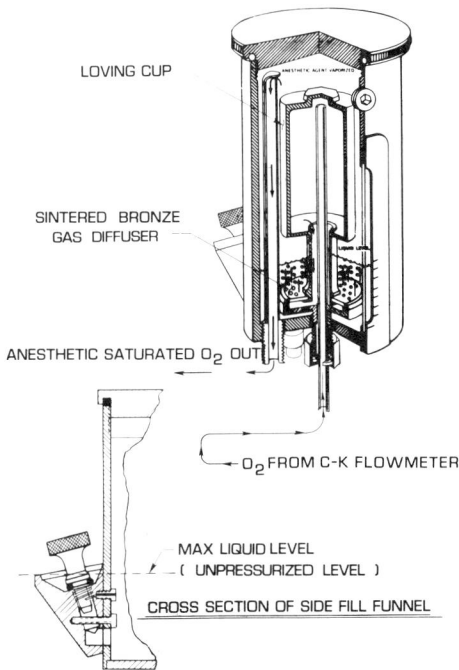

Figure 6-5. The Copper Kettle. The copper container plays an important role as a source of heat and in transfer of heat from room air and metal parts of the gas machine to the liquid to be vaporized. Gas flowing through the liquid is finely dispersed by passing through a sintered bronze (Porex) disc. The tiny bubbles produce maximal vaporization efficiency by providing a large surface for the liquid-gas interface. The disc conducts the heat required for vaporization directly to the liquid. Filling port is placed on the side to prevent overfilling. (Reproduced with permission from Morris LE: Anesthesiology 13:587, 1952.)

The concentration of vapor delivered to the breathing system is the volume of vapor delivered per minute divided by the total gas flow.

$$\text{per cent delivered} = \frac{\text{ml vapor}}{\text{total gas flow}} \times 100$$

Total gas flow includes the flow from the kettle as well as the direct flow of oxygen and nitrous oxide. A rapid means of calculating the delivered concentration of halothane utilizes the approximate vapor pressure of halothane, which is one-third atmosphere at room temperature. One third of the gas exiting from a kettle will be halothane vapor and two thirds oxygen; that is, each 2 ml of oxygen that enters the kettle will add 1 ml of vapor, delivering 3 ml of gas. Similar calculations can be made for enflurane, with the vapor pressure about one-fourth atmosphere, or methoxyflurane, with the vapor pressure about one-thirtieth atmosphere. The delivered percentage of vapor may also be read from a graph or slide rule that provides values for liquid temperature, metered oxygen, and total gas flow or from a specially calibrated flowmeter.

Although the Copper Kettle antedated the introduction of the halogenated agents, it was readily adapted to vaporization of these volatile liquids. The Vernitrol is of similar design, incorporating a separate oxygen flow which is saturated on passage through the vaporizer. Other vaporizers (Fluotec, Pentec, Fluomatic, Pentomatic, Dräger Vapor) are made for specific agents and provide relatively constant vapor concentrations over wide variations in flow rate (Fig. 6–6). These vaporizers, which function outside the breathing circuit, divert a portion of the total gas flow into a vaporizing chamber where a wick saturated with anesthetic provides a large gas-liquid interface for vaporization. The gas-vapor mixture exits from the chamber and rejoins the main gas stream. The proportion of gas diverted to the chamber is controlled by a calibrated dial, whose settings are accurate only within the flow range specified for the device. Calibration should be verified periodically in a laboratory or by the manufacturer. Unless compensation is made, back pressure from the breathing circuit may build up and alter pressure in the vaporizing chamber, causing surges of anesthetic-laden gas. The vaporizers mentioned minimize change in temperature both by having a large heat capacity (mass) and by compensation with temperature-sensitive ports that alter the proportion of gas flows.

While some agent-specific vaporizers (Fluotec Mark III) have an indexed filling port that accepts a tube specific for a bottle of that anesthetic,

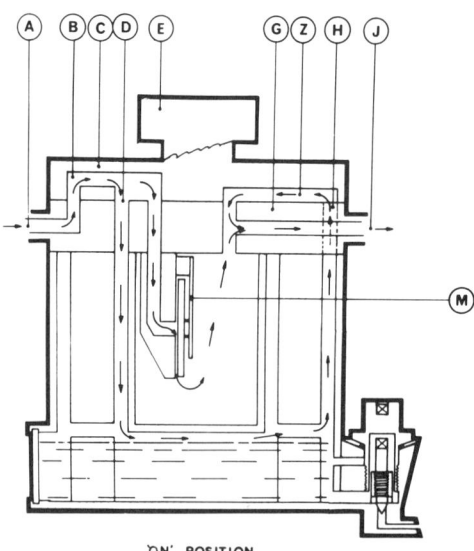

Figure 6–6. Fluotec Mark III agent-specific vaporizer. When control knob E is rotated clockwise, the vaporizer is ON. In this position, oxygen enters at A, passes through channel B into the vaporizing chamber at the bottom, and thence through channels H and Z to outlet J. Wicks saturated with halothane in the vaporizing chamber assure a large gas-liquid interface for efficient vaporization. Oxygen also flows through temperature-sensitive valve M and joins the halothane-laden stream from H to exit at J. The position of the control knob regulates the size of the opening of channel H and thus the flow through it. In the OFF position, with knob E fully counterclockwise, oxygen flows directly from A to J and ports D and H are occluded. Indexed filler port and drain are lower right.

most vaporizers can be filled with any agent. For this reason, vaporizers should be filled with the same care used in handling other potent drugs and clearly labeled to indicate their contents.

When two or more vaporizers are mounted in series, the anesthetic from the upstream one can condense and contaminate that in the downstream vaporizer. To prevent this, only one vaporizer should be used at a time and all turned off when not in use. Since the downstream vaporizer is the one contaminated it should contain the more potent agent; addition of a less potent agent provides a lesser risk.

Preservatives such as the thymol in halothane can accumulate in a vaporizer with time because of differences in vapor pressure. While these residues do not appear to be harmful, excessive quantities may interfere with the functioning of the vaporizer. Some recommend that the contents of vaporizers be drained and discarded every two weeks, but we consider this a wasteful procedure. A more rational approach is to discard the liquid if it is discolored. The vaporizer can be rinsed with a fresh charge of the agent. Ether can also be used to rinse vaporizers, taking the usual precautions for flammable agents and thoroughly airing the vaporizer before returning to service.

CARBON DIOXIDE ABSORBERS

In a rebreathing system, an absorbent is necessary to remove exhaled carbon dioxide (Fig. 6-1). To assure that all of the exhaled gas passes through the absorber, directional valves are incorporated (Fig. 6-1). Before anesthesia is begun, the valves should be tested to assure unidirectional flow through the absorber. Thus the anesthetist should inhale and exhale through the system to determine competency, and during anesthesia should observe the action of the valves as well as the patient for signs of carbon dioxide accumulation. Among other things, duration of efficient action of an absorber depends upon carbon dioxide output, tidal volume, respiratory rate, flow rate of fresh gases, capacity and shape of the canister, surface area, water content, porosity of the absorbent granules, and the chemicals used for absorption. When used with high fresh gas flows modern canisters may be efficient for 16 to 18 hours of use. Some clinicians change absorbents on a weekly or biweekly schedule. Others prefer to rely upon color change. In any case, the anesthetist should observe any change in color of the indicator dye or any accumulation of heat as a rough index of carbon dioxide absorption. Fresh granules of soda lime crumble easily, whereas the exhausted material is quite hard.

CHEMICAL ABSORPTION OF CARBON DIOXIDE

Carbon dioxide combines with the hydroxides of sodium, calcium, or barium. Two mixtures are commercially available:
1. Soda lime (SL) (USP): 5 per cent NaOH and 95 per cent $Ca(OH)_2$.

2. Baralyme (BL): 20 per cent $Ba(OH)_2 \cdot 8H_2O$ and 80 per cent $Ca(OH)_2$.

For practical use, the combined substances are supplied in granules sufficiently hard to resist crumbling and formation of dust, which is a respiratory tract irritant. Water is incorporated for the neutralization reaction; Baralyme contains water as the octahydrate of $Ba(OH)_2$. Water constitutes 15 to 19 per cent of the total weight of soda lime. When not present in chemical combination the water can evaporate, thus reducing the effectiveness of the soda lime. Soda lime should be stored in sealed containers and exposed to some degree of moisture when in use.

Absorbents incorporate dyes (ethyl violet—SL and Clayton yellow—BL) which change color as the reaction of neutralization proceeds. Regardless of the color of the absorbent, carbon dioxide can still be channeled through a canister into the inspired gas. Since the color change is not completely reliable, evidence of carbon dioxide retention in the patient must be sought. Neutralization reactions for the two absorbents are as follows.

Soda lime:

$$H_2CO_3 + 2\,NaOH \rightarrow Na_2CO_3 + 2H_2O \text{ (rapid)}$$
$$H_2CO_3 + Ca(OH)_2 \rightarrow CaCO_3\downarrow + 2H_2O \text{ (slower)}$$

Baralyme:

$$H_2CO_3 + Ba(OH)_2 \rightarrow BaCO_3\downarrow + 2H_2O \text{ (fairly rapid)}$$
$$H_2CO_3 + Ca(OH)_2 \rightarrow CaCO_3\downarrow + 2H_2O \text{ (slower)}$$

In each case the fundamental reaction is that of neutralization:

$$H^+ + OH^- \rightarrow H_2O$$

The heat of neutralization, 13.7 kcal per mole of water formed, is liberated during this reaction. As carbon dioxide is absorbed, therefore, the canister becomes warm to touch. The reaction itself does not require addition of heat, for canisters at 0, 28, or 100° C absorb effectively.

The larger the surface area of absorbent exposed to expired gas, the more rapid and efficient is the absorption of carbon dioxide. An irregular granule offers a larger surface area than a cylindrical pellet. While surface area also increases as granule size decreases, granules that are too small increase resistance to gas flow. The common soda lime granule is approximately 8 mesh, 2.5 mm, in size.

Optimal absorptive conditions provide that at least one tidal volume be accommodated entirely within the air space of the canister. When flow of expired gases ceases during inspiration, the tidal volume remains in contact with the absorbent. About half the volume of a properly packed canister consists of intergranular space or voids.

CARBON DIOXIDE ABSORPTION SYSTEMS

There are two kinds of closed carbon dioxide absorption systems: the circle and the to-and-fro. In the first, valves so direct the flow of gas that it passes through the absorber in one direction only. In the second, now rarely used, respired gas passes to and from the reservoir bag through the absorber to the patient; valves are not needed. As gas passes through either system, absorption first takes place near the inlet, next along the sides of the canister, and finally at the outlet. With obstruction to gas flow, or because of areas of lesser resistance, channeling can occur; the gas follows the path of least resistance, bypassing the bulk of absorbent. The absorbent should, therefore, be tightly packed and held in place with screens, while baffles are used to disperse gas flow uniformly. Because of these variables, only about half of the theoretical capacity will have been used at the time of failure of a single charge of absorbent.

Trichloroethylene reacts with soda lime or Baralyme to form the explosive and neurotoxic dichloroacetylene and the respiratory tract irritant, phosgene; heat hastens both reactions. Rubber or plastic goods used with trichloroethylene should be thoroughly aired before subsequent use in a closed circuit system and several hours, or preferably longer, should elapse before a patient who has breathed trichloroethylene should be allowed to breathe from a circuit containing absorbent.

Soda lime and Baralyme are both strongly alkaline and corrosive to skin and mucous membranes; barium hydroxide is toxic if ingested. If granules of these substances are in contact with tissues for any length of time, chemical burns result. The water of exhalation which condenses and accumulates in a canister dissolves alkali, forming a caustic solution that has caused burns in both patient and anesthetist.

CONDUCTING TUBES AND FACE MASK

Gases are led from the machine to the breathing system, which incorporates a circle absorber as shown in Figure 6–1 or some other kind (Chapter 12). Tubing carrying gas from the machine to the breathing system is of small bore, but tubing through which the patient breathes must be nonkinkable and of wide bore to minimize resistance. Corrugated, black conductive rubber tubing with an inside diameter of 22 mm is commonly used. However, sterile disposable sets containing breathing tubes, face mask, Y-connecter and reservoir bag are available in both conductive and nonconductive materials. Some sets incorporate a bacterial filter. Disposable sets are appropriately used in bacteriologically contaminated patients or those unduly susceptible to infection.

An appropriate face mask is chosen; the best fit is attained by testing prior to induction. Poor fit delays induction of anesthesia and thwarts application of positive pressure breathing when needed. In applying the mask, excessive pressure on the face, nose, or eyes must be avoided.

ESCAPE VALVES AND SCAVENGER SYSTEMS

Techniques that supply gases in amounts larger than required to meet the metabolic need for oxygen and uptake of anesthetic result in an excess of gas, which must be vented through an escape valve (Fig. 6–1). For example, during nitrous oxide anesthesia, in order to provide a safe concentration of oxygen and yet give an effective percentage of nitrous oxide, gas flows of 4 liters or more per minute are often used; this also facilitates denitrogenation of the lungs and body tissues. Unless nitrogen can escape from the system, the partial anesthetic effect of nitrous oxide will not be achieved. High gas flows also assist in carbon dioxide elimination and avoidance of heat retention. If the gas volume supplied exceeds the minute volume of ventilation, there is little likelihood of carbon dioxide retention.

Formerly, excess gas was vented through an escape valve into the surrounding atmosphere; now there is evidence indicating that long-term exposure to traces of anesthetic gases may cause an increase in spontaneous abortions, fetal malformations, and malignancies in operating room personnel. Cognitive and motor skills may also be impaired during exposure. Many anesthetists use total gas flows of 3 to 7 L per minute, far in excess of the amount taken up by the patient. When a mixture of nitrous oxide, oxygen in 50 per cent concentration, and halothane, 1 per cent, is used at such flows in an air-conditioned operating room, the atmosphere may contain 10 parts per million (ppm) (0.0001 vol per cent) of halothane and 500 ppm of nitrous oxide. By the use of scavenger equipment and avoidance of leaks, the concentrations can be reduced more than tenfold.

Waste gases from the escape valve must be eliminated without increasing risk to the patient or others. Gases may be vented to an air-conditioning exhaust duct, but only if all exhaust air is vented to the outside. Alternatively, the gases can be drawn into the suction system or removed via a separate pump, but not if explosive gases are in use. Finally, the gases can be directly vented to the outside if an exterior wall is nearby. Gas must be removed from the escape valve without pressure build up or without causing negative pressure in the breathing circuit. The scavenger valve, tubing, and system must accommodate the maximal flows used. Finally, the exhaust tubing must be protected from kinking or occlusion.

The kind of scavenger system used depends on the anesthetic technique; systems have been adapted to the open, semi-open, and circle techniques. A scavenger valve to replace the escape valve of an anesthesia circle is shown in Figure 6–7. Others are described in Chapter 24.

Additional pollution of the operating room atmosphere occurs while

Anesthesia Equipment

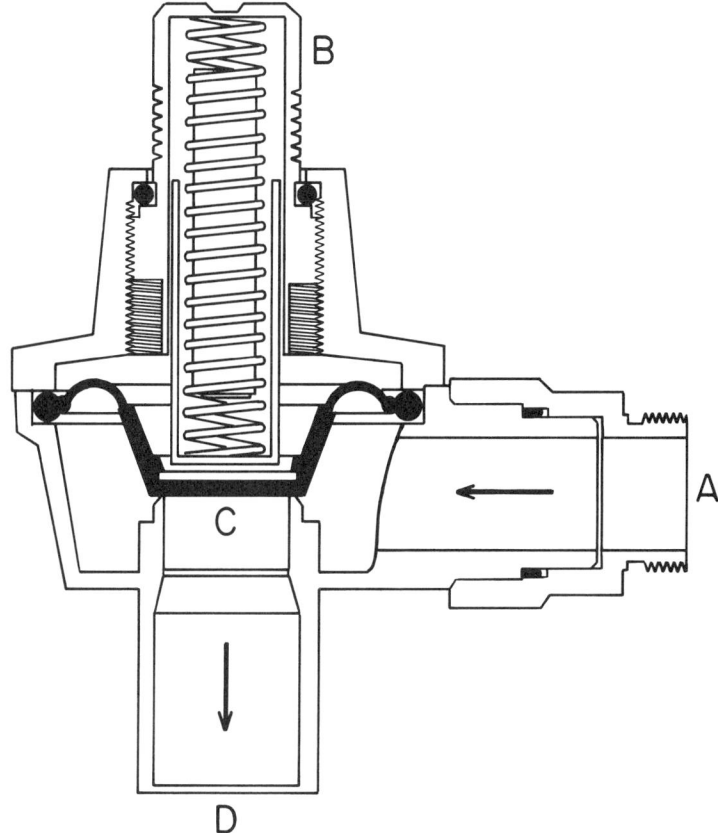

Figure 6–7. Waste gas scavenger valve. The waste gas scavenger valve is a modification of the exhaust valve which allows the excess gases to be collected and removed from the operating room. The valve replaces the exhaust valve, and is fitted to the machine via the thread at (A). Gases in excess of those needed by the patient enter at (A), raise the diaphragm (C), and exit at (D). The pressure required to raise the diaphragm is adjusted by rotating knob (B). The exiting gases are led through wide-bore tubing to the outside atmosphere through the air-conditioning exhaust duct, hospital suction, or directly through an outside wall. Appropriate precautions must be taken to avoid pressure or vacuum build up in the exhaust line. (Redrawn, with permission from Ohio Medical Products, Airco Inc.)

filling vaporizers, and if there are leaks from breathing circuit connections as well as high and low pressure gas leaks within the machine. Mechanical ventilators may cause the same kinds of contamination.

USE OF MECHANICAL VENTILATORS ON ANESTHESIA MACHINES

The use of a mechanical ventilator during anesthesia to assist or control respiration allows the anesthetist to attend to parenteral fluid therapy, monitoring, and other matters essential to the care of patients. However, their use can also divert attention from the patient and lead to complacency. A ventilator powered by a compressed gas supply can be mounted directly on the anesthesia machine, the bellows of the ventilator thereby replacing the reservoir bag in the breathing circuit. A simplified diagram of a compressed gas–driven ventilator is shown in Figure 6–8. Ventilators for adult use should be able to deliver tidal volumes up to 1500 ml at pressures up to 50 mm Hg, with controls to vary the rate and volume of respiration. Other controls for inspiratory and expiratory flow rate and for expiratory pause are useful in providing a ventilatory pattern with minimal circulatory depression. Safety devices should be incorporated to prevent overpressurization of the lungs (a pressure relief valve) and a bypass to permit the

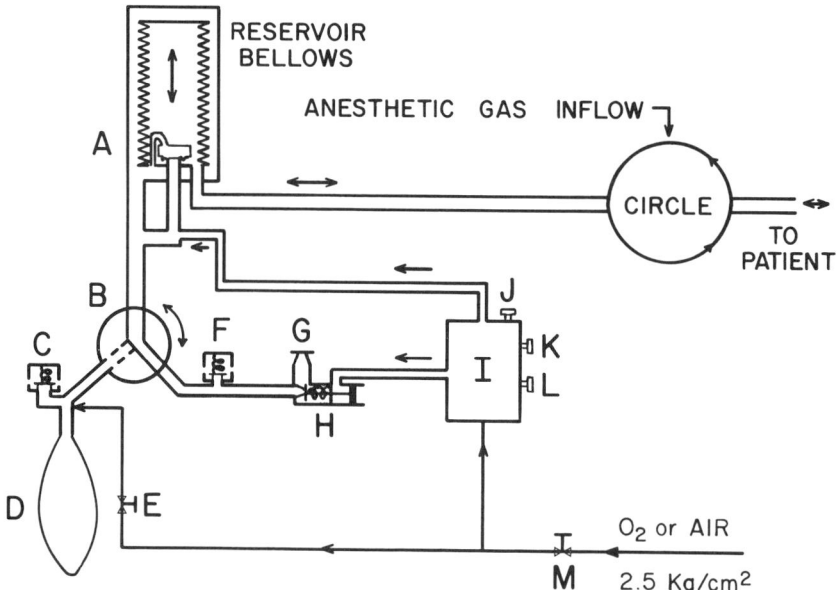

Figure 6–8. Gas-driven mechanical ventilator. The **Reservoir bellows** replaces the reservoir bag of the anesthesia breathing system. Respired gases enter the bellows from the anesthesia machine, through the anesthesia **circle**. The bellows, contained in a transparent closed vessel, is compressed by oxygen (or compressed air) entering the vessel from the respiratory cycle controller (*I*). At the end of inspiratory phase, this oxygen flow ceases, the exhalation valve (*H*) is opened by a second flow from the controller, and the oxygen exits at valve (*G*). Following exhalation, the cycle repeats itself. Volume of respiration as well as inspiratory and expiratory times and pauses are governed by the settings (*J*, *K*, *L*) of the controller. Excessive positive pressure is prevented by the relief valve (*F*). The overflow valve (*A*) dumps excess gas if the bellows is overfilled. Manual-assisted or controlled respiration may be selected by connecting the manual bag (*D*) to the exterior of the bellows using the selector valve (*B*), after filling the bag through the valve (*E*). Alternatively, the ventilator may be disconnected from the machine and replaced by a reservoir bag. The ventilator is turned on by opening valve (*M*). The oxygen (or compressed air) used to drive the ventilator serves only that purpose and does not enter the breathing system. The Venturi negative expiratory pressure generator and the airway pressure sensor for assisted respiration are not shown. (Redrawn from the Ventimeter/Ventilator circuit with permission of Air-Shields, Inc., a Narch Health Company.)

patient to breathe in case the bellows empties. The ventilator should permit rapid change to manual control of respiration with a reservoir bag.

Assisted or controlled respiration during anesthesia is best conducted by manual compression of the reservoir bag. By this means, changes in pulmonary compliance can be detected instantly, periodic hyperinflation of the lungs is more readily accomplished, and the anesthetist's attention is focused constantly on the patient. Mechanical ventilation is of greatest value to the anesthetist who must work without assistance.

HAZARDS OF ANESTHESIA MACHINES

In spite of many advances in the design and incorporation of safety features in anesthesia machines, hazards are still associated with their use. The two greatest dangers are inadvertent administration of an hypoxic gas mixture or of an overdose of anesthetic. Either of these errors may result from carelessness on the part of the anesthetist, improper mechanical design or malfunction of the machine, or a combination of both. Delivery of an inadequate amount of oxygen may be caused by many faults: an empty oxygen cylinder or failure to open the valve, loose connections, clogged lines, sticking flowmeters, or failure or faulty installation of the service oxygen supply. Prior to use, newly installed or repaired oxygen or nitrous oxide supply lines should be tested to insure the identity and purity of the gases as well as the adequacy of flow. Central supply systems must be checked regularly by the hospital engineering service. Overdose of anesthetic can result from unobserved changes in oxygen flow, failure to add diluting oxygen when using a kettle vaporizer, sticking flowmeters, inadvertent use of several agents caused by leaking valves or malfunctioning flowmeters, failure to turn off the Kettle vaporizer, use of a wrong agent or a mixture of agents in the vaporizer, or an overfilled Kettle vaporizer. Steps have been taken in machine design to reduce the possibility of human error or mechanical failure. The pin-index system prevents incorrect installation of cylinders. Fail-safe systems should eliminate the possibility of administering hypoxic gas mixtures; however, not all machines are so equipped. Most machines now incorporate color-coded flowmeters, scales, and needle-valve knobs, and distinctively shaped knobs and other features calculated to reduce error. Newer agent-specific vaporizers offer indexed filling ports. Ultimately, however, proper use of an anesthesia machine rests with the anesthetist; there is no mechanical substitute for vigilance.

Machines should be checked routinely for leaks, sticking, or cracked flowmeters, defective needle valves, loose or worn components, and other evidence of wear or breakage. While every anesthetist should understand the principles, parts, and functioning of machines, unless technical personnel in the hospital are skilled in the maintenance and repair of such machines, all but minor repairs should be left to trained servicemen. The best policy is to have the machines serviced by the manufacturer or a qualified technician on a regular basis.

ANESTHESIA CHECKLIST

Prior to induction of anesthesia, the anesthesia machine and its contents should be readied for use. All parts of the machine should be in good working order and all accessory equipment and necessary supplies on hand. After completion of anesthesia, the gas tanks should be turned off, expended items replaced, and the machine cleaned and readied for use. The following checklist is useful as an aid in preparing for anesthesia.

ANESTHESIA MACHINE CHECKLIST

Prior to Induction

A. Inspection for presence of
  1. Tank wrench
  2. Reservoir bag
  3. Breathing tubes
  4. Mask and connector
  5. Scavenger system
  6. Head strap
  7. Vaporizers filled, caps and drains closed
B. Gases
  1. Tanks on proper yokes
  2. Central oxygen and nitrous oxide lines properly connected
  3. Turn on nitrous oxide, check pressure; turn on nitrous oxide flowmeter (if gas flows, fail-safe is not functioning). Turn off flowmeter
  4. Turn on oxygen, check pressure; turn on oxygen flowmeter, check flow
  5. Turn on nitrous oxide flowmeter—gas should flow; turn off nitrous oxide cylinder, turn on flowmeter and vent
C. Carbon dioxide absorber
  1. Soda lime: present? functional?
  2. Replace if necessary and secure canister properly
D. Breathing circuit
  1. Fill bag with oxygen, occlude outflow and compress bag, investigate cause of leaks
  2. Breathe through circle filter, investigate:
     a. Undue resistance
     b. Presence of irritating gas
     c. Competence of directional valves

After Anesthesia

A. Turn off gas cylinders; allow pressure gauges to come to zero
B. Close flowmeter knobs gently so that valve seats are not damaged

C. Replace empty cylinders; disconnect central oxygen and nitrous oxide
D. Remove face mask, breathing tubes, and reservoir bag for cleaning
E. If machine is defective, remove from use and notify responsible individuals

REFERENCES

Brown ES, Seniff AM, Elam JO: Carbon dioxide elimination in semiclosed systems. Anesthesiology 25:31, 1964.

Bruce DL, Bach MJ, Arbit J: Trace anesthetic effects on perceptive, cognitive and motor skills. Anesthesiology 40:453, 1974.

Compressed Gas Association, 500 Fifth Avenue, New York, NY 10036. Pamphlets:
   G-4: Oxygen.
   M-1: Standard for 22 mm Anesthesia Breathing Circuit Connectors.
   P-2: Characteristics and Safe Handling of Medical Gases.
   P-2.1: Standard for Medical-Surgical Vacuum Systems in Hospitals.
   V-1: American National-Canadian Standard Compressed Gas Cylinder Valve Outlet and Inlet Connections.

Compressed Gas Association, Handbook of Compressed Gases. New York, Reinhold Publishing Corporation, 1966.

Dorsch JA, Dorsch SE: Understanding Anesthesia Equipment. Baltimore, The Williams & Wilkins Company, 1975.

Epstein RM, Rackow H, Lee A St J, et al: Prevention of accidental breathing of anoxic gas mixtures during anesthesia. Anesthesiology 23:1, 1962.

Feeley TW, Hedley-Whyte J: Bulk oxygen and nitrous oxide delivery systems: Design and dangers. Anesthesiology 44:301, 1976.

Macintosh RR, Mushin WW, Epstein HG: Physics for the Anaesthetist. 3rd ed, Philadelphia, F. A. Davis Company, 1963.

Matteo RS, Gissen A, Lee A St J: Safety in the use of nitrous oxide: A modification of standard anesthetic machine to eliminate sources of human error and system failure. Anesthesiology 31:361, 1969.

Morris LE: A new vaporizer for liquid anesthetic agents. Anesthesiology 13:587, 1952.

National Fire Protection Association, 40 Atlantic Avenue, Boston, Mass 02110.
   NFPA No. 56A: Inhalation Anesthetics, 1973.
   NFPA No. 56F: Nonflammable Medical Gases, 1974.
   NFPA No. 76A: Essential Electrical Systems for Health Care Facilities, 1975.

Occupational Disease Among Operating Room Personnel: A national study. Report of an ad hoc committee on the effects of trace anesthetics on the health of operating room personnel. Anesthesiology 41:321, 1974.

Rendell-Baker L: Some gas machine hazards and their elimination. Anesth Analg 55:26, 1976.

Witcher C, Piziali R, Sher R, et al: Development and Evaluation of Methods for the Elimination of Waste Anesthetic Gases and Vapors in Hospitals. HEW Publication No. (NIOSH) 73-137, Washington DC, US Government Printing Office, 1975.

Chapter 7

AN APPROACH TO ASEPSIS IN ANESTHESIA

In the operating room and special care units, the patient, attending personnel, the apparatus used, and air conditioning and housecleaning methods all may play a role in the contraction and spread of nosocomial infections. Traditionally, anesthetists have remained aloof from these problems, concerning themselves primarily with cleaning their own equipment. Few internal controls have been instituted and there has been little surveillance of the adequacy of aseptic techniques. As the risks for patients increase, anesthetists must share in the responsibility of preventing infection, just as they at one time adopted measures to prevent anesthetic explosions. Perhaps the same standards of antisepsis should be applied to the work of the anesthetist as to that of the surgeon.

The anesthetist not only cares for patients in the operating room, but for others in recovery and intensive care units. Patients with infections, whether overtly ill or healthy carriers, may act as sources of infection for others. Thus, anesthetists in their many contacts may act as vectors in the spread of infection, as several well-documented reports have shown. Subsequent entry into the operating room may determine whether wound infection or bronchopneumonia will follow a clean operative procedure. Furthermore, asymptomatic carriers of the hepatitis B surface antigen (HB_S antigen) may transmit the disease in the course of their work or contract it from a patient. Although the following discussion is addressed to the anesthetist, all concerned should take notice. Initial suggestions will be followed by an analysis of procedures for sterilizing equipment, a more obvious source of trouble. The terms used are defined as follows: antiseptics are agents that destroy all microorganisms on animate surfaces; sterilization implies death of all forms of microbial life.

PERSONAL HYGIENE AND BEHAVIOR

Operating room garments should be changed and shoes cleaned with disinfectant after exposure to infection. Operating room clothing and shoes should not be worn outside the operating area. Face masks saturated with exhaled vapor should be discarded after several hours of use, not continually worn about the neck. Conversation during operation, although difficult to contain, should be minimal, since droplet nuclei containing bacteria multiply with talking. A physician with an acute respiratory infection should not enter the operating room; the presence of virulent bacteria can be determined by throat culture. The hands must be kept clean. Repeated washing throughout the day with detergent bactericidal soaps or pHisoHex (hexachlorophene in detergent) reduces transient bacterial flora. In addition, the anesthetist should help to enforce aseptic discipline and be conversant with accepted housekeeping methods in the operating area.

CARE OF THE PATIENT

Theoretically, the patient should wear a cap and mask, as does any other person in the operating room. Although a mask is seldom worn, a cap is useful to contain the hair and any shed products of the scalp. A patient with sepsis should be masked until the anesthesia face mask is applied, the anesthetist in turn being protected by a gown and gloves. Bedding on litters and bed clothes should be clean and not agitated unnecessarily, as bacterial flora in the air will be increased. Upon return to the recovery area, a patient with infection is placed in isolation so as not to endanger others. Similar precautions are followed in those prone to infection: the premature infant, the tracheostomized or burned patient, a patient with uremia, and those with bone marrow suppression. Ultraviolet light barriers help to protect these people and should be used in any area where airborne infection must be kept at a minimum. The wavelength of ultraviolet light emanating from a cold cathode low pressure mercury lamp is 2537 Å. The optimal intensity at the level of an operating table is 25 $\mu w/cm^2$, which results in an intensity at eye level of 46 $\mu w/cm^2$. Unless the patient is protected by an antisunburn lotion or cream, a painless skin erythema appears at six to ten hours, after ten minutes of exposure. Although the retina is not affected, an annoying conjunctivitis and photophobia appear after exposure. Thus a protective eye shield should be worn. Another approach in the high-risk situation is the use of laminar flow techniques whereby potentially contaminated air currents are directed away from the patient.

ANESTHESIA TECHNIQUE

There is nothing more indicative of a poor clinician than a chaotic, unclean anesthesia table and machine. Equipment should be arranged in an orderly manner and waste containers used for disposable objects; contaminated equipment such as endotracheal tubes and suction catheters should be wrapped in towels and kept separate from clean material. A disinfectant could well be used to clean the surface of the anesthesia machine and work table upon completion of each procedure. Any piece of apparatus used in conjunction with anesthesia, whether a blood pressure cuff or a cooling blanket, should be scrupulously clean.

INJECTIONS AND INTRAVENOUS THERAPY

This subject is discussed in Chapters 21 and 22. The infectious hazard of these procedures lies not only in careless preparation of the injection site, but also in the contamination of the equipment and the fluids used. Multiple dose vials should be carefully handled to avoid contamination. When closed liquid containers have been autoclaved, a vacuum should be demonstrable upon opening, an index of sterility. Dates of sterilization and sterilization indicators are checked, even though the latter are not infallible. In administering whole blood or its products, the possibility of massive bacterial contamination or transmission of serum hepatitis must be borne in mind. An excellent preventive against infection is the use of disposable sterilized equipment whenever practicable; however, costs of these items run high.

PREPARATION FOR NERVE BLOCKS AND PERCUTANEOUS PROCEDURES

Although needle puncture is not the equivalent of a surgical incision, preparation of the skin should be done carefully, especially in spinal and peridural anesthesia. Though there is no such thing as sterilization of the skin without destruction of the skin itself, a bacteriologically clean surface can be prepared. Transient bacterial flora can largely be removed by washing with soap and water and the bacteria killed with antiseptics. Resident flora, consisting for the most part of *Staphylococcus albus* and about 5 per cent other pathogenic bacteria, require scrubbing and chemical treatment for removal. Deep or hidden bacteria in hair pits and orifices of sebaceous glands cannot be removed but these are mostly nonpathogenic. Because transient and resident bacteria multiply after the skin is injured, it is best to shave the skin just before a procedure rather than the night before.

The bactericidal activity of an antiseptic depends upon its concentration, the temperature of the solvent, and the degree and duration of contact. Dirt and grease are removed beforehand with a detergent or triethylene glycol. The most effective skin antiseptics are ethyl or isopropyl alcohol in 70 per cent concentration by weight, the iodophors, and tincture of benzalkonium (Zephiran) 1:1000 in 70 per cent alcohol. Iodine 2 per cent in 70 per cent alcohol is likewise effective but has the disadvantage of causing burns and allergic reactions. All these are bactericidal if sufficient contact and duration of action are allowed. Alcohols, the iodophors (Betadine, Wescodyne), and Zephiran are nontoxic to skin, nonallergenic, relatively inexpensive, and easily stored. For asepsis, one of the alcohols, suitably colored to indicate the area covered, is effective with one application. If the skin is obviously contaminated, a more thorough surgical scrub is employed.

STERILIZATION OF EQUIPMENT FOR ANESTHESIA AND INHALATION THERAPY

Equipment used for inhalation should be so cared for that the possibility of transmission of infection from one patient to another is avoided. The esthetic aspects of providing clean equipment require no comment; deterioration of equipment that can result from cleaning must be only a secondary consideration in the important matter of preventing infection. Reports concerning transmission of disease via anesthesia apparatus are confusing at best; to our knowledge a complete epidemiologic study has not yet been done. However, it is well known that mechanical ventilators and humidifiers used in respiratory therapy can be responsible for crossinfection. It is also important to note that pathogenic bacteria have been cultured from equipment at the termination of anesthesia in infected persons. For this reason we follow the practice of treating anesthesia apparatus as if it were always contaminated. A corollary of this approach is that sufficient equipment must be on hand so that apparatus can be properly cleaned while others are in use.

Infective organisms comprise the nonsporulating vegetative bacteria, fungi, tubercle bacillus, viruses, protozoa, and bacterial spores. The method of sterilization chosen depends upon the nature of the material to be sterilized and the degree of sanitation sought. The following procedures are applicable to anesthesia apparatus.

HEAT STERILIZATION

Moist heat is the most dependable means of killing pathogenic organisms. Moisture increases cellular permeability, and heat destroys by coagulating protein. Elevated pressures permit utilization of higher temperatures; no living organism can withstand ten to 15 minutes exposure at a temperature of 105° C and 6.8 kg pressure as applied in an autoclave. Material thus treated is properly wrapped beforehand to allow penetration of heat and subsequent handling and storage without contamination. The package is considered sterile up to four weeks. Dating of a package and sterilization markers indicate that the material has been treated but not necessarily that it is sterile. Athough autoclaving eliminates the hazard of allergic reaction and irritation from chemical germicides, deterioration of rubber and plastics is hastened and sharp instruments become dull and discolored.

Other methods of heat sterilization include boiling in water for 15 minutes, offering only a bactericidal effect, and dry heat treatment at 160° C for one hour, useful for powders, greases, oils, and glass syringes.

CHEMICAL STERILIZATION

Solutions or gases are used for sterilizing objects that cannot be treated with heat, the incorporated chemicals killing organisms by coagulation or alkylation of protein. The time required for action depends upon the nature of the material to be sterilized, the degree and nature of the contamination, and the temperature, concentration of the chemical, and its effectiveness as a bactericidal agent. Nonsporulating vegetative bacteria, common viruses, the tubercle bacillus, and spores are increasingly resistant to destruction, in the order named. The disadvantage of most chemicals is that they act only at exposed surfaces, some reacting with metals, while others impregnate materials and remain as a source of irritation. Rubber is particularly susceptible to deterioration because of its adsorptive porosity and the chemicals used in its manufacture. Mineral and vegetable oils, ethers, esters, oxidizing acids, and hydrocarbon solvents cause swelling, tackiness, and more or less rapid destruction of rubber. Phenols and cresols are not only destructive but may cause cutaneous burns if the rubber becomes impregnated. Water, alkalis, and salts of mercury do little harm. Plastics are especially susceptible to destruction by strong chemicals. The agents discussed in the next section are commonly used for sterilization.

Liquid Germicides

Phenols. These are tuberculocides and viricides but not sporicides, ordinarily used in 1 to 3 per cent concentration to clean surfaces of furniture and apparatus. Some of the proprietary phenols are Staphene, Amphyl, and O-Syl. These should never be used on equipment that comes in contact with patients.

Halogens

CHLORINE. Agents incorporating chlorine usually provide only a light tuberculocidal and sporicidal action; they are often used in the operating area to clean floors. Metals are corroded. Clorox is a commonly used proprietary preparation.

IODINE. When used in 0.5 to 2.0 per cent concentration in alcohol, iodine is bactericidal and tuberculocidal. Disadvantages in cleansing skin are staining of fabrics, irritation, burns, and allergic reactions. Combination of iodine with detergents, quaternaries, and macromolecules to form iodophors eliminates these faults; Wescodyne and Betadine are nonirritating, do not stain, and are nonallergenic. Iodophors can be used instead of aqueous and alcoholic solutions of iodine, being useful for topical application and irrigation of mucous membranes and on surfaces of apparatus as well as for cleaning floors and walls.

Quaternary Ammonium Compounds. These have soaplike properties and are effective against ordinary vegetative bacteria. Viricidal activity is limited and there is no tuberculocidal effect. Zephiran, a nonirritating compound, is effective in 1:1000 aqueous solution. Quaternaries are inactivated by organic matter, milk, serum, disinfectants, and hard water and are adsorbed on surfaces. For these reasons these germicides have been largely abandoned.

Alcohols. Ethyl and isopropyl alcohol in 70 to 90 per cent concentration not only kill vegetative bacteria readily but are tuberculocidal as well. These solutions have been underrated for sterilization purposes. The combination of alcohol with other germicides renders the latter more effective.

Hexachlorophene. Preparations of hexachlorophene have become popular, but justification for their use is questionable. This substance is insoluble in water, but is one of the few antiseptics that does not lose antibacterial potency in the presence of soap. It is used in the form of hexachlorophene soap or in combination with a detergent in preparations like pHisoHex.

GAS STERILIZATION

Ethylene Oxide

The trend toward use of disposable equipment has led manufacturers to seek nondestructive methods of sterilization. Ethylene oxide (EO), a colorless gas with a pleasant ethereal odor, is an excellent bactericdal agent for this purpose. Major advantages include excellent penetration and the fact that few materials are harmed; practically any object or piece of apparatus can be treated without damage. However, EO lacks rapidity of action even though it is effective against all organisms. The gas is extremely flammable so that mixture is necessary with carbon dioxide or Freon, both flame-quenching substances. Humidification, elevated temperature, increased pressure, creation of a vacuum beforehand, and thorough airing afterward are essential steps in the procedure. The inhalation toxicity of EO is approximately equivalent to that of ammonia, and a vesicant action is demonstrable if it is allowed to remain in contact with skin. The long time for sterilization, eight to 24 hours for the complete process, the special equipment required, and the need for dilution with carbon dioxide or Freon result in a time-consuming and costly method of sterilization. The major hazard is inadequate aeration. Residual EO and its by-products, ethylene glycol and ethylene chlorohydrin, are highly irritant to tissues and have caused tracheal inflammation as well as facial burns. A properly designed aerator supplies adequate aeration upon 12 hours' exposure at 50°C. Plastic or rubber materials, if stored at room temperature, should perhaps not be used until a minimum of several days has elapsed after sterilization.

PRACTICAL POINTS IN CLEANING EQUIPMENT

Contaminated anesthesia apparatus includes face masks, airways, laryngoscope blades, suction catheters, breathing tubes, reservoir bags, and, in the anesthesia machine, directional valves, the carbon dioxide absorber, and certain types of vaporization bottles. Before sterilization, apparatus should be washed with soap and hot water to remove gross debris, although ordinary soap is not bacteriostatic. Immediate immersion of apparatus in cleaning solutions prevents crusting and drying of secretions that are difficult to remove. Scrubbing of equipment is a hazard to personnel if pathogenic bacteria are present. For this reason we suggest that disinfection of apparatus be carried out initially with a solution of Wescodyne, a detergent-iodine complex (1½ oz in a pail of water), which is tuberculocidal and viricidal. Immersion in this solution should be complete and should last at least three minutes. Scrubbing can be performed in the solution without hazard. An alternate antiseptic is Cidex, an activated buffered solution of glutaraldehyde, which is bactericidal, sporocidal, and viricidal. Fortunately this solution is good for treatment of metal objects and instruments, offering rust-resisting properties as well. The interior of tracheal and pharyngeal airways should be cleaned with tight-fitting, stiff-bristled malleable brushes. Pipe cleaners can be used for finer apertures. Other equipment is scrubbed with a brush, particular attention being paid to crevices and angles that accumulate dirt and secretions. This is probably the single most important aspect of equipment sterilization. Brushes, too, should be sterilized periodically. Suction catheters and metal suction tips are rinsed with water under pressure; adhesive tape and oily lubricants are removed with acetone. At the termination of mechanical cleansing, the parts should be thoroughly rinsed in tap water. Certain pieces of apparatus such as the reservoir bag, delivery tubes, and face masks, if not used for patients with obvious transmissible disease, may be hung to drain and dry, then used again.

Once equipment has been cleaned, sterilization can be performed in various ways. The best procedure is to package the items, and then expose them to EO sterilization. In a large department of anesthesia it would be advantageous to have an EO sterilizer large enough to accommodate an anesthesia machine. Smaller sterilizers are available and are used for spinal anesthetic ampules and ophthalmic operating instruments. However, the smaller devices are not infallible, especially if not leakproof.

In a bacteriologic study performed by one of us, considerable contamination of presumably sterile tracheal tubes was found just before introduction into the trachea. Further study revealed that the method of handling equipment was just as important as the initial sterilization. Therefore, the following procedure has been followed: with the exception of the anesthesia machine, all items of equipment are sterilized with EO. Equipment must be handled properly in order to avoid transmission of disease. Breathing valves of the anesthesia machine are tested for competency by breathing through them with corrugated tubing kept on each machine. Before removal of sterile goods from containers, the hands are rinsed in a lubricating germicide* provided in a plastic squeeze bottle. The breathing system, once assembled, is tested for leakage of gas without breathing through the apparatus. Oral and nasal airways are placed in a basin of sterile saline. Endotracheal cuffs are tested for leakage without removal from the plastic sheath. The tracheal tube is removed just prior to intubation and lubricated with sterile saline from the basin. Suction catheters are kept packaged until ready for use.

SPECIAL PRECAUTIONS IN VIRULENT INFECTIONS

In the presence of tuberculosis or other infection with virulent pathogens, everything used during the anesthesia procedure must be sterilized. If closed system anesthesia is selected, disposable equipment, a to-and-fro technique or nonrebreathing system is used, because a circle filter is difficult to sterilize. If the patient has a pulmonary infection a mask should be worn before induction of anesthesia. At the termination, the patient is then isolated from others. The anesthetist should wear a gown, and some may wish to wear gloves as well. At completion of the procedure the anesthetist's gown is placed in a "dirty linen" bag to be sterilized in the autoclave along with other material from the operating room. Gloves and soda lime are decontaminated in O-Syl soluton and the soda lime then discarded. All metal parts of the anesthesia equipment are autoclaved. Rubber and plastic parts are boiled in water for 15 minutes; the rubber cushion on the face mask is deflated before subjecting it to heat. The anesthesia machine is scrubbed with a sporicidal chemical. The following disinfectants have been shown to be effective against the tubercle bacillus: ethyl alcohol, 70 per cent; isopropyl alcohol, 70 per cent; cresol solution saponated, N.F. XIII; orthophenyl phenol; *p-tert*-amylphenol, 2 per cent (O-Syl); and Cidex.

---

*Lubricating germicide: benzalkonium chloride, 17 per cent 30 ml; cetyl alcohol, 100 gm; isopropanol, 99 per cent 2660 ml; distilled water, *q.s. ad* 4000 ml.

REFERENCES

Albrecht WH, Dryden GE: Five year experience with the development of an individually clean anesthesia system. Anesth Analg 53:24, 1974.

Berry FA Jr: Comparison of bacteremia occurring with nasotracheal and orotracheal intubation. Anesth Analg 52:873, 1973.

Dryden GE: Uncleaned anesthesia equipment. JAMA 233:1298, 1975.

Stetson JB, Whitbourne JE, Eastman C: Ethylene oxide degassing of rubber and plastic materials. Anesthesiology 44:174, 1976.

Symposium on Infection: Br J Anaesth 48:1-47, 1976.

Chapter 8

MONITORING

Anesthetists administer potent depressant drugs to patients whose physiologic reserves may already be compromised; therefore they must unremittingly observe the patient's condition. Adjustments in therapy must be made, sometimes rapidly, because of alterations in physiologic function or surgical requirements. Constant vigilance is essential for safe care.

The primary resources for monitoring are the anesthetist's sense of sight, sound, and touch. Color of the patient's skin, tissues, and blood gives crude but useful clues to performance of the cardiovascular and respiratory systems. Observation of movement of the abdomen and chest provides information regarding volume of ventilation. Distended superficial veins may indicate inadequate myocardial function or overzealous infusion of fluids or blood. Divergent gaze, tearing, swallowing, and grimace are valuable indicators of light anesthesia. Dilated pupils might indicate either shallow or excessively deep anesthesia, or, more compellingly, a sign of life-threatening cerebral hypoxia.

These simple observations for evaluating the condition of the patient are sufficiently dependable and useful that they should not be abandoned even when more sophisticated methods are used. On the other hand, the use of mechanical and electronic devices substantially enlarges the breadth of patient monitoring during anesthesia and permits increased vigilance from the standpoint of the quantitative information derived.

CIRCULATION

HEART BEAT

The pulse in a superficial artery, commonly the temporal, radial, or femoral, provides information on rate, rhythm, and strength of the heart beat. Continuous auscultation of the chest not only provides these data, but also information on adequacy of the airway and quality of the breath sounds. An esophageal stethoscope or a weighted stethoscope bell on the chest or in the suprasternal notch can be used (Fig. 8–1). Using a monaural earpiece fashioned from a piece of latex rubber tubing or molded especially

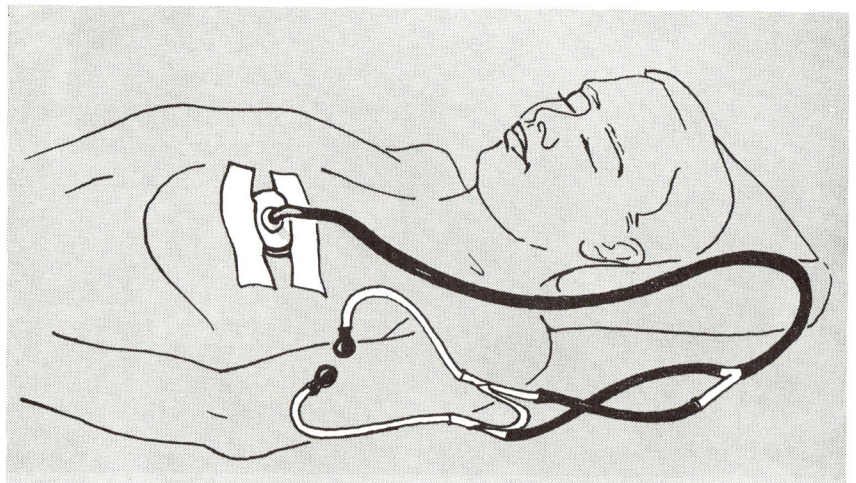

Figure 8–1. The precordial stethoscope, an excellent monitor of cardiac rate and rhythm in infants, children, and adults. If desired the binaural stethoscope attachment can be replaced by a single hearing aid consisting of an individually molded earpiece or the wide, soft end of a Foley catheter.

for this purpose, the anesthetist can maintain continuous auditory contact with the patient yet freely communicate with other operating room personnel. The earpiece can also be connected to the stethoscope for measuring blood pressure so that by turning a three-way stopcock, blood pressure can be taken. A commercially available valve automatically switches from one stethoscope to the other when the blood pressure cuff is inflated.

INDIRECT MEASUREMENT OF ARTERIAL PRESSURE

It is customary to measure blood pressure every 5 minutes while the patient is anesthetized, although during periods of cardiovascular instability more frequent measurements must be made. The familiar indirect sphygmomanometric method introduced by Riva-Rocci in 1896 is usually used. A cuff of appropriate width should be chosen so that the pressure transmitted to the major arteries of the arm is approximated by that measured in the cuff. Normally, this is accomplished when width of the cuff exceeds the diameter of the limb by 20 per cent. A higher pressure is required to occlude the arteries when the cuff is narrow or the arm corpulent, yielding an artificially high pressure reading.

The blood pressure cuff is ordinarily placed on the arm contralateral to that in which the intravenous infusion is begun. When the operation is to be performed in the axilla or on the arm, both intravenous infusion and blood pressure cuff may be placed on the same extremity. During operation on both upper extremities, an extra-wide blood pressure cuff is applied to the thigh.

Measuring blood pressure in the leg is sometimes preferable in the very obese patient.

Use of a stethoscope or other sound transducer over a major artery in the limb permits detection of Korotkoff sounds to estimate systolic and diastolic pressures. Palpation of return of the pulse or flushing of previously exsanguinated tissues distal to the deflating cuff only gives an estimate of systolic blood pressure. A less accurate method for estimating systolic blood pressure involves judging the point at which the manometer indicator begins to bounce with each pulse.

The bounce technique is refined through use of the oscillotonometer, which is made of two adjacent cuffs and uses an aneroid manometer to read pressure in the proximal cuff; oscillations in the distal cuff are estimated through a sensitive pneumatic-mechanical linkage. As pressure in the cuffs is reduced below systolic, a lever is intermittently depressed to display oscillations from the distal cuff. When the oscillations suddenly increase in amplitude, pressure in the proximal cuff (read when the lever is released) provides an indirect measurement of systolic pressure. A marked decrease in amplitude of oscillations during further cuff deflation indicates the diastolic pressure. The instrument is most accurate in the normal or low ranges of blood pressure.

In certain patients, especially when hypotension or hypothermia and sometimes obesity are present, Korotkoff sounds cannot be heard and even the oscillotonometric technique may fail. A particularly useful device under these circumstances is the Doppler flowmeter, an electronic instrument that transmits a high frequency vibratory signal toward the artery from a small crystal placed on the overlying skin. The frequency of the signal changes as it is reflected from the moving bloodstream. A receiving crystal detects the reflected signal, which is then amplified and monitored through headphones. The Doppler transducer can be positioned over the radial or dorsalis pedis artery to detect the presence or absence of blood flow during deflation of a conventional blood pressure cuff. A special application of the Doppler principle identifies pulsation of the arterial wall rather than motion of blood, permitting measurement of both systolic and diastolic blood pressures; the Doppler shifts are detectable through headphones or automatically via an electronic device that digitally displays systolic and diastolic pressures.

Difficulty in hearing Korotkoff sounds can be caused by hypotension, vasoconstriction, or malfunction of the apparatus. When there is an absence of sounds the novice is more likely to try to readjust the apparatus, whereas the experienced anesthetist promptly estimates arterial blood pressure by another means such as strength of the radial, carotid, or femoral pulse. Additional problems are introduced when pulse pressure is narrow, especially when accompanied by bradycardia. Under these circumstances the cuff must be deflated slowly to detect sounds, since the pulse pressure is transversed.

ELECTROCARDIOGRAM

The availability of reasonably priced compact electrocardiogram (ECG) monitors encourages routine monitoring of the ECG, as does the use of disposable electrodes containing adhesive patches incorporating small sponges soaked with conductive gel. A convenient pattern of electrode placement is to apply the positive lead (color-coded black) in the left midaxillary line, the negative lead (white) on the right shoulder, and the indifferent lead (usually green) on the left shoulder. When other electrode arrangements are required for certain operations, one should try to position the electrodes so that the main electric axis of the heart is directed toward the positive and away from the negative electrodes.

Every operating room should be equipped with an oscilloscopic display. In addition, there should be a recording device so that when problems arise, the ECG pattern can be recorded for later comparison with preoperative tracings. Storage devices are available to permit retrieval of transient ECG abnormalities. Cardiotachometers for continuous display of heart rate commonly are incorporated into the ECG monitor, as are audible signals coupled with the QRS complex. Most ECG monitors also offer audible or visual alarms to indicate bradyarrhythmias or tachyarrhythmias.

Failure to obtain a clear ECG tracing is most often caused by inadequate electric continuity between the skin and the ECG amplifier. Removal of oil and dry skin by rubbing the site of electrode placement with a gauze sponge sometimes helps to correct this. A broken wire or cable also will result in failure to obtain an acceptable ECG tracing; malfunction of the electronic device is less likely.

CENTRAL VENOUS PRESSURE

Adequacy of replacement of circulating blood volume relative to cardiac competence can be evaluated by measuring central venous pressure (CVP), normally 3 to 10 cm H_2O. In general, if arterial blood pressure, urine output, and CVP are all low, the circulating blood volume is probably inadequate or the venous capacity excessive. On the other hand, a low arterial blood pressure and oliguria combined with an elevated CVP (above 15 cm H_2O) is suggestive of a weak myocardium, and use of an inotropic agent should be considered (see Chapter 22). CVP alone is not a reliable guide to adequacy of blood volume. During rapid infusion of blood or fluids, the CVP often rises transiently above normal limits, only to fall with equilibration of fluid in the body compartments. Causes of increased CVP other than those discussed include pericardial tamponade, superior vena cava obstruction, and tension pneumothorax.

CVP can be approximated by lifting the arm of the patient until the veins of the dorsum of the hand collapse; the height of the hand above the right atrium is taken as CVP. Height of the drip chamber of an intravenous infusion set can be lowered until blood returns from the vein.

A more reliable index of CVP is obtained with a catheter positioned so that the tip lies in the vena cava or right atrium. The catheter is introduced percutaneously through the internal jugular, subclavian, or basilic vein. The basilic route is probably safest but difficulty often is encountered in passing the catheter through the axilla. Catheterization of the subclavian vein carries a relatively high risk of inducing pneumothorax. Percutaneous puncture of the internal jugular vein, however, is not difficult to perform, is usually successful, and is safe when carefully done. Proper technique requires that the patient be supine, with neck fully extended and the head sharply rotated away from the vein to be punctured. The right side usually is chosen because the right internal jugular vein has a relatively straight course to the right atrium. The operating room table is adjusted to a 20-degree head-down position in order to distend the vein. Puncture is initially made with a 22-gauge 4.3-cm needle attached to a 5-ml syringe containing 2 ml of 1 per cent lidocaine. The needle should enter the skin near the junction of the two heads of the sternocleidomastoid muscle, about 5 cm superior to the clavicle. After anesthetization of the skin in the conscious patient, slight negative pressure is applied to the plunger as the needle is advanced in a direction slightly lateral to the midline at an angle of about 30 degrees to the skin. When the vein is identified by appearance of venous blood, the 22-gauge needle is withdrawn and replaced with a 14-gauge needle through which a 30-cm 16-gauge radiopaque catheter is threaded. After the larger needle is beneath the skin, a small bolus of lidocaine is injected to expel any cored tissue and the needle is advanced along the pathway traversed by the smaller needle. When the vein is again punctured, the syringe is removed and the catheter threaded about 20 cm beyond the needle, usually sufficient for the tip to enter the right atrium. After the needle is withdrawn from the skin, pressure is applied to prevent bleeding, a shield is placed over the tip of the needle to prevent shearing of the catheter, a sterile dressing with antibiotic ointment is applied, and the needle and catheter are secured with adhesive tape or suture.

The reference level at which CVP is measured is that of the right atrium, usually considered to be 5-cm posterior to the sternum in the supine position (Figure 8–2). To adjust the CVP scale, which is attached to an intravenous pole, a meter stick to which a bubble level is attached may be used. One end of the stick is placed on the manubrium at the second intercostal space, and, after the bubble is brought to the center of the level, the vertical CVP scale is adjusted to read 5 cm at the other end of the meter stick.

PULMONARY WEDGE PRESSURE

When it is important to have a precise assessment of left ventricular function, a method for estimating left atrial pressure is desirable. A catheter with a small inflated balloon at its tip (Swan-Ganz) can be floated through the right side of the heart into the pulmonary artery. The catheter is inserted by cutdown or percutaneously through a large-bore needle. The balloon serves three functions: it provides a relatively large surface area to assist in flow-directed advance of the catheter; the tip of the catheter is recessed within a fold in the inflated balloon, tending to minimize arrhythmogenic irritation of the right ventricular wall; and inflation of the balloon when the catheter tip is in a small pulmonary artery establishes continuity

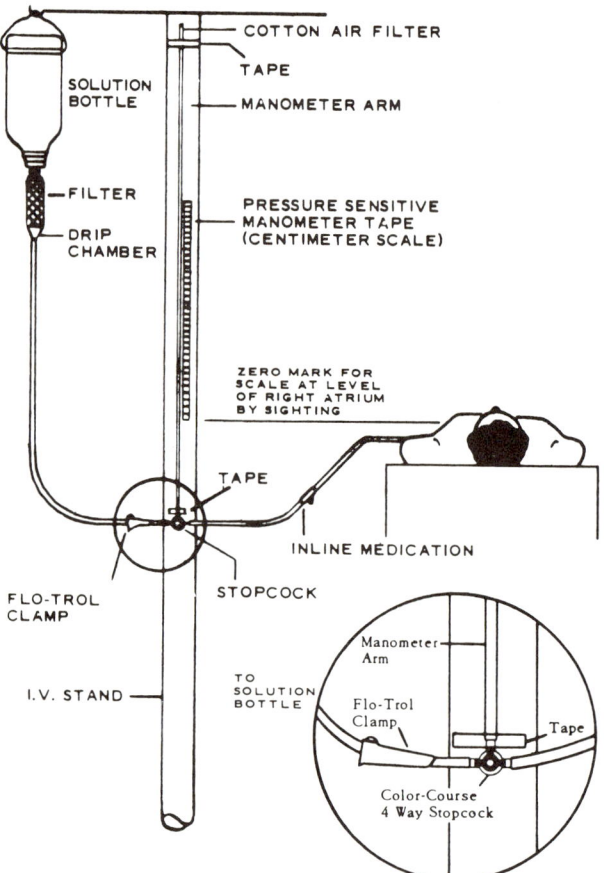

Figure 8-2. Constant monitoring of central venous pressure. Inset shows detail of circled area. (Reproduced with permission of the Fenwal Co.)

between the catheter lumen and the left atrium through the pulmonary capillaries. This permits indirect measurement of mean left atrial pressure ("wedge pressure").

CARDIAC OUTPUT

Special triple lumen flow-directed catheters embodying a thermistor near the tip are available for measuring cardiac output (CO) using the principle of thermal dilution. After a cool thermal marker has been injected through the proximal lumen (located near the right atrium), the curve describing dilution of the marker as blood flows to the thermistor in the pulmonary artery can be translated with analog or digital computation into a value for CO. Frequent measurements of CO are possible with this system, but the value of the information obtained must be appraised relative to potential complications of pulmonary artery catheterization: pulmonary infarction, cardiac arrhythmias, thromboembolism, balloon rupture, and catheter knotting.

DIRECT MEASUREMENT OF ARTERIAL BLOOD PRESSURE

For major operations and in seriously ill patients, it is desirable to measure the arterial blood pressure continuously through a cannula inserted into a peripheral artery. The same cannula can be used for intermittent sampling of arterial blood for measurement of Po_2, Pco_2, and pH.

The radial artery is usually chosen over the brachial artery because the latter is an "end-artery" which, when interrupted, might result in ischemia; both radial and ulnar arteries perfuse the hand. To assure adequacy of circulation in the event of thrombosis of the radial artery, a modification of Allen's test is recommended to evaluate ulnar arterial blood flow. The patient makes a tight fist to partially exsanguinate the hand while the anesthetist occludes both radial and ulnar arteries with digital pressure. If release of pressure over the ulnar artery does not lead to postischemic hyperemia, the contralateral ulnar artery should be similarly evaluated. If ulnar circulation is insufficient bilaterally, the benefits of arterial monitoring should be reassessed relative to the increased risk. In the absence of adequate ulnar circulation, thrombosis of the radial artery can lead to ischemia of the fingers.

Radial artery cannulation is preceded by positioning the wrist in slight hyperextension with a small folded towel behind it and taping the hand and the forearm to a rigid arm board. The skin is prepared with antiseptic. Sterile gloves are unnecessary so long as that portion of the cannula entering the artery and the site of puncture is not touched. A wheal of local anesthetic is raised over the point of maximal arterial pulsation, usually 1 to 2 cm proximal to the crease at the wrist, and the skin incised with an 18-gauge steel needle to facilitate passage of the cannula. With the index finger of the operator's nondominant hand palpating the artery proximal to the site of puncture, an 18-gauge plastic cannula-over-needle is inserted parallel to the axis of the artery, angled 30 to 45 degrees to the surface. The operator's hypothenar eminence is supported on the palm of the patient's supinated hand, while the hub of the cannula-needle is grasped between thumb and index finger. The barrel of a plastic syringe with plunger discarded, may be inserted into the needle hub to provide a convenient grip as well as a small reservoir to contain spurting blood as the artery is entered.

The intent is to puncture the arterial wall cleanly with a single insertion. To help assure that the back wall of the artery is not inadvertently punctured, the bevel of the needle is held downward. When brisk spurting of blood indicates puncture, the steel needle is held firmly while the overlying plastic cannula is advanced full length (3 to 6 cm) into the artery. If arterial blood flow is not encountered during insertion, the inner needle should be withdrawn before the catheter is removed, because successful puncture is sometimes evident during withdrawal rather than during insertion. After the cannula has been inserted, firm digital pressure at the tip of the cannula will halt blood flow while a three-way stopcock is attached to the hub. The procedure is completed by flushing the cannula with heparinized saline (500 U/500 ml), fixing it with tape or suture and applying antibiotic ointment and a sterile dressing.

Standard connecting tubing, preferably with locking fittings to avoid inadvertent separation, is used to connect the arterial cannula to a strain-gauge transducer. A manifold is interposed to permit flushing of the cannula with heparinized saline without opening the system to air and to obtain samples of arterial blood. Air bubbles must be meticulously removed from the tubing to avoid injecting air into the artery during flushing. When the strain gauge, amplifier, and oscilloscope have been calibrated with a mercury manometer, display of the arterial pressure waveform permits the reading of systolic and diastolic pressures as well as mean pressure when the signal is electronically damped.

When a strain gauge is unavailable or not chosen, saline-filled tubing can be connected from the stopcock to a length of air-filled tubing attached to an aneroid or mercury manometer. The cannula is flushed through the stopcock, while the manometer is protected from damage by the air column. Inertia permits only the reading of mean arterial blood pressure, and frequent flushing is required to prevent clotting as blood refluxes into the cannula.

MEASUREMENT OF BLOOD LOSS

The anesthetist should evaluate blood loss continuously, recording a cumulative estimate on the anesthesia record every 15 minutes. Sponges should be inspected and blood content estimated to the nearest 5 ml. Accuracy improves with practice; outdated bank blood can be used to make sample sponges containing known blood volumes. When major blood loss is expected, sponges discarded from the operative field are weighed and the dry weight subtracted to assess blood content. The weight of 1 ml of blood is assumed to be 1 gm. The volume thus determined is added to that in the suction bottle after subtraction of estimated volume of irrigating solutions, and added to that estimated to be present on the drapes.

Blood volume measurement using serum albumin or erythrocytes tagged with a radioactive indicator is feasible, but because of complexity it is seldom used in practice. Serial determinations of hematocrit or hemoglobin concentration often assist in evaluating adequacy of blood replacement. Arterial blood pressure, heart rate, CVP, skin color, and urine output remain the most valuable clinical indicators of the adequacy of blood and fluid replacement (see Chapter 22).

AIR EMBOLISM

The danger of air embolism exists when veins with intraluminal pressures that are negative in relation to the atmosphere are opened, such as during intracranial operations in the sitting patient. Under such circumstances, special monitoring techniques are indicated. A CVP catheter is advanced into the right atrium so that if air has been entrained, negative pressure can be applied to the catheter to diagnose the presence of air and to remove as much of it as possible. Location of the catheter tip in the right atrium should be confirmed radiographically. A Doppler transducer applied precordially or an esophageal stethoscope is a useful adjunct to the CVP catheter for diagnosing air embolism.

RESPIRATION

Continuous observation of the chest wall, abdomen, suprasternal notch, and the lungs in the open chest helps in assessing the adequacy of pulmonary ventilation. Continuous auscultation of breath sounds through an esophageal or precordial stethoscope adds to the information obtained. When trouble is suspected, thorough auscultation of the entire chest is indicated.

RESPIRATORY FREQUENCY, TIDAL VOLUME, AND MINUTE VOLUME

Respiratory rate is easily counted. With spontaneous breathing, tidal exchange can be observed for signs of obstruction of the airway and depth of anesthesia—irregular, rapid breathing in light planes or regular breathing in deep anesthesia. Tidal volume is difficult to estimate and is usually depressed by volatile anesthetics. Effective alveolar exchange may be further reduced by an increased physiologic dead space during inhalation anesthesia. The combination of tachypnea, reduced tidal volume, and increased dead space reduces alveolar ventilation. Incompletely blocked surgical stimuli during light planes of anesthesia often induce hyperventilation.

Spirometry can be used to measure average tidal volume (V_T); by subtracting estimated dead space (V_D) and multiplying by respiratory frequency (f), one obtains an estimate of alveolar ventilation: $\dot{V}_A = (V_T - V_D) \times$ f. (See Chapter 33.) Physiologic dead space does not remain static, increasing with depth of anesthesia, especially with intermittent positive pressure ventilation, sometimes approaching values up to one-half of tidal volume. Alveolar ventilation of about 60 ml/min/kg body weight is usually adequate under basal conditions. Many commercially available spirometers are available for monitoring the anesthetized patient. Some, like the one shown in Figure 8–3, are mechanically activated, indicating gas flow by transferring motion of a rotor to a pointer on a dial. The delicate rotor of such a device may not be designed to withstand the high flows generated during vital capacity maneuvers nor the humidity of closed circuit breathing systems. Other spirometers combine the mechanical aspects of a rotor-stator with electronic analysis and display; some of these can be used not only for measuring volumes during quiet breathing but also for measuring forced vital capacity during preanesthetic evaluation. The pneumotachograph, with which gas flow can be measured by recording the pressure drop

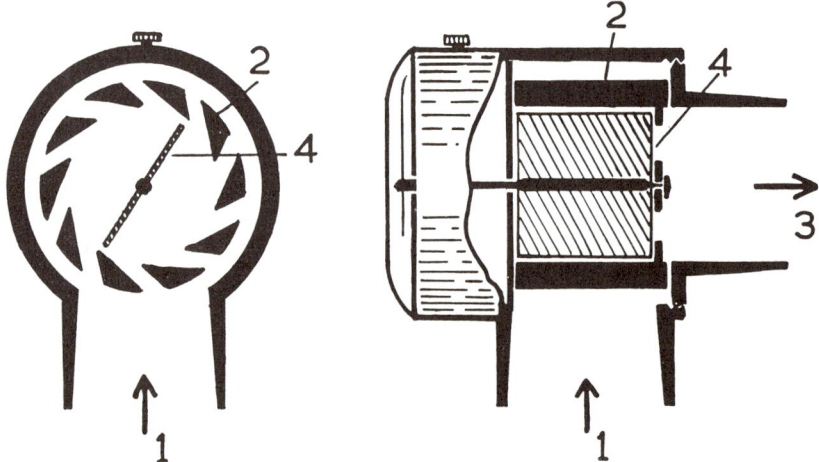

Figure 8–3. The Wright anemometer. Air enters the instrument at (*1*) and, having passed through 10 tangential slots in a cylindrical stator ring (*2*), escapes through the outlet (*3*). Within the stator ring (*2*) a flat, two-bladed rotor (*4*) is turned by the passing air at a speed proportional to the air flow through the instrument. (Reproduced with permission from Mushin, Rendell-Baker, and Thompson: Automatic Ventilation of the Lungs. Oxford, Blackwell Scientific Publications, 1959.)

across a small fixed resistance, can be used during general anesthesia. However, to obtain volume of ventilation, the flow signal must be integrated and the cost of such a system may not be justified for routine monitoring.

Pitfalls exist when a spirometric device is incorporated into the anesthesia circuit to measure ventilation. When the spirometer is placed between the fresh gas inlet and the "popoff" valve, fresh gas inflow as well as the patient's ventilation is measured. Mathematic corrections can be made; gas flow can be turned off for brief measurement; or the spirometer can be placed between the patient and the breathing circuit so that only gases passing to and from the patient are measured. If spirometry is performed while agents such as nitrous oxide are being absorbed by or excreted from the lungs in appreciable quantities, this also influences the readings obtained. Anesthetics can also alter the calibration of some spirometric devices. Because the condensation of exhaled water vapor interferes with the function of mechanical spirometers, intermittent rather than continuous measurement is advisable when the instrument is near the patient's airway.

OXYGENATION

The adequacy of oxygenation of arterial blood has traditionally been estimated by looking for cyanosis; at least 5 gm of deoxygenated hemoglobin in each 100 ml of blood must be present for the dusky blue coloration to appear. Because the appearance of the skin is influenced by both venous and arterial blood, conditions such as hypothermia and hypotension, as well as pigmentation of the skin and intensity and color of incident light, all interfere with the use of cyanosis as a reliable sign of oxygenation of arterial blood. Color of the oral mucous membranes or of blood in the surgical field is a more dependable indicator.

Measurement of Pa_{O_2} is the most readily available method for accurate assessment of oxygenation. As with carbon dioxide, the P_{O_2} in an end-tidal gas sample (PET_{O_2}) can be analyzed with the oxygen electrode on a blood gas analyzer. PET_{O_2}, however, may provide only a poor estimate of Pa_{O_2} because of the limited degree to which PET_{O_2} approaches PA_{O_2}, as well as the degree to which the PA_{O_2} reflects Pa_{O_2}.

Oximetry has been used for evaluation of oxygenation of arterial blood perfusing the pinna of the ear, but the technique is unreliable. Recent technologic advances utilizing fiberoptic light transmission and computer analysis now permit automatic compensation for factors such as skin pigmentation and ear thickness; calibration is possible without blood sampling, and thus clinical use of the ear oximeter is more feasible. The cost of the device is sufficiently high, however, to preclude routine use. But the technique has potential as a noninvasive substitute for blood gas analysis during assessment of oxygenation.

CARBON DIOXIDE

The ultimate measure of adequacy of pulmonary ventilation is Pa_{CO_2}. Therefore, when there is concern over the possibility of respiratory acidosis, arterial blood should be analyzed for P_{CO_2} and pH. To this end, the radial artery is usually punctured with a 22- or 23-gauge needle, although sometimes the brachial artery is more accessible.

If a rapid-acting carbon dioxide analyzer is available, Pa_{CO_2} can be estimated from end-tidal P_{CO_2} (PET_{CO_2}). However, at least two problems arise: although there may be no gradient for P_{CO_2} between an alveolus and its pulmonary capillary, the exhaled gas from underperfused alveoli can exert a dilutional effect leading to a PET_{CO_2} as much as 10 torr lower than Pa_{CO_2}, a gradient that can be doubled in an emphysematous patient; the second problem occurs during shallow breathing when it is difficult to obtain a representative end-tidal plateau.

Mass spectrometers or analyzers based upon the absorption of infrared energy by carbon dioxide, although rapid enough for on-line measurement of PET_{CO_2}, are expensive and seldom used clinically. An inexpensive alternative entails sampling end-tidal gas in a syringe and analyzing it for P_{CO_2} with the appropriate electrode in a blood gas analyzer.

RENAL FUNCTION

The urinary bladder should be catheterized during major operations in order to observe the flow of urine. This provides an opportunity to measure urine output, a valuable indicator of the adequacy of blood and fluid replacement. Urine flows greater than 30 to 40 ml per hour are usually judged compatible with normovolemia. Oliguria can result from a reduced circulating blood volume, the antidiuretic effects of anesthetics, the stress of operation, or acute renal failure. If infusion of blood or fluid restores blood pressure and CVP to acceptable values but does not result in adequate urine flow, one may choose to administer a 10-mg intravenous test dose of furosemide (Lasix) to show that the kidneys can respond. When this is done, however, some of the subsequent value of using urine output to judge adequacy of volume replacement is lost. Monitoring urine output also permits visual evidence of hemoglobinuria, which is sometimes the first and occasionally the only sign of an incompatible blood transfusion.

THE NEUROMUSCULAR JUNCTION

Muscle tone is usually judged by observation of the surgical field, by noting the amount of positive pressure required to fill the lungs with a given volume of gas, and by testing the tension of jaw muscles by manually opening the mouth of the anesthetized patient. A nerve stimulator is a useful adjunct. The use, interpretation, and limitation of this device are described in Chapter 14.

THE CENTRAL NERVOUS SYSTEM

Although central nervous system (CNS) depression is an expected component of general anesthesia, the anesthetist should unremittingly watch for signs of pathologic CNS depression owing to hypoxemia, excessively deep anesthesia, embolization, or stroke. The appearance of the eyes gives valuable clues: fixed, dilated pupils usually indicate profound CNS depression and demand immediate reassessment of the patient's condition; unequal pupils suggest embolization or stroke (see Chapter 16.)

Electroencephalography has been used to evaluate CNS function during extracorporeal circulation and to help gauge depth of anesthesia. Although seldom used for these purposes today (see Chapter 16), electroencephalography is thought useful by some surgeons for giving early warning of cerebral hypoxia during carotid artery surgery.

BODY TEMPERATURE

Thermal regulatory function is depressed by most inhalation anesthetics. Therefore, body temperature often falls during general anesthesia, especially if the operation is long, requires large amounts of blood and fluid administration, and the chest or abdomen is opened. Infants, who have a large surface area to body mass ratio, are particularly subject to hypothermia during anesthesia (see Chapter 24). Hyperthermia, although less common, can also occur in the infant or adult anesthetized patient owing to the thermal insulation of sterile drapes and a pharmacologic loss of thermal regulatory capacity secondary to use of atropine and inhalation anesthetics. Some patients are febrile before anesthesia is induced. Hyperthermia of unknown origin can appear without warning and be malignant and potentially fatal (see Chapter 28.) Fever from any cause increases the requirement for uptake of oxygen and excretion of carbon dioxide. For all these reasons, routine monitoring of body temperature is necessary during anesthesia.

Temperature can be measured at many sites: esophagus, nasopharynx, rectum, skin, and tympanic membrane. Esophageal measurement at the level of the heart provides the best estimate of core temperature. Tympanic membrane temperature approximates the temperature of the brain, but it is possible to damage the membrane. Thermal probes carry heat away from organs with small heat capacity, a common problem in all thermometry and especially troublesome when measuring tympanic membrane or skin temperature.

Electronic devices for thermometry usually incorporate a thermistor or a thermocouple. In the thermistor, a change in temperature alters the electric resistance of a ceramiclike metallic bead, while in the thermocouple a change in temperature alters the potential difference between two dissimilar metals. Both devices respond quickly so that readings closely follow temperature even when it is rapidly changing. Probes are of various shapes and sizes and are available to accommodate thermal measurement at different sites. Thermistors and thermocouples require electronic circuitry to process information from the probes; the circuitry is factory calibrated, but requires calibration checks by the user for continued high-quality performance. Testing is easily done by simultaneously measuring a series of water temperatures with the electronic device and a dependable mercury thermometer. Although less convenient than the electronic method, a clinical thermometer can be used to record temperature in the rectum, nasopharynx, or axilla of the anesthetized patient.

MISCELLANEOUS MONITORING DEVICES

For patient safety, it is sometimes useful to measure variables unrelated to organ function. For example, oxygen tension can be monitored within the anesthesia circuit, even though it is not financially feasible to measure the patient's end-tidal P_{O_2} continuously. Most oxygen monitors used in anesthesia circuits today are battery powered and have polarographic or fuel-cell electrodes. Some older models employ the paramagnetic principle. The design assumes that zero drift will be insignificant, leaving only the gain to be adjusted during calibration. Room air is usually adequate as a calibrating gas, although a check with 100 per cent oxygen is desirable. Calibration should be done before application of each anesthetic and rechecked whenever there is apparent discrepancy between the analyzer reading and setting of flowmeters or the condition of the patient.

Instruments are available for analysis of the concentrations of gases in the anesthesia circuit but are seldom used because anesthesia flowmeters are quite accurate. On occasion, however, a halothane or nitrous oxide analyzer can prove useful for trouble-shooting when a problem is suspected with a machine or vaporizer. Mass spectrometers and infra-red analyzers are expensive but provide accurate and rapid analysis of anesthetic concentrations.

Because of potential occupational hazards (see Chapter 11), continuous monitoring of trace concentrations of anesthetic which escape into an operating room has been proposed, even though a closed anesthetic circuit or a scavenger system is used. Whether or not this propsoal gains favor will depend upon data yet to come.

Pressure within the anesthesia circuit is easily monitored with an aneroid manometer, available on most anesthesia machines. This is useful in aiding the anesthetist to assure that pressures applied to the patient's airway are within safe limits. Airway pressure generated when the lungs are inflated with a fixed volume of gas is a measure of pulmonary compliance, useful as a rough indicator of adequacy of neuromuscular blockade. Decreased compliance can also signal the onset of bronchospasm or pulmonary edema.

REFERENCES

Ali H, Savarese J: Monitoring of neuromuscular junction. Anesthesiology 45:216, 1976.
Buchbinder N, Ganz W: Hemodynamic monitoring: Invasive techniques. Anesthesiology 45:146, 1976.
Burton GW: Measurement of inspired and expired oxygen and carbon dioxide. Br J Anaesth 41:723, 1969.
Cooper EA: The measurement of ventilation. Br J Anaesth 41:718, 1969.

Chapter 9

THE ANESTHESIA RECORD

Although anesthetics had been given since 1846 and many important clinical observations had been made by individuals like John Snow, the first formal records of anesthetic administration were not kept until the year 1895. At that time Harvey Cushing and Amory Codman, then second-year Harvard medical students, began to keep "ether" charts. They recorded pulse rate, respiration, depth of anesthesia, and amount of ether given in an effort to give safer anesthesia; they realized full well the dangers. Subsequently, in 1902, Cushing introduced the Riva-Rocci method of measuring blood pressure; this was added to the anesthesia record.

Anesthesia records are of undeniable value to patient, anesthetist, surgeon, and nursing staff. If pulse rate, respiration, blood pressure, and other pertinent findings have been recorded at frequent intervals, the patient's condition can be assessed at any moment. A good anesthesia record also is of help if a patient must be anesthetized again. There are cogent medicolegal reasons for keeping accurate records, since review can establish the course of events more convincingly than recourse to memory. In an article on prevention of malpractice claims, J. B. Dillon stated that in a 10-year experience of reviewing cases of alleged malpractice, he had yet to see one in which record of the anesthetic course was complete. If one engages in the simplest clinical research, anesthesia records are the key to the collection of data, but it must be emphasized that conclusions from data are only as reliable as the original records. Furthermore, governmental supervision of medical practice and reimbursement for services will require the evidence provided by records.

A fine record is of little value if anesthesia is poor; in other words, care of the patient should never be sacrificed for the sake of a record. There are times when the patient demands complete attention. It would be foolhardy at these times to withdraw one's attention in order to complete the record. In the majority of cases, however, one should be able to keep a full and detailed account of any procedure.

Examples of suitable records are shown in Figures 9–1 and 9–2.

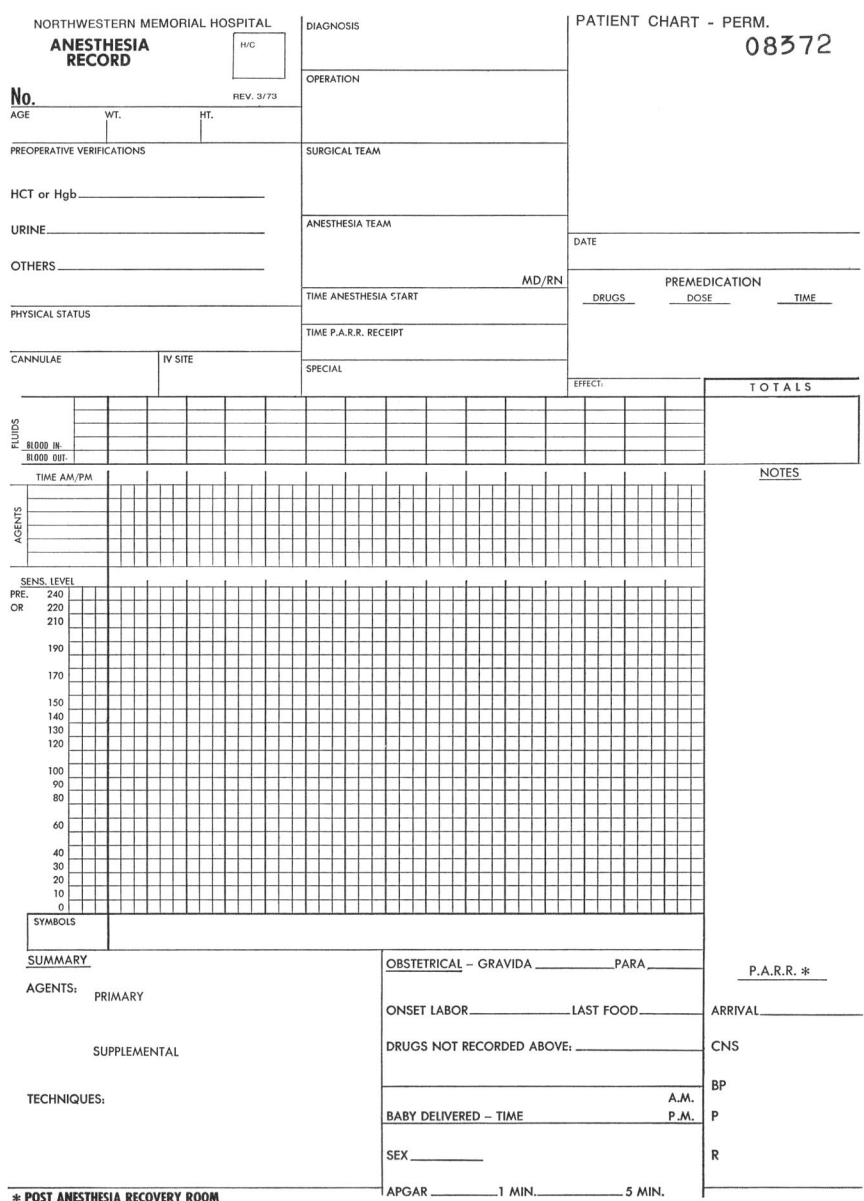

Figure 9–1. Anesthesia record.

Records should be kept in duplicate—one for the hospital chart, the other for departmental files and analysis. A third copy is sometimes kept for the anesthetist's own files, while parts of the record may be used for billing purposes.

The Anesthesia Record

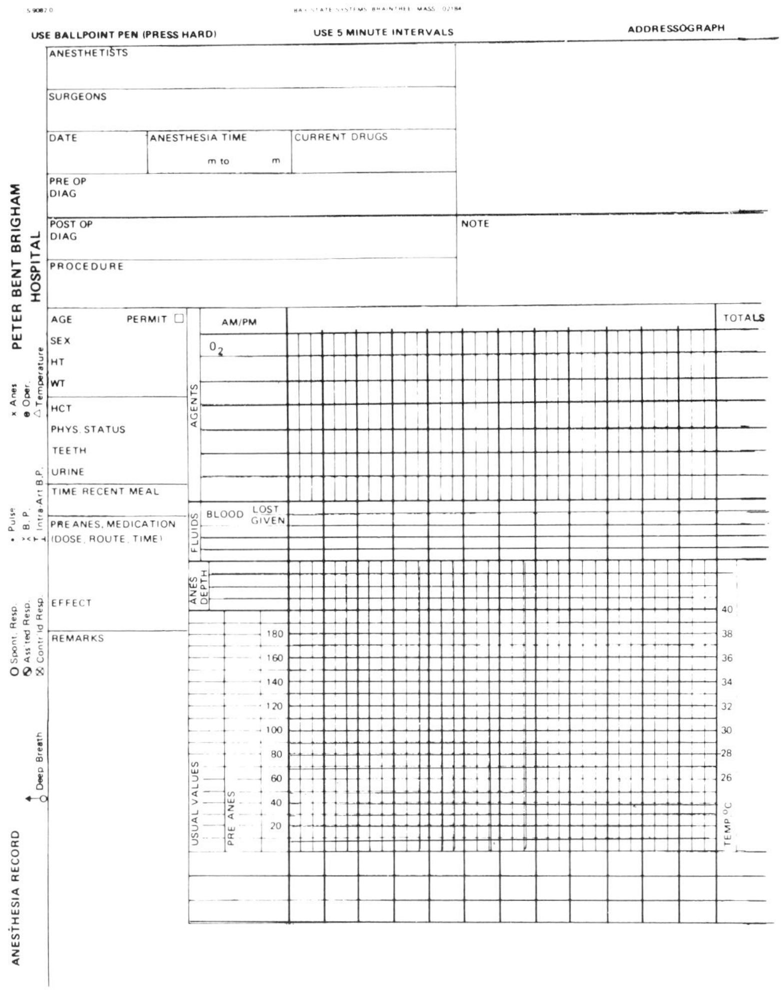

THE ANESTHESIA RECORD

Figure 9-2. Anesthesia record.

INFORMATION DERIVED FROM ANESTHESIA RECORDS

The instructions given here apply to any anesthesia chart and should improve the quality of information gained. Notations should be entered in ballpoint pen, pressing down firmly.

FACE OF THE RECORD

Name. The patient's name is printed legibly, family name first. Address and telephone number are useful for follow-up studies and for business purposes. These items can be stamped on the chart with an addressograph plate.

Age. Age is written in years for adults and for the infant in terms of months, weeks, or days.

Height. Height is written in inches or centimeters; if not known, an estimate should be made.

Weight. Weight is given in pounds or kilograms; if unknown, an estimate should be made.

Recent Meal. The patient is asked when last food or drink was ingested. "No" is entered if the patient has had nothing by mouth for at least six hours; otherwise "yes" is written and a description given of oral intake. At the same time, the patient is asked about removal of false teeth and of chewing gum or tobacco. Infants and young children usually will have been fed within four hours of operation; injury, shock, emotional tension, or alcohol ingestion almost always delay emptying of the stomach. Parturients often have a full stomach.

Physical Status. See Chapter 2 for numerical rating.

Premedication. The amount, time, route of administration, and effect of preanesthetic drugs are recorded. Note is made as to whether sedation is adequate or if untoward effects have occurred. If no medication was given, "none" is written.

Information of Vital Importance. There should be a place at the top of an anesthesia record to call attention to information of special importance. If a patient has myasthenia gravis, active tuberculosis, or major allergy, this is of vital importance. Some may choose to indicate whether the patient has accepted or is a suitable candidate for the anesthesia planned.

Operative Permit. The patient should have granted permission in writing for performance of anesthesia and operation. This is essential in the case of minors, for whom the parent or legal guardian should grant permission. Individual states vary in their legal requirements, and anesthetists should be familiar with the law in their communities.

Drug History. As indicated in Chapter 3, many therapeutic drugs adversely affect the course of anesthesia. Questions should be asked and note made on any drugs the patient has been taking.

L. P. This refers to spinal or peridural anesthesia. In evaluating the cause of untoward sequelae of spinal anesthesia, it is important to have an idea of the trauma caused by lumbar puncture. One should record needle gauge; spinal level of insertion; kind of lumbar puncture, whether midline or lateral; number of insertions; absence of paresthesias or location when produced; character of cerebrospinal fluid (CSF), whether clear or bloodstained; ease of aspiration or flow of CSF. When using a catheter for serial spinal or peridural anesthesia, estimated length of catheter inserted is noted.

Induction: S.U. If induction is satisfactory, "S" is circled; if unsatisfactory, the "U," and reasons are given. Common components of unsatisfactory induction include vomiting, retching, cough, soft tissue obstruction, laryngospasm, excessive mucus, excitement, slow uptake of inhalation agents, apnea, respiratory depression, hypotension, cyanosis, and ECG irregularities.

Airway. Details of airway insertion during anesthesia are recorded in this space. When an airway is placed in the pharynx through the mouth or nose, "oropharyngeal" or "nasopharyngeal" is written. It should be indicated whether insertion was accompanied by trauma, such as bleeding from the gums or nose, damage to teeth, or injury to lips. Information regarding trauma is likewise recorded when a catheter is passed into the trachea. In addition, "endotracheal" should be circled and the following data supplied:

The Anesthesia Record

1. Route of intubation: orotracheal or nasotracheal (right or left).

2. Number of attempts at intubation: each insertion of the laryngoscope or each time the tube is passed beyond the epiglottis is counted as an attempt. When intubating blindly, an attempt is each time the tube is advanced with the expectation of entering the larynx.

3. Diameter of tube; use of stylet.

4. Method of intubation; unless otherwise noted it is assumed that intubation was performed under direct vision with a laryngoscope. If a laryngoscope was not used, "blind" is written.

5. Note is made if the tube is cuffed (also when the cuff was inflated and how much air was used) or if a pharyngeal pack was placed.

Maintenance. This space is for recording important happenings during anesthesia. As experience increases, the anesthetist is better able to select which observations should be recorded. The simplest method is to number the observations 1, 2, 3 – chronologically, writing the same number below the graphic chart with the remark made. Here comments are made on aspects of the patient's condition other than pulse, respiration, or blood pressure; for example, excessive secretions, laryngospasm, hiccough, fever, tremor, muscle twitching, or convulsions. Notes are made concerning the conduct of anesthesia that cannot be shown on the graphic chart: respiratory obstruction, cyanosis, and wearing off of spinal or regional anesthesia. An anesthesia record should have a place for recording esophageal or rectal temperature, central venous and pulmonary artery pressure, blood loss, and fluid replacement. It is important to note reasons for changing the anesthetic or method and to record the time at which the patient's position is changed, because alterations in respiration or circulation often appear.

Treatment given during the procedure that is not recorded elsewhere should be noted here: for example, tracheobronchial toilet (abbreviated TBT); aspiration of mucus or other material from trachea or bronchi; dose and route of administration of drugs. When transfusion is given, positive identification of each unit of blood is made.

Details should be written of surgical manipulation that may be significant physiologically or affect the conduct of anesthesia. For example, traction on the gallbladder may cause a fall in blood pressure.

Technique. The technique by which an anesthetic is given is written directly below the agent. More than one method may be used for the same agent during anesthesia; any change is recorded. The several techniques of inhalation anesthesia are described in Chapter 12.

Controlled Respiration (CR). This signifies that the anesthetist "breathes" for the patient, controlling both rate and depth of respiration after apnea has been produced by hyperventilation, administration of drugs which depress activity of the respiratory center, or administration of a neuromuscular blocker.

Assisted Respiration (AR). This technique is used to improve ventilation and to minimize movements of the mediastinum or diaphragm as the patient continues to make respiratory efforts. The anesthetist supplies positive pressure to the reservoir bag just during inspiration; expiration occurs passively at ambient pressure.

Position. The appropriate term for position of the patient during operation is indicated. Symbols may be used.

Fluids. Amounts of solution given during anesthesia are written in the designated space.

THE CHART

Anesthetics. Anesthetics, analgetics, and adjuvants are listed. The amount or concentration of agent is included even in the case of agents administered by inhalation. In general, the main agent is that with which the greatest depth of anesthesia is obtained (except when a potent agent has been used only for induction). When a local anesthetic for spinal or regional anesthesia is given with the idea of performing the operation using this method alone, it is considered the main agent even if the block fails and another anesthetic technique is substituted; however, the new agent must also be listed. In spinal or peridural anesthesia, volume of anesthetic injected is recorded as well as drug and concentration used.

Depth of Anesthesia. Although not a simple matter with modern inhalation anesthetics, the estimated level of narcosis is charted in the space labeled "Plane of 3rd Stage" each time vital signs are recorded.

Level of Spinal or Peridural Anesthesia. Space is provided for the level of sensory block. Levels should be determined as frequently as practicable, but especially at the beginning and end of the procedure.

Pulse Rate, Blood Pressure, and Respiratory Rate. A filled in circle is used to indicate pulse rate, an open circle for respiratory rate, v for systolic and $\wedge$ for diastolic pressure. A dash (—) may be used to record mean pressure. Pulse, respiratory rate, and blood pressure should be determined and recorded at least every five minutes.

Along the bottom of the graph, symbols are placed denoting beginning and termination of anesthesia and operation.

Start of anesthesia — X
Start of operation — •
End of anesthesia and operation — ⊗

REVERSE OF RECORD

The back of an anesthesia record can provide space for a summary of the patient's preoperative condition as well as room for postoperative notes. Conscientious analysis and recording of significant events of the postoperative course provide valuable data. It is common to hear expressions of opinion as to the incidence of a particular complication. Unless reliable data have been gathered, such opinions merit little credence.

Notes for the record are obtained from the patient and the hospital chart, the nurse's notes, the surgeon's notes, and the anesthetist's physical examination. Every patient should be seen within the first 24 hours of operation, and again on the second, fourth, and sixth postoperative days, the frequency of visits relating to the patient's condition. Sufficiently close contact should be maintained during the patient's stay in the hospital to enable recording of such delayed phenomena as pulmonary embolism, wound disruption, or postlumbar puncture (LP) headache. Any of these complications may take place as late as the seventh to tenth postoperative day. The number of days of observation should be recorded.

Although the form of the anesthesia chart may vary, there are certain fundamentals of anesthesia and surgical convalescence which should be recorded. These are described according to systems.

Nervous System

HEADACHE. Adequate description of headache includes time of onset; when patient sat up or got out of bed; duration; location; severity; the patient's psychologic or emotional make-up; presence of nausea, vomiting, stiff neck, or dizziness; disturbances of hearing or vision; and relation to posture — a nonpostural LP headache with stiff neck suggests a meningeal reaction. Dimness, blurring of vision, or diplopia are noted. "Blocking of the ears," diminution in hearing, and tinnitus may relate to changes in CSF pressure transmitted to the internal ear. These details are important in describing LP headache.

DISTURBANCE OF SENSATION. Under this heading one lists hyperesthesia or hypoesthesia, that is, increased or decreased perception of any sensory modality (touch, pain, temperature, vibration, or position sense). Patients given spinal or other kinds of regional anesthesia are questioned specifically about the presence of numbness, tingling, or paresthesia. Backache can be recorded under the heading of sensory disturbance.

DISTURBANCES OF MOTOR AND VISCERAL FUNCTION. Paresis or complete paralysis should be recorded, including any subjective or objective evidence of weakness, change in gait, or abnormalities of bowel or bladder function.

MENTAL STATE. One of the complications of general anesthesia and operation may be development of a toxic psychosis. The elderly are likely to show mental disturbance of varying degree in the early postoperative days. Disorientation may also occur as a result of administration of opioids—a reaction common in the aged. Emergence delirium and excitement in the immediate postoperative period should be recorded in detail and treatment noted. Delayed recovery of consciousness or occurrence of convulsions is listed.

Respiratory Tract

SEQUELAE OF TRACHEAL INTUBATION. These include evidence of trauma to nose, mouth, pharynx, or larynx. One also records presence of edema, obstruction to respiration, infection, subcutaneous emphysema, mediastinal emphysema, hoarseness, sore throat, or cough.

MAJOR RESPIRATORY COMPLICATIONS. Development of atelectasis is not uncommon. Diagnosis of pneumonia may be made if the clinical course is prolonged, a febrile reaction subsides slowly, toxemia is evident, and there are physical and x-ray signs of consolidation. Miscellaneous respiratory complications include hiccough, pleural effusion, pneumothorax, and aspiration pneumonitis.

Circulatory System

Complications such as shock, hemorrhage, cardiac arrhythmias, thrombophlebitis, pulmonary edema, and embolism are recorded. Sequelae related to anesthetic management, like low blood pressure and bradycardia, and prolonged hypertension or tachycardia related to vasopressor drugs, should also be noted.

If cardiac failure and pulmonary edema occur, one evaluates the role of parenteral fluid therapy, hypoxia, respiratory obstruction, hypertension, or hypotension as causative factors. If signs of coronary insufficiency or infarction develop, similar evaluation is made.

Gastrointestinal Tract

NAUSEA AND VOMITING. Although it is difficult to analyze the causes of nausea or vomiting in the postoperative period, a beginning can be made in this direction if certain details are recorded. These are time of onset, duration, severity, presence of abdominal distention, relation to administration of opioids, or prior history of these sequelae.

Liver

Evidence of hepatic damage is recorded and the role of anesthetic management evaluated.

Kidney and Bladder

Prime concerns are oliguria, anuria, and urinary retention. Hypotension, incompatible transfusion, and drugs given are evaluated as possible causes. Treatment of sequelae is noted. The nature of retention can be evaluated best by recording the number of catheterizations. If an indwelling catheter is in place, this is stated.

NOTES ON THE PATIENT'S HOSPITAL CHART

In addition to the preoperative notes and data written on the back of the anesthesia record, notes should be made on the patient's permanent hospital record. Significant facts concerning the postoperative course are recorded over the signature of the anesthetist. Headache, pulmonary, cardiovascular, gastrointestinal, and urinary tract complications are analyzed from the standpoint of anesthesia.

USE OF RECORDS FOR STATISTICAL PURPOSES

If every anesthesia chart contained sufficient information, many aspects of anesthesia subject to erroneous impression might be described with reasonable accuracy. Even if this were accomplished, however, the ordinary anesthesia record does not lend itself readily to the gathering of facts for analysis. For this reason, several systems have been devised to facilitate accumulation of data of statistical value. We describe several techniques here because not all anesthetists have access to computer-based systems.

The least complicated method of gathering data is the use of a punch card system. The chart is made of lightweight cardboard, with rows of holes at the edges of the card. Each group of holes pertains to an item of interest, such as anesthetic used or operation performed. During conduct of anesthesia the usual information is recorded on the chart. Subsequently, the holes at the edges are cut with a punch. For example, if halothane had been used the hole opposite "halothane" would be punched so that it extended to the edge of the card. Eventually, in obtaining data on halothane anesthesia, all of the records would be stacked and a sorting needle passed through the holes punched. All unpunched charts would be carried away, leaving only the halothane charts for counting and analysis. Such charts can be "combed" with one or two needles or a hand-operated mechanical device containing as many as six needles. This kind of card can be used for many purposes, such as the study of nerve blocks or inhalation therapy. Advantages of this system are that the anesthesia chart and statistical record are one and the same, and sorting of information is simply performed by hand. Disadvantages include the limitation in the number of variables available for analysis, the initial higher cost of the card, and the increased time and complexity involved in sorting large numbers of records. The limiting factor in the usefulness of any record, particularly the punch card type, is the reliability of the individual making the initial observations and, subsequently, the individual who punches the record.

In another system increasingly used, code numbers are substituted for items of interest on the anesthesia chart. Numbers may be printed directly on the chart for encirclement or printed on a second sheet. In either case code numbers are transferred to a final record card, a small oblong cardboard with vertical and horizontal spacings. This card, too, is punched, the perforations corresponding to code numbers of the variables studied. Initial punching and final sorting as well as duplication and checking for errors are accomplished by machine. Advantages of this system are the low cost of the record card, the large number of variables coded, and the accuracy, rapidity, and ease of recording and collecting information. On the other hand, a code book is required and extra personnel are needed to perform intermediate steps before the final record card is punched. In the long run this system proves to be more expensive, and the apparatus needed for sorting is not always readily available.

Data gathered from any system of record keeping can be used as input to a computer-based system and stored on permanent magnetic tape. Depending upon the computer program adopted, hospital reports can be prepared, billing done, or research and case follow-ups accomplished with the data automatically recovered and assembled by the computer.

We have presented this brief discussion of statistical systems because we believe this to be an important aspect of anesthesia. Obviously an anesthesia department will have to assess the advantages and disadvantages of the several anesthesia charts available before adopting one for use. Whatever the statistical system selected, the user should remember the dictum that the record is only as good as the individual who keeps it. Nevertheless, little progress can be made toward safer administration of anesthetics unless clinical practice is under continuous unbiased scrutiny. Record keeping and statistical systems discussed in this chapter represent a step in this direction.

DEATH REPORTS

The conscientious anesthetist will analyze carefully the circumstances surrounding the death of every patient who has received an anesthetic. After discussion among supervising staff, a decision is reached as to whether a written summary of the events should be prepared. If anesthesia management viewed in its broadest aspects appears not to have contributed to the death, a report is not written. In the United States the joint committee on residency training programs insists on an analysis of every surgical death occurring within 24 hours of anesthetic administration. If anesthesia is judged to be an obvious contributing factor, detailed analysis is indicated.

In some instances a cause and effect relation between anesthesia and death is less certain, but suggestive. Examples follow:

1. A patient, having retched violently in the postoperative period, ruptures an abdominal incision and dies as a result of this complication.
2. Severe hypotension occurs during operation, and a cerebral or coronary vascular accident is responsible for death 24 to 36 hours later.
3. Hepatic failure follows a prolonged period of hypotension during or after operation.
4. Delayed death from pneumonia or lung abscess results from aspiration of gastrointestinal contents during or following anesthesia.

These cases deserve as careful an analysis as those in which death can be attributed directly to the anesthetic. Careful preparation of a report is of considerable educational value to the individual who administered the anesthetic. Discussion of reports at departmental conferences or by anesthesia study commissions is also enlightening. In the aggregate, such information can be used to assess the many factors that contribute to a fatal outcome. We believe that preparation of death reports is an essential feature of the teaching and practice of anesthesia. An anesthetist or a department not resorting to analyses overlooks an opportunity for self-appraisal and improvement. The death report should include:

1. Name—last, first. Race, sex, age, physical status.
2. Date of admission.
3. Date of last anesthesia.
4. Date of death.
5. Hospital number.
6. Family and past history, including previous anesthesias.
7. Present illness, physical examination, and laboratory findings. Course in hospital prior to operation.
8. Surgical diagnosis and proposed operation.
9. Anesthesia—complete description including premedication, time given, effect, technique, course, complications, and recovery.
10. Operation—surgeon, surgical procedure, and surgical complications. Anesthetist's opinion of surgical contribution to death.
11. Recovery room record (see Chapter 31).
12. Postoperative course and treatment, including kind and amount of fluids, opioids, oxygen, and vasopressor drugs.
13. Death—date, time after operation, and description (if during anesthesia or operation, include under 10).
14. Discussion of probable causes of death.
15. Cause of death according to anesthetist who gave the anesthetic.
16. Cause of death according to supervising anesthetist and departmental staff.
17. Moral to be drawn.
18. Additional notes, with references.
19. Autopsy findings, autopsy number.
20. Cause of death according to pathologist.
21. Final decision on causes of death (anesthesia, condition of patient, operation, etc.).

Items 9 through 13 should be written within 24 hours of death and discussed with the supervising anesthetist as soon as possible.

APPRAISAL

To a beginning resident, an intern, or a student, record keeping may seem a mundane aspect of anesthesia. However, its importance is stressed by far too few. Problems that have arisen as a result of inadequate record keeping include:

1. A patient fails to recover as expected from anesthesia. Was there anything that happened during the operation to provide a clue as to when and how the problem occurred?

2. The elapsed time between induction of anesthesia and beginning of operation is long. Are there data available to prove that preparation time was too slow?

3. A medicolegal suit against an anesthesiologist ends up in a court of law. The court asks the defendant for the written proof on which the defense is based.

4. An anesthetist claims that his or her patients experience postlumbar puncture headache in only one of 100 cases. Where is the documentation for this statement?

Accurate record keeping is a discipline; if taught and mastered early it is likely to be followed throughout one's professional life. If not, it may never be practiced until a case discussion before peers requires proof of a statement that is not available; or a court of law seeks documentation that the defendant cannot produce; or a research project fails because of lack of acceptable data.

Learn from those who have experienced or witnessed all examples given. Accurate record keeping is necessary!

REFERENCES

Beecher HK: The first anesthesia records. Surg Gynecol Obstet 71:689, 1940.
Borje H: Computerized anesthestic record keeping. Acta Anaesthesiol Scand (Suppl) 52, 1973.
Committee on Clinical Anesthesia Study, American Society of Anesthesiologists, Inc.: A comprehensive simple anesthesia record. Anesthesiology, 21:557, 1960.
Lindberg DAB: The Computer and Medical Care. Springfield, Ill., Charles C Thomas, 1968.
Moore DC, Bridenbaugh LD, Bagdi, PA, et al: Tabulation of anesthetic data: An improved system. Anesthesiology 29:595, 1968.

Section 3

ANESTHESIA AND OPERATION

Part A

INHALATION ANESTHESIA

Chapter 10

FUNDAMENTALS OF INHALATION ANESTHESIA

In order to produce a desired pharmacologic effect with any class of drugs, an adequate dose of a compound of sufficient potency must be administered and delivered to the effective site of action. Usually, the oral or parental route of administration is utilized in therapy. However, the inhalation anesthetics are unique in that the respiratory tract is utilized as a means of entry to the body. The special characteristics of this mode of administration are considered in the section on Uptake and Distribution. Factors altering dose requirements are considered under Minimal Anesthetic Concentration.

UPTAKE AND DISTRIBUTION OF INHALATION ANESTHETICS

Although the precise mode of action of anesthetics is not completely understood, it is clearly recognized that the primary site of action is the brain. The aim in clinical anesthesia is to achieve an adequate partial pressure of anesthetic in the brain so that it may exert the desired effect. The effect varies according to the concentration developed in the brain (Fig.

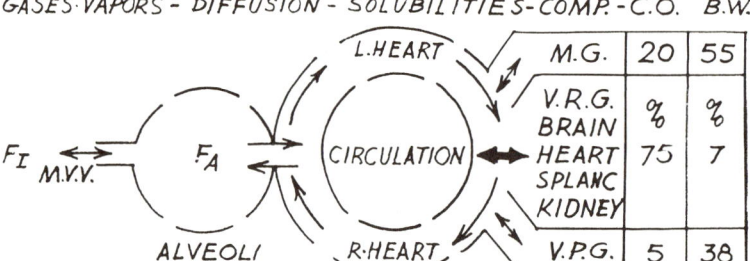

Figure 10-1. Schematic diagram of uptake and distribution of inhalation anesthetics. The inspired concentration, F_I or fraction inspired, of anesthetic is under direct control of the anesthetist. F_I is delivered to the alveoli by the minute volume of ventilation ($M.V.V.$). The alveolar concentration, F_A or fraction in alveoli, regulates tension (partial pressure) of anesthetic agent in arterial blood. The four tissue groups or compartments ($COMP.$), the vessel rich group ($V.R.G.$), the muscle group ($M.G.$), and the vessel poor group ($V.P.G.$) tend toward equilibration with anesthetic tension in arterial blood but reach that equilibrium at rates determined by the volume of blood flow to each tissue. The brain is the site of action. $C.O.$ = cardiac output and $B.W.$ = body weight, both expressed in per cent. $SPLANC$ = splanchnic circulation.

10-1). Concentration in tissues is the product of the solubility and partial pressure of the anesthetic in that tissue. The solubility of an anesthetic is for all practical purposes considered a constant, but the partial pressure is changeable, therefore controlling the concentration of anesthetic present. The partial pressure of anesthetic in the brain is indirectly controlled through the composition of the inhaled gas mixture.

The concentration of a gas in a mixture is proportional to its partial pressure. The terms partial pressure (torr) and concentration (vol per cent) are used interchangeably to describe the dosage of inhaled anesthetics:

$$\frac{PP_A}{\text{Total P}} = \text{concentration, vol per cent}$$

Where PP_A = partial pressure of anesthetic, and P = pressure

The term "tension" is used synonymously with partial pressure, and is applicable both to gas mixtures and to body tissues.

By controlling the composition of the inspired gas mixture, a pressure gradient is created between the inspired atmosphere and the blood circulating to the brain so that the anesthetic flows into or out of the brain, with the respiratory and circulatory systems as conduits. During induction of anesthesia, a chosen concentration of anesthetic is introduced via the inspired mixture. As the anesthetic reaches the alveoli a gradually decreasing pressure gradient is created between the inspired mixture and alveolar gas, then to the arterial blood and the brain. During recovery, as the anesthetic is allowed to escape to the atmosphere a reversal of the pressure

Fundamentals of Inhalation Anesthesia

gradient occurs, and the anesthetic moves down the gradient from brain, to blood, to alveolar gas, and finally to the external atmosphere. During the period between induction and recovery, the partial pressure of anesthetic in the brain is controlled indirectly by discrete manipulations of the inspired concentration.

The brain and other body tissues tend to equilibrate with the partial pressure of anesthetic drug delivered to them by arterial blood; the blood, in turn, tends to equilibrate with the alveolar partial pressure of anesthetic. The alveolar tension of anesthetic is paramount because it determines the tension of anesthetic in blood perfusing the brain and other body tissues. Factors that indirectly affect the alveolar partial pressure regulate the concentration of anesthetic in blood, brain, and other tissues. These factors must be clearly understood (Fig. 10–1).

FACTORS AFFECTING ALVEOLAR TENSION

The partial pressure of anesthetic in alveolar gas represents the algebraic sum of factors that deliver and remove anesthetic from the alveoli. Increasing the inspired concentration and augmentation of minute volume of ventilation increase delivery of total mass of anesthetic and cause alveolar partial pressure to rise (Table 10–1). Conversely, decreased inspired tension or decreased minute volume of ventilation reduces alveolar tension. A high pressure gradient between venous blood and alveolar gas enhances removal of anesthetic and ultimately reduces alveolar tension. Similarly, an increase in cardiac output or increase in the solubility of an anesthetic tends to increase removal from alveolar gas and to reduce the partial pressure of anesthetic in the alveolus. Alternatively, reducing any of these variables reduces uptake and tends to cause a rise in alveolar partial pressure of anesthetic (Table 10–1).

The effects on alveolar anesthetic tension of alterations in inspired tension, ventilation, and cardiac output are obvious and need no further explanation. The mixed alveolar-venous tension gradient of anesthetic relates to removal of the anesthetic from the circulating blood by tissues, or to addition of anesthetic to the blood from the tissues during recovery. Over a given period uptake of anesthetic from the lung must equal the sum of up-

Table 10–1. FACTORS PROMOTING INCREASE IN ALVEOLAR ANESTHETIC TENSION

Increased Delivery
    Increased inspired tension of anesthetic
    Increased minute volume of ventilation

Decreased Removal
    Decreased cardiac output
    Decreased alveolar–venous anesthetic gradient
    Decreased solubility of anesthetic

take by the various body tissues (Fig. 10-1). An agent of high solubility is taken up rapidly from the lungs and the rise of anesthetic tension is slowed both in alveolar gas and in blood. This in turn limits the rise in partial pressure in the brain and results in a slow rate of induction. Conversely, with an anesthetic of low solubility not so much is removed from the lungs. Alveolar tension of anesthetic therefore rises quickly and alveolar gas, blood, and brain equilibrate rapidly, facilitating the onset of anesthesia.

The solubility of anesthetics is expressed in terms of blood:gas or tissue:blood partition coefficients. Anesthetic gases and vapors equilibrate between two phases, according to pressure gradients. At equilibrium the partial pressure of anesthetics is the same in both phases. An agent with a blood:gas partition coefficient of 2 will reach twice the concentration (in vol per cent) in the blood phase as in the gas phase at equilibrium, but the partial pressure will be the same in both phases. Similarly, an agent with a brain:blood partition coefficient of 2 will reach twice the concentration of anesthetic in the brain as in the blood at equilibrium, but the partial pressure in brain and blood will be equal. Table 10-2 lists the currently employed anesthetics in decreasing order of blood solubility and hence according to increasing rapidity of induction of anesthesia. Also shown are tissue solubilities of these agents. Tissue solubility regulates tissue uptake of anesthetic, thus governing depletion of anesthetic from capillary blood. As a result the partial pressure of anesthetic is thereby lowered, influencing the alveolar-venous concentration gradient, and in turn affecting alveolar tension.

THE RELATIONSHIP BETWEEN INSPIRED AND ALVEOLAR TENSION

At a constant inspired tension of anesthetic, alveolar tension tends to approach that inspired until total body equilibrium is reached. At equilibrium, the inspired alveolar, blood, and tissue tensions are equal and no

Table 10-2. PARTITION COEFFICIENTS OF ANESTHETICS AT BODY TEMPERATURE $37 \pm 0.5°C$* (OSTWALD)

| Anesthetic | Blood/Gas | Tissue/Blood | | | Oil/Gas |
		Brain/Blood	Muscle/Blood	Fat/Blood	
Methoxyflurane	13.0	2.0	1.8	63	970
Ether	12.1	1.1	0.9	5	65
Trichloroethylene	9.15				960
Halothane	2.3	2.6	2.5	60	224
Enflurane	1.8	2.6	1.7	105	98
Isoflurane	1.4	3.7	4.0	45	98
Nitrous oxide	0.47	1.1	1.2	3	1.4
Cyclopropane	0.46	1.3	1.2	21	11.8

*Average values gathered from the literature.

Fundamentals of Inhalation Anesthesia

exchange of anesthetic occurs across the alveolar-capillary membrane. With most anesthetics, this state is rarely reached. The curves describing the rate at which alveolar tension approaches equilibrium have a uniform shape, each divided into three portions: an initial steeply rising slope, a midportion starting where the knee of the curve occurs, and a final, relatively flat slope slowly rising toward an ultimate equilibrium. The steep rise represents initial uptake of anesthetic from the alveoli; the midportion represents approaching equilibration of the rapidly perfused vessel-rich group of tissues—brain, heart, kidneys, liver, and the final portion represents the slower equilibration of the remaining more poorly perfused tissues (Figure 10-2). These curves lie in inverse order to the solubility of the anesthetic, that is, the least soluble approaches equilibrium fastest. These curves also faithfully represent the manner in which anesthetic in arterial blood approaches an ultimate steady state, since arterial blood is in equilibrium with the alveolar tension upon each perfusion of the lung. Also these curves depict the partial pressures at which the brain approaches equilibration.

To summarize, during administration of an inhalation anesthetic, alveolar tension at first rapidly rises toward that of inspired gas, then more slowly. Arterial tension follows the alveolar tension as pulmonary blood equilibrates with alveolar gas. Then tissue tensions rise, approaching the arterial level. The vessel-rich group of tissues, including the brain, equilibrates most rapidly while the remaining body tissues equilibrate more slowly. As a rule the administration of anesthesia is completed before al-

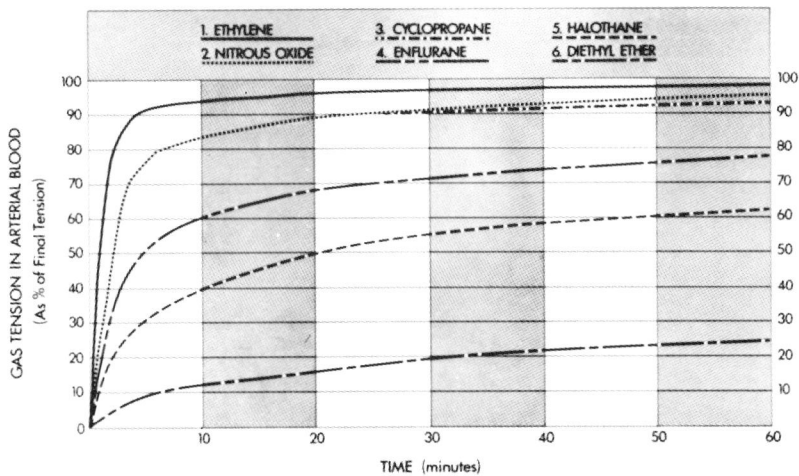

Figure 10-2. The rate of rise of tension of anesthetic in arterial blood with different agents administered at a constant inspired tension.

veolar gas tension has reached the inspired tension. When the anesthetic is removed from inspired gas diffusion from the alveoli occurs, subsequently reflected in the blood and tissues. The same physical and biologic factors regulating uptake also affect the rate of elimination of anesthetics.

PHYSICAL CONSEQUENCES OF ANESTHETIC UPTAKE

Normally gas is moved in and out of the lungs solely by the mechanical activity of ventilation. This, however, is not quite true during induction and recovery from anesthesia. During induction, uptake by the blood of anesthetic from an inhaled gas mixture tends to reduce the volume of gas in the alveoli. This causes a mass movement of inspired gas mixture into the alveoli from the tracheobronchial tree and into the tracheobronchial tree from the inspired source, in effect augmenting the volume of gas inspired. During recovery, anesthetic moves from blood to alveoli, increasing the volume of alveolar gas and inducing a mass movement of gas out of alveoli into tracheobronchial tree and out of the respiratory system. This augments the volume of gas exhaled. The consequences of these effects are of practical importance during administration of those anesthetics (nitrous oxide, ether, cyclopropane, and fluroxene) that are taken up in significant volume when inhaled at high concentrations even though some are poorly soluble. The more potent agents (methoxyflurane, halothane, enflurane, and isoflurane) are administered in such low concentrations that the volume uptake is limited even though some are highly soluble.

The *concentration effect* is caused by two factors: the ventilatory augmentation action and the concentrating action, which operate when anesthetics are taken in significant volume during induction. The higher the concentration of anesthetic administered the greater the uptake and the greater the augmentation of inspired volume. Increased volume of ventilation promotes an increase in alveolar partial pressure (Table 10–1) and tends to offset the fall in partial pressure induced by pulmonary capillary uptake; thus a more rapid induction of anesthesia results. A concentrating action also contributes to the concentration effect. Removal of half the nitrous oxide from a lung filled with 50 per cent concentration (50 parts in 100 parts total) produces 33 1/3 per cent nitrous oxide (25 parts in 75 parts total) instead of halving the concentration to 25 per cent. At lower concentrations such as 1 per cent (1 part in 100 parts total), the removal of half the anesthetic reduces the concentration by nearly half (0.5 parts in 99.5 parts total). Higher inspired partial pressures tend to concentrate the anesthetic and blunt the effect of uptake. The concentration effect implies that the higher the inspired concentration, the more rapid is the rise in alveolar partial pressure and the induction of anesthesia.

The *second gas effect* occurs when two anesthetics are administered concurrently; this results from the same two factors that produce the concentration effect—ventilatory augmentation and a concentrating action owing to anesthetic uptake. Uptake of a large volume of a "first gas," usually nitrous oxide, in a gas mixture, augments inspired volume and increases alveolar delivery of the "second gas" in the mixture, more than would be expected in the absence of the first gas. Moreover, uptake of the first gas tends to increase the alveolar concentration of the second gas by a concentrating phenomenon similar to that described previously for nitrous oxide. The result is a more rapid rise in alveolar partial pressure of the second gas in the presence of, rather than in the absence of, the first gas, and thus a more rapid induction of anesthesia.

Augmentation of exhaled volume may occur as anesthetic gases are eliminated. Diffusion hypoxia may occur owing to rapid diffusion of nitrous oxide from pulmonary capillary blood into alveolar gas at the termination of a nitrous oxide anesthetic. The resulting reduction in partial pressure of both oxygen and carbon dioxide can be prevented and the patient protected from hypoxemia by administration of an enriched oxygen atmosphere for the first two or three minutes following termination of nitrous oxide anesthesia.

THE MINIMUM ALVEOLAR CONCENTRATION – A MEASURE OF POTENCY

The relationship between the administered dose and the quantitative effect produced is an expression of drug potency. By itself, potency is a relatively unimportant property of an anesthetic, as the sole limitation placed on the inhaled partial pressure is the need for an adequate oxygen content in the inhaled gas mixture. Only in the case of nitrous oxide is potency a meaningful limitation. The ability to assess potency, however, is important in evaluating factors that alter patient response to anesthetics and in the study of mechanisms of anesthesia.

The pharmacologic concept of the median effective dose has been adapted by Eger to fill this need. He has defined *minimum alveolar concentration* (MAC) as the anesthetic concentration at 1 atm which produces im-

Table 10–3. MEASURES OF ANESTHETIC POTENCY (VOL PER CENT)

Agent	MAC	Induction Concentration	Maintenance Concentration
Methoxyflurane	0.16	Up to 3	0.2–1.0
Halothane	0.76	2–4	0.5–2.0
Isoflurane	1.12	2–4	1.0–3.0
Enflurane	1.68	2–5	1.5–3.0
Ether	1.92	10–30	4–15
Cyclopropane	9.2	20–50	10–20
Nitrous oxide	105.0	Up to 80	Up to 80

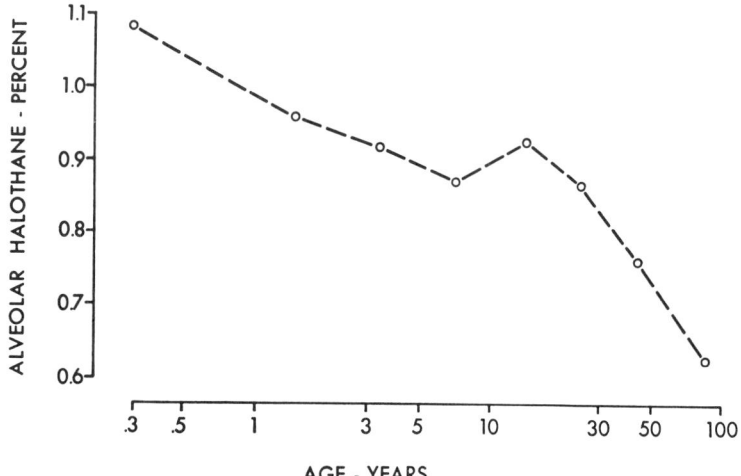

Figure 10-3. Halothane MAC (vertical axis) constantly decreases with age, with the possible exception of a slight increase at puberty. (From Gregory GA, Eger EI II, Munson ES: Anesthesiology 30:488, 1969.)

mobility in 50 per cent of subjects exposed to a noxious stimulus (Table 10-3). The concept has been criticized because it measures only a single point—abolition of a muscular response—on a continuum of responses that represents a graded dose response curve to anesthetics. The concept neglects consideration of the importance of slope of the response curve.

Analysis of a second point in the anesthetic dose response curve, the point at which response to verbal command returns ("MAC AWAKE"), permits the inference that the curves for methoxyflurane, halothane, ether, and fluroxene are parallel, since the ratios of MAC AWAKE to MAC are constant. Moreover, the MAC concept is applicable to all inhalation anesthetics and no satisfactory alternate method is available. Thus MAC has been used extensively to evaluate factors that influence anesthetic requirements.

The variability of MAC in a single species is small and the correlation of MAC values for measurements in man and in all other species studied shows a remarkable consistency. Based on measurements of MAC, it appears that patient susceptibility to anesthetics is not altered significantly by gender, duration of anesthesia, thyroid function, variations in Pa_{CO_2} between 10 and 90 torr, metabolic alkalosis or acidosis, variations in Pa_{O_2} between 40 and 500 torr, or moderate anemia or hypertension. A slight circadian variation has been demonstrated in the rat.

Increased susceptibility to anesthetic depression occurs with marked hypercarbia, severe anemia or hypoxemia, increasing age (Fig. 10-3), decreasing body temperature (Table 10-4), depletion of brain catecholamines, and exposure to other central nervous system depressants.

Measurement of MAC has allowed quantitative evaluation of patient

Table 10-4. EFFECT OF LOWERING BODY TEMPERATURE ON MAC

Agent	Number of Dogs	MAC at $37°C$	Change in $MAC/10°C$*	Decrease in $MAC/10°C(\%)$
Cyclopropane	6	15.9 ± 3.6	3.0 ± 1.5	20 ± 9
Diethyl ether	5	3.3 ± 0.7	1.2 ± 0.5	38 ± 11
Fluroxene	8	6.6 ± 0.8	2.8 ± 1.2	42 ± 15
Methoxyflurane	7	0.24 ± 0.03	0.13 ± 0.03	52 ± 11
Halothane	6	0.87 ± 0.11	0.44 ± 0.88	53 ± 8

*The change in MAC/10°C indicates the decrease in absolute per cent gas concentration required to prevent movement in response to tail clamp per 10°C lowering of body temperature from 37°C. Values are the average ± one standard deviation. (From Regan MJ and Eger EI II: Anesthesiology 28:689, 1967.)

responses to combinations of cerebral depressants. Opioid premedication reduces MAC in a dose-related manner. Each increase in dose is accompanied by a proportional decrease in the amount of inhalation anesthetic required to reach the desired level of anesthesia. Diazepam also reduces anesthetic requirements. The additive effect of mixtures of inhaled anesthetics has also been documented. Antagonism of anesthetics by central stimulants, such as amphetamine, has likewise been verified. Thus an awareness has developed among anesthesiologists of the quantitative nature of anesthetic potency and of the factors that may alter it.

Anesthetists have long recognized the resistance of the infant and the relative susceptibility of the elderly to anesthetic depression. A progressive decrease in anesthetic requirement from infancy to old age, except for a slight increase at puberty, has now been documented. The clinical impression that hypothermia reduces anesthetic requirements has also been verified and the variability in the interaction of hypothermia with different anesthetics has been documented (Table 10-4).

MECHANISM OF ACTION OF ANESTHETICS

The manner in which chemical compounds interact with living structures to produce the anesthetic state has intrigued scientists and clinicians ever since the phenomenon of anesthesia was first observed over 130 years ago.

Any theory of anesthetic action must be able to explain a perplexing series of facts relating to narcosis:

1. An extensive array of unrelated chemical structures produces general anesthesia. They seem to share no common structure-activity relationship.
2. During narcosis, alterations of function occur in virtually all systems of the body. Physiologic, metabolic, and structural changes have been described and must be explained.

3. Lipid solubility of anesthetics seems to be of importance, since the wide range of effective concentrations is reduced to a very small range when solubility in body lipids is calculated.
4. The phenomenon of pressure reversal of general anesthesia occurs and must be explained by any mechanistic theory.

Heretofore attempts at an explanation of narcosis based on chemical, physical, physiochemical, neurophysiologic, biochemical, and neurochemical interactions have all been wanting. Over the last decade, however, there has been a revival of interest in and an application of newer techniques to this still unsolved problem. Approaches that hold promise focus on physiochemical interactions of anesthetics with biologic membranes and on the resultant alterations in membrane function.

The interested reader is referred to any standard textbook of pharmacology for an extensive discussion of theories of historical interest. These were proposed by some of the outstanding biologic scientists of the last century. The following discussion focuses primarily on molecular interactions of current interest, although reference to older approaches is made when applicable.

PHYSICOCHEMICAL MECHANISMS

The basic principle postulated by Meyer and Overton (1899–1901) that lipid solubility of anesthetics controls anesthetic action remains viable. Specifically, the narcotic action of a drug has been shown to correlate strongly with its solubility in biologic membranes. Interactions of anesthetics with biologic membranes have been shown to cause expansion of the membrane. Membrane expansion by a critical volume of 0.4 per cent results in anesthesia, and both expansion and anesthesia are reversed by hyperbaric pressure (40 to 100 atm). Membrane expansion in protein-containing biologic membranes is ten times greater than predicted solely on the basis of the amount of anesthetic present in the lipid phase, and the expansion of the pure lipid membranes of liposomes is of the predicted order of magnitude. This suggests an interaction between anesthetic molecules and membrane protein. Evidence is available to show that anesthetics selectively combine with hydrophobic groups in biologic protein, whether purified or membrane associated. Perhaps these alterations in membrane structure affect synaptic transmission in the brain to give rise to the clinical phenomenon of anesthesia.

Eyring has postulated that anesthetics induce changes in the tertiary structure of membrane protein which could alter cation flux through membrane pores, thereby depressing membrane excitability. Long before this, Lillie, in 1909, demonstrated anesthetic-induced alterations in membrane permeability, but there is no reason to postulate that anesthetics selectively alter only plasma membranes. The membranes in mitochondrial and endoplasmic reticulum cannot be disregarded as sites of anesthetic action. Functions of mitochondria in regulating intracellular calcium levels

NEUROPHYSIOLOGIC AND BIOCHEMICAL MECHANISMS

The classic experiments of Larrabee and Posternak suggested assignment of the primary site of anesthetic action to the synapse. C. P. Richards has demonstrated synaptic inhibition by all anesthetics studied (halothane, ether, methoxyflurane, enflurane, trichloroethylene, and chloroform), but it is not clear whether this action is pre- or postsynaptic. If acting presynaptically, a decreased release of the excitatory neurotransmitter, acetylcholine, or increased release of the inhibitory neurotransmitter, α-aminobutyric acid, could be responsible. Both events occur upon experimental exposure to anesthetics. If the anesthetic is acting postsynaptically, reduced sensitivity to acetylcholine or hyperpolarization of the postsynaptic membrane could occur; both phenomena have been observed. Therefore, depressed excitation or increased inhibition in cerebral synaptic areas must be considered separate viable mechanisms for anesthetic action.

Inhibition of synaptic transmission could result from all other kinds of cerebral metabolic actions of the anesthetics. The anesthetized brain is rich in energy, and older theories of anesthetic action based on reduced cellular respiration or deficiencies in energy stores are inconsistent with current observations. Anesthetic inhibition of metabolism of mitochondrial energy has been demonstrated but lacks linkage to a causative mechanism of narcosis. The concomitant depression of calcium uptake by brain mitochondria implies elevations of intracellular Ca^{++} which should reduce release of transmitter and stabilize postsynaptic membranes. Both actions depress synaptic transmission and lead to depression of central nervous system function.

The several mechanisms discussed here are not necessarily exclusive of one another. It is possible that the basic underlying event in anesthetic action is an alteration of membranous structure within the cell by anesthetic molecules. Subsequent events may involve metabolic or neurophysiologic alterations which depress synaptic transmission, thus resulting in anesthesia. All other alterations associated with anesthesia could then take place. Alternatively, a unitary theory of anesthetic action may not explain the actions of all drugs that give rise to anesthesia. In fact, there may be several ways in which the anesthetic state is induced.

PRACTICAL POINTS
INDUCTION

Induction of anesthesia is accomplished either by intravenous administration of an ultra short-acting barbiturate or other intravenous agents, or by inhalation of an appropriate mixture of anesthetic and oxygen. The anesthetic potency of the gas mixture initially administered nearly always exceeds that needed for maintenance, frequently approaching 5 MAC (see Table 10–3). This is called overpressure, a stratagem used to overcome the delays in induction imposed by anesthetic solubility in blood and the need successively to equilibrate alveolar gas and circulatory blood in order to deliver anesthetic to brain. If this is not done, induction may be relatively prolonged and sometimes dangerous if excitement occurs. When the expedient of overpressure is adopted, induction is relatively rapid.

As the mask is applied and unconsciousness is approached encouragement and gentle suggestion should lull the patient into a state of security. It is better not to concentrate attention upon physiologic processes such as breathing, but to explain quietly what is happening and to suggest a tranquil induction and safe emergence from anesthesia. This kind of hypnotic suggestion adds considerably to the ease and smoothness of induction.

AIRWAY AND RESPIRATORY PROBLEMS

The most troublesome problems in inhalation anesthesia involve the airways and adequacy of respiration. In probable order of development, these may be encountered as follows:

Mask Fit

If a mask is poorly fitted to the patient's face, the effective concentration of anesthetic is diluted by admixture with room air. A good mask fit is not easily achieved in the edentulous patient, in the patient with a prominent nose or receding jaw, or in the patient who needs gastrointestinal drainage tubes. A poorly fitted mask creates difficulty in applying positive pressure ventilation to the lungs. On the other hand, excessive pressure by the mask may injure the trigeminal or facial nerve, eyes, or skin.

Depressed Respiration

If during induction respiration is depressed by premedicants or inhalation agents, the alveolar concentration of anesthetic may not readily approach that needed to provide anesthesia. Overdosage with premedication, especially with the opioids, is a common cause. Depression of respiration may not be evident until the first few breaths of anesthetic are taken. Large doses of intravenous barbiturates used for induction, or the too early administration of a neuromuscular blocker, both of which reduce alveolar ventilation, also delay induction. Whenever respiration is depressed, assisted or controlled breathing is necessary not only to facilitate induction of anesthesia but to prevent hypoxia and hypercarbia.

Abnormal Respiratory Patterns and Pulmonary Disease

Rapid shallow breathing or tachypnea may not provide the alveolar ventilation required for uptake of anesthetic. Tachypnea is common during induction, not the result of stimulation of the Hering-Breuer receptors as once thought, but probably resulting from a central effect of the anesthetic. Abnormalities of the lung characterized by poor mixing of gases and unequal distribution, or slow diffusion of gases across the pulmonary membrane, also interfere with attainment of anesthesia. Certain kinds of heart disease with associated diminution in respiratory function also exert the same effect.

Respiratory Obstruction

Almost as soon as a patient loses consciousness in the supine position, the lower jaw relaxes and recedes; or during the excitement of the second stage, the jaws may be clenched tight. In either case the tongue may cause obstruction as it is sucked against the hard palate during inspiration or when it falls back into the pharynx; this is indicated by stertorous sounds. Such obstruction may be sensed by the hand holding the mask or detected by listening over the breathing tubes. Respiratory obstruction is best discovered, however, by observing the rise and fall of the chest rather than movement of the reservoir bag. In the presence of obstruction, the chest retracts as the diaphragm descends instead of expanding as it should; this gives rise to a characteristic rocking motion indicating that descent of the diaphragm is not followed by free inflow of air. Although movement of the reservoir bag does not indicate adequacy of pulmonary ventilation, failure of the bag to move with respiration implies that the anesthetic is not being breathed.

Respiratory obstruction must be corrected as soon as practicable. When obstruction is diagnosed the jaw should be lifted upward, moving the tongue with it. Extension of the cervical spine or turning the head to the side may help. The most effective means of lifting the jaw is to place the fingers behind the vertical ramus of the mandible (Fig. 10-4). This maneuver is one of the most difficult to teach the beginner; when applied it should be maintained for as short a time as possible, as soreness and swelling may result. A pharyngeal airway should be inserted as soon as possible.

It is possible beforehand to single out the person who may develop soft tissue obstruction when unconscious, usually the individual who has a short thick neck or is obese. Some workers apply topical anesthesia to the mucous membranes of the nose and pharynx to facilitate early placement of an airway. There are two kinds of airway, oropharyngeal and nasopharyngeal (Fig. 10-5). Their purpose is to displace the tongue anteriorly; the patient then breathes through or around the airway. The oral airway is more efficient, but if obstruction takes place before the jaw relaxes it may be impossible to open the mouth. In this situation, a soft, well-lubricated

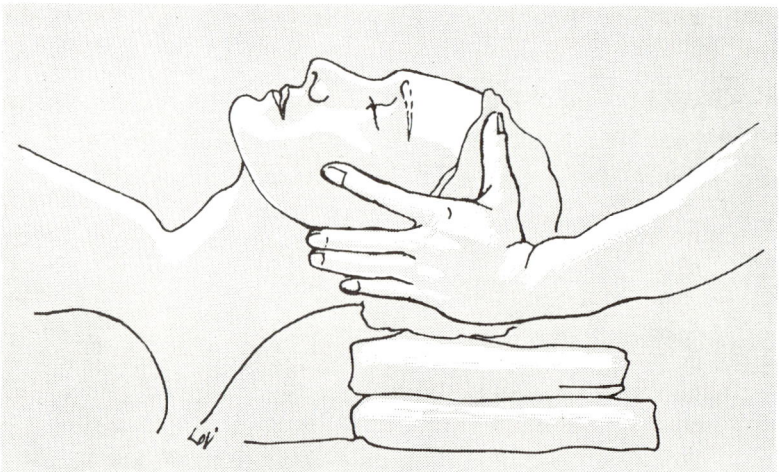

Figure 10-4. Technique of lifting jaw with fingers behind the mandible to overcome respiratory soft tissue obstruction.

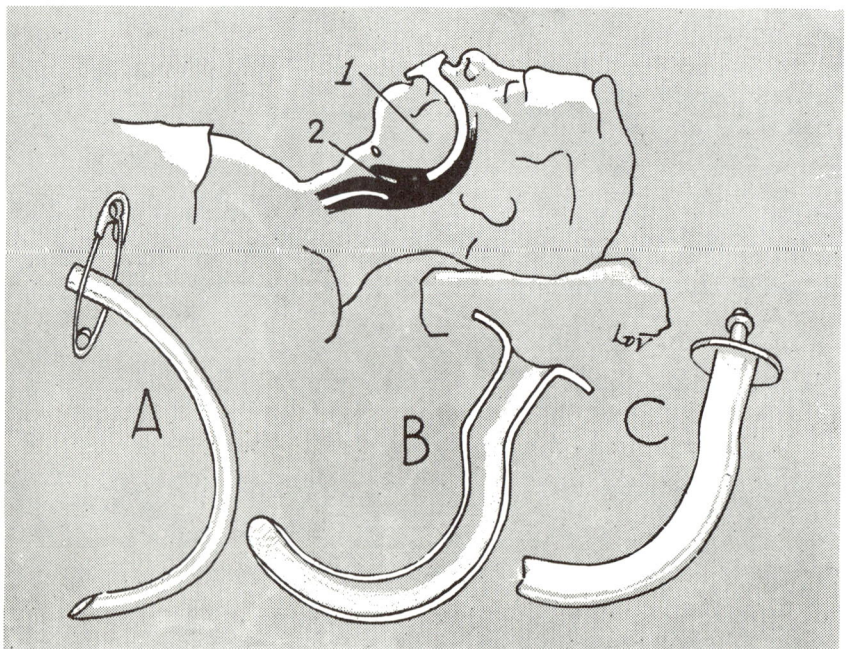

Figure 10-5. Pharyngeal airways. Oropharyngeal airway displacing tongue (*1*) forward and upward from the pharynx (*2*). *A*–Nasopharyngeal airway of soft rubber tubing. *B*–Plastic oropharyngeal airway. *C*–Hard rubber oropharyngeal airway with nipple for oxygen insufflation.

Fundamentals of Inhalation Anesthesia

nasopharyngeal tube should be passed; care must be taken to avoid injury to the highly vascular mucous membrane of the nose, as hemorrhage can be severe. Similarly, the oral airway should be placed carefully to avoid injury to lips and teeth, and is more easily inserted if lubricated. Placement of an airway must be done deftly; haste is essential so that the partial pressure of anesthetic in the lungs is not reduced while the face mask is removed. At the same time, the reservoir bag should not be allowed to empty because it will require refilling with oxygen, thereby offering a lower anesthetic concentration.

Cough and Laryngospasm

Cough sometimes follows placement of an airway, usually caused by pharyngeal irritation by a high concentration of anesthetic delivered after the airway is cleared. Irritation can be avoided by temporarily decreasing the concentration of anesthetic after airway insertion, then increasing it slowly. Cough is overcome by gradually deepening anesthesia and assisting the inspiratory phase following cough, by pressure on the reservoir bag.

Laryngospasm is a serious complication at any time but possibly of greatest consequence during induction of anesthesia. Laryngospasm occurs most frequently at light levels of anethesia when there is direct pharyngeal, laryngeal, or peripheral painful stimulation. All manner of laryngospasm may occur, from a minor degree indicated by a high-pitched crowing sound to complete, impassable closure of the glottis. Sustained moderate pressure on the reservoir bag helps to facilitate ventilation and overcome the spasm. An assistant should keep a finger on the pulse to detect signs of failing circulation when anoxia develops, often indicated by progressive slowing and loss of amplitude of the pulse. If laryngospasm is complete and lasts as long as a minute, an intravenous or intramuscular injection of a small dose of succinylcholine, 20 mg, will relax the striated muscles of the larynx.

The halogenated hydrocarbons are associated with less cough and laryngospasm than encountered with the older, more irritating anesthetics. Cough and laryngospasm are also more frequent in the heavy smoker or the patient with chronic bronchitis. The increased risk of laryngospasm in those with excessive secretions may be adequate justification for postponement of an elective operation.

Mucous and Salivary Secretions

Accumulation of secretions in the air passages can result in obstruction. Increase in secretions may be part of the initial neurologic stimulant phase of general anesthesia or the result of irritation from the anesthetic, further increased by hypoxia and retention of carbon dioxide during a difficult induction. The halogenated hydrocarbons pose fewer problems with secretions and pharyngeal irritability than the others; thus many clinicians now eliminate atropine in premedication when a halogenated anesthetic is administered. Diminution of parasympathetic activity with atropine or scopolamine eliminates the profuse, watery kind of secretion, leaving a sparse, viscid substance. If secretions are troublesome, the patient's head can be turned to the side and lowered in order to allow their escape through the side of the mouth. When the problem is more serious, suction of the pharynx should be performed, preferably in a deeper plane of anesthesia to avoid laryngospasm or vomiting.

Retching and Vomiting

Stimulation of the vomiting center frequently occurs during induction and emergence from anesthesia. Opioid premedicants, movement of the patient, persistent attempts at pharyngeal suction, and too early placement of an airway contribute to this complication. Postoperatively the incidence is higher in women, particularly during the third and fourth weeks of the menstrual cycle, in patients given cyclopropane or ether, after prolonged deep anesthesia, and following intra-abdominal operations.

Anesthetists should be on the alert for premonitory signs such as repetitive swallowing. The sequence of swallowing, retching, and vomiting can sometimes be interrupted if care is taken to avoid partial respiratory obstruction, which seems to precipitate the problem. Unfortunately, fluid and particulate matter may well up into the pharynx without warning, and silent aspiration during general anesthesia of at least some gastric material is more common than realized. So long as gastric contents are not carried into the respiratory tract, little harm is done. The head is lowered and turned to the side and vomitus wiped out or suctioned. This should be done in stages, with intermittent administration of oxygen. Once assured that aspiration has not occurred, induction should then proceed rapidly as the risk of vomiting is reduced at a deeper level of anesthesia. If regurgitation or vomiting occurs during recovery, the patient should be turned to the lateral position and closely observed until able to protect the airway. The treatment of aspiration of stomach contents is discussed in Chapter 28.

The aforementioned complications may be encountered in rapid succession during induction of anesthesia, in addition to prolonged excitement with vigorous muscle movement and breath-holding. Considerable experience is required to avoid these complications as well as to manage them.

MAINTENANCE

Induction of anesthesia should be followed by the start of operation without delay. Patients fully anesthetized by potent anesthetics in current use may become hypotensive when not stimulated surgically. Usually, the patient will show some mild response such as pupillary dilation, increase in heart rate, depth of respiration, or breath-holding as the incision is made. Slight movement, if it does not affect the surgical field, is not objectionable. If in doubt, it is better to reach a plane somewhat deeper than necessary before the incision is made. It is easier to lighten anesthesia than to deepen it once the complications of light anesthesia have appeared. Subsequently, the inspired concentration of anesthetics can be decreased.

Once a satisfactory level has been reached, the lightest level of anesthesia compatible with good operating conditions is maintained. The smaller the amount of drug administered the better, but too little anesthesia defeats the purpose, prolongs operation, and often leads to excessive administration later on. When muscle relaxation is required, such as during closure of the peritoneum, the need is anticipated and anesthesia deepened at the time.

An anesthetist can obtain valuable information by observing the surgical field throughout operation. The following observations are significant: (1) Adequacy of oxygenation, as indicated by the color of arterial blood in the wound, is a good means of detecting hypoxemia, especially in dark-skinned persons. (2) Comparison of the color of venous and arterial blood is of value in estimation of cardiovascular function. Dark venous blood suggests inadequate tissue perfusion; continuous ooze may signify a clotting defect or transfusion reaction; continued brisk arterial or venous bleeding suggests the need for transfusion. (3) A competent anesthetist should observe surgical manipulations, understand operative procedure, and be able to anticipate the surgeon's next step. Only then is one able adequately to prepare for sequential manipulations, essential because alterations in depth of anesthesia involve a certain time lag. Placement of surgical packs, traction on viscera, and rapid decompression of the abdomen may all lead to precipitous hypotension. (4) Degree of muscular relaxation should be watched carefully. More or less relaxation may be needed at different stages of the operation. The caliber and tone of the bowel and its extrusion from the peritoneal cavity are indicative of depth of anesthesia. Progressive loss of tone and dilation of bowel occur with deepening anesthesia; extrusion usually suggests inadequate muscle relaxation. A surgeon should not be expected to inform an anesthetist that better relaxation is needed; the anesthetist can anticipate the need by observation of the field or by sensing chest wall compliance during manual ventilatory control.

EMERGENCE

It is best to have a patient as nearly awake as possible at the termination of operation. When laryngeal and pharyngeal reflexes have been recovered, the patient is less likely to develop respiratory obstruction or to aspirate gastric contents. However, the need to have a patient awake should not lead to administration of so little anesthesia that restraint is necessary as the last sutures are placed, or fascial closure is disrupted; this too, is hazardous.

During emergence the complications described under induction of anesthesia may reappear. When it is considered safe to move the patient, transfer to bed or litter is done gently to avoid strain on ligaments and muscles in the relaxed individual. If still unconscious, the patient is placed in the lateral decubitus position to protect against airway obstruction and aspiration of vomitus. Before the anesthetist leaves the patient, vital signs should be obtained and all information relating to treatment transmitted to the recovery room nurse.

APPRAISAL

The theoretic and practical aspects of inhalation anesthesia have been treated in this chapter. Inhalation anesthesia is a controllable technique because the lungs act as the avenue of entrance and escape for the anesthetic. The patient's respiratory efforts or the anesthetist's artificial control of respiration influence the level of anesthesia from moment to moment. Premedication must be chosen with a view to disturbing respiration and circulation least. Respiratory obstruction owing to soft tissue, excessive secretions, or laryngospasm must be avoided and treated promptly if induction of anesthesia is to be rapid and safe. Abnormalities of pulmonary ventilation and diffusion must be detected, because they markedly influence the course of anesthesia. The role of the circulation and the body tissues as relates to the partial pressure of anesthetic in the brain must be kept clearly in mind. Physical properties of the gases relating to solubility and diffusion must be understood. In spite of all the knowledge required, we believe that inhalation is still the best technique to teach the beginner.

REFERENCES

Eger EI: Anesthetic Uptake and Action. Baltimore, Williams & Wilkins Co, 1974.
Eyring H: Untangling biological reactions. Science, 154:1609, 1966.
Goodman LS, Gilman A: The Pharmacological Basis of Therapeutics. 5th ed, New York, Macmillan Publishing Co, 1975.
Halsey MJ, Miller RA, Sutton JA (eds): Molecular Mechanisms in General Anaesthesia. Edinburgh, Churchill-Livingstone, 1974.
Miller KW, Paton WDM, Smith RA, et al: The pressure reversal of general anaesthesia and the initial volume hypothesis. Mol Pharmacol 9:131, 1973.
Seeman P: The membrane actions of anesthetics and tranquilizers. Pharmacol Rev 24:583, 1972.

Chapter 11

INHALATION ANESTHETICS

Most classifications of neurotropic drugs include only two groups: the central nervous system depressants and the stimulants. Anesthetics are classified as depressants in this one-dimensional scale of neurophysiologic function. The actual properties of neuropharmacologic agents are inadequately described by this simplistic approach. Some drugs, including most anesthetics, combine neurodepressant and neuroexcitatory effects; others, such as pentylenetetrazol (Metrazol), exert only stimulant effects; still others, such as pentobarbital, are primarily depressants. Winters has examined the behavioral and neurophysiologic correlates of neurotropic drug action and has postulated a two-dimensional continuum of central nervous system response to stimulants and depressants (Figure 11–1). It is likely that each of these responses involves a different membrane site in the central nervous system and that drug exposure may activate either the activating site, or the depressive site, or both. Some anesthetics, such as enflurane, have more prominent excitatory effects than others, for example, the barbiturates, but most activate both sites and result in an electroencephalogram (EEG) which progresses through successive stages toward a seizure pattern. Most anesthetics diverge from this pattern before seizure activity is manifest, while inducing a pattern of suppression and periods of electric silence.

THE ELECTROENCEPHALOGRAM

The effects of anesthetics on the EEG of humans were described more than 30 years ago. Since then much effort has been devoted to correlating EEG activity with blood concentrations of anesthetics, and attempts have been made to establish a characteristic progression of EEG tracings indicating sequential levels of anesthesia.

It has become evident, particularly through recent work of Clark and his colleagues, that the effects of anesthetics on the EEG differ widely. Cyclopropane stands at one end of a spectrum, causing progressive slowing

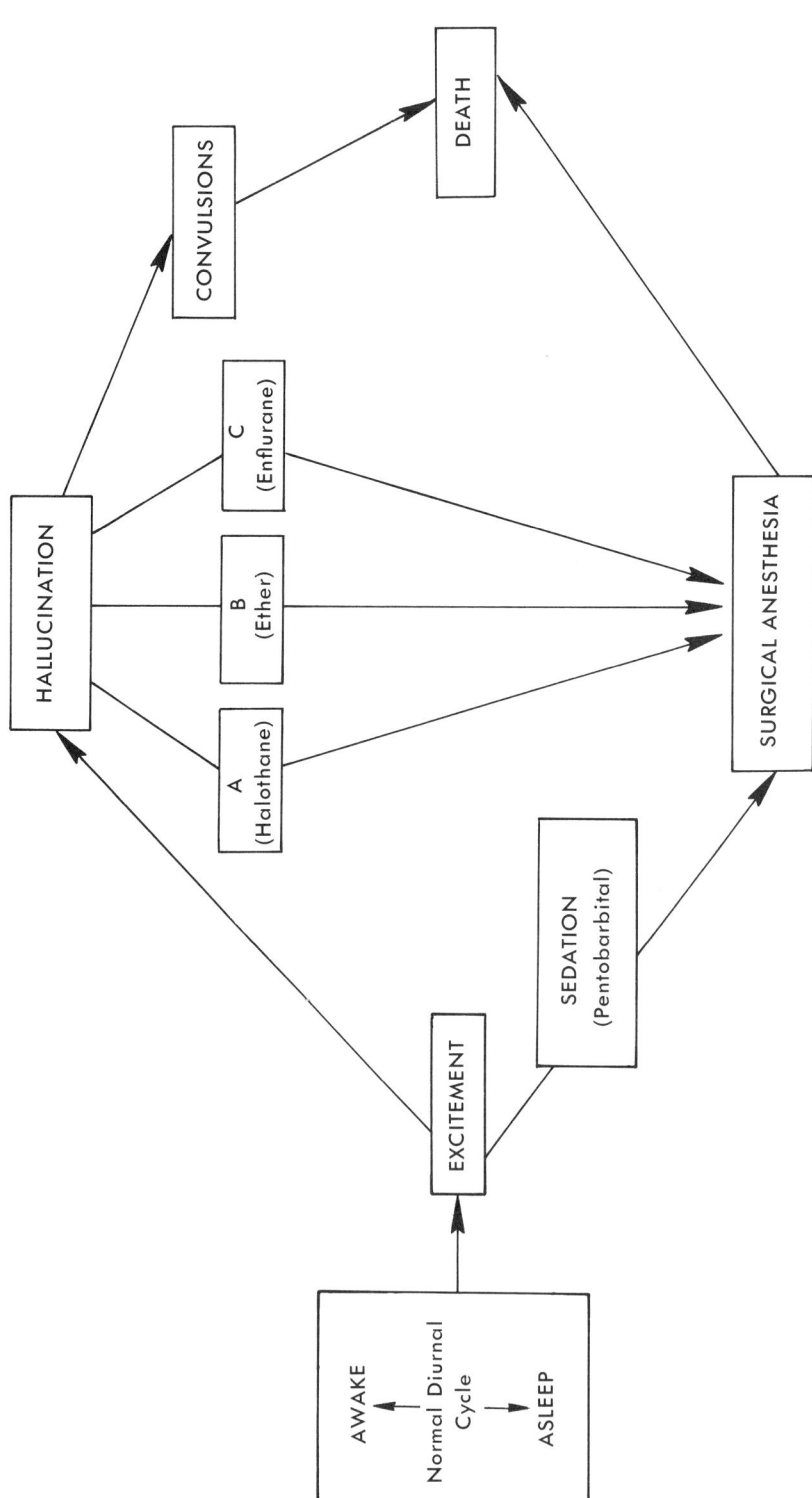

Figure 11-1. After Winters' scheme of drug-induced CNS excitation and depression as shown by gross behavior and EEG recordings. (Winters WD: Neurophysiological classification of psychoactive drugs. *In* Kales A (ed): Sleep: Physiology and Pathology. Philadelphia, JB Lippincott Co, 1969).

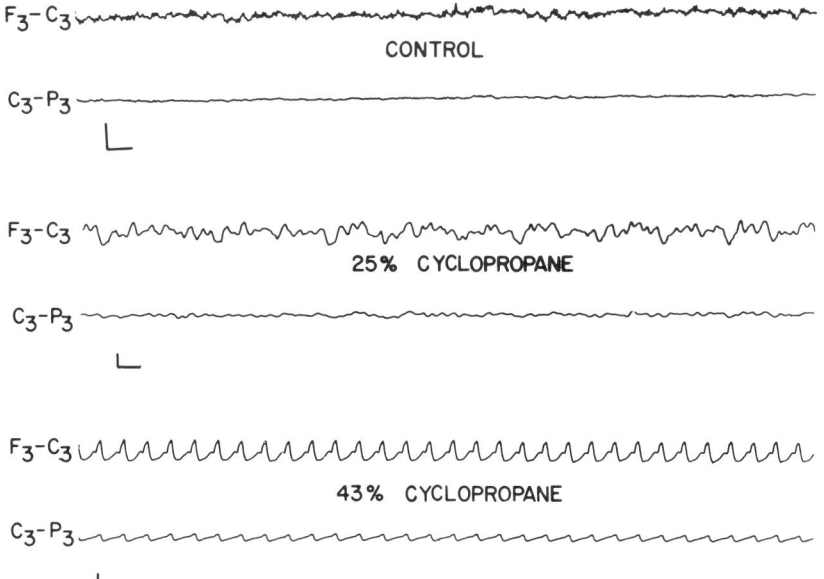

Figure 11-2. Effect of cyclopropane on EEG. Electrode placements designated in accordance with 1-20 system. F = frontal, C = central, P = parietal, 3 = on left. Calibration: 1 sec and 100 μv. See text for description. (Reproduced with permission from Clark DL, Rosner BS, Beck C: J Appl Physiol 28:802, 1970.)

with increasing depth of anesthesia until, at approximately 40 per cent inhaled concentration, a clocklike regularity is established at about 1 Hz (Figure 11-2). Enflurane lies at the opposite end of the scale, producing 14 to 18 Hz activity, then progressing to spike-dome complexes alternating with periods of electric silence, and ultimately resulting in frank seizure activity (Figure 11-3). Nitrous oxide and ether provide intermediate patterns (Figure 11-4).

A rigorous EEG comparison of agents at various levels of anesthesia is not possible because of differences in arterial pressure produced. Cyclopropane can be inhaled in concentrations five times greater than required for surgical anesthesia without causing hypotension, but methoxyflurane, halothane, and enflurane in much lesser amounts cause severe hypotension. Carbon dioxide accumulation alone can slow the EEG and when respiratory acidosis develops during general anesthesia, slowing is also evident. Thus, the EEG must be interpreted for the anesthetic used and the physiologic changes induced.

GENERAL CHARACTERISTICS OF THE INHALATION ANESTHETICS

Ideally, one should be able to regulate the partial pressure or concentration of general anesthetic agent in the blood from moment to moment, as

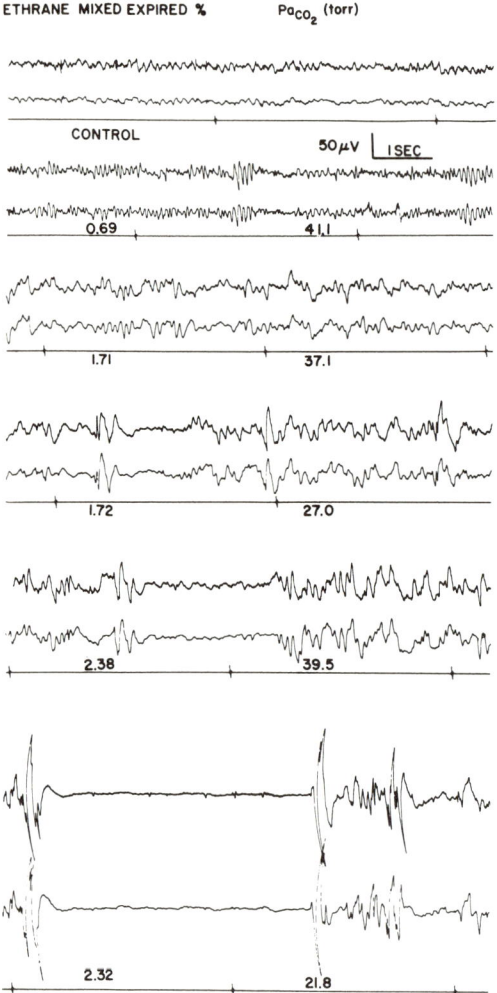

Figure 11-3. Effect of increasing depth of enflurane and change in Pa_{CO_2} on EEG in man. (Reproduced with permission from Clark DL, Hosick EC, Rosner BS: J Appl Physiol 31:884, 1971.)

the central nervous system tends to equilibrate with the partial pressure of anesthetic in blood. If more is needed, the concentration should be amenable to prompt increase; if overdose is evident, one should be able to reduce the concentration just as promptly.

The three methods of producing anesthesia—rectal, intravenous, and inhalation—vary considerably in controllability. Blood levels following intravenous administration remain more or less under control, since injection is made directly into the circulation. Because of the enormous absorptive surface of the lungs, changes in alveolar anesthetic concentration are rapidly reflected in blood, but the residual gas volume in the lung serves as a buffer to retard changes in alveolar concentration when inspired anesthetic tension is altered. Absorption into the blood from the rectum and colon is unpredictable.

Inhalation Anesthetics

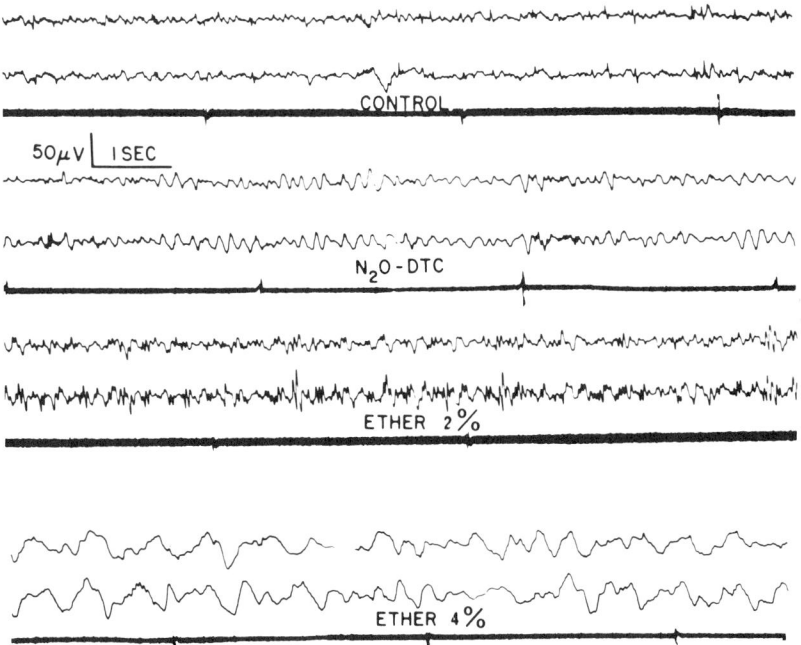

Figure 11-4. Effect of nitrous oxide 80 per cent in ether-oxygen on EEG (different subjects at 2 per cent and 4 per cent ether). (Reproduced with permission from Clark DL, Hosick EC, Rosner BS: J Appl Physiol 31:884, 1971.)

From the standpoint of elimination, the majority of drugs used for intravenous anesthesia undergo metabolic change in the body, and are thus rendered inactive in varying degrees by oxidation, reduction, hydrolysis, or conjugation. The ultimate safety of these substances therefore is related to the totality of their metabolism. Although subject to careful titration, once an injected drug enters the circulation there is no way of prompt removal. Urinary excretion is both slow and unpredictable. On the other hand, although inhalation anesthetics also are metabolized in varying degree, their uptake and elimination are accomplished primarily by alveolar ventilation. Therefore this is the most controllable method used to produce general anesthesia.

PHYSICAL AND CHEMICAL PROPERTIES

VAPOR PRESSURE AND BOILING POINT OF LIQUIDS

The physical properties of anesthetic gases and volatile liquids determine how they are supplied by the manufacturer, suggest the systems used in their administration, and influence both uptake and distribution in the body after inhalation. The basis of these phenomena is the molecular na-

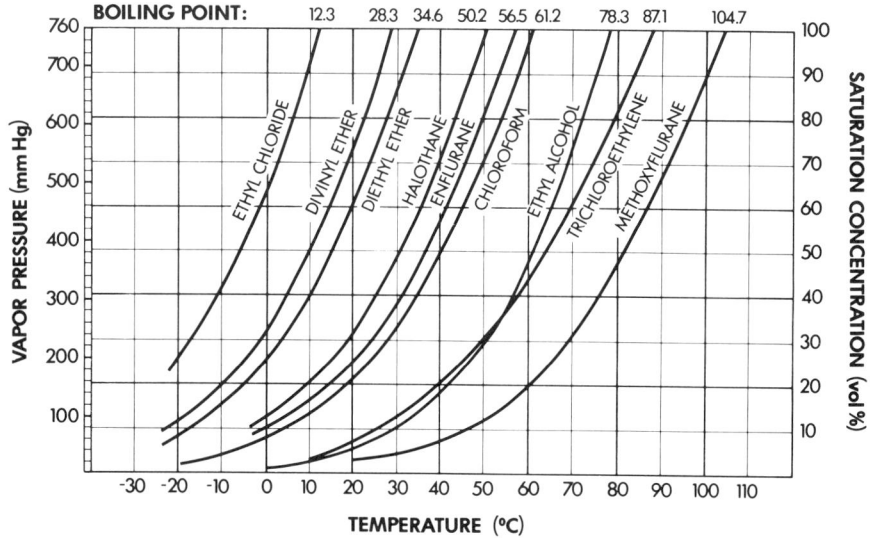

Figure 11-5. Vapor pressure curves of some volatile liquids.

ture of the matter and the general laws of physics which govern diffusion, solubility in body fluids, and the relations among pressure, volume, and temperature. Anesthetists should bear these concepts in mind as they administer anesthesia. For this reason, the vapor pressure curves of some of the volatile liquids are shown in Figure 11-5, and various other physical and chemical properties are listed in Table 11-1. The ideal volatile liquid would be that compound easily vaporized at ambient temperatures with a very low boiling point that could result in rapid evaporation. Heat of vaporization should be minimal so that the liquid is not markedly cooled as vaporization takes place, and the vapor pressure is sufficient to provide enough molecules for an anesthetic effect.

REACTIVITY AND STABILITY

Anesthetics are soluble in the conductive rubber parts of breathing systems in proportion to their concentration and the rubber-gas partition coefficient (Table 11-2). Not only may the rubber undergo deterioration, but considerable amounts of anesthetic may be given a second patient who breathes through the same apparatus. The solubility of these agents is less in polyethylene but deformation of plastic equipment occurs after prolonged exposure. Halothane plus water vapor corrodes brass, solder, and aluminum. In the presence of heat, trichloroethylene reacts with the alkali of carbon dioxide absorbents to form dichloroacetylene and phosgene, both quite toxic. Ether must be stored in copper-lined containers to prevent peroxide formation. Phenylnaphthylamine is added both to divinyl ether and

Table 11-1. Some Physical and Chemical Properties of the Inhalation Anesthetics*

Agent	Formula	Boiling Point (°C)	Vapor Pressure (20°C-Torr)	Latent Heat of Vaporization (Cal/Gm)	Useful Inspired Concentrations (Per Cent)		MAC
					Induction	Maintenance	
Water†	H_2O	100.0	21	537			
Nitrous oxide	N_2O	−89		90	60–80	50–70	101.0
Cyclopropane	C_3H_6	−33		114	25–50	10–20	9.2
Diethyl ether	$(C_2H_5)_2O$	35	450	87.5	10–30	5–15	1.92
Halothane	$CF_3CHBrCl$	50.2	243	35	1–4	0.5–2	0.77
Methoxyflurane	$CH_3OCF_2CCl_2H$	104.6	22.5	49	3	0.25–1	0.16
Trichloroethylene	$CHCl:CCl_2$	86–88	60	57.2	2.5	1.0–1.5	
Enflurane	$CFHCl \cdot CF_2 \cdot O \cdot CHF_2$	56.5	180	42	2–5	1.5–3.0	1.68
Forane‡	$CF_3 \cdot CHCl \cdot O \cdot CHF_2$	48.5	250	44	1–4	0.8–2.0	1.2

*In many instances the figures given are approximate; some data are lacking.
†Water is included for reference purposes.
‡Agent under investigation.

Table 11-2. SOLUBILITY OF ANESTHETIC AGENTS IN CONDUCTIVE RUBBER

Agent	Rubber-Gas Partition Coefficient (25°C)
Nitrous oxide	1.2
Cyclopropane	6.6
Fluroxene	20
Divinyl ether	45
Diethyl ether	58
Enflurane	74
Halothane	120
Chloroform	300
Methoxyflurane	635
Trichloroethylene	840

fluroxene to prevent polymerization, while thymol is added to trichloroethylene, and halothane and butylated hydroxytoluene to methoxyflurane to prevent decomposition. Most of these anesthetics are supplied in tinted glass bottles to minimize decomposition by light.

FLAMMABILITY

With few exceptions, most of the older anesthetics are flammable and therefore liable to be ignited and to cause explosions when mixed with oxygen or nitrous oxide. The emphasis in development of new agents therefore focused on nonflammability. Advances in fluorine chemistry allowed the synthesis of partially fluorinated ethers and hydrocarbons, which are potent nonflammable anesthetics. This group of agents has virtually supplanted all the older anesthetics with the exception of nitrous oxide.

PHARMACOLOGIC CHARACTERISTICS

POTENCY

The intensity of action of a drug can be expressed by means of a dose response curve and the potency suggested by the location of the effective dose on this curve. However, efficacy and potency, or dose required, are not necessarily related, and it usually makes little difference whether the effective dose is large or small, barring expense or problems in administration. What is important is the slope of the curve, which to some extent indicates the margin of safety as well as the median effective dose (ED_{50}). Eger and his associates defined the potency of anesthetics in terms of the minimum alveolar concentration (MAC) required to prevent movement in one half of the patients exposed to a painful stimulus. MAC is now used extensively in pharmacologic studies as an expression of equipotent doses of different anesthetics; the concept is discussed more fully in Chapter 10.

BIOTRANSFORMATION

For many years it had been assumed that, except for trichloroethylene, the inhalation anesthetics were inert, that is, excreted by the lungs and not metabolized in the body. Using radioactive labeled compounds, Van Dyke and his colleagues (1965) found that inhalation anesthetics are converted to carbon dioxide and the metabolites excreted by the kidneys, suggesting that these agents may owe part of their pharmacologic properties to chemical reactivity. Subsequent studies have shown that the majority of inhalation anesthetics are metabolized to the extent of 10 to 20 per cent of the administered dose, while the methoxyflurane absorbed is 50 per cent changed. Anesthetics are altered in the microsomal fraction of liver and other organs, where they may not only induce or accelerate their own rate of metabolism but likewise may be influenced by microsomal-inducing drugs such as phenobarbital (see Chapter 3). The metabolic products may be inert or toxic, perhaps causing destruction of the hepatocyte or malfunction of renal tubular epithelium, as noted in the discussions on halothane and methoxyflurane.

RESPIRATION

Anesthetics alter the normal respiratory pattern and interfere with the normal mechanisms of gas exchange. Various respiratory patterns ranging from apnea, through breath-holding and irregular breathing, to a predictable rhythmic pattern or tachypnea may be seen during anesthesia. Breath-holding and irregular respiratory patterns are common during induction with most anesthetics, especially at presurgical levels. The onset of surgical anesthesia is often heralded by regular rhythmic respiration. Tachypnea may be observed during attempts to increase the depth of anesthesia with any of the volatile anesthetics but trichloroethylene, particularly, causes marked elevations in respiratory rate, sometimes approaching 60 breaths per minute. With tachypnea, the tidal volume is sharply reduced, alveolar ventilation becomes inadequate, and respiratory acidosis results. During cyclopropane anesthesia tachypnea is not so prominent, but the progressive decrease in tidal volume with increasing depth of anesthesia results in hypoventilation. Halothane, methoxyflurane, enflurane, and isoflurane induce significant degrees of hypoventilation during surgical anesthesia.

An unmedicated individual at rest generally takes regular breaths of nearly equal tidal volumes, a pattern interrupted periodically by a breath two or three times the normal volume. This serves to prevent development of microatelectasis and is thought to be mediated by stretch receptors at the root of the lung. The opioids and general anesthetics depress this sighing mechanism and therefore predispose to development of atelectasis and hypoxemia.

Ventilation can be described in terms of removal of carbon dioxide from arterial blood. The relationship between CO_2 and ventilation is a reciprocal one because ventilation is stimulated by CO_2 and CO_2 is eliminated by ventilation, best described by a CO_2 *ventilation diagram* (Figure 11-6). Two kinds of curve, each representing one variety of relationship between CO_2 and ventilation, can be plotted on the $\dot{V}_E$ and Pa_{CO_2} axes: the CO_2 excretion hyperbola (curve A), and the CO_2 *ventilatory response curve* (curve B); these describe the spontaneous ventilatory response to alterations in Pa_{CO_2}. The latter curve is displaced to the right both by opioids (curve C) and anesthetics in a dose-related manner. Normally, curve B is nearly a straight line with the slope increasing about 2 L in terms of $\dot{V}_E$ for each torr increase in CO_2, with considerable variation among individuals. The slope becomes steeper with hypoxia and catecholamine stimulation and flattens with loss of consciousness or onset of anesthesia. Thus it is reduced by one third to one half in light anesthesia (curve D) and reaches a plateau in deep anesthesia (curve E). Agents which stimulate the sympathetic nervous system (e.g., cyclopropane, diethyl ether, and nitrous oxide) do not result in as much depression of the slope.

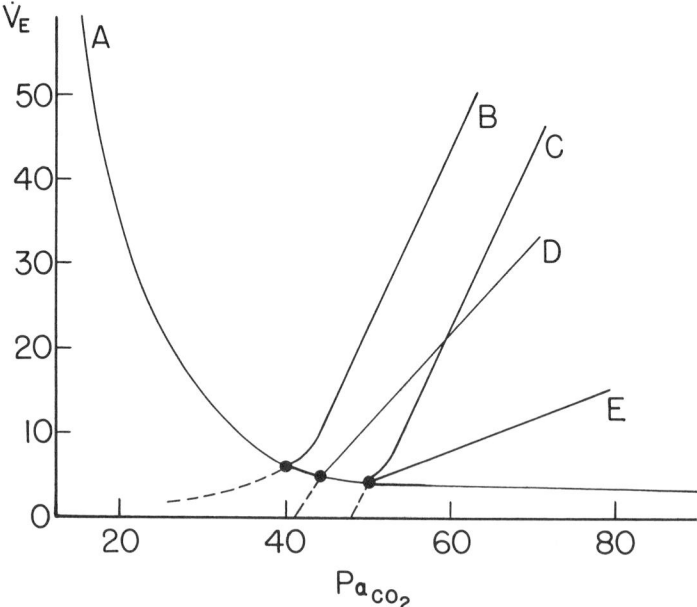

Figure 11-6. Ventilation—carbon dioxide diagram. *A* represents the CO_2 excretion hyperbola, *B* the CO_2 ventilatory response curve, and *C*, *D*, and *E* represent the shift of the CO_2 ventilatory response curve occurring with opioids and light and deep anesthesia, respectively.

The mechanisms responsible for the respiratory changes noted during general anesthesia are imperfectly understood, but all of these compounds diminish the ventilatory response to CO_2, presumably reflecting depression of the central nervous system response to the intracellular effect of H^+ on cells of the respiratory centers.

CIRCULATION

The electrocardiogram and arterial blood pressure measured directly or indirectly are utilized to evaluate the state of the cardiovascular system during anesthesia. Measurements of central venous pressure and pulmonary wedge pressure are also used in seriously ill patients. These pressures are the resultant of the many factors that determine both the cardiac output and the regional vascular resistance in various circulatory beds. Effective concentrations of most anesthetics alter blood flow significantly. The effects on several vascular beds will be considered separately, since alterations in flow result from local mechanisms and cannot be predicted on the basis of changes in arterial pressure alone.

Cerebral Circulation

Anesthetics affect cerebral circulation both directly and indirectly, the indirect actions mediated by ventilatory depression and accumulation of CO_2, which is a potent cerebral vasodilator, and by depression of cerebral metabolism which may affect local metabolic control mechanisms for cerebral perfusion. Anesthetics directly affect smooth muscle of the cerebral vessels. All inhalation anesthetics are direct cerebral vasodilators but differences among them are not distinctive enough to justify further detail. Increases in intracranial pressure taken as indices of cerebral vasodilation have been reported with all the commonly used inhalation anesthetics. It has been suggested that the direct effect on vascular smooth muscle may not be the principal cause of cerebral vasodilation but rather the result of uncoupling of metabolic control of the cerebral circulation. Recently, it has been shown that cerebral autoregulation is depressed by halothane, and by inference this is considered a property of all volatile anesthetics.

Coronary Circulation

The relationships among coronary blood flow, blood pressure, and myocardial metabolism are discussed in Chapter 27. Halothane, isoflurane, methoxyflurane, and diethyl ether all reduce coronary blood flow and myocardial oxygen consumption, apparently resulting from a decreased myocardial need for oxygen.

Splanchnic Circulation

The splanchnic circulation comprises the circulation to the gastrointestinal tract, pancreas, liver, and spleen. Cyclopropane, halothane, methoxyflurane, and isoflurane all reduce splanchnic blood flow, but not by the same mechanism. Despite a rise in blood pressure, cyclopropane induces a marked increase in splanchnic vascular resistance. Halothane leaves resistance unaltered while reducing perfusion pressure. Methoxyflurane acts by a combination of both mechanisms. Nitrous oxide does not significantly alter splanchnic hemodynamics.

Renal Circulation

Renal blood flow is reduced by anesthetics independent of alterations in arterial pressure. Cyclopropane, nitrous oxide, halothane, enflurane, diethyl ether, and isoflurane all increase renal vascular resistance and decrease renal blood flow. These effects are easily explained for agents stimulating the sympathetic nervous system but hardly account for the renal vasoconstriction with halothane. Reductions in glomerular filtration rate (GFR, inulin clearance) ranging from 19 to 55 per cent and in renal plasma flow (RPF, PAH clearance) from 36 to 67 per cent have been reported at surgical planes of anesthesia. In general, higher reductions in GFR and RPF are associated with deeper levels. The filtration fraction (GFR/RPF) and calculated renal vascular resistance are consistently increased, suggesting that increased efferent arteriolar tone maintains glomerular filtration pressure.

Circulation to Skin and Muscle

Diethyl ether, cyclopropane, fluroxene, isoflurane, halothane, and nitrous oxide all dilate the cutaneous vessels, probably owing to a central inhibitory action on thalamic temperature-regulating mechanisms thus allowing vasodilation to occur at onset of anesthesia. Increased flow persists at deep anesthetic levels of cyclopropane, ether, isoflurane, and methoxyflurane, but with fluroxene and halothane there is a return toward normal flow as depth of anesthesia is increased. Neither nitrous oxide nor diethyl ether significantly alters muscle blood flow; however, both cyclopropane and halothane diminish it, the former by increasing muscle vascular resistance and the latter by decreasing perfusion pressure.

Cardiac Effects

All commonly used potent anesthetics exert a direct depressant effect on myocardial contractility (Figure 11–7). In the isolated heart exposed to 1 MAC concentration of any potent anesthetic, this depression is approximately equivalent to that seen in uncompensated congestive heart failure.

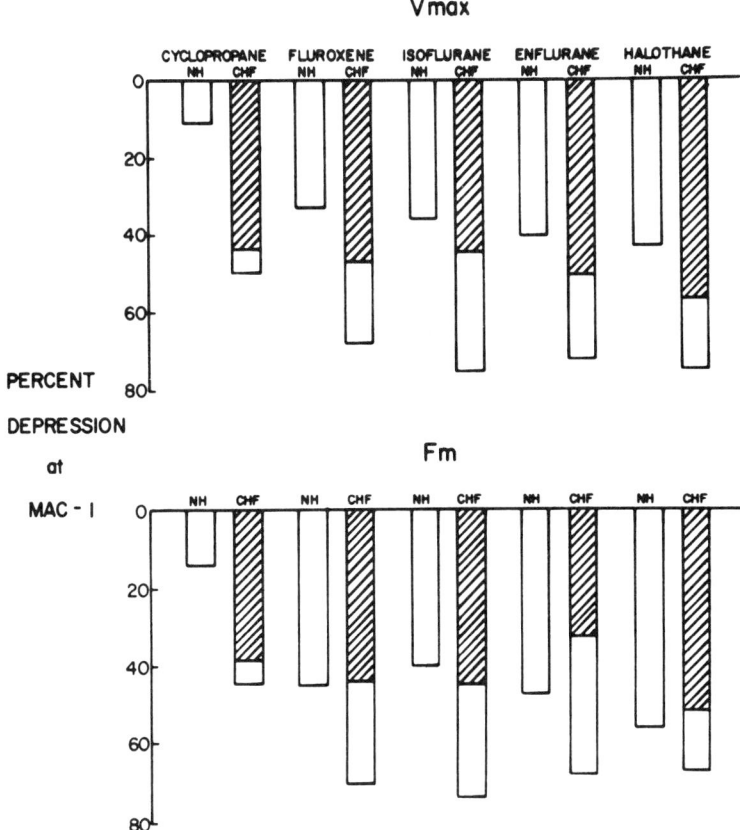

Figure 11-7. Percentage depressions of V_{max} and F_m by five anesthetics at equipotent concentrations (1 MAC) in muscles from normal hearts and muscles from hearts after congestive heart failure. Percentage depressions were calculated from the preanesthetic control values for normal hearts. Hatched areas of bars for cardiac failure values represent the depression caused by cardiac failure alone. (Reproduced with permission from Kemmotsu O, Hashimoto Y, Shimosato S: Anesthesiology 40:252, 1974.)

During clinical anesthesia with fluroxene, cyclopropane, diethyl ether, and isoflurane, cardiac output, stroke volume, and mean arterial pressure are maintained at or above normal owing to stimulation of sympathetic nervous activity. Halothane, methoxyflurane, and enflurane, by contrast, lack sympathetic stimulation and cardiovascular depression is evidenced by a dose-dependent decrease in arterial pressure, stroke volume, and cardiac output. Prolonged anesthetic administration partially reverses the depressant effect of halothane and increases the stimulant effects of agents activating the sympathetic nervous system. These changes may result from increased beta-sympathetic activity, since Price has shown that propranolol blocks the phenomenon.

RENAL EFFECTS

General anesthesia results in an antidiuresis characterized by a marked reduction in urine volume, 60 to 70 per cent, increased urine osmolality, and reabsorption of water by the renal tubules in excess of solute, resulting in a negative free water clearance. Partial reversal of the antidiuresis by intravenous administration of ethanol suggests that antidiuretic hormone (ADH) is released during general anesthesia, which is in part responsible for the antidiuresis. Reduction in GFR also contributes to the oliguria observed. Sodium and potassium excretion are reduced as a result of the reduction in GFR, possibly because of hormonal factors acting on the renal circulation. Increased amounts of renin sampled in the renal vein during cyclopropane and halothane anesthesia suggest that activation of the renin-angiotensin-aldosterone system may, in part, be responsible for renal vasoconstriction as well as for sodium retention.

The antidiuresis resulting from anesthesia, together with that from operative trauma and the use of opioids, may result in a persistent oliguria and postoperative fluid retention. Administration of large quantities of fluid in the immediate perioperative period may result in dilutional hyponatremia and water intoxication, particularly among patients in the geriatric age group.

The clinical significance of anesthetic effects on renal function is not clear. In most patients without renal disease, changes in hemodynamics and water and electrolyte excretion are transitory and return to normal in the postanesthetic period. Renal effects of general anesthetics in patients with preexisting renal disease have not been thoroughly assessed. A toxic nephrogenic effect of methoxyflurane is discussed further on.

MUSCLE RELAXATION

Many of the inhalation anesthetics cause muscle relaxation. Diethyl ether provides excellent relaxation at doses that allow ventilatory volume and blood pressure to be maintained near normal. The relaxant effect of ether may result in part from depression of sensitivity to acetylcholine at the postjunctional membrane of the neuromuscular junction, and in part from depression of central nervous system and spinal reflex activity. Methoxyflurane demonstrates similar effects. At least part of the relaxant effect of halothane, ether, enflurane, and isoflurane has been shown to be exerted at a stage subsequent to the acetylcholine receptor. Other anesthetics such as nitrous oxide and trichloroethylene do not produce muscle relaxation, and low concentrations of cyclopropane have been shown to increase contractility of skeletal muscle. Halothane, enflurane, and isoflurane at anesthetic concentrations produce muscle relaxation but are often combined with nondepolarizing neuromuscular blockers. See Chapter 14 for a discussion of the interaction of general anesthetics and neuromuscular blockers.

ANALGESIA

It is not easy to assess the degree of analgesia produced by anesthetic levels of inhalation agents, for the anesthetized subject cannot report on the experience. One is tempted to interpret such signs as movement, rise in pulse rate or arterial pressure, tachypnea, or sweating as evidence of inadequate analgesia, but there may be other causes for these reactions. Nevertheless, the MAC at which a subject does not move in response to a painful stimulus is employed as a measure of analgetic potency, although MAC involves variables other than analgesia. Use of the tibial pressure method to assess subanesthetic doses of anesthetics suggested to Dundee that methoxyflurane produces minimal analgesia, while trichloroethylene and ether are more potent. Considerable analgesia is present in the first plane of ether anesthesia after some degree of tissue saturation has taken place. During early phases of anesthesia with halothane or enflurane in oxygen, analgesia may be inadequate even at inspired concentrations that result in cardiovascular depression. The addition of nitrous oxide frequently counteracts the cardiovascular depression, because it acts as a mild sympathetic stimulant while simultaneously providing the analgesia needed.

TOXICITY OF INHALATION ANESTHETICS

The inhalation anesthetics are potential protoplasmic poisons, thus affecting cellular function. Nitrous oxide inhaled in subanesthetic concentrations over a period of several days results in depression of cell division in bone marrow granulocytes. Halothane inhibits both leukocyte motility and phagocytosis. Epidemiologic studies both in Europe and the United States indicate that women working in operating rooms have a high incidence of spontaneous abortion and delivery of infants with a significant increase in congenital anomalies. Exposure of pregnant rats to trace concentrations of halothane produces embryotoxic effects manifest as structural changes in brain, liver, and kidney. Both epidemiologic studies in humans and animal experiments provide presumptive evidence that some anesthetics may be carcinogenic. A committee of the American Society of Anesthesiologists has recommended adequate pollution control in all anesthetizing locations to protect exposed personnel (see Chapter 6).

RENAL TOXICITY

High dose methoxyflurane anesthesia causes nephrotoxicity characterized by vasopressin-resistant polyuria and azotemia. Methoxyflurane is metabolized in the liver to free fluoride and oxalate, both nephrotoxic. Inorganic fluoride inhibits some of the enzymes essential for fluid and electrolyte exchange in the loop of Henle, the proximal convoluted tubule, and the collecting ducts. At serum levels of fluoride greater than 50 μM polyuria is usually evident and the tubular effect may be irreversible with prolonged high levels. The syndrome is further characterized by a high serum osmolality and low urine osmolality. In some patients renal failure has been irreversible, requiring chronic dialysis, and several patients have undergone renal transplantation. Enflurane and isoflurane both are metabolized *in vivo* to inorganic fluoride but the resulting serum levels are much lower than those found with methoxyflurane; the risk of renal toxicity is probably nonexistent for isoflurane and minimal for enflurane.

LIVER TOXICITY

Halogenated hydrocarbons have been suspect as hepatotoxins because of the uniformly toxic action of chloroform and carbon tetrachloride, causing acute yellow atrophy of the liver. Before its introduction to clinical use halothane was carefully screened in small groups of normal subjects for hepatotoxicity, and reversible alterations of liver function were found similar to those seen with other anesthetics. No evidence of halothane-induced liver damage was found. Sporadic reports of halothane hepatitis began to appear in 1958, and in 1963 the mounting number of cases caused a committee of the National Research Council to undertake the National Halothane Study. This was a retrospective study of over 850,000 anesthetics administered between 1958 and 1962, in 34 institutions. Fatal postoperative massive hepatic necrosis was rare and usually associated with shock, sepsis, massive blood transfusion, or prior hepatic disease. Coincident development of viral hepatitis could not be ruled out. Today it is to some extent possible to identify at least one kind of viral hepatitis through identification of the hepatitis B surface antigen (HB_sAg). The anesthetics given may have played a role in a few cases, but not in a sufficient number to permit meaningful conclusions. The possibility of a rare occurrence of halothane-induced hepatic necrosis, in the range of one in 10,000 anesthetics administered, could not be ruled out. The incidence of nonfatal or nonicteric hepatic disease is unknown. However, halothane compared favorably with the other general anesthetics in overall death rates, and in death rates adjusted for variations in age, sex, preoperative physical status, and operation. No evidence was uncovered to support the imputed risk of halothane in operations performed on the gallbladder or bile ducts and in craniotomy procedures. Administration of methoxyflurane, fluoroxene, and enflurane has also been associated with the occurrence of postsurgical jaundice.

The clinical picture of fever, eosinophilia, and, occasionally, skin rash plus their appearance after repeated halothane administration suggested that postanesthetic hepatic necrosis might represent a sensitivity or immune reaction. Supporting evidence for this thesis is lacking. More cogent is the similarity of postanesthetic necrosis to that produced by carbon tetrachloride. In the process of metabolism in hepatic microsomes, carbon tetrachloride is broken down into highly reactive chlorine-containing groups which activate lipid peroxidases, thereby destroying cell membranes. This phenomenon has been observed in the rat exposed to halothane after microsomal enzyme induction with phenobarbital (see Chapter 3). In humans, halothane in low concentration can induce its own metabolism. Thus, it would seem wise to avoid unnecessary repeated administration of halothane, and before use to question the patient carefully on prior exposure to other drugs known to be microsomal enzyme inducers (phenobarbital, certain carcinogens, and steroid hormones). Development of unexplained fever or jaundice after a previous exposure to a halogenated anesthetic would seem to interdict repeated exposure. If the entity of halothane-induced hepatic necrosis exists, the complications may result from an unusual combination of circumstances, including abnormal enzymatic responses.

THE GASEOUS ANESTHETICS

NITROUS OXIDE

Nitrous oxide (N_2O) was first prepared by Priestley in 1776, and its anesthetic properties were described by Humphrey Davy in 1799. Davy's suggestion that this inorganic gas might "be used with advantage during surgical operations" passed unheeded until 1844, when Gardner Quincy Colton administered nitrous oxide to Horace Wells while a fellow dentist extracted one of Wells' teeth. It was not until 1868 that Andrews combined oxygen with nitrous oxide to lay the foundation for present-day use. Nitrous oxide supports combustion, the combination with oxygen increasing the range over which an anesthetic explosion may occur. Although impurities inherent in the manufacturing process have largely been eliminated, the possible presence of nitric oxide and nitrogen dioxide, highly pulmonary toxic substances, should be noted.

Today more techniques of general anesthesia are based upon the use of nitrous oxide than upon any other agent. This is so despite the fact that the highest concentration of nitrous oxide that can be given safely for maintenance of anesthesia ranges from 75 to 80 per cent, concentrations that will not anesthetize a fit subject. However, lack of potency is overcome by the addition of drugs of various kinds. Analgesia is enhanced by prior intramuscular injection followed by intermittent intravenous use of opioids. Anesthesia is aided by the use of thiopental for narcosis, and skeletal muscle relaxation is provided by a neuromuscular blocker. In many instances anesthesia obtained with halothane or enflurane entails the use of low concentrations of these volatile liquids in conjunction with the analgetic property of nitrous oxide; if the latter were eliminated, anesthesia would be inadequate. This is not to say that nitrous oxide must be given whenever the volatile liquids are used, but experience indicates that nitrous oxide can be combined with minimal amounts of other vapors for surgical anesthesia, a concept supported by measurement of MAC. One cannot claim that supplementation with nitrous oxide is preferable to administration of a potent, all-purpose anesthetic such as ether, but clinical impression suggests that the combination provides a more satisfactory intraoperative and postanesthetic course. Excessive depth of anesthesia is avoided, and circulatory and respiratory depression with the more potent agents is lessened and even counteracted by the mild sympathetic stimulating effect of nitrous oxide.

For the patient in profound shock, or the debilitated or the desperately ill from a variety of causes, nitrous oxide in concentrations as low as 40 to 50 per cent may provide adequate anesthesia even for intra-abdominal procedures. The susceptibility of these patients to depressant drugs is reflected in serious signs of overdose when normal concentrations of the potent anesthetics are given.

Although it is commonly held that nitrous oxide in the absence of hypoxia has no adverse actions, this is not strictly true. Price and Helrich showed that 80 per cent nitrous oxide in oxygen exerts a mild, direct depressant action on myocardial contractile force. Inhalation of nitrous oxide after thiopental induction is associated with reduction in the respiratory stimulant response to carbon dioxide, more than that attributed to the barbiturate alone. The incidence of nausea and vomiting after nitrous oxide anesthesia is low but not negligible.

The high partial pressure of nitrous oxide in blood and its low blood-gas partition coefficient cause it to diffuse into air-containing body cavities until equilibrium is approached, the volume increasing because of the lesser solubility of nitrogen in blood. This can cause considerable distention of the bowel during prolonged anesthesia at high inspired concentrations. Pneumothorax likewise increases in volume (Figure 11-8), as will other air pockets such as lung cysts or air in the middle ear; use of nitrous oxide has been shown to displace a tympanoplasty graft. During pneumoencephalography, inhalation of nitrous oxide can increase intracranial pressure through diffusion; if necessary, nitrous oxide can be used as the contrast medium. Lastly, nitrous oxide dissolved in blood can enlarge the volume of air emboli, increasing their lethality proportionately. These sequelae may occur after inhalation of any relatively insoluble agent given at high partial pressures.

During induction of anesthesia with nitrous oxide, the PA_{O_2} increases above the inspired pressure because, despite the relative insolubility of the anesthetic in blood, a large amount is rapidly taken up (Figure 11-9). This offers a modest margin of safety for a few minutes if high concentrations (90 per cent) of nitrous oxide are given to healthy patients to facilitate induction. During maintenance a large volume, as much as 30 L of nitrous oxide, may be taken up by the lungs over the first 20 minutes for distribution to body tissues. At termination of anesthesia, if the patient is abruptly

Inhalation Anesthetics   151

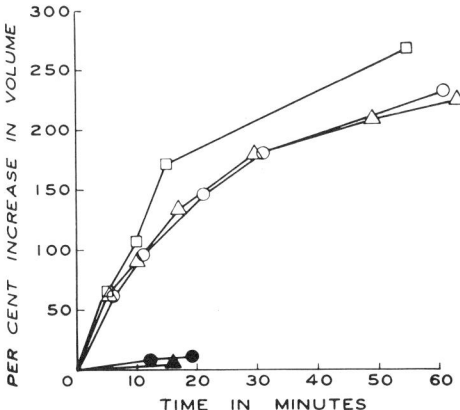

Figure 11-8. Increase in intrapleural gas volume on administration of nitrous oxide (*open squares, circles,* and *triangles*) as opposed to change in volume on administration of oxygen, plus halothane (*filled circles* and *triangle*). (Reproduced with permission from Eger EI, Saidman, LJ: Anesthesiology 26:61, 1965.)

permitted to breathe room air, a correspondingly large volume of nitrous oxide diffuses outward; this lower $P_{A_{O_2}}$, temporarily causing hypoxemia (diffusion hypoxia). At the same time $P_{A_{CO_2}}$ is lowered, causing respiratory depression. The sequence is avoided by administration of 100 per cent oxygen for a few minutes before removing the face mask.

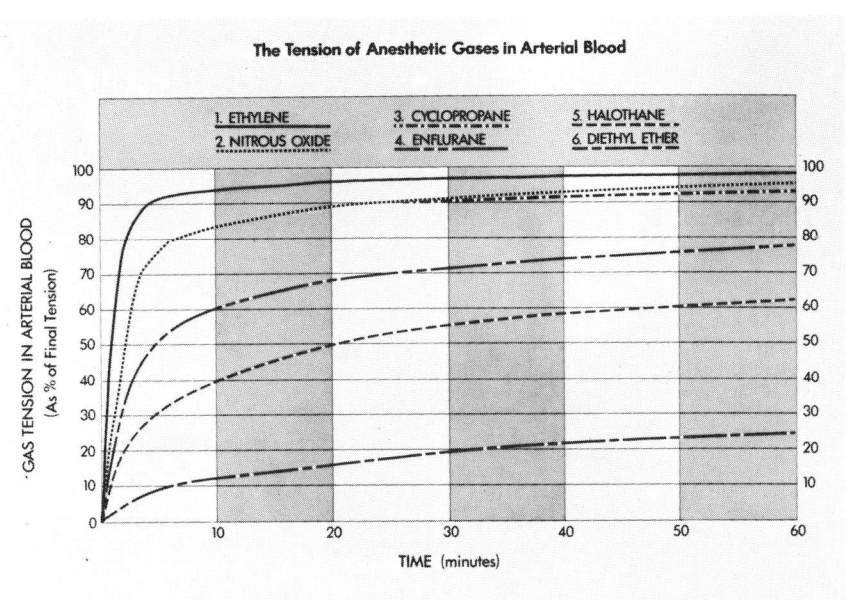

Figure 11-9. Total uptake of ether, enflurane, and halothane is illustrated here for alveolar concentrations (as indicated). When combined with 56% alveolar nitrous oxide (equals 60% inspired nitrous oxide), these are sufficient to produce surgical anesthesia. The shape of each curve is similar but their positions differ: a lower potency or higher solubility raises the position of the curve. Thus we see nitrous oxide (low potency) and diethyl ether (high solubility) as the uppermost graphs. (Reproduced with permission from Eger EI II, Uptake, Distribution and Elimination of Enflurane. Madison Wisc, Ohio Medical Products, 1975.)

CYCLOPROPANE

Cyclopropane, or trimethylene, is a simple cyclic hydrocarbon which is flammable because of the unstable state of the C-C bonds. First prepared by von Freund in 1882, its anesthetic properties were not appreciated until studies were undertaken by Lucas and Henderson in 1929; in 1934 the drug was then introduced to clinical practice by Waters. Cyclopropane has been almost entirely abandoned since the introduction of the nonexplosive halogenated hydrocarbon anesthetics. Nonetheless, we discuss the agent because of the pharmacologic principles involved.

In terms of MAC, cyclopropane is the most potent of the anesthetic gases. A wide range of safety is found between anesthetic and lethal dose, and the concentration required for anesthesia is so low that the oxygen content of the anesthetic mixture can always be well above 20 per cent. A closed carbon dioxide absorption breathing circuit is usually used because the gas is highly flammable as well as expensive. Induction is rapid, although in high concentration the gas is moderately irritating to the respiratory tract. When the desired plane of anesthesia is reached, the flow of cyclopropane often is discontinued intermittently.

Tidal volume diminishes steadily as anesthetic depth increases. Absence of peripheral stimulatory reflexes permits relatively easy control of respiration by modest hyperventilation, an effect enhanced by prior use of an opioid. Most clinicians do not permit spontaneous respiration, attempting to prevent respiratory acidosis by assisted or controlled breathing throughout operation.

The modest elevation in arterial blood pressure seen during cyclopropane anesthesia is attributed to direct activation of vasomotor and vasopressor centers in the hindbrain. As a result, sympathetic tone and peripheral vascular resistance are increased throughout the body. A reduction in blood pressure occasionally seen at the termination of cyclopropane anesthesia has been thought to result from cessation of sympathetic stimulation or diminution in circulating plasma volume, a mechanism similar to that found after discontinuation of an infusion of norepinephrine.

Myocardial contractile force is well maintained as a result of increased sympathetic activity, effectively antagonizing the direct depressant action of cyclopropane upon the heart. Cardiac output does not diminish until deep anesthesia is reached because the heart remains competent and venoconstriction serves to augment venous return. Because cardiac output is normal or increased while total peripheral resistance rises, cardiac work increases and central venous pressure rises to maintain a filling pressure sufficient to support the afterload. Increases in central venous pressure of 5 cm H_2O or more are not uncommon, probably contributing to the slight reduction in plasma volume following inhalation of cyclopropane.

Heart rate remains unchanged or tends to fall, although premedication with morphine, in addition to causing a reduction in cardiac output, frequently causes bradycardia. With cyclopropane alone, bradycardia is the result of increased vagal activity. Cyclopropane thus enhances both sympathetic and parasympathetic activity.

A variety of arrhythmias may occur during inhalation of cyclopropane, increasing with depth of anesthesia. Respiratory acidosis increases the number and severity of ventricular arrhythmias, since cyclopropane sensitizies the myocardium to the action of catecholamines. This leads to ventricular irregularities, most commonly A-V nodal rhythm and ventricular extrasystoles, but except in the case of accidental catecholamine injection, ventricular fibrillation does not occur in humans. It is best to avoid cyclopropane in the presence of pheochromocytoma or thyrotoxicosis, in which catecholamine activity is prominent. Injection of epinephrine is also best avoided during cyclopropane anesthesia.

Treatment of cyclopropane-induced arrhythmias consists of decreasing the depth of anesthesia and augmenting ventilation to correct respiratory acidosis. If the arrhythmia persists, a change is made to another anesthetic. Lidocaine in doses from 50 to 100 mg given intravenously reduces the excitability of the specialized conducting tissues of the heart and is therefore used to treat the arrhythmia.

With return of consciousness the concentration of cyclopropane in expired air approaches 1 per cent, while only traces are found several hours after termination of anesthesia. Excitement during emergence is common, and can be lessened by administration of a small dose of opioid intramuscularly toward the end of anesthesia. Nausea, vomiting, and headache are frequent although probably not to the extent seen after ether. Deleterious metabolic effects are unusual; hepatic and renal function are only transiently affected.

VOLATILE LIQUIDS

DIETHYL ETHER

In the 15th century Paracelsus distilled a mixture of sulfuric acid and alcohol, presumably forming ether, which he termed "sweet oil of vitriol." Of this he said, "It has associated with it such a sweetness that it is taken even by chickens, and they fall asleep from it for a while but awaken later without harm." Use of this substance for surgical anesthesia awaited the concept of administration of drugs by inhalation—made possible around the turn of the 19th century by Priestley, Beddoes, Davy, and others. It is agreed that C. W. Long of Georgia first gave ether for a minor surgical operation in March of 1842, while W. T. G. Morton subsequently gave the definitive public demonstration in Boston, on October 16, 1846.

Diethyl ether (C_2H_5-O-C_2H_5) is an excellent anesthetic, safer perhaps than any other. In thinking about anesthesia the average patient intuitively objects to ether because of the more pleasant induction with intravenous barbiturates, but more so because ether as given decades ago was so unpleasant. Induction was difficult, with salivary secretions, vomiting, and laryngospasm; excessive depths were produced; and fluid and electrolyte disorders were untreated in those days, while the postoperative course was accompanied by headache, nausea, vomiting, and dehydration. Today, ether given to a patient otherwise well managed need not be followed by these grim events; nevertheless, the agent is seldom used.

Analgesia rather than surgical anesthesia is useful for certain operations. With peripheral venous blood levels of ether as low as 10 to 15 mg per cent, pain relief can be provided together with adequate operative conditions for major operations on the heart. Analgesia is best reached by return to the first stage after deepening anesthesia for a brief period.

In the isolated heart-lung preparation, ether in concentrations that produce first or second plane anesthesia in the intact animal diminishes contractile force of the heart. In intact man or animal, this effect is opposed by increased activity of the sympathetic nervous system. Cardiac output and arterial pressure usually remain at normal levels, with heart rate tending to remain elevated into the deeper planes of anesthesia. Tachycardia may, in part, be related to vagal blockade. In patients unable to respond with increased sympathetic activity, as in prior thoracolumbar sympathectomy or norepinephrine depletion resulting from drug therapy, a progressive decline in blood pressure may be noted from the outset. Ether does not sensitize the myocardium to the action of catecholamines. Early in the course of anesthesia cutaneous blood flow increases, as with other anesthetics. Splanchnic and renal blood flow decline, and a strong antidiuretic action is seen owing in part to antidiuretic hormone secretion.

Ether provides profound muscle relaxation. The mechanisms responsible are several but primarily involve the central nervous system, centering around depression at synaptic pathways in the spinal cord. Neuromuscular transmission is decreased at deeper planes of anesthesia, an alteration differing qualitatively from that produced by d-tubocurarine. However, the effects of curare are augmented, dictating a lower dose of the blocking agent. Similarly, ether augments the neuromuscular blocking properties of antibiotics such as neomycin (see Chapter 14). As part of the action on the autonomic nervous system ether results in bronchodilation, which caused it to be used both therapeutically and for general anesthesia in patients with bronchial asthma. Spontaneous respiration remains adequate throughout deeper levels of anesthesia, even though the response of respiratory centers to CO_2 is reduced. This suggests that respiration is maintained reflexly by excitation at peripheral sites.

Mobilization of hepatic glycogen and a moderate rise in blood sugar level are noted upon administration of ether, probably as manifestations of sympathetic discharge. In the presence of acidosis, dehydration, and fever, especially in children, ether may produce convulsions. Preoperative correction of fluid and electrolyte imbalance, reduction of elevated body temperature, omission of atropine premedication, and avoidance of closed-system techniques combine to reduce the incidence of this complication.

HALOTHANE (FLUOTHANE)

During the years 1951 to 1956 halothane ($CF_3CHBrCl$) was synthesized by Suckling as the possible ideal anesthetic, conceived largely on theoretic principles. Primary features built into the molecule were chemical stability, nonflammability, and potency. Toxicity is related to chemical reactivity, since an inert compound is unlikely to enter into, and therefore to alter, metabolic processes. The CF_3 group is not only inert but confers stability on adjacent carbon atoms, decreasing the reactivity of chlorine and bromine. Halogenated hydrocarbons are also nonflammable if the percentage of hydrogen in the molecule is as low as that in halothane.

In terms of theoretic criteria preparation of halothane was successful, but in terms of the ideal anesthetic, there are deficiencies. Halothane is overly depressant to the cardiovascular system; it needs to be stabilized against photochemical decomposition both by addition of thymol and storage in tinted glass bottles; it exerts undesirable effects upon rubber, plastics, and some metals; and the initial costs were high. In spite of these failings, however, halothane represented a remarkable advance. Raventos first studied its pharmacologic properties in animals; Johnstone then reported on his clinical experience.

Induction of anesthesia is more rapid than with ether but slower than with agents of lesser solubility in blood, such as nitrous oxide and cyclopropane. Irritability of the larynx is reduced, spasm is rare, and respiratory tract secretions are not stimulated. Return to consciousness is not so rapid as with other substances of comparable blood-gas partition coefficients because of the higher blood-tissue solubility coefficient and the considerable uptake in fat, which delay elimination of halothane for many hours. Emergence from anesthesia is frequently accompanied by pyramidal tract signs and shivering, probably of neurologic origin rather than the result of the lowered body temperature commonly found. Shivering can be eliminated by administration of methylphenidate (Ritalin). Halothane produces relatively poor relaxation of abdominal muscles; hence it is frequently used with a neuromuscular blocker.

Halothane is highly soluble in rubber (Table 11-2) with the following implications: Induction of anesthesia may be slow because of uptake of halothane in rubber parts of the breathing circuit, exaggerated at low flows but almost eliminated at high flow rates. During prolonged administration, halothane is retained in rubber and eliminated over a period of hours at termination of anesthesia. A second patient anesthetized with the same apparatus is therefore exposed to trace amounts of the agent.

Halothane decreases arterial blood pressure, myocardial contractile force, and heart rate. Measurements of cardiac dynamics indicate that the

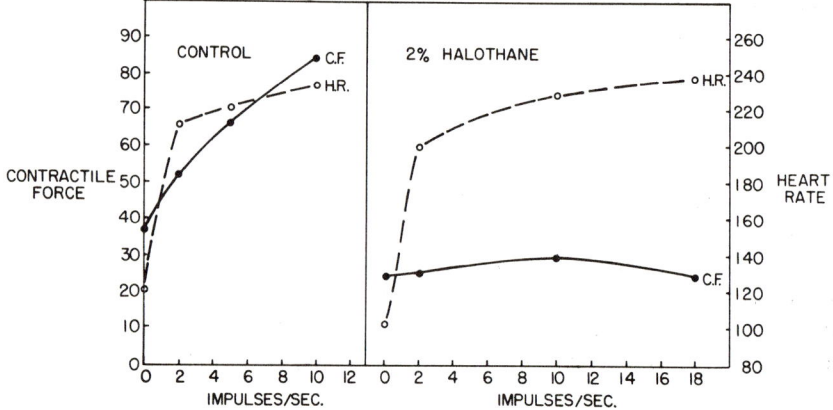

Figure 11-10. Effects of 2 per cent halothane (inspired) on responses of cardiac rate and contractile force in the dog to graded poststellate ganglionic stimulation. Contractile force is in arbitrary units, rate in beats per minute. (From Price HL, Price ML: Anesthesiology 37:764, 1966.)

ejection rate is reduced less than contractile force by virtue of an increase in diastolic volume of the heart that tends to restore stroke volume toward normal. Another factor tending to preserve stroke volume is the marked reduction in mean aortic pressure with consequent decrease in afterload and work. Halothane interferes with neither axonal conduction nor release of norepinephrine within the myocardium, nor does it affect beta-adrenergic receptors with which the neurotransmitter combines. However, supramaximal poststellate ganglionic stimulation in the dog breathing 2 per cent halothane fails to increase the contractile force (Figure 11-10) and heart rate is unaltered. Thus, some aspect of the contractile mechanism of excitation-contraction linkage appears to be affected.

There is no predominant action to account for the circulatory depression produced by halothane. The combination of central autonomic inhibition, ganglionic blockade, and suppression of the peripheral response to norepinephrine effectively robs sympathetic mechanisms of their compensatory action, permitting unantagonized depression of cardiac action and vasodilation peripherally. Muscle blood flow, therefore, decreases not as a result of vasoconstriction but as a result of reduction in perfusion pressure. The altered balance between pressure and perfusion also accounts for the diminution in splanchnic and renal blood flow. Cerebral circulation, on the other hand, increases because of vasodilation.

Ventricular arrhythmias are rare during halothane anesthesia if respiratory acidosis and hypoxia are avoided, but nodal rhythm is common, often accounting for sudden episodes of hypotension. The drug sensitizes the heart to catecholamines; thus, indiscriminate injection of these substances is unwise. Local infiltration of epinephrine is permissible if ventilation is adequate and the total dose in the adult does not exceed 100 μg (10 ml of a 1:100,000 solution) over a 10-minute period or more than 300 µg per hour.

Halothane seems to cause bronchodilation, perhaps through stimulation of beta-adrenergic receptors, for in the dog the decreased airway resistance created by halothane is eliminated by beta-blocking drugs. However, there is little evidence for a direct bronchodilating action in humans. Respiration is depressed at all anesthetic concentrations, the central effects unopposed by the peripheral reflex stimulation seen with ether. Whatever the mechanism, the drug is useful in the anesthetic management of patients with bronchial asthma.

METHOXYFLURANE (PENTHRANE)

Methoxyflurane (CH_3-O-CF-CCl_2H), synthesized by Larsen in 1958 and introduced into practice by Artusio in 1959, is the most potent and the least volatile of the liquid anesthetics. Saturated vapor pressure at room temperature is only 22 to 25 torr, and the saturated concentration is 3 per cent, the maximum concentration reached unless the liquid temperature is raised. Effective anesthetic concentrations are well below the flammable range.

Methoxyflurane usage is markedly limited because of a dose-related nephrotoxicity (see page 147). Use is now restricted to low concentrations of short duration in nonobese patients. Exposures of more than 2 MAC hours should be avoided. Many centers no longer employ this drug but some prefer it for analgesia in the first stage of labor.

Because of the high blood-gas solubility coefficient, induction with methoxyflurane is slow. Its high solubility in rubber (Table 11-2) causes loss of large amounts of the drug into rubber goods, further slowing induction. High fat solubility slows emergence but this is countered by early termination of anesthetic administration.

Myocardial contractile force and cardiac output are progressively reduced upon increasing depth of anesthesia, with no compensating increase in sympathetic activity. With time, myocardial contractile force returns toward normal. Pulse rate is reasonably stable and cardiac arrhythmias are rare, as with all of the anesthetic ethers.

The drug is a potent respiratory depressant, decreasing both rate and volume of ventilation. Good muscle relaxation is produced, additive to the action of competitive neuromuscular blockers. The analgesia persisting into the postoperative period is a manifestation of slow elimination. Renal and hepatic toxicity are described on pages 147 and 148.

FLUROXENE (FLUOROMAR)

Fluroxene (F_3C-H_2C-O-CH = CH_2) is a fluorinated combination of ethyl and vinyl ether, one of a series of compounds synthesized by Krantz and introduced to practice in 1954. It has been withdrawn from the market by the manufacturer because of limited use. The drug is flammable at concentrations used for induction and lacks sufficient potency for rapid induction. Emergence is associated with a high incidence of nausea and vomiting. As with cyclopropane, it activates the sympathetic nervous system. Use of the drug was popular at a time when clinicians were searching for an alternate to halothane to avoid the implication of "halothane hepatitis," but since the introduction of enflurane it has been little used.

TRICHLOROETHYLENE (TRILENE)

Trichloroethylene ($CHCl=CCl_2$) was first prepared by Fisher in 1864. Intoxication of those who used this chemical as an industrial solvent was occasionally reported, as were irreversible neurologic sequelae, but it was not until 1934 that Jackson used the drug as a general anesthetic. Because of a high blood-gas partition coefficient, induction of anesthesia is slow, as is emergence. The drug is therefore combined with thiopental and nitrous oxide to provide anesthesia for minor surgical procedures. The vapor may be self-administered by means of simple inhalers for analgesia during the first stage of labor and for operations such as cystoscopy; the inhaled concentration achieved approaches 0.25 to 0.75 vol per cent. Deep planes of anesthesia are not attempted with trichloroethylene because tachypnea and cardiac arrhythmias appear.

The circulatory effects of the drug are benign during light anesthesia except for spontaneous occurrence of cardiac arrhythmias. With deeper planes of anesthesia, A-V nodal rhythm, ventricular extrasystoles, and ventricular tachycardia may develop since trichloroethylene sensitizes the heart to catecholamines. Recent data suggest, however, that if hypoventilation is avoided, if the inspired concentration of the anesthetic is less than 0.6 per cent, and the total dose of injected epinephrine does not exceed 0.5 mg, the vasoconstrictor may be used for local infiltration during operation.

Trichloroethylene reacts with soda lime warmed in the reaction with CO_2 to form dichloroacetylene, which is particularly toxic to the cranial nerves. The drug is therefore administered in nonrebreathing systems, commonly via the Magill circuit. The question is sometimes asked if it is safe to give anesthesia in a closed system to a patient recovering from trichloroethylene anesthesia, even after a day or two. If, as stated, the critical temperature for the breakdown of trichloroethylene by soda lime is 60° C, a temperature of 40° C usually found in today's large carbon dioxide absorbent canisters would seem insufficient to cause degradation. High gas flows, 4 to 6 L per minute, further limit the possibility of development of high temperatures. Because considerable amounts of trichloroethylene are absorbed by rubber in breathing systems (Table 11-2), the apparatus should be permitted to air for some time before use in other patients. Chemicals related to trichloroethylene are carcinogenic, so the question of carcinogenicity of trichloroethylene has been raised. However, no currently used anesthetic has been adequately tested to eliminate the possibility of carcinogenicity.

ENFLURANE (ETHRANE)

Because of emerging disadvantages with all the available anesthetics, chemists continue to search for better compounds. Interest has focused on the ethers because investigations of Krantz and others suggested the greatest rewards. In 1963, Terrell synthesized enflurane (Ethrane) ($CFHCl-CF_2-O-CHF_2$) and in 1965 its isomer, isoflurane (Forane) ($CF_3-CHCl-O-CHF_2$). Enflurane was introduced to clinical trial in 1963 and released for general use in 1972. Isoflurane was brought to clinical trial in 1969, studied extensively, and temporarily withdrawn by the manufacturer because of reports implying it had carcinogenic properties when used in the rat. Investigations are still in progress, but it is anticipated that several years will be required to solve the problem.

Enflurane is a stable, nonflammable liquid, somewhat less volatile than halothane, which produces rapid induction of anesthesia, easy maintenance, and rapid recovery. Cardiac rhythm tends to be stable and there is only mild sensitization of the heart to epinephrine.

Anesthesia with enflurane is accompanied in about 2 per cent of patients by signs of motor hyperactivity such as twitching of the muscles of the jaw, face, neck, or extremities. These signs are accompanied by the appearance of EEG seizure patterns, more likely at high concentrations of ethrane and at low levels of Pa_{CO_2}. Seizures have not been associated with evidence of cerebral hypoxia and are not accompanied by permanent sequelae.

Ventilatory depression parallels anesthetic depth. The decrease in slope of the ventilatory response to CO_2 with both enflurane and isoflurane is similar to that seen with comparable MAC equivalents of halothane. Assisted or controlled ventilation at surgical depths of anesthesia thus is indicated.

Cardiac output is well maintained during enflurane anesthesia, and the cardiac responses to hypercarbia are similar to those seen in awake persons (markedly increased cardiac output). Cardiac output is not altered by hypocarbia. These changes probably reflect intact cardiac sympathetic control mechanisms activated by CO_2. Enflurane depresses myocardial contractility (Table 11–3) in a dose-related and reversible manner. Arterial hypotension occurs as a result of a fall in peripheral resistance. Cardiovascular reflexes remain intact.

Muscle relaxation also occurs in a dose-related manner, with surgical depths of anesthesia adding to the effects of the competitive-type neuromuscular blockers. In general, small doses of either tubocurarine or pancuronium are administered to permit lighter levels of anesthesia.

Enflurane is metabolized in the liver by defluorination to produce free fluoride, but serum fluoride levels are far lower than those found with methoxyflurane. A relative contraindication to the use of enflurane exists in patients with renal failure and in those with decreased urinary output. Isoflurane is metabolized only slightly and poses no such prohibition.

Table 11-3. Δ DECREASES IN MYOCARDIAL MECHANICS AT MAC-1 (%)*

	V_{max}	F_m	Max Power	Max Work	Max dF/dt
Enflurane	12	36	44	50	37
Methoxyflurane	31	40	55	51	43
Halothane	39	35	51	52	45

*Reprinted with permission from Shimosato S.: The effects of Ēthrane (correspondence). Anesthesiology 31:386, 1969.)

ISOFLURANE (FORANE)

It is unlikely that isoflurane will be released for clinical use until the issue of carcinogenicity is settled. The compound does not cause central nervous system excitation or seizure activity, as does ethrane. Vasodilation is produced, but cardiac performance is well maintained even at deep levels of anesthesia. Arterial pressure falls because of a decrease in peripheral vascular resistance, but perfusion in all vascular beds is well maintained. Isoflurane is a profound respiratory depressant and provides excellent muscle relaxation. The action of competitive neuromuscular blockers is markedly enhanced. This drug could become the most useful anesthetic of all.

APPRAISAL

We have adopted a historical approach in this discussion of the inhalation anesthetics. Of the older agents only nitrous oxide enjoys wide usage. Ether and cyclopropane have been gradually abandoned not only because of the potential hazards of anesthetic explosions, but because the effects of these agents, as the sole drugs for surgical anesthesia, were highly unpleasant for patients thus treated. It is probable, however, that if ether or cyclopropane were employed today with the balanced techniques used for the newer agents, the effects would not be nearly as unpleasant. Perhaps we have gone down the wrong road in continuing to synthesize inhalation agents patterned after the old, for new and unforeseen problems have arisen in the way of circulatory and respiratory depression and toxicity. All the while intravenous agents have appeared and disappeared, none approaching the long-sought ideal general anesthetic. It would seem that little further progress can be made along these lines until we have a better understanding of central nervous system activity, particularly in relation to neural transmission. Then, perhaps, we can find specific agonists or antagonists to produce the anesthetic effect, unaccompanied by adverse reactions.

REFERENCES

Bunker JP, Forrest WH, Mosteller F, et al (eds.): The National Halothane Study. A Study of the Possible Association Between Halothane Anesthesia and Postoperative Hepatic Necrosis. Bethesda, Md., U.S. Government Printing Office, 1969.

Brown BR Jr: Hepatic microsomal lipoperoxidation and inhalation anesthetics: A biochemical and morphologic study in the rat. Anesthesiology 36:458, 1972.

Cascorbi HF, Blake DA, Helrich M: Differences in biotransformation of halothane in man. Anesthesiology 32:119, 1970.

Cohen EN, Trudell JR, Edmunds HN, et al.: Urinary metabolites of halothane in man. Anesthesiology 43:392, 1975.

Cohen EN: Occupational disease among operating room personnel: A national study. Report of an ad hoc committee on the effects of trace anesthetics on the health of operating room personnel. American Society of Anesthesiologists. Anesthesiology 41:321, 1974.

Cromwell TH, Stevens WC, Eger EI II, et al: The cardiovascular effects of compound 469 (Forane) during spontaneous ventilation and CO_2 challenge in man. Anesthesiology 35:17, 1971.

Eger EI II, Smith NT, Cullen DJ, et al: A comparison of the cardiovascular effects of halothane, fluroxene, ether and cyclopropane in man. Anesthesiology 34:25, 1971.

Eger EI II: Anesthetic Uptake and Action. Baltimore. The Williams & Wilkins Co., 1974.

Kemmotsu O, Hashimoto Y, Shimosato S: Inotropic effects of isoflurance on mechanics of contraction in isolated cat papillary muscles from normal and failing hearts. Anesthesiology 39:470, 1973.

Mazze RI, Cousins MJ: Renal toxicity of anesthetics: With specific reference to the nephrotoxicity of methoxyflurane. Can. Anaesth. Soc. J. 20:64, 1973.

Mazze RI, Cousins MJ, Barr GA: Renal effects and metabolism of isoflurane in man. Anesthesiology 40:536, 1974.

Miletich DJ, Ivankovich AD, Albrecht RF, et al: Absence of autoregulation of cerebral blood flow during halothane and enflurane anesthesia. Anesth. Analg. 55:100, 1976.

Stevens WC, Cromwell TH, Halsey MJ, et al: The cardiovascular effects of a new inhalation anesthetic, Forane, in human volunteers at constant carbon dioxide tension. Anesthesiology 35:8, 1971.

Theye RA, Michenfelder JD: Individual organ contributions to the decrease in whole-body V_{O_2} with isoflurane. Anesthesiology 42:35, 1975.

Van Dyke RA: Metabolism of halothane (editorial). Anesthesiology 43:386, 1975.

Waud BE, Waud DR: The effects of diethyl ether, enflurane and isoflurane at the neuromuscular junction. Anesthesiology 42:275, 1975.

Winters WD: Neurophysiological classification of psychoactive drugs. In Kales A. (ed.): Sleep, Physiology and Pathology. A symposium. Philadelphia, J. B. Lippincott Co., 1969.

Chapter 12

TECHNIQUES OF INHALATION ANESTHESIA

Techniques of inhalation anesthesia are classified according to the presence or absence of (1) a reservoir bag in the breathing circuit, (2) rebreathing of expired gases, (3) an absorber to remove expired carbon dioxide, and (4) directional valves in the breathing circuit. The reservoir bag and absorber have been discussed in Chapter 6 and will be considered here only as they relate to the techniques described.

REBREATHING OF EXPIRED GASES

At end expiration, that part of the tidal volume remaining in the tracheobronchial tree, pharynx, and mouth is returned to the alveoli as inspiration begins; some rebreathing is therefore inevitable. Inhalation techniques may increase rebreathing to a varying degree. The least rebreathing is associated with insufflation, in which large volumes of fresh gas are continuously delivered to the mouth or trachea. The higher the flow of gas, the greater the displacement of expired air and the less rebreathing. Insufflation was used in the early days of thoracic surgery as a means of providing positive pressure to counteract pneumothorax, but it was abandoned because it depressed blood pressure and resulted in an accumulation of carbon dioxide.

In the "open" or, as it is often somewhat incorrectly called, "nonrebreathing" technique, a valve directs the expired gas to the atmosphere. At the beginning of inspiration, if the valve is competent, the only gas rebreathed, excluding that in the respiratory dead space, is the gas between the valve and the mouth or nose. At expiration all the gas is delivered to the atmosphere. The volume rebreathed increases if the valve is attached to a mask rather than a tracheal tube. Higher degrees of rebreathing occur with the semiopen and semiclosed techniques even though valves are used, while complete rebreathing characterizes a closed system.

Directional valves may be made of rubber, metal, mica, or plastic; they must seat properly to be competent and should offer minimal resistance to breathing. They should be tested periodically for competence and cleaned, in order to hold resistance to a minimum. The presence and location of the valves are of importance. If absent in a closed system, a high inspired concentration of carbon dioxide will result even though a carbon dioxide absorber is present. If the valves are located close to the reservoir bag, inspired carbon dioxide levels will be higher than if they are near the mouth. Nonetheless, in most circle systems the valves are near the reservoir bag, on the expiratory side.

Various combinations of the four factors listed earlier are incorporated in the several techniques of inhalation anesthesia (Table 12–1); brief descriptions follow.

Table 12–1. Techniques of Inhalation Anesthesia

	Reservoir Bag	Rebreathing of Expired Gases	Chemical Absorption of Expired CO_2	Directional Valves
Insufflation	No	Least	No	No
Open (nonrebreathing)				
Demand (McKesson)	No	Minimal	No	Two
Leigh, Fink, Ruben Stephen-Slater, or Frumin valve	Yes	Minimal	No	Two
Semiopen				
Open drop	No	Partial	No	None
Ayre technique	No	Partial	No	None
Magill attachment	Yes	Partial	No	One
Semiclosed	Yes	Partial	Yes	Two
Closed				
To-and-fro	Yes	Complete	Yes	None
Circle	Yes	Complete	Yes	Two

INSUFFLATION

With this technique, anesthetic gases and oxygen are delivered at varying flow rates to the mouth via a metal hook, or directly into the trachea. Valves are not required nor is a carbon dioxide absorber or reservoir bag necessary. If 8 to 10 L of gas per minute are delivered into the trachea at the level of the carina, there is little rebreathing. During inspiration the inhaled mixture is composed of gas coming from the delivery tube plus room air breathed through the nose or mouth. Dead space in the tracheobronchial tree and apparatus is minimal. The technique is rarely used today, but offers the advantages of posing minimal resistance to breathing and of not requiring complex equipment. Disadvantages include waste of gas; inability to assist respiration in the absence of a reservoir bag; variable dilution of the anesthetic by room air, highest during peak inspiratory flow rates (the composition of the inspired gases is thus unpredictable); and drying of the tracheal mucosa with loss of water and heat. In addition, anesthetics are spread throughout the operating room, exposing those present to potential toxic effects and an explosive hazard if ether is used. Some of these disadvantages characterize other techniques as well.

OPEN OR NONREBREATHING SYSTEMS

These systems permit the patient to inhale only the anesthetic mixture delivered from the machine (Fig. 12-1). The composition of the inspired

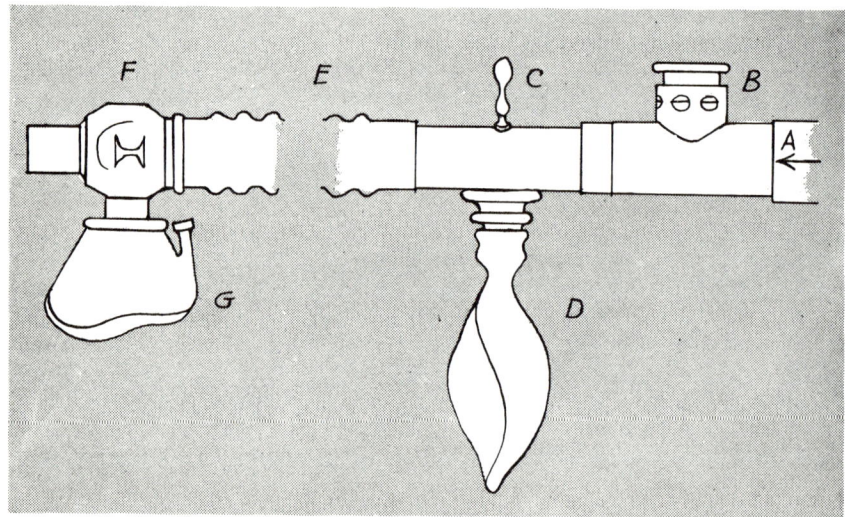

Figure 12-1. One type of nonrebreathing system: A—gas supply; B—pop-off valve; C—obturator for reservoir bag; D—reservoir bag; E—corrugated conducting tubing; F—nonrebreathing valve of the Ruben type; G—face mask.

mixture can therefore be determined precisely. Each expired breath goes directly into the surrounding air, as with the Ruben or Fink valves. With this technique and normal ventilation, residual nitrogen in the lungs can essentially be washed out in three minutes; this minimizes the dilutional effect of nitrogen and increases the partial pressure in the alveoli of anesthetics such as nitrous oxide. Induction of anesthesia is thus hastened. If a reservoir bag is not used, the inspiratory valve must be capable of supplying a high flow of gas upon demand.

The disadvantages of the technique are: high flows of gases are necessary, water vapor and heat are lost, anesthetic gases are not confined to the breathing system, and resistance to breathing varies with the efficiency of the valves and both the diameter and total length of the delivery tubing. Unless the inspired gases are humidified, the technique is ill-advised in children or for long operations in adults.

SEMIOPEN SYSTEMS

The system that we call semiopen is characterized by the British as "semiclosed without carbon dioxide absorption technique." A semiopen system allows exhaled gas to pass into the surrounding air with some return to the inspiratory limb of the apparatus for rebreathing, the degree of return being determined by the volume of flow of fresh gas. If the flow is great enough, rebreathing can almost be eliminated. The rate of flow required to achieve this depends upon the design of the system. There is little need for chemical absorption of carbon dioxide.

THE OPEN DROP METHOD

This is the simplest of the inhalation techniques, requiring the least equipment. A volatile anesthetic is dropped upon gauze stretched over a wire frame or onto a gauze mask held over the nose and mouth (Fig. 12-2). There are no valves or delivery tubing; therefore resistance to respiration is minimal. Dead space is determined by the firmness of fit of the face mask, or by the thickness of the gauze placed about the mask to prevent escape of the anesthetic. Measures taken to increase the concentration of anesthetic result simultaneously in an increase in dead space, a reduction in oxygen tension beneath the mask, and an increase in carbon dioxide and water vapor. If room air is breathed, a lower Pa_{O_2} results but is corrected by flowing 500 ml of oxygen per minute beneath the mask; however, the higher the flow of oxygen, the lower the concentration of anesthetic.

An important aspect of this technique is the effect of mask temperature on the vaporization of liquid anesthetics, particularly ether. Thermocouples placed between the layers of gauze on the mask indicate that the temperature is quickly lowered to the vicinity of 0° C. At room temperature the vapor pressure of ether is about 500 torr, but at 0° C it approaches 100 torr. The effect of cooling in retarding induction of anesthesia is obvious; closed system techniques do not share this limitation.

Finally, condensation of water vapor on the gauze interferes with vaporization of the anesthetic. The colder the gauze, the more rapid the con-

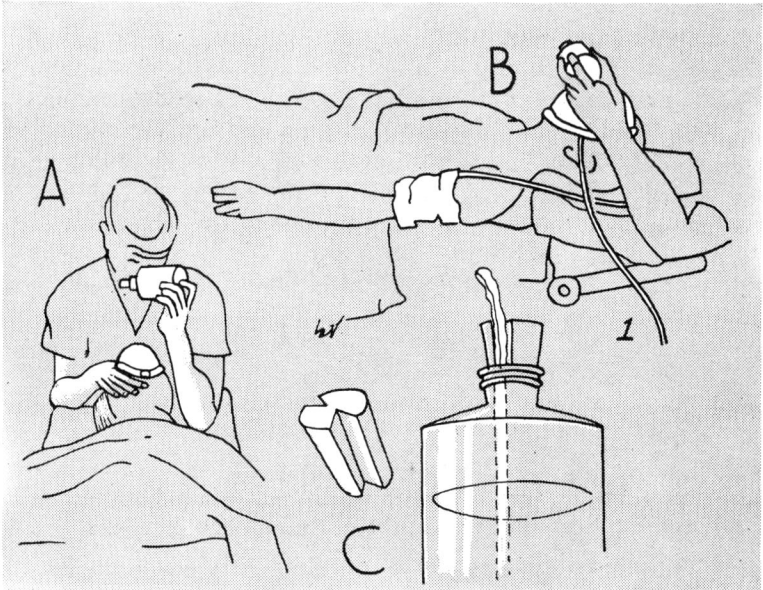

Figure 12–2. Technique of "open drop" anesthesia. *A* — method of supporting the head with the arms. *B* — lateral view showing support of head and insufflation of oxygen (*1*) beneath the mask. *C* — Cork cut and wick in place to drip ether.

densation of moisture in the expired air. Often the gauze becomes saturated with water, further increasing the dead space and leading to accumulation of carbon dioxide. Therefore, one should replace wet gauze to correct the impaired evaporation caused by moisture as well as by low temperature.

The open drop method is seldom used in modern practice, although some find it useful with halothane for brief anesthesia in children for eye examination or myringotomy.

AYRE'S T-PIECE

This device was introduced primarily for use during endotracheal anesthesia in infants and young children undergoing repair of harelip and cleft palate. The T-piece consists of a metal tube 1 cm in diameter into which gases and vapors are "injected" through a small inlet tube at a right angle to the main limb (Fig. 12–3). One end of the T-piece is connected to the endotracheal tube, the other is open to air. Rubber tubing can be attached to the open end to constitute a reservoir for the anesthetic gases, most of which would otherwise escape to the air. If the capacity of the reservoir is equal to one third the respiratory tidal volume, the total flow of gas into the

Techniques of Inhalation Anesthesia

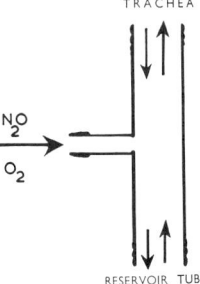

Figure 12–3. The Ayre T-piece. Nitrous oxide and oxygen supplemented with ether enter through the side tube. The tracheal end of the T-piece is connected to the endotracheal tube. The end marked "reservoir tube" is open to the air. (From Ayre, P: Br J Anesth 28:520, 1956.)

system to prevent dilution of the inspired anesthetic mixture should be about twice the respiratory minute volume. This flow rate minimizes accumulation of carbon dioxide. Since reservoir bag and valves are absent, resistance to respiration is minimal.

The technique is often modified. Some use a Y-piece rather than the T-piece, substituting corrugated tubing for the reservoir and adding a reservoir bag or escape valve. The reservoir bag permits assisted respiration, thereby conferring greater versatility (Fig. 24–3). The technique is appropriate for the infant and small child if high gas flows are used, but again the drying effect on the respiratory mucosa and the potential toxic effects of waste anesthetics on operating room personnel must be considered. The original technique, however, remains simple and useful, particularly for children up to the age of four.

THE MAGILL ATTACHMENT

In this attachment the expiratory valve is close to the face mask or tracheal tube, separated from the reservoir bag by corrugated tubing (Fig. 12–4). Gas enters the system from the supply source at a constant flow rate. The expiratory valve opens when pressure in the system is slightly higher than that of the atmosphere. During the early phase of expiration, fresh gas flows directly into the bag while expired gas flows back into the corrugated tubing, forcing gas from the tubing into the bag. When the pressure in the bag equals the opening pressure of the expiratory valve, the valve opens and expired gas escapes. Fresh gas continues to flow into the corrugated tubing, thus eliminating via the valve expired gas that had previously entered at the onset of expiration.

With inspiration, gas is drawn from the system faster than it is supplied from the machine; therefore, additional gas must be drawn from the reservoir, thereby decreasing its volume. The corresponding reduction of pressure in the system causes the expiratory valve to close. The bag empties slowly until the inspiratory flow rate falls below that of fresh gas. Mapleson (1954) has found that if the flow of fresh gas into the system is at least equal to the patient's respiratory minute volume, rebreathing will not occur. Mapleson's adaptation of this system offers a combination of the Ayre and Magill principles.

The Magill system is a relatively simple means of administering inhalation anesthetics with less dependence upon the competency of valves than in the purely open technique and gas flows are lower. However, problems remain in the loss of water vapor and heat, the dissemination of flammable gas, and possible toxic effects on personnel.

SEMICLOSED SYSTEMS

In a semiclosed system, exhaled gas passes into the atmosphere or mingles with fresh gases and is rebreathed, but a chemical absorber is placed in the breathing circuit. Because of the absorber, carbon dioxide accumulation is less of a problem than in the semiopen system and maintenance of an adequate oxygen supply is the dominant factor. With semiclosed systems, denitrogenation is accomplished more slowly and induction of anesthesia therefore is delayed. Total gas flow should at least equal respiratory minute volume if the proportion of oxygen in inspired gas is equal to that of atmospheric air as shown on the flowmeter. If a lower flow rate is selected, rebreathing increases and a larger proportion of the fresh gas must be oxygen.

Inhaled gases are humidified to a greater extent in such a system and loss of heat and water vapor is less than with the techniques previously described. The reservoir bag permits assisted respiration—not only constituting a convenience but becoming a true "reservoir" and providing maximal flow rate at peak inspiration. Semiclosed systems are probably the most commonly used systems today.

CLOSED SYSTEMS

Complete rebreathing of expired gas takes place in a closed system with practically all of the carbon dioxide chemically absorbed. Oxygen is added in amounts sufficient to supply metabolic demand. In the to-and-fro technique, the gases pass back and forth through a chemical absorber without interposition of valves, a most efficient method of absorption because the gases pass through the absorber twice. However, because of the chemical reaction and low flow of fresh gas, accumulation of heat is greater than with any other system. Channeling of gas through the absorber with the possibility of accumulation of carbon dioxide may occur, and the possibility of inhalation of soda lime dust is another hazard. The canister is

Techniques of Inhalation Anesthesia

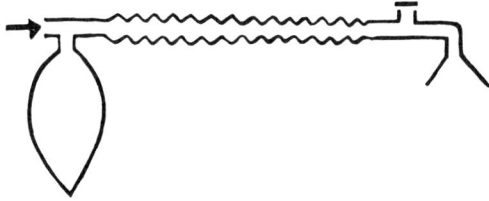

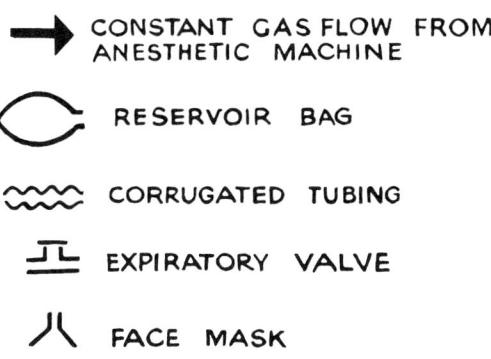

Figure 12-4. The Magill attachment. See text for description of operation of system.

heavy and needs to be supported close to the patient's face. Most find the system too clumsy to use. The chief value of the to-and-fro system lies in the minimal resistance to breathing and the ease of sterilization after use in anesthetizing a patient with communicable disease.

In the circle system with inspiratory and expiratory valves, gas flow is directed so that a single passage is made in one direction through the absorber. A closed system is achieved only when it is impervious to leaks, that is, when the expiratory valve is closed and the mask fit is tight. A total flow rate of over 500 ml per minute suggests that the system is not truly closed. From the equipment standpoint this method is convenient (see Chapter 6) and conservation of heat and moisture is maximal. The cost of gases is reduced, as they are confined to the system, and the potential for explosions and disagreeable odors is less than when semiclosed or open techniques are employed. Resistance to breathing is enhanced, however, because of turbulent flow through valves, the absorber, and the tubing and connectors.

With a constant flow rate and no need for escape valve adjustment, the closed system aids in determination of depth of anesthesia by suggesting changes in chest wall and lung compliance as respiration is assisted or controlled. With the advent of highly potent halogenated agents, closed systems, while economical, are hazardous without constant monitoring of inspired anesthetic concentrations.

FLOW RATES IN ANESTHESIA SYSTEMS

During inhalation anesthesia several considerations dictate the rate of gas flow. The volume of gas delivered to the breathing system is considered to have one or more functions: (1) achievement or maintenance of a specified alveolar concentration of anesthetic; (2) compensation for losses from the breathing circuit resulting from variations in absorption and leakage; (3) dilution or elimination of other gases in the breathing circuit and from the lungs; (4) the use of additional gas as a vehicle for volatile anesthetic; and, finally, (5) matters of practicality.

ACHIEVEMENT AND MAINTENANCE OF ALVEOLAR GAS CONCENTRATION

In a nonrebreathing system, a change in flowmeter setting alters the inspired gas concentration immediately. However, in a closed circle system, especially one of large internal volume, change in flow alters the inspired concentration only slowly. The speed of induction of anesthesia, therefore, relates in some measure to the characteristics of the anesthesia system used. A patient breathing cyclopropane via a to-and-fro canister and a 2-L reservoir bag will lose consciousness in a minute or two. The same gas flows in a circle system with a large canister and 4-L bag might not anesthetize the patient for several minutes.

LOSSES FROM THE BREATHING CIRCUIT

Flow rate of gases is set according to losses from the system. These include: rate of metabolism of the anesthetic; absorption of gas by tissues; losses by diffusion through rubber, skin, and surgical incision and into body cavities; and leakage from the system, including escape valves, poor connections, and undetected perforations in rubber goods. Absorption of halothane, enflurane, and methoxyflurane by rubber is significant and continues long after induction of anesthesia; the gas is then slowly released.

The metabolic demand for oxygen is high. An adult of 1.7 sq m body surface requires approximately 240 ml oxygen per minute. Most general anesthetics decrease the metabolic rate by 10 to 15 per cent while lowered body temperature reduces metabolic rate and fever increases it. The metabolism of anesthetics is low when compared with the large volumes absorbed in body tissues, but up to 30 per cent may be metabolized. The uptake, distribution, and metabolism of inhalation anesthetics are considered in Chapter 10.

Planned loss via escape valves or leakage as a result of ill-fitting connections and perforations in rubber must be made up by higher delivery of gas. In high flow techniques the effect of leaks is negligible, but in low flow systems the effect is considerable. Leaks should be sought and corrected prior to induction.

DILUTION OR WASHOUT OF GAS

When nitrous oxide, a weak anesthetic effective only at high partial pressures, is used, a high initial flow rate is necessary to wash out residual lung nitrogen and replace it with the anesthetic mixture. At the conclusion of anesthesia, high flows of oxygen or nitrous oxide in oxygen may be used to eliminate a more soluble agent such as halothane or enflurane, thus hastening emergence. However, conversion to an open system or breathing of room air is likely to be more effective in this regard. High flows are also used to diminish carbon dioxide accumulation, as in the Magill system.

VAPORIZATION OF VOLATILE ANESTHETICS

When volatile anesthetics are administered, the characteristics of both the vaporizer and the agent influence the selection of gas flows. Some vaporizers yield the stated concentration only at specified flow rates. The Fluotec vaporizer, for example, requires at least a 4-L flow to deliver the concentrations indicated on the dial. Divergence from indicated concentration is greatest below 1 L and above 10 L per minute flow.

Methoxyflurane typifies an anesthetic for which a specific gas flow is necessary for adequate effect. For example, at room temperature an efficient vaporizer will saturate the carrier gas to deliver a 3.3 per cent concentration of methoxyflurane. If 500 ml of oxygen per minute pass through a Copper Kettle vaporizer, the effluent yields less than 17 ml of methoxyflurane vapor per minute, insufficient to anesthetize the patient, since early in the course of anesthesia as much as 30 ml of methoxyflurane per minute may be required. Similar considerations apply when methoxyflurane is used as an adjuvant to nitrous oxide. Let us suppose that 8 L of 80 per cent nitrous oxide per minute are delivered during induction and all of the oxygen so provided, approximately 1.6 L, passes through the vaporizer flowmeter. The ensuing concentration of methoxyflurane would be 0.6 per cent, resulting in a slow induction of anesthesia. If the nitrous oxide were discontinued abruptly, and only oxygen continued to pass through the vaporizer, alveolar nitrous oxide concentration would decrease owing to absorptive uptake and washout. Anesthesia might then lighten and the patient awaken before enough methoxyflurane had been inhaled. Delivering all the oxygen required through the vaporizer is a potentially dangerous maneuver if the anesthetist is forgetful and shunts the vaporizer out of the system. Oxygen is a carrier mixture which should always be supplied via a flowmeter other than that to the vaporizer. These are common problems when the vaporizer is outside the circle system; if within the system, all inspired gases pass through the vaporizer. In this circumstance an inefficient vaporizer may produce a higher concentration of anesthetic than an efficient one.

MATTERS OF PRACTICALITY

Simplicity of Calculations. With efficient vaporizers the concentration of anesthetic delivered is easily calculated; certain flow rates simplify the mathematics. For instance, at ambient temperature if total gas flow is 5 L per minute, comprising 1.5 L of oxygen and 3.5 L of nitrous oxide, approximately 1 per cent halothane will be delivered for each 100 ml of oxygen going through the Copper Kettle or Vernitrol vaporizer. An easier method is offered on some machines in which oxygen flows through the Copper Kettle are set according to temperature. When the bypass oxygen flow has been set according to the Kettle temperature, flow of oxygen through the Kettle can be adjusted to deliver a specific concentration of halothane as indicated by a scale. Perhaps the best technique is to have on hand a graphic representation of concentration of anesthetic delivered according to temperature, total gas flow, and gas flow through the vaporizer.

The Escape Valve. Another factor in choice of flow rate is the adjustment of the escape valve. It should be possible to adjust the valve during controlled or assisted respiration so that pressure on the breathing bag first inflates the lungs and then vents excess gas. Some valves are not so easily adjusted; with these it may be more convenient to empty the bag periodically, at other times leaving the valve closed. Some find it difficult to judge adequacy of ventilation unless the escape valve is closed.

Dictates of the Operation. Circumstances during operation may require changes in gas flow. For example, during a thoracotomy in which a bronchus has been divided, high flows are necessary to compensate for leakage as suturing is done. A closed cyclopropane anesthesia circuit may require conversion to a semiclosed system with nitrous oxide, oxygen, and curare when the cautery must be used.

Mechanical Limitations of Equipment. Some vaporizers impose limitations on flow for optimal vaporization and therefore cannot be relied upon for accurate concentrations of anesthetics at all flow rates, as in the Fluotec device with low vaporizer flow. Rotameters are often more accurate in the upper two thirds of the scale than in the lower third. A Vernitrol vaporizer designed for ether offers a flowmeter range of flows up to 1300 ml per minute; this flowmeter cannot be relied upon to deliver exactly 100 ml of oxygen per minute in order to vaporize halothane or enflurane.

Economy. For prolonged procedures, considerable saving in the cost of anesthetics is made possible by use of a semiclosed breathing circuit with low flows, or a closed system. By definition a semiclosed system is one in which fresh gas inflow is low in order to provide considerable rebreathing. Many use high flows for the first 30 to 60 minutes and convert to low flows for the duration of a long operation.

Environmental Contamination. Appreciable quantities of anesthetics are detectable in the operating room environment, the concentration varying with distance from the anesthesia machine, total gas flow, concentration of volatile agents, and patterns of room ventilation. The evidence suggests that chronic inhalation of trace amounts of anesthetics may be harmful, a matter discussed elsewhere (Chapter 6).

REFERENCES

Ayre P: The T-piece technique. Br J Anaesth. 28:520, 1956.
Fitton EP: A theoretical investigation of oxygen concentrations in gases inspired from various semi-closed anaesthetic systems. Br J Anaesth, 30:269, 1958.
Linde HW, Bruce DL: Occupational exposure of anesthetists to halothane, nitrous oxide and radiation. Anesthesiology 30:363, 1969.
Macintosh RR, Mushin WW, Epstein HG: Physics for the Anaesthetist. 3rd ed. Philadelphia. FA Davis. 1963.
Mapleson WW: The elimination of rebreathing in various semi-closed anaesthetic systems. Br J Anaesth, 26:323, 1954.
Noble WH: Accuracy of halothane vaporizers in clinical use. Can Anaesth Soc J. 17:135, 1970.
Smith TC: Nitrous oxide and low inflow circle system. Anesthesiology. 27:266, 1966.
Tayyab MA, Ambiavagar M, Chalon J: Water nebulization in non-rebreathing systems during anesthesia. Can Anaesth Soc J, 20:728, 1973.

Part B

INTRAVENOUS ANESTHESIA AND TRACHEAL INTUBATION

Chapter 13

INTRAVENOUS ANESTHESIA

Early efforts at producing insensibility by means of intravenous injection of opioids were made in 1665. Oré published the results of a trial of administration of chloral hydrate by vein in 1875. However, it was not until the introduction of the rapidly acting barbiturates in the 1930s that the intravenous method achieved popularity.

Induction of anesthesia by intravenous administration of a rapidly acting barbiturate is not an unpleasant experience. A patient who has been anesthetized this way usually prefers it to all others. In addition, because many surgeons promise their patients intravenous anesthesia, an increasing demand for the method is created. It is difficult to avoid starting general anesthesia with a barbiturate given intravenously regardless of the anesthetic subsequently used for maintenance. Since the technique is simple, it appeals to individuals not qualified by experience or training to use it safely. It has been aptly said that thiopental is fatally easy to give.

This chapter outlines the principles involved in the safe use of intravenous anesthetics. The barbiturate most commonly used is thiopental. Another of the thiobarbiturates is thiamylal (Surital); the oxybarbiturates include methohexital (Brevital) and hexobarbital (Evipal) (Fig. 13-1). All

Intravenous Anesthesia

are similar in action and will be treated together. The chapter also describes the use of other anesthetics given by the intravenous route, including neuroleptics, ketamine, diazepam, morphine, and steroids.

BARBITURIC ACID DERIVATIVES

THEORETIC CONSIDERATIONS

Controllability

Barbiturate anesthesia differs from that produced by inhalation agents in that once the barbiturate has been injected, there is little the anesthetist can do to facilitate its removal. Dissipation of effects, as will be shown, depends upon redistribution of the drug from brain to other tissues and to a lesser extent upon biotransformation. With halothane, nitrous oxide, or other vapors or gases, the partial pressure in blood can be altered at will by varying the concentration of agent in the respired air. With overdosage of an inhalation agent, concentration can be diminished rapidly by ventilating the lungs with oxygen or air. Opioid injection can be countered by the use of antagonists. Controllability with intravenous barbiturates is improved by the use of solutions varying from 0.2 to 2.5 per cent, the more dilute solutions given by continuous infusion and the higher concentrations injected intermittently. Theoretically, the lower the concentration or total quantity injected per unit of time, the greater the controllability of the level of anesthesia; but practically, with a continuous infusion there is danger that frequent adjustment of the rate of flow may distract the anesthetist's atten-

CHEMICAL CONFIGURATION OF THE BARBITURATES USED INTRAVENOUSLY FOR GENERAL ANESTHESIA

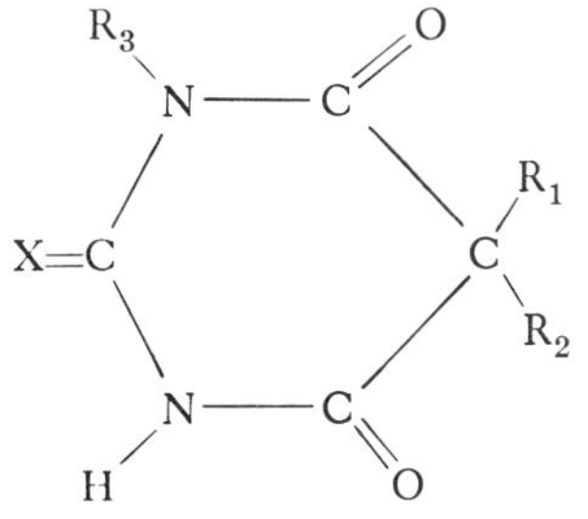

GENERAL FORMULA

	R_1	R_2	R_3	X
Thiopental (Pentothal)	Ethyl	1 methylbutyl	H	S
Thiamylal (Surital)	Allyl	1 methylbutyl	H	S
Methohexital (Brevital)	Allyl	1 methyl 2 pentynyl	CH_3	O
Hexobarbital (Evipal)	Methyl	1-cyclohexen-1-yl	CH_3	O

Figure 13–1. Chemical configuration of the barbiturates used intravenously for general anesthesia.

tion from the patient. Often the infusion is forgotten during stress; overdosage is therefore more likely to occur. We do not recommend continuous infusion of barbiturates.

Fat in the Body

The intravenous barbiturates are metabolized and the products of metabolism excreted. Interestingly, though, it is nót biotransformation that terminates their action, but rather redistribution in the body. As an illustration we shall follow the course of a single injection of thiopental.

Initially, upon intravenous injection the drug is diluted in the central pool of blood in the heart and lungs, passing then in high concentration to the organs of highest blood flow—the brain, heart, liver, and kidneys. Cerebral concentration rises rapidly, peak concentration being reached in approximately 50 seconds, and unconsciousness ensues. With recirculation, as equilibration with lean tissues begins, thiopental is removed from the brain and the plasma concentration declines. Muscle, skin, bone, and finally fat begin to take up thiopental, 15 to 30 minutes being required for equilibration with the first three, while equilibration with fat takes several hours (Fig. 13-2).

Through redistribution, the cerebral concentration decreases sufficiently so that the patient awakens, often within five to 10 minutes of injection, despite the fact that only a small amount of the drug has undergone biotransformation. Although the exact amount is currently a matter of con-

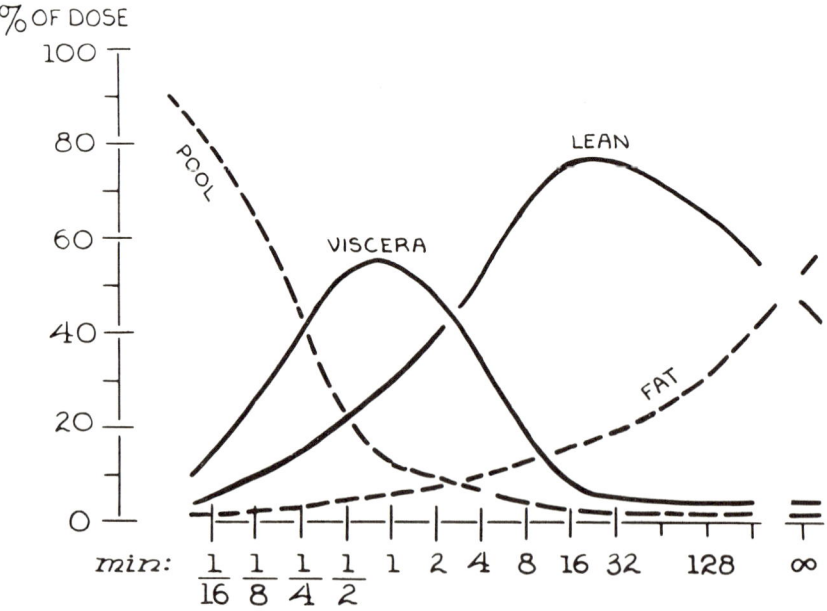

Figure 13-2. Distribution of thiopental in different body tissues and organs at various times after intravenous injection. (Reproduced with permission from Price HL, Linde HW, Price ML: Clin Pharmacol Ther 1:298, 1960.)

troversy, the rate of this process is taken as 10 to 15 per cent per hour of the total dose injected.

If instead of a single injection multiple injections are made, more drug is stored in the body and large total doses may lead to saturation of lean as well as fatty tissues. Under these conditions even small additional doses may be excessive and caution must be exercised. Largely because of the slow release of drug stored in fat, recovery is slow.

Considerable quantities of barbiturate are bound to plasma protein, particularly the albumin moiety. The tissues come into equilibrium only with the unbound fraction, since the bound part is not readily available for diffusion. Equilibration between tissues and the unbound portion is dependent in part upon the hydrogen ion concentration of blood. Acidosis reduces protein binding of the drug, tending to increase cell penetration; acidosis also increases the amount of undissociated drug present. For both these reasons the acidosis resulting from carbon dioxide retention causes plasma thiopental levels to decline and anesthetic depth to increase. Respiratory alkalosis has a reverse action.

The rate at which barbiturates penetrate the central nervous system can be correlated with the lipid solubility of the un-ionized molecules—or the partition coefficient between lipid solvents and aqueous buffer. For example, the onset of hypnotic action following the intravenous administration of pentobarbital is slower than that following comparable doses of thiopental. While thiopental is largely non-ionized at pH 7.4, it has a very high partition coefficient (3.3). Pentobarbital, on the other hand, is even less ionized and much less protein bound, but it has a far lower partition coefficient (0.05); thus its penetration and hypnotic action are slow.

The thiobarbiturates undergo metabolic degradation by desulfuration and oxidation, principally in the liver, with some biotransformation occurring in the brain and kidney as well. Inactive metabolites are excreted via the kidneys except for the drug methohexital, a significant amount of which is eliminated in feces. Biotransformation of the oxybarbiturates occurs only in the liver. Narcosis with the latter, therefore, can be expected to last somewhat longer in patients with liver decompensation.

Acute tolerance to the thiobarbiturates can develop. A patient given 2 gm of thiopental in increments, following an initial dose of 500 mg, may regain consciousness with a blood level of about 20 mg per 100 ml. Another patient given only 1 gm of barbiturate with an initial dose of 250 mg may regain consciousness with a blood level of about 10 mg per 100 ml. The time of awakening differs little between the two subjects. Viewed in practical terms, individuals given large initial doses of thiobarbiturates will require larger increments to maintain anesthesia than those who receive smaller doses for induction. The mechanism of acute tolerance is unknown.

Alkalinity of Solutions

Solutions of thiopental, thiamylal, and methohexital are highly alkaline, the pH of 2.5 per cent solutions in distilled water being about 10.6. As a result, intravenous injection of the barbiturate may be followed by thrombophlebitis, or, in the event of extravasation, by nerve injury or tissue necrosis. If a thiobarbiturate is injected into the tubing of an intravenous infusion, these complications are less likely to occur. Accidental intra-arterial injection has led to arterial spasm, gangrene, and loss of an extremity when the concentration exceeded 2.5 per cent.

This alkalinity was once thought to lend "self-sterilizing" properties. Solutions were kept for weeks or until precipitation occurred. We now know that solutions of the intravenous barbiturates can and do support bacterial growth, so it is recommended that all solutions unused within 24 hours be discarded.

Anesthetic Action

Intravenous barbiturates can produce any degree of central nervous system depression, ranging from mild sedation to coma. The totality of effect is dependent upon the extent of excitability at the time of administration and any tolerance that may have been induced by prior exposure. The mode of action of barbiturates is believed to involve depression of the short synaptic pathways in the central reticular core of the brain stem, sparing direct spino-lemnisco-thalamic pathways. For these reasons, barbiturates differ from inhalation anesthetics such as ether in their lesser ability to block afferent sensory impulses. An antianalgetic action has been alleged for the thiobarbiturates, but its clinical significance is unclear.

Recognition of these fundamental differences among the anesthetics is essential for the rational use of intravenous barbiturates. Healthy muscular individuals may require excessive doses for adequate anesthesia. Often the degree of anesthesia appears adequate, but with surgical stimulation movement or struggling occurs, responses indicative of poor afferent blockade. Minor pharyngeal stimulation often precipitates laryngospasm or cough. This is so common that it is said that thiopental sensitizes vagal nerve endings, leading to laryngospasm. We believe this is further evidence that afferent pathways are unblocked.

RESPIRATORY EFFECTS

The respiratory effects of thiobarbiturates are the result of direct depression of the medullary and pontine representations for respiratory control. Actions on pulmonary stretch receptors, afferent and efferent nerves concerned in respiration, and neuromuscular junctions are negligible. Immediately following injection, respiratory depression may be pronounced for the reasons cited. Central stimulatory responses to carbon dioxide are depressed at all levels of anesthesia and ultimately abolished as anesthesia deepens. Responses to peripheral chemoreceptor excitation persist longer but are also extinguished at profound depths of anesthesia. At ordinary levels of anesthesia, tidal volume is diminished, respiratory rate is increased, and the thorax tends to assume the end-expiratory position.

CIRCULATORY EFFECTS

The barbiturates depress the activity of hypothalamic autonomic centers regulating the force of cardiac contraction. Myocardial contractility is reduced, while vascular tone is increased by direct action. Baroreceptor reflexes, conduction in autonomic nerves, and sympathetic ganglion transmission are little affected. The end result of these actions is that cardiac output is reduced while total peripheral resistance increases. The barbiturates used for anesthesia do not sensitize the autonomic tissues of the heart to the arrhythmic effect of the catecholamines to any significant extent.

CENTRAL NERVOUS SYSTEM EFFECTS

Thiopental reduces cerebral metabolism and oxygen consumption. There is evidence that these reductions in metabolic activity lead to parallel reductions in cerebral blood flow. Because of the slower flow (as much as one third in light anesthesia and up to one half in deep anesthesia) cerebral blood volume and spinal fluid pressure diminish—thus use of the barbiturates is recommended in patients with increased intracranial pressure.

CLINICAL USE OF INTRAVENOUS BARBITURATES

Selection of Patients

Intravenous barbiturate anesthesia is not suitable for all patients. Caution is advised in those with severe bronchial asthma. Individuals with poor superficial veins are unsuitable choices merely because of technical problems. Patients with tumors or other lesions encroaching upon the air passages may become hypoxic with loss of consciousness and relaxation and engorgement of cervical tissues, unless a satisfactory airway is first established, as by tracheal intubation following topical anesthesia. Individuals with acute or chronic respiratory infections often react poorly to barbiturate anesthesia, developing chest spasm and cough. The method is unsuited to muscular individuals for other than brief operations unless supplementation with a potent analgetic or inhalation agent is planned. Patients suffering from acute intermittent porphyria may undergo exacerbation of symptoms following barbiturate administration; a rapidly progressive fatal course has been described.

Intravenous anesthesia *per se* with a barbiturate is not adequate for many types of operations even when nitrous oxide is inhaled. If this combination is chosen, the anesthetist must be certain that surgical conditions are adequate without danger of overdosage. For operations requiring muscle relaxation, a thiobarbiturate is frequently used for induction, with analgesia provided by nitrous oxide and an analgetic and relaxation achieved with a neuromuscular blocker.

Rapid induction of anesthesia for tracheal intubation has become popular; 3 to 6 mg of tubocurarine are given intravenously to prevent or lessen fasciculations caused by the depolarizing neuromuscular blocker while the patient is given 100 per cent oxygen to facilitate nitrogen washout. This is followed by 250 to 500 mg of barbiturate, administered simultaneously with, or followed by, a paralyzing dose of a depolarizing muscle blocker. The technique is hazardous, since a high blood concentration of anesthetic is produced in a short time. If used in the poor risk patient with cardiovascular disease or with acute upper intestinal tract obstruction, mortality may be high. We have seen death, cerebrovascular accident, and myocardial infarction resulting from hypotension following this procedure, as well as aspiration of vomitus. If tracheal intubation follows use of succinylcholine, cough and bronchospasm may appear upon recovery of respiratory reflexes because of the irritant effect of the tracheal tube in an essentially unanesthetized patient. Furthermore, subsequent overdose with an inhalation anesthetic may result from attempts to quiet the patient.

Management of Anesthesia

Patients are prepared as for any general anesthetic. If opioids are administered for premedication, and they are an essential part of a balanced technique, the anesthetist can anticipate a greater degree of respiratory depression following injection of an intravenous barbiturate. Anesthesia should never be induced with a barbiturate unless an anesthesia machine is at hand, with oxygen ready and the usual assortment of resuscitative equipment available.

Patients with excessive nasal, pharyngeal, or bronchial secretions should be asked to clear their passages before induction, in order to minimize the laryngospasm and cough so often initiated by the presence of secretions after induction of anesthesia.

We prefer to inject the barbiturate into the tubing of an intravenous infusion, but some patients have venous constriction upon arrival in the operating room. Under these circumstances the anesthetist should not persist in attempts at venipuncture. There is no excuse for exposing a patient to painful, multiple needle punctures in an effort to provide a seemingly pleasant induction of anesthesia. It is sensible to abandon the intravenous route and use one of the rapidly acting inhalation agents for induction.

Induction of Anesthesia

A test dose of not more than 50 mg should be given at first. Pain at the site of injection suggests extravasation of the drug, but more commonly is the result of venospasm caused by the high pH of the solution. Ordinarily drowsiness occurs soon after initial injection. Failure of the patient to become drowsy usually suggests either that considerable quantities of barbiturate may be needed or that something has gone wrong with the injection. If loss of consciousness follows the initial dose, the amount of drug subsequently needed for anesthesia is likely to be relatively small. Generally, incremental doses are preferable and safer than single high doses.

When the initial injection of barbiturate is to be followed by inhalation anesthesia, sufficient time should elapse to permit placement of the mask without the patient's awareness. If too much barbiturate is given, the resulting respiratory depression will delay induction of inhalation anesthesia.

An intravenous barbiturate is used as the sole anesthetic only for brief surgical procedures such as closed reduction of a fracture or dislocation, or incision and drainage of an abscess. When combined with nitrous oxide, longer operations not requiring relaxation can be accomplished. The amount of barbiturate required is reduced and a more steady state of anesthesia provided, but time is required for saturation with nitrous oxide. During maintenance, nitrous oxide can be used with equal parts of oxygen or as high as four parts to one of oxygen. A total gas flow of 6 to 8 L per minute is supplied for the first three to five minutes to denitrogenate the lungs, subsequently reduced to 2 to 3 L per minute. If respiration is depressed by the initial injection of barbiturate, assistance is provided until the tidal volume returns to normal levels.

Maintenance

The amount of barbiturate required depends upon the physical condition of the patient, the premedication given, and the nature and duration of operation. Persistent tachycardia, pupillary dilation, sweating, tachypnea, movement, and arterial hypertension are manifestations of pain perception and inadequate depth of anesthesia. Under such conditions, if a considerable quantity of barbiturate has already been given, the anesthetist may elect to change to a more potent anesthetic or to inject small doses of analgetic intravenously (morphine 1 to 2 mg, meperidine 10 to 25 mg, fentanyl 0.05 to 0.1 mg). Assisted or controlled respiration is necessary if the patient is given a neuromuscular blocker, with tracheal intubation to facilitate respiratory control. The signs of anesthesia are more elusive in the presence of muscle paralysis.

Barbiturates and neuromuscular blockers have been given in combination from the same syringe. Because of chemical incompatibilities that result in precipitation, the choice of drugs is limited. Separate use of the agents allow for more accurate titration in relation to need.

COMPLICATIONS

Extravascular Injection

In the conscious patient this complication is indicated by pain at the site of injection, but in the anesthetized patient it can be detected only by careful observation. If extravasation occurs, treatment consists of injection of 5 to 10 ml of 1 per cent procaine into the involved area to dilute and neutralize the barbiturate solution and to prevent vasospasm; otherwise neuritis or ulceration of the skin may result.

Intra-arterial Injection

This is most likely to occur with injection at the antecubital space, but can take place at any site where artery and vein are in proximity or where the artery is superficial. Arteries, particularly the radial artery, often follow an anomalous course. Intra-arterial injection is detected by the sudden onset of severe pain described as hot or scalding. The pathologic lesion seen after intra-arterial injection is a chemical endarteritis that destroys endothelial and subendothelial layers of the arterial wall. In severe cases the muscle layers may also be involved, with diffuse thrombosis. Injury takes place immediately, requiring only brief contact, the degree varying with the concentration and amount of drug injected. The necrotizing effect is a property of the drug itself and not related to alkalinity. Experimental work suggests local endogenous release of norepinephrine, which is perhaps the cause of the arterial spasm. Other work proposes that gangrene results from precipitation of thiopental crystals with occlusion of capillaries on the venous side. The ultimate results are not likely to be disastrous unless concentrations greater than 2.5 per cent are used; to our knowledge, gangrene has not been reported following the use of 2.5 per cent thiopental.

No single regimen has proved effective in treatment. However, any or all of the following measures may be tried: If possible, the needle should be left in place and 10 ml of 1 per cent procaine injected. Procaine dilutes and neutralizes the barbiturate solution. Local heparinization has been advised and local injection of phentolamine, an alpha-adrenergic blocker, is theoretically justified. Stellate ganglion block or general anesthesia with halothane may be elected to promote vasodilation. If arterial thrombosis occurs, amputation may ultimately be necessary. Some patients have recovered completely without treatment and others have developed gangrene in spite of therapy.

Cough and Laryngospasm

Together these constitute the most common complications of intravenous barbiturate anesthesia. Often the explanation is poor choice of anesthetic. One is not likely to forget the development of cough, chest wall and laryngeal spasm, anoxia, and cyanosis in a patient with bronchial asthma or chronic bronchitis. Blood within the pharynx, early stimulation of the pharynx or trachea by airway insertion, movement of head or neck, or painful peripheral stimuli also may be precipitating events. Should cough or laryngospasm appear, treatment depends upon the precipitating factor. If secretions are at fault, they should be aspirated after more barbiturate has been injected to diminish reflexes, When an airway causes cough, it is removed and anesthesia deepened before replacement. Laryngospasm usually can be overcome by steady, positive airway pressure. Should spasm persist and cyanosis appear, intravenous injection of succinylcholine (50 mg in the adult) followed by ventilation with oxygen is indicated.

Vomiting

This is uncommon during intravenous barbiturate anesthesia unless there has been irritation of the pharynx, or the patient has been allowed to emerge into the second stage, has recently eaten, or has a distended stomach.

POSTANESTHETIC COURSE

As a rule, recovery from barbiturate anesthesia is gradual and uneventful. The time of awakening depends upon the total dose of drug given and upon the muscular development and physical condition of the patient. Some individuals appear to awaken quickly, only to return to the anesthetized state when undisturbed. Others, believing themselves completely recovered, request to sit up or stand. If allowed to do so they may develop vertigo and fall. An attendant should be present the first time a patient gets out of bed after intravenous barbiturate anesthesia.

Patients recovering from barbiturate anesthesia may occasionally show muscle fasciculation and rigidity, stertorous respiration, and slight cyanosis. This syndrome is poorly understood; it is possibly of neurologic origin, but in most cases appears to be related to temporary derangement of body temperature control. It is more commonly seen when the environmental temperature is low; rectal temperature is often in the vicinity of 36° C. Treatment consists of warming. If cyanosis causes concern, oxygen may be given even though the cyanosis is more a manifestation of vasoconstriction than of lowered Sa_{O_2}.

NEUROLEPTANESTHESIA

The designation "neuroleptic" characterizes a drug that reduces motor activity, diminishes anxiety, and produces a state of indifference during which the individual can respond appropriately to command. These substances are also adrenolytic, antiemetic, and antifibrillatory; they block ganglionic transmission and are anticonvulsant as well.

First used in the 1950s, the "lytic cocktail" of Laborit and Huguenard consisted of meperidine, chlorpromazine, and promethazine. This resulted in a form of "neuroplegia," wherein there was major blockade of the autonomic nervous system, which led to marked circulatory depression. When combined with physical cooling, a type of artificial hibernation resulted. The lytic cocktail achieved transient popularity. It was succeeded a decade later by "neuroleptanesthesia," consisting of the intravenous administration of one of the butyrophenone series (similar to the phenothiazine group) and a powerful opioid, either in fixed combination or individually, together with inhalation of nitrous oxide. When the latter is omitted the resulting state is termed neuroleptanalgesia. One ml of the fixed combination called Innovar contains 2.5 mg droperidol (Inapsine) and 0.05 mg of fentanyl (Sublimaze), the former a butyrophenone and the latter an opioid chemically related to meperidine (Fig. 13-3).

PHARMACOLOGIC ACTIONS

Central Nervous System

Droperidol produces marked tranquilization and some amnesia, adding to the effect of other central nervous system depressants, barbiturates, analgetics, anesthetics, and other tranquilizers. Therefore, these compounds should be used in reduced amounts when combined with droperidol. Moderate antiemetic action may last as long as seven hours postinjection. The incidence of extrapyramidal effects consisting of akathisia, dystonia, or parkinsonlike responses has been as low as 1 per cent in adults but up to 15 per cent in children. Such responses may be enhanced in the presence of pyridoxine (vitamin B_6) ingestion.

Fentanyl is a potent analgetic with a brief duration of action, 70 times more potent than morphine. Effects can be seen within four minutes of intravenous injection, with maximal intensity in ten to 15 minutes and duration of satisfactory action from 45 to 60 minutes. Fentanyl has little emetic effect in humans, the incidence being about 3 per cent. Miosis, bradycardia, and bronchoconstriction are also seen.

Respiration

Droperidol has weak respiratory actions, causing a slight reduction in respiratory rate but with a compensating increase in tidal volume. Fentanyl reduces both tidal volume and respiratory rate, and as is the case with all opioids, respiratory depression occurs in equianalgetic doses. The carbon dioxide response curve is shifted to the right, the slope remaining essen-

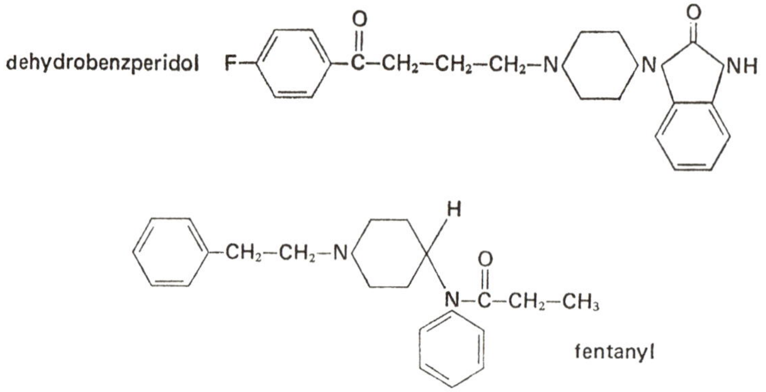

Figure 13-3. Structural formulas of droperidol and fentanyl.

tially unchanged. The effect of droperidol is not additive to that of fentanyl. It is well to remember that the respiratory depressant effect of the combination or of fentanyl alone outlasts that of analgesia, which is of relatively brief duration.

Cardiovascular System

Droperidol causes mild hypotension secondary to alpha-adrenergic blockade and peripheral vasodilation. The threshold to epinephrine-induced arrhythmias is raised by as much as 75 per cent in both dogs and humans. There is little evidence of myocardial depression. Fentanyl in average doses also produces mild hypotension and bradycardia, representing a parasympathomimetic stimulant effect that is blocked by atropine.

Musculoskeletal System

Droperidol has little or no action on this system in man. Fentanyl can produce skeletal muscle rigidity when given in large doses or if given rapidly by vein. Neuromuscular transmission is unaffected and the rigidity can be eliminated by a neuromuscular blocker or an opioid antagonist.

CLINICAL USE

Although respiratory tract secretions are rarely a problem, a belladonna derivative is desirable because of the increased vagal tone induced by the combination of the sympatholytic action of droperidol and the parasympathomimetic stimulant properties of fentanyl. One to 2 ml of Innovar may be given intramuscularly for premedication if sedation is desired. Despite what may appear to be adequate sedation, about 10 per cent of patients complain of restlessness or vague feelings of dysphoria, a reaction often delayed as long as 60 to 90 minutes after administration.

Induction of anesthesia may be accomplished by a slow, continuous intravenous infusion of Innovar, with the calculated dose added to 250 ml of 5 per cent dextrose in water and the drip titrated to the patient's reaction. In general, 1 ml of Innovar per 10 to 15 kg is given, the larger dose used in young, healthier individuals. Care must be taken not to give the induction dose too rapidly lest skeletal muscle rigidity result. To avoid this, many prefer to use droperidol and fentanyl separately, giving the droperidol to produce sedation and allowing for a slower, more controlled injection of the opioid. In either event we recommend individualizing the dose to the patient's requirements. The induction dose is given over a period of five to six minutes. Gradually the patient becomes sleepy, and spontaneous eye closure occurs; the patient may appear to be asleep but still responds to oral commands. As sedation increases respiratory effort decreases, and at times the patient may indeed forget to breathe, but does so if asked to. Oxygen by mask should be given as soon as tidal volume begins to diminish. Cardiovascular signs remain stable as long as the patient is not moved or tilted head up. When patient response becomes markedly depressed, nitrous oxide and oxygen are added and consciousness is rapidly lost.

We must emphasize that the reported cases of cardiac arrest associated with the administration of Innovar have resulted from overdose and lack of recognition of the potential for respiratory and circulatory depression.

If muscle relaxation is needed, any of the neuromuscular blockers can be used. Owing to the long duration of action of droperidol (seven to 12 hours), droperidol or Innovar is rarely given after induction. Supplemental injections of fentanyl are given for any of the following indications: tachycardia, increase in blood pressure, sweating, grimacing, or muscle movement. Early in the course of anesthesia a tracheal tube is poorly tolerated; this can be overcome by topical local anesthesia prior to intubation.

Anesthesia is terminated by discontinuing nitrous oxide and allowing the patient to breathe oxygen first, then room air. As a rule consciousness returns within a few minutes, although amnesia may persist for another 30 to 60 minutes.

POSTOPERATIVE COURSE

A patient who has been anesthetized with Innovar can easily be neglected in the recovery room or on the ward; uncomplaining, his or her condition alternates between being awake and asleep. The patient is easily aroused but not alert, and takes deep breaths or coughs on command. Analgetic requirements in the immediate postoperative period are reduced. This results in part from the sedation of droperidol. Nausea (5 per cent) and vomiting (1 per cent) are uncommon. The chief postoperative complaint is confusion, inability to concentrate, and mental depression. The most annoying consequence is the development of extrapyramidal signs; the incidence is low and control is possible with 0.5 mg of atropine, 25 mg of diphenhydramine (Benadryl), 1 to 2 mg of benztropine (Cogentin), or 1 to 2 mg of physostigmine.

APPRAISAL

Neuroleptanesthesia is a safe, simple technique that has thus far had no demonstrable toxic effects on the liver or kidneys. The cardiovascular system remains stable unless the patient is hypovolemic or change in position occurs. The method has proved useful in aged and poor risk patients. Tracheal intubation using topical anesthesia in the patient with a full stomach is greatly facilitated by the injection of small amounts of Innovar or droperidol. Tranquilization produced by droperidol renders the patient cooperative and receptive to suggestion. The droperidol-fentanyl mixture without nitrous oxide can be used for diagnostic procedures including bronchoscopy, pneumoencephalography, and carotid arteriography, as well as to provide sedation and analgesia for simple surgical procedures such as burn dressings. As with any potent narcotic or tranquilizer that produces marked depression and sedation (unconsciousness with overdosage), the patient must be observed continuously, and the means for providing life support must be at hand.

Drugs other than droperidol and fentanyl have been used for neuroleptanesthesia. Chlorpromazine has proved an unsatisfactory substitute for droperidol in that inadequate sedation is produced. Diazepam, on the other hand, has aroused considerable interest, having the advantages of absence of extrapyramidal tract reactions and distinctly lessening the incidence of dysphoria. Substitutes for fentanyl include alphaprodine (Nisentil), meperidine, pentazocine, and morphine. While muscle rigidity may accompany rapid intravenous administration of single doses of most opioids, the amount necessary to produce that occasionally seen after fentanyl is usually quite high.

DISSOCIATIVE ANESTHESIA

Anesthetic drugs with actions at specific sites in the central nervous system have been sought for a long time as alternatives to the general anesthetics, which have far-reaching effects on the brain. The most successful of these to date has been ketamine (Fig. 13–4), a substance permitting surgical operations on patients who at first glance appear to be awake in that movement may occur and the eyes remain open. So far as recollection or awareness is concerned, however, the individuals are anesthetized.

Ketamine is chemically related to the hallucinogens, so that unpleasant dreams during awakening, not uncommonly extending into the postoperative period, constitute a drawback. Characteristics of ketamine anesthesia include profound analgesia, near normal pharyngeal and laryngeal reflexes,

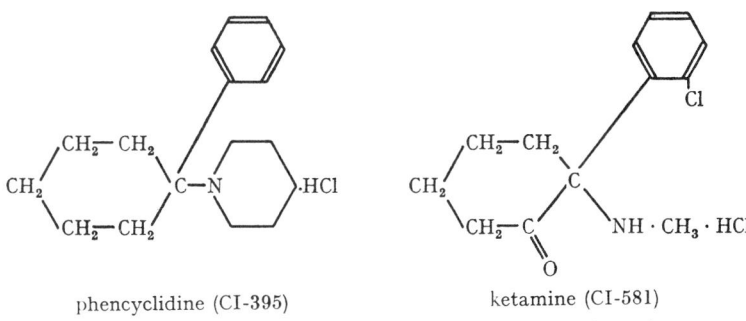

Figure 13–4. Structural formulas of phencyclidine and ketamine.

normal to increased skeletal muscle tone, circulatory stimulation evidenced by hypertension and tachycardia, and an increase in CSF pressure. Some but certainly not all of these are highly desirable effects. The airway is usually easily maintained. Respirations tend to become rapid and shallow for a few minutes after injection but thereafter return to normal. Airway obstruction and severe respiratory depression can occur in all age groups but are most common in the adult, probably representing overdose. In patients with moderate to severe bronchospastic disease, decreases in airway resistance have been demonstrated after ketamine injection. The changes are dose-related, attributed by some to endogenous release of catecholamines. Similar changes are not seen in normal patients.

Current thinking vis-à-vis the mechanism of action of the drug implicates interruption of cerebral association pathways, relative sparing of the reticular activating and limbic systems, and depression of the thalamoneocortical system. Data underlying these assumptions are incomplete, however. The cardiovascular responses, which can be reduced by alpha-adrenergic or sympathetic ganglionic blockade, are thought to be secondary to inhibition of baroreceptor reflexes. It has been shown that myocardial oxygen consumption is increased with ketamine and thus its use in patients with severe coronary artery disease may be inadvisable.

CLINICAL MANAGEMENT

Premedication should include a belladonna drug to reduce salivary secretions. Many believe that an opioid lessens the total dose of ketamine required. Induction via the intravenous route is accomplished with 2 mg ketamine per kg injected over a 60-second period. Within 30 to 40 seconds the patient becomes unconscious and is usually ready for operation. Some individuals show purposeless movements, nystagmus, eye opening, or vocalization. Blood pressure and pulse may rise as little as 10 or as much as 50 per cent. The airway is usually well maintained in children and young adults, but older patients may require airway correction, ranging from elevation of the mandible to placement of an oral airway. Complete airway obstruction is usually indicative of overdose. Maintenance of anesthesia is achieved by repeated injection of 30 to 50 per cent of the induction dose as often as every five to seven minutes. Induction may also be achieved by the intramuscular route. Three to 5 mg per kg are injected, with operation begun within three to five minutes. Maintenance doses are usually given intravenously for better control.

Indications for additional drug are based primarily on the response to surgical stimulation. Movement, however, may occur in response to a stimulus but not of the purposeless type normally seen in some patients given ketamine.

Although the drug produces profound analgesia, it does little to block visceral pain; hence it is not useful for intra-abdominal or intrathoracic procedures unless supplemented by nitrous oxide or other inhalation agents. The increase in muscle tone that results from ketamine requires administration of a neuromuscular blocker when relaxation is needed. Increase in intraocular pressure seen after ketamine is probably the result of increased tone in the extraocular muscles.

POSTOPERATIVE COURSE

Time of recovery from ketamine depends upon the total dose given. An aggregate large dose with repeated injections for maintenance results in a prolonged awakening time. Recovery is frequently complicated by vivid dreams, and in 10 to 15 per cent of patients the dreaming is accompanied by psychomotor activity of varying degree. Such emergence delirium can be terminated by the intravenous injection of thiopental 50 to 75 mg or diazepam 5 to 10 mg. In an effort to decrease emergence phenomena, many anesthetists substitute a tranquilizer for the last ketamine dose or resort to an opioid-tranquilizer combination; recovery is more tranquil but correspondingly prolonged. Skillful neglect, that is, allowing the patient to awaken undisturbed and unstimulated, is also attended by a more peaceful course.

INDICATIONS

Ketamine has proved useful in diagnostic procedures, especially in neuroradiology, as well as for superficial operations of short duration. The compound has found its chief use in the anesthetic management of children and young adults. Finally, it is quite effective as an induction agent for general anesthesia in the poor risk patient and in hypovolemic states.

CONTRAINDICATIONS

Ketamine is contraindicated in patients with hypertension, prior cerebrovascular accident, psychiatric disorders, increased intracranial pressure, and upper respiratory infection, as well as in those who have demonstrated sensitivity to the drug. Some believe that many of the problems seen with ketamine represent overdose; dosage should be based on lean body mass (1.9 mg/kg) rather than on body weight. With this technique, circulatory changes are minimal and emergence delirium is reduced. Others feel strongly that the use of ketamine should be restricted to children and patients under 30 years of age.

Experience with the use of this drug has indeed shown that careful selection of dose and patient results in fewer complications and increases the effectiveness of the agent.

STEROID ANESTHESIA

In 1927 Cashin and Moravek reported that large doses of cholesterol produce general anesthesia, while Hans Selye some 30 years ago found that progesterone, desoxycorticosterone, and pregnanedione also caused general anesthesia. In 1955 hydroxydione (Viadril), a pregnanedione derivative described as endocrinologically inactive, was introduced as an anesthetic; this achieved only modest success, in part because of local irritation upon intravenous injection. The most recent addition consists of a mixture of two pregnanediones (Fig. 13-5). With the mixture (Glaxo CT 1341 – Althesin) anesthesia is characterized by rapid induction, brief duration, and a rapid, clear-headed recovery. At present its prime role is as an alternative to the commonly used intravenous barbiturates but the compound has not been approved for use in the United States.

Since the mechanism of action of commonly used general anesthetics is unknown, it is not surprising that the same is true for the steroids, some of which produce convulsions. We mention this type of compound primarily to indicate the wide spectrum of substances that can produce loss of consciousness and immobility in response to stimuli.

OTHER INTRAVENOUS AGENTS

DIAZEPAM

Diazepam (Valium) (Fig. 13-6) is a tranquilizer of the benzodiazepine series, an anticonvulsant, a muscle relaxant, and an amnesic. The amnesic action is anterograde and involves the input or "consolidation" process rather than retrieval of information.

Diazepam causes slight respiratory depression—chiefly in reduction of tidal volume. Elevations in Pa_{CO_2} have been found but patients are usually capable of adequate respiratory exchange.

Circulatory changes are minimal; the slight fall in blood pressure may

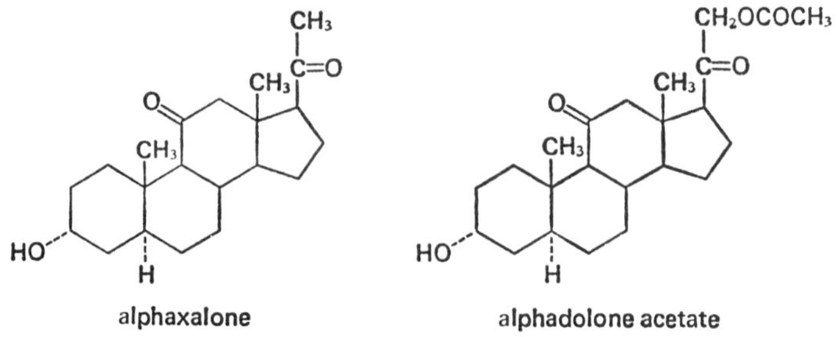

Figure 13-5. Structural formulas of the two steroids constituting Althesin.

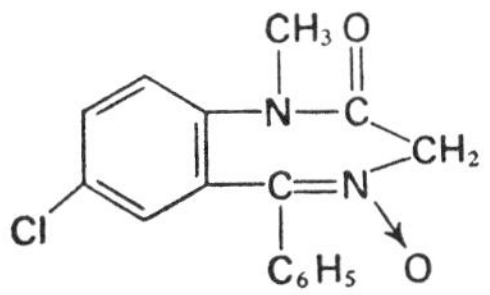

Intravenous Anesthesia

Figure 13-6. Structural formula of diazepam.

be partly or wholly explained by simple sedation. There may also be some direct or reflex vasodilatory effect on the peripheral vessels.

Compared with thiopental for induction, diazepam causes less hypotension and bradycardia. If heart rate and mean aortic pressure are constant, diazepam significantly improves left ventricular function. The mechanism of this effect is unknown, but it may be the result of a decrease in coronary vascular resistance with subsequent increase in coronary artery flow.

Diazepam is a highly effective anticonvulsant drug and good for controlling muscle rigidity and spasm in patients with tetanus and cerebral palsy. This action seems to be at spinal reflex pathways but a more peripheral action also has been implicated. The drug provides useful sedation if the trachea is to be intubated in the awake patient.

MORPHINE

Lowenstein's report in 1969 on the use of large doses of morphine to produce anesthesia for open heart operations triggered a wave of popularity for the technique, still evident today. As experience with the technique accumulated, it was used for all kinds of critically ill patients. Doses ranging from 0.5 to 3.0 mg per kg given intravenously over a 15 to 20 minute period produce unconsciousness and analgesia, which is supplemented by nitrous oxide and a neuromuscular blocker. The drug is usually injected slowly, 10 mg per ml, $1/2$ ml per minute.

Respiratory Effects

All opioids depress respiration as a result of action on the respiratory center in the medulla. Thus the respiratory response to a carbon dioxide challenge is greatly reduced, while the hypoxic drive is enhanced. Death owing to overdose is almost always the result of respiratory arrest.

Circulatory Effects

Cardiac index and stroke volume index increase but total peripheral resistance decreases. The hypotension occasionally seen in the supine position may result from sleep or diminished physical activity; decreased respiratory drive with hypercapnia resulting in peripheral vasodilation; histamine release; and centrally mediated peripheral vasodilation.

The increased capacity of the peripheral venous system reduces venous return to the heart and lowers cardiac output and systemic blood pressure. Elevating the legs and giving intravenous fluids and peripheral vasoconstrictors usually reverse the hypotension. After the initial hypotension, alpha-adrenergic activity is stimulated resulting in increased peripheral resistance and hypertension, which increase the afterload on the heart.

Postoperative Management

The use of large doses of morphine leads to other concerns for the anesthetist. Before the patient becomes unconscious the desire to breathe is lost, necessitating reminders to breathe. Chest wall and cogwheel rigidity occur frequently enough to dictate early use of a neuromuscular blocker followed by tracheal intubation and the addition of nitrous oxide and oxygen. The technique presupposes the use of mechanical ventilation for at least 24 hours, since depression of respiratory drive lasts at least that long after a morphine anesthetic.

The availability of naloxone prompted attempts at "turning off" the morphine after the operation was completed. However, the duration of action of naloxone is much shorter than the respiratory depressant action of morphine. Repeated doses of naloxone are required and constant observation is mandatory. Mechanical ventilatory support is a more practical solution.

PROPANIDID

Eugenol is the chief constituent of oil of cloves and cinnamon leaf oil. Several of the eugenols possess anesthetic properties differing from those used in common practice.

Propanidid (Fig. 13–7) is the only eugenol currently used in anesthetic practice, mostly in Europe. The onset of action is comparable to thiopental or methohexital and may be accompanied by involuntary muscle move-

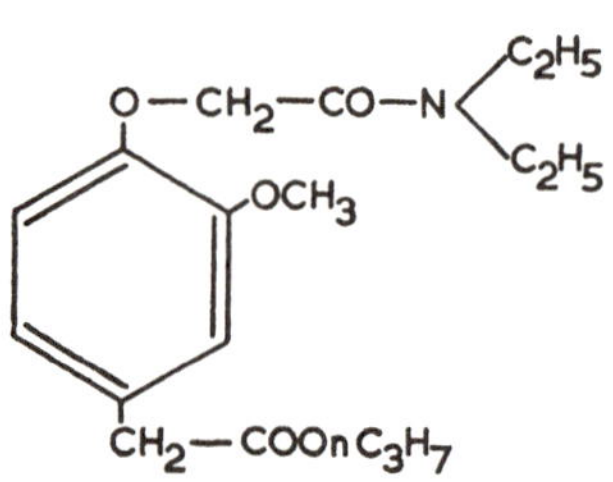

propanidid

Figure 13–7. Structural formula of propanidid.

ments. Recovery is rapid owing to enzymatic breakdown of the compound by plasma pseudocholinesterase.

Profound and precipitous hypotension has followed overdose with propanidid. Hyperventilation is common and may relate to stimulation of the carotid chemoreceptors. The period of apnea that usually follows hyperventilation also appears to be dose-related. Propanidid is not available in the United States.

REFERENCES

Barbiturates

Saidman LJ, Eger EI II: The effect of thiopental metabolism on duration of anesthesia. Anesthesiology 27:118, 1966.

Skovsted P, Price ML, Price HL: The effects of short-acting barbiturates on arterial pressure, preganglionic sympathetic activity and barostatic reflexes. Anesthesiology 33:10, 1970.

Neuroleptics

Corssen G, Domino EF, Sweet RB: Neuroleptanalgesia and anesthesia. Anesth Analg 43: 748, 1964.

Finch JS, DeKornfeld TJ: Clinical investigation of the analgesic potency and respiratory depressant activity of fentanyl, a new narcotic analgesic. J Clin Pharmacol 7:46, 1967.

Martin JS, Murphy JD, Colliton RJ et al: Clinical studies with Innovar. Anesthesiology 28: 458, 1967.

Nilsson E, Janssen P: Neurolept-analgesia – an alternative to general anesthesia. Acta Anaesth Scand 5:73, 1961.

Ketamine

Ferrer-Allado T, Brechner VL, Dymond A et al: Ketamine-induced electroconvulsive phenomena in the human limbic and thalamic regions. Anesthesiology 38:333, 1973.

Huber FC, Reves JG, Gutierrez J, Corssen G: Ketamine: Its effect on airway resistance in man. South Med J 65:1176, 1972.

Lanning CF, Harmel MH: Ketamine anesthesia. Ann Rev Med 26:137, 1975.

Tweed WA, Minuck M, Mymin D: Circulatory responses to ketamine anesthesia. Anesthesiology 37:613, 1972.

Wulfsohn NL: Ketamine dosage for induction based on lean body mass. Anesth Analg 51: 299, 1972.

Steroid Anesthesia

Carson IW: Group trial of althesin as an intravenous anesthetic. Postgrad Med J *Suppl* 2, 48: 108, 1972.

Heuser G: Induction of anesthesia, seizures and sleep by steroid hormones. Anesthesiology 28:173, 1967.

Tammisto T, Takki S, Tigerstedt I, Kauste A: A comparison of althesin and thiopentone in induction of anesthesia. J Anaesth 45:179, 1973.

Diazepam

Abel RM, Staroscik RN, Reis RL: Effects of diazepam (Valium) on left ventricular function and systemic vascular resistance. J Pharmacol Exp Ther 173:364, 1970.

Catchlove R, Kafer E: The effects of diazepam on the ventilatory response to carbon dioxide and on steady state gas exchange. Anesthesiology 34:9, 1971.

Dalen J, Evans G, Banas J: The hemodynamic and respiratory effects of diazepam (Valium). Anesthesiology 30:259, 1969.

Morphine

Johnstone R, Jobes D, Kennell E et al: Reversal of morphine anesthesia with naloxone. Anesthesiology 41:361, 1974.

Lowenstein E: Morphine "anesthesia" – A perspective. Anesthesiology 35:563, 1971.

Lowenstein E, Hallowell P, Levine F et al: Cardiovascular response to large doses of morphine in man. N Engl J Med 281:1389, 1969.

Wong K, Martin W, Hornbein T et al: Cardiovascular effects of morphine sulfate with oxygen and nitrous oxide in man. Anesthesiology 38:542, 1973.

Propanidid

Conway CM, Ellis DB: Propanidid. Br J Anesth 42:249, 1970.

Doenicke A: General pharmacology of propanidid. Acta Anesth Scand (Suppl) 17:21, 1965.

Wyant GM, Zoerb DL: Propanidid–a new nonbarbiturate intravenous anaesthetic. Can Anaesth Soc J 12:569, 1965.

Chapter 14

NEUROMUSCULAR BLOCKING AGENTS

There is more to anesthesia than simply rendering a patient unconscious and free from pain. In order to provide an optimal surgical field, an anesthetist must also control muscle tone. Since one of the major objectives in the use of neuromuscular blocking agents is suppression of muscle tone, a review of these agents is in order.

Skeletal muscle functions most effectively if the resting muscle is not limp, so that when a sudden response is required time is not wasted in taking up the slack. Since a voluntary muscle cell responds in an all-or-none fashion, all the muscle cells cannot be partially activated to produce the background tone. Rather, the motor centers produce a continual random discharge such that only a small fraction of the cells contracts at any moment. It is this background activity that the anesthetist must control to provide convenient access for the surgeon during operation.

One way to suppress tone is to abolish it at its origin with deep anesthesia. However, this has the disadvantage of requiring high concentrations of agents that are far from innocuous. A second option is to block the signals as they traverse the vertebral canal, as is done with spinal and peridural anesthesia. The third approach, that discussed here, became available in 1942 with the introduction by Griffith and Johnson of neuromuscular blockers to clinical anesthesia. These agents, as exemplified by tubocurarine, interfere selectively with the transmission of signals from the motor nerve to the voluntary muscle cell. Their use leads to a division of labor such that the anesthetic need be used only to produce unconsciousness and analgesia and therefore can be administered at lower and safer concentrations. Skeletal muscle contraction can then be controlled separately with a neuromuscular blocker. To use these drugs properly, one must understand how they act.

NEUROMUSCULAR PHARMACOLOGY AND PHYSIOLOGY

In order to understand the mechanisms of action of neuromuscular blockers, one must first appreciate the physiology of the nerve, the muscle, and the neuromuscular junction. This subject is far too extensive for the present discussion, so the reader should review the background elsewhere. The physiology is presented in B. Katz, *Nerve, Muscle and Synapse,* while a recent review by Waud and Waud in the monograph *Muscle Relaxants* introduces the pharmacology. In particular, the reader should be familiar with the following points before proceeding further:

1. The resting membrane of nerve or muscle is polarized with the inside negatively charged. This voltage difference, the "membrane potential," results from the presence of a semipermeable membrane between solutions of different ionic concentrations on the inside and outside of the muscle cell.

2. Excitable membranes may be divided into two classes: those that are electrically excitable, that is, respond to the passage of an electric current outward through the cell membrane, and those that are chemically excitable, that is, respond to the presence of a chemical agent. Chemically excitable membranes are found at the end-plate region of striated muscle, while the remainder of muscle membrane and nerve membrane is electrically excitable.

3. The resting polarized state of an electrically excitable membrane can be altered by application of an electric current. If a positive charge is injected into the cell, the membrane potential rises toward zero and the membrane is said to be depolarized.

4. In an electrically excitable membrane, small depolarizations can be graded. However, as the stimulus increases, a degree of depolarization is reached ("threshold") that creates an all-or-none process ("action potential"). The nature of the underlying mechanism is such that not only is the internal negativity abolished, but the membrane actually reverses polarity so that the inside of the cell becomes positive ("overshoot").

5. The electric charge associated with the passage of an impulse along a nerve or muscle is self-propagating. Movement of Na^+ across the membrane produces a flow of positive charges into the cell. Since charges cannot accumulate at one point, the positive current flows along the core of the nerve or muscle cell and then outward through an adjacent part of the membrane ("local action current"). This outward current is the electric stimulation needed to depolarize the adjacent membrane. Thus the process is propagated along the cell.

6. Electrically excitable membranes show "accommodation." Normally, the stimulus activating a nerve or muscle membrane is a pulse that results in a single action potential. If, however, the stimulus is a steady current, an action potential can be recorded only when the stimulus is first applied. Although the current continues to flow through the membrane, further activity in the membrane cannot be seen, even when a stronger stimulus is applied. In other words, the electrically excitable membrane becomes inexcitable in the presence of a steady depolarization.

7. Chemically excitable membranes are activated by compounds typically bearing positively charged quaternary nitrogen groups. When exposed

to these compounds, the membrane potential shifts in a positive direction. However, in contrast to the electrically excitable membrane, the chemically excitable membrane does not reverse its potential, but seeks a level at which the inside is still slightly negative. Also, the response of the chemically excitable membrane is continuously graded and not an all-or-none process.

8. Just as the electrically excitable membrane behaves differently when a prolonged stimulus is applied, so, too, does the chemically excitable membrane. Prolonged application of an agonist is associated with a decreased degree of depolarization ("desensitization"). Note, however, that the time scale is quite different. Accommodation can appear within the duration of a single action potential, that is within milliseconds, whereas desensitization may take hours to develop.

Accommodation and desensitization appear to underlie the two types of neuromuscular blocks seen with depolarizing blockers.

9. Within the axon the combination of choline and acetate, catalyzed by choline acetylase, forms acetylcholine, which is stored in vesicles in the nerve terminals as a readily available store and a more slowly mobilized reserve supply. When a nerve action potential reaches the nerve ending, the electric charge releases calcium inside the nerve ending with the result that the stored transmitter is released into the synaptic cleft—the area between the nerve ending and the end-plate region of muscle.

10. The released transmitter reacts with specialized sites ("receptors") on the end-plate region of muscle membrane, leading to depolarization of the end plate ("end-plate potential").

11. Released acetylcholine is eliminated both by diffusion away from the end-plate region and by enzymatic destruction by cholinesterase, which is located around the synaptic cleft.

A useful and convenient frame of reference when examining neuromuscular transmission is shown in Table 14–1. The table indicates the sites of action of various classes of agents that interfere with the whole signalling system. We shall focus here on the neuromuscular blockers proper, that is, those drugs reacting directly with the postsynaptic receptor for the transmitter. Muscle relaxation can result from interference at any of the steps along the motor pathway.

Neuromuscular blockers are divided into two groups: those that combine with the acetylcholine receptor and cause depolarization of the end-plate region—the depolarizing agents—and those that combine with the acetylcholine receptor to prevent depolarization—the competitive agents.

ACTION OF DEPOLARIZING AGENTS

This group includes succinylcholine (Anectine, Quelicin) and decamethonium. Depolarizing blockers exhibit two phases of action; each of these is discussed in turn.

Table 14-1. SITES OF ACTION OF CHEMICAL COMPOUNDS THAT AFFECT NEUROMUSCULAR TRANSMISSION

Physiologic Process	Blocking Agents
Initiation of signal in CNS	Volatile anesthetics
Nerve action potential	Volatile anesthetics Local anesthetics
Acetylcholine release	Hemicholinium Antibiotics Botulinum toxin
Acetylcholine-receptor combination	d-Tubocurarine Pancuronium Gallamine
Depolarization of end-plate	Volatile anesthetics
Muscle action potential	Succinylcholine* Decamethonium* Local anesthetics Volatile anesthetics Tetrodotoxin
Muscle contraction	Calcium chelating agents

*The assignment of succinylcholine and decamethonium reflects the fact that, although both drugs act at the acetylcholine receptor, the actual block of neuromuscular transmission is the result of accommodation of the electrically excitable membrane around the end plate.

PHASE I BLOCK

Depolarizing neuromuscular blockers have the same action at the neuromuscular junction as acetylcholine, that is, they react with the receptors at the end-plate region of muscle and lead to depolarization of the chemically excitable membrane. Depolarization of the end plate, in turn, leads to local action currents that spread to and depolarize the adjacent electrically excitable membrane, thus causing muscle contraction. Clinically this is seen as fasciculation, an uncoordinated contraction of muscles, a phenomenon that may cause the patient to complain of stiff, sore muscles in the postoperative period. Because succinylcholine and decamethonium are not as rapidly eliminated as acetylcholine, depolarization of the end-plate region persists. Unlike a brief stimulus, continuous passage of local action currents leads to inexcitability in the electrically excitable muscle membrane adjacent to the end plate. Neuromuscular block ensues. The block is not at the end plate but rather in the area of the electrically excitable membrane around the end plate.

PHASE II BLOCK

M. Zaimis first showed that with time, the neuromuscular block produced by decamethonium changes its characteristics. For example, a tetanus became less well sustained, and the block could be antagonized rather than aggravated by neostigmine. The depolarizing agents were said to have "changed their mode of action," to have a "dual mode of action," or to have passed into phase II block. Speculation as to the nature of this change has been considerable.

What is known about the changing action of depolarizing agents? As a starting point, remember that the action of depolarizing agents is to depolarize the end plate. Muscle contraction, or muscle block, or both are secondary effects resulting from the depolarization. If we focus on the depolarizing effects of these agents, we find that although stable drugs can produce a depolarization that is prolonged, the effect is not of infinite duration. This reduction of depolarization that occurs with prolonged exposure is called "desensitization," and the degree of reduced effect and the duration of exposure needed to bring it about vary among animal species and muscle groups.

Next, if we compare the relationship between depolarization and twitch response, we find that, with repeated exposure to a depolarizing drug, less and less depolarization is needed to cause complete block (Fig. 14–1) until finally, exposure to the drug causes complete block without any depolarization. Thus, with time, something other than depolarization must be responsible for the block. The actual cause is unknown. There is, however, no reason to consider phase II block to be competitive in nature.

In summary, we can only say that phase II block exists, it is associated with a reduced contribution of depolarization to the block, and it occurs in situations such as prolonged or repeated exposures that predispose to desensitization. There appears to be no close relationship between the degree of phase II block and indices that can be measured clinically such as tetanic fade or posttetanic facilitation (see comments in connection with monitoring, pages 210 et seq.).

ACTION OF COMPETITIVE AGENTS

This group includes tubocurarine, dimethyltubocurarine (Metubine), gallamine (Flaxedil), and pancuronium (Pavulon). These drugs combine with acetylcholine receptors but do not activate them. However, their presence on the receptor prevents access of the transmitter. The larger the dose of blocking agent, the more receptors occluded and the fewer receptors available for reaction with the transmitter. Decreasing the receptors available to acetylcholine progressively reduces the height of the end-plate potential until it no longer reaches threshold for excitation of the adjacent electrically excitable muscle membrane; neuromuscular block ensues.

What fraction of the receptors must be blocked before neuromuscular transmission fails? On teleologic grounds one would expect that more acetylcholine receptors are available than are necessary barely to initiate an action potential in the muscle membrane; that is, that there would be a

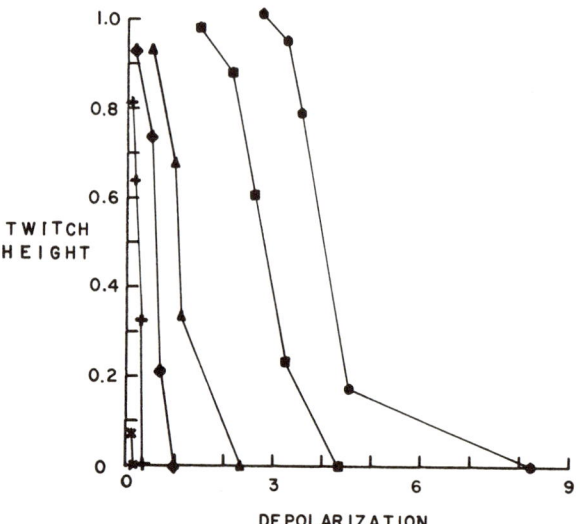

Figure 14-1. Changing mode of action of succinylcholine. Measurements from the dog tibialis anticus muscle. Ordinates: strength of muscle twitch in response to a single shock applied to the motor nerve (relative to control response). Abscissae: intensity of depolarization of end-plate region (millivolts, recorded with external electrodes). Single doses of succinylcholine 0.1 mg/kg were given at half-hourly intervals. During onset and offset of neuromuscular block a series of paired observations of twitch response and depolarization was made. For simplicity, only the recovery limbs are presented. The righthand curve (*full circles*) was obtained with the first injection. Note that about 8 mv of depolarization produced complete block. As the depolarization fell, the twitch gradually recovered. This is the typical picture of depolarization block. The remaining five curves were obtained following the second, fourth, sixth, eighth, and tenth injections. Note that with each succeeding dose, progressively less depolarization is associated with block, until at the last dose, complete block was associated with a barely measurable electrical effect, that is, something other than depolarization was producing the block. The shift from the first to the last curve illustrates the development of phase II block.

margin of safety. Figure 14-2 shows the experimentally observed relationship between the fraction of receptors blocked and the twitch response following motor nerve stimulation. It can be seen that until 75 to 80 per cent of the receptors are blocked, no interference with the twitch response can be measured, and that transmission fails in all fibers when 90 to 95 per cent of the receptors are occluded. In other words, the more resistant fibers respond with less than one tenth of the receptor pool available, and all fibers function when only one fifth to one fourth of the receptors are free. As was expected, there is a large margin of safety in neuromuscular transmission.

Clinically, we may view the action of competitive antagonists as resembling an iceberg (Fig. 14-3). Because most of the receptors must be blocked before there is any decrease in twitch response, the first dose of an agent must be a relatively large one. The anesthetist works at the top 20 to 25 per cent of the iceberg, and it is only this small fraction of receptors

Neuromuscular Blocking Agents

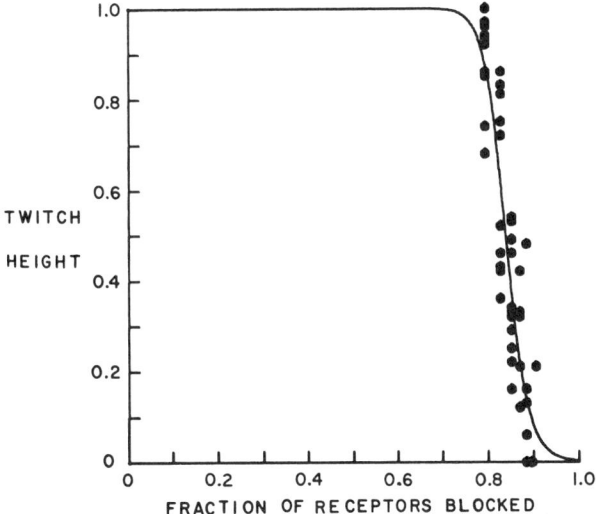

Figure 14-2. Illustration of the margin of safety of neuromuscular transmission. Ordinates: fractional twitch height. Abscissae: fraction of receptors blocked by tubocurarine. Note that neuromuscular transmission is normal until about 80 per cent of the receptors have been blocked, while 90 per cent must be occluded before the most resistant fibers fail. (The reader will note a family resemblance of Figure 14-1 to Figures 14-2, 14-3, 14-4, and 14-5. This reflects the fact that response of a muscle to nerve stimulation represents the standard measure of neuromuscular transmission, while intensity of depolarization (Figure 14-1) or receptor blockade (Figures 14-2, 14-4, 14-5) represent the direct effect of depolarizing and competitive agents, respectively.)

that must be reblocked as the antagonist is eliminated. Subsequent doses, therefore, are smaller. The problems of surveying the bottom of the iceberg will be considered later.

The preceding description of the postsynaptic action of neuromuscular blocking agents is the classic view. Another opinion holds that these drugs exert some or most of their effect presynaptically, that is, at the nerve endings. It is possible, however, to explain the initiation of presynaptic effects by the action of a drug acting postsynaptically. Also, drugs such as tubocurarine display the kinetics compatible with competitive antagonism. The question might then be "are the acetylcholine receptors presynaptic or postsynaptic?" Recently, it has become possible to separate the nerve endings from the end-plate region. By doing so, Kuffler has been able to show that acetylcholine receptors are situated primarily in the postsynaptic membrane of the end-plate region. Thus, presynaptic events are at most a side issue in the action of neuromuscular blocking agents.

EFFECTS ON OTHER ORGANS

Although neuromuscular blockers are reasonably specific in their action, there are some side effects that deserve mention.

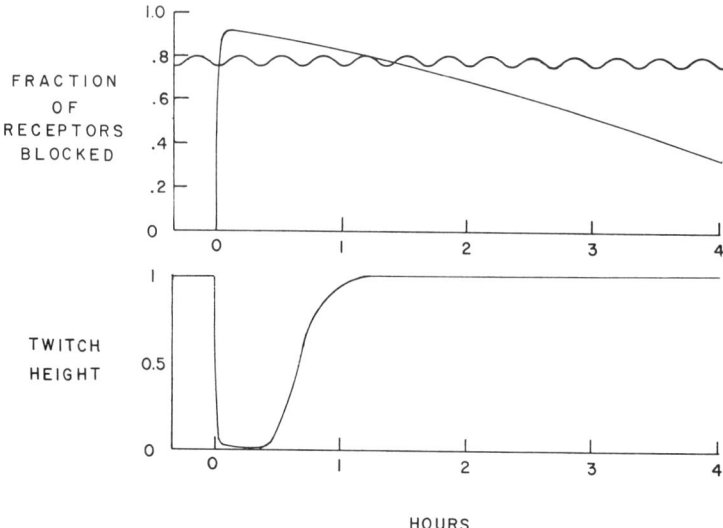

Figure 14-3. Diagrammatic representation of events during administration of a single dose of tubocurarine sufficient to produce maximal or near maximal relaxation at its peak effect. *Top:* Calculated fraction of receptors blocked as a function of time. As drug concentration rises in the muscle, receptors are quickly blocked; then, as the drug is slowly eliminated (*concentration* falls with a half-life of one hour), receptors gradually become free. *Bottom:* Corresponding twitch response calculated on the basis of results such as those in Figure 14-2, that is, when receptor occupancy reaches 75 to 80 per cent the twitch begins to fall, and by 90 per cent receptor occlusion, the twitch is essentially abolished. As receptors again become free, the twitch response recovers and returns to normal when the receptor occupancy has fallen to 75 to 80 per cent. Note that the twitch response reflects only changes in receptor occlusion that occur above the 75 to 80 per cent level (*wavy line*). Thus monitoring the twitch allows one to examine only the tip of the iceberg, above this level.

SUCCINYLCHOLINE

In addition to its effect at the neuromuscular junction, succinylcholine displays, to some extent, the actions of acetylcholine at other receptor sites. Thus, a patient may develop hypertension and tachycardia from stimulation of autonomic ganglia, or bradycardia, salivation, and increased bronchial secretions from a muscarinic action. These effects are more common upon repeated intravenous injection and are seen most frequently in children. Incidents of cardiac arrest have been reported. The decreased heart rate following a second dose of succinylcholine may be attenuated by the prior administration of atropine, tubocurarine, or pancuronium. It has been suggested that the bradycardia results from a reflex response of the autonomic nervous system or from sensitization of the heart by the metabolic products of succinylcholine (succinylmonocholine or choline). Neither of these hypotheses has been verified.

Depolarizing agents can increase intraocular pressure, an effect usually attributed to contracture of the extraocular muscles. Extraocular muscles have many end-plate regions per muscle fiber. The distribution of chemically excitable muscle membrane all along the muscle fiber leads to a generalized depolarization of the muscle membrane by passive electrotonic spread. Contraction of these muscles, then, can occur without the presence of an action potential. Katz and Eakins have shown that in cats an increase in intraocular pressure occurs after the extraocular muscles have been cut, and they believe that contraction of the smooth muscles of the orbit is also involved. In any case, since the duration of the increase in intraocular pressure is brief following a single dose of succinylcholine, there seems to be no contraindication to its use for endotracheal intubation in patients with glaucoma. Succinylcholine should not be used, however, in patients with penetrating eye wounds, when even a transient increase in intraocular pressure could lead to loss of vitreous humor.

It is generally believed that depolarizing agents, by causing fasciculation of the abdominal muscles, can produce an increase in intragastric pressure sufficient to open the gastroesophageal sphincter. Miller and Way showed that the rise in pressure is proportional to the intensity of fasciculations. This phenomenon becomes important in patients who are in danger of aspirating gastric contents. The succinylcholine-induced increase in intragastric pressure may be diminished by the prior administration of a small dose of a competitive agent (for example, 3 mg tubocurarine).

A common complaint from patients who have received a depolarizing agent is muscle pain. This problem occurs most frequently in young patients who undergo minor operations and early ambulation. Although occurrence of pain cannot be related to the degree of fasciculation observed, most investigators believe that uncoordinated muscle contraction is the cause. Suggested mechanisms of the pain include local damage to muscle fibers, damage to muscle spindles, lactic acid production, and potassium flux. Fasciculation and the ensuing muscle pain can be eliminated by prior administration of a competitive agent.

TUBOCURARINE

The most common side effect of tubocurarine is a dose-related fall in arterial pressure. Although the cause of the hypotension is still controversial, the two mechanisms most frequently suggested are ganglionic block and histamine release. Tubocurarine is an active ganglionic blocking agent. However, because its potency at the neuromuscular junction is greater than at the ganglia, there is some doubt that a clinical concentration of tubocurarine is sufficient to cause hypotension. Tubocurarine certainly liberates histamine in experimental animals. There is no convincing evidence, however, that histamine is the cause of hypotension in humans. In any case, if a patient is already hypotensive, or if hypotension may become a problem, an anesthetist should consider using another blocking agent.

Histamine release has also been blamed for bronchospasm following administration of tubocurarine. Again, no direct proof has been shown. It is difficult, as well, to determine from clinical reports whether the bronchospasm in question is even the result of tubocurarine administration, as opposed to some other factor such as light anesthesia. The possibility of bronchospasm is not of major importance in the choice of blocking agent.

GALLAMINE

Gallamine causes tachycardia and an increase in arterial pressure. The tachycardia has been attributed to a combination of vagolytic effect and a tyraminelike effect whereby norepinephrine is released from sympathetic nerve endings. Another neuromuscular blocking agent would be preferable in the presence of tachycardia and hypertension.

PANCURONIUM

Pancuronium also causes an increase in arterial pressure and heart rate, although both effects are less pronounced than those seen with gallamine. The mechanism has not been clearly explained.

UPTAKE, DISTRIBUTION, AND ELIMINATION

The uptake and distribution of the neuromuscular blockers are not remarkable; they behave according to the general principles of pharmacokinetics. The easiest way to approach the matter is to consider first the simplest case and then superimpose any perturbations relevant to each specific agent. Decamethonium, which is not metabolized, is a good model. Thus one starts by picturing a charged compound, not metabolized and restricted to the extracellular space. Since the neuromuscular blockers are typically administered by rapid intravenous injection, their kinetics can be subdivided into two phases: that of redistribution and that of elimination.

REDISTRIBUTION

Immediately after injection, there is a high local concentration in venous blood flowing from the site of injection toward the heart. As this blood mixes with blood returning from other parts of the body, the drug is diluted. Passage through the lung spreads the drug through a still greater volume. Next the already somewhat attenuated bolus is swept out to the various tissues and the drug begins to be mixed throughout the entire extracellular space. During this period, the concentration in the arterial flow to muscle exceeds the concentration in the extracellular space around the end-plate region of muscle, so the drug diffuses from muscle capillaries to the site of action. While general redistribution from plasma to extracellular space can take a considerable time, particularly in poorly perfused tissues, it is essentially over in about ten minutes as far as the muscle end plate is concerned. After this time, the end-plate concentration follows the plasma concentration closely. Thus, to picture the further course of the concentration at the end plate, we need only follow the plasma concentration. This brings us to the second phase of the distributional process.

ELIMINATION

The course of subsequent events can be deduced easily for the charged, unmetabolized drug. The major portal of exit is the kidney. Every minute, the glomeruli filter 120 ml of plasma, that is, 120 ml of extracellular fluid are put into the renal tubules. Since all the drugs used as clinical neuromuscular blocking agents carry a permanent charge, they cannot diffuse back across the renal tubular membrane and hence are eliminated in the urine. Thus, the 12 L of extracellular space through which the drug is distributed are cleared of drug at a rate of 120 ml or 1 per cent per minute. This amounts to saying that the extracellular concentration will fall with a half-life of a little over an hour. (If the concentration fell linearly at the rate of 1 per cent per minute, then it would fall 50 per cent in 50 minutes and the half-life would be 50 minutes. However, as the elimination proceeds, each 120 ml of glomerular filtrate contains progressively less drug, and the rate at which the concentration falls slows with time; that is, the concentration falls exponentially. The effect of this is to make the half-life longer than 50 minutes. The actual theoretic value works out to be 69.3 minutes.)

In summary then, the basic picture is a concentration at the site of action which rises for about ten minutes, levels off, and passes into an exponential decay with a half-life of a little over an hour. Variants can now be superimposed on this scheme.

BINDING TO PLASMA PROTEINS

At clinical concentrations, about half of tubocurarine in plasma is bound to plasma proteins. The effect of this is to make the plasma volume appear twice as big as it is, and thus the drug appears to be distributed through more than 12 L. The exponential elimination might be expected to be slowed slightly, but hardly enough to be perceptible clinically. The binding of pancuronium (about 20 per cent) and gallamine is so low as to have a negligible effect on the kinetics.

METABOLISM

If the drug is metabolized, then the rate of elimination will be accelerated. Metabolism appears to be negligible with gallamine, tubocurarine, and decamethonium. Pancuronium is deacetylated at either the 3 position, the 17 position, or both, to give metabolites, two of which show neuromuscular blocking activity. To further complicate the picture, the extent of any of the reactions involved is not known in humans. However, the metabolism does appear to contribute to the elimination of pancuronium, that is, its half-life appears to be on the short side of an hour. Succinylcholine is metabolized extremely rapidly to succinylmonocholine and choline (see further on).

BILIARY EXCRETION

Tubocurarine but not gallamine is excreted through the bile. This feature may appear trivial until a patient with no renal function is concerned. In such an individual, the half-life of tubocurarine will be greatly prolonged, but eventually the drug will be eliminated. On the other hand, the effect of gallamine can last so long that artificial dialysis may be required.

ULTRARAPID ONSET OF ACTION

A good example of very rapid onset of action is succinylcholine, which has already been noted to undergo rapid metabolic destruction. This implies a brief duration of action, but the clinical significance relates not so much to rapid *offset* as to rapid *onset,* which facilitates rapid endotracheal intubation and therefore minimizes the interval during which a patient is unconscious with an unprotected airway. This feature gives succinylcholine its prominent position in anesthesia. That rapid destruction should imply rapid onset of action may at first appear to represent a paradox. However, on reflection it may be seen that this trick has a biologic basis. Cholinesterase, which accelerates destruction of the transmitter, is placed at nerve endings to permit faster transmission of the signal. To get a rapid onset of action, one can give an overdose and get away with it if the drug is rapidly destroyed. Thus, in the usual clinical setting, when an intravenous bolus of succinylcholine is injected, an intentional overdose is given to achieve a rapid onset with the expectation of rapid curtailment of drug action by plasma cholinesterase.

This brings us to another peculiarity relevant to the pharmacokinetics of succinylcholine. Rarely, patients have an atypical pseudocholinesterase. In these individuals the overdose aspect is prominent since the drug effect is not abbreviated by rapid metabolism. Thus one ends up with "prolonged apnea"—a direct expression of overdose. The genetic aspects and diagnosis of this condition are discussed further on.

PLACENTAL TRANSFER

While this can have little effect on duration of action in the mother, it might have important implications for the newborn's ability to breathe. However, neuromuscular blockers do not appear to cross the placenta in significant amounts.

FACTORS INFLUENCING ACTION OF NEUROMUSCULAR BLOCKERS

ABNORMAL PSEUDOCHOLINESTERASE ACTIVITY

Genetic. Under normal conditions, succinylcholine is metabolized by serum cholinesterase to succinylmonocholine and choline. Serum cholinesterase is determined genetically by allelic genes, four of which have been identified: the normal (N), the dibucaine-resistant (D), the fluoride-resistant (F), and the silent (S). These four genes can combine to form ten genotypes; of these, six (D-D, F-F, S-S, D-F, D-S, F-S) show a marked decrease in their ability to metabolize succinylcholine. An individual with such a genetic makeup will show a greatly prolonged effect from succinylcholine — the "overdose" mentioned previously. There is no danger to the patient as long as the condition is recognized and proper care instituted. The best treatment is controlled ventilation until the drug is eliminated.

Acquired

LIVER DISEASE. Serum cholinesterase is synthesized in the liver. Foldes has shown that even moderate liver disease can reduce serum cholinesterase by 50 per cent and double the duration of action of succinylcholine.

ORGANOPHOSPHOROUS COMPOUNDS. Organophosphorous compounds such as echothiophate are irreversible cholinesterase inhibitors used as eye drops for the treatment of glaucoma. Systemic absorption has been shown to decrease cholinesterase activity significantly and prolonged responses to succinylcholine have been reported.

SYSTEMIC DISEASES

Patients with myasthenia gravis are markedly sensitive to the actions of competitive agents. Depolarizing agents can be used, but tend to reach phase II sooner than in normal individuals. The "myasthenic" syndrome associated with small-cell carcinoma of the lung (Lambert-Eaton syndrome) is also associated with increased sensitivity to both depolarizing and nondepolarizing agents. Although in theory one could handle the increased sensitivity to blocking agents by scaling down the dose, in practice, the nature of myasthenia is such that a blocker is seldom necessary and if possible should be avoided.

Patients with myotonia congenita and myotonia dystrophica respond to depolarizing agents with muscle contracture rather than relaxation. The muscle spasm may be so intense that ventilation, either spontaneous or controlled, is impossible. The mechanism is not known.

Depolarizing neuromuscular blockers cause an increase in serum potassium of about 0.5 mEq per L in normal individuals. However, in patients with burns, massive trauma, tetanus, injury to the central nervous system, or lower motor neuron lesions, the serum potassium elevation is greatly exaggerated and may lead to cardiac arrest. It is unknown whether this increased release of potassium associated with depolarization is caused by injury to the muscle membrane or is the result of an increase in the extent of chemically excitable membrane similar to that seen following chronic denervation. The period of greatest risk lasts from a few days to six months following the injury. The exaggerated potassium release may be diminished by prior administration of a competitive antagonist, but the effect is not predictable. It is therefore wiser to avoid depolarizing agents entirely in such patients.

Individuals with renal failure obviously should not be given drugs such as decamethonium or gallamine that are eliminated solely via the kidneys. Other agents such as tubocurarine and pancuronium may be used safely if it is remembered that the half-life will be prolonged.

ANTIBIOTICS

Antibiotics like streptomycin, neomycin, polymyxin A and B, gentamicin, kanamycin, colistin, and lincomycin have neuromuscular blocking effects that are synergistic with both depolarizing and nondepolarizing neuromuscular blockers. The mechanism appears to be presynaptic. Patients receiving these drugs may be considered to have a reduced margin of safety.

OTHER DRUGS

Drugs other than antibiotics that patients may be taking and that may increase the effect of neuromuscular blockers include ganglionic blocking agents, cholinesterase inhibitors, local anesthetics, and antiarrhythmic drugs (quinidine, procainamide, and phenytoin).

ACID-BASE BALANCE

There is an extensive literature concerning the effect of acid-base balance on the potency of neuromuscular blockers. Investigators differ in their opinions and in the design of their experiments. Also, it is not known whether differences in the extent of neuromuscular block are the result of pH changes *per se* or of alterations caused by acid-base imbalance (e.g., changes in blood flow, serum electrolytes, or protein binding).

TEMPERATURE

Classically, lowering the temperature is said to strengthen a depolarizing block and to antagonize a competitive block. Recently the latter response has been questioned by investigators who have shown that tubocurarine induced neuromuscular block is also enhanced by hypothermia.

INHALATION ANESTHETICS

All the inhalation anesthetics increase the effects of neuromuscular blockers. As suggested by Table 14-1, the possible sites of action are numerous. In clinical concentrations, general anesthetics do not depress nerve conduction nor do they interfere with the acetylcholine-receptor combination. Some anesthetics, cyclopropane, for example, have been shown to have an effect on the motor nerve terminals, but the importance of this on muscle relaxation is unknown. Volatile anesthetics have been shown to increase the twitch response to both direct and indirect stimulation—if anything, an "antirelaxant" effect. Inhalation anesthetics have their greatest effect at synapses. In this regard, their effect on spinal cord motor neurons and the neuromuscular junction appears to be similar.

At the neuromuscular junction the volatile anesthetics halothane, isoflurane, methoxyflurane, diethyl ether, fluroxene, and enflurane depress chemically-induced depolarization of the end-plate region. Unlike neuromuscular blockers which depress depolarization by combining with the acetylcholine receptor, the action of volatile anesthetics is on the muscle membrane distal to the receptor. The higher the anesthetic concentration, the greater is the depression of depolarization. Only when depolarization is depressed by 50 per cent (2.5 to 3.0 MAC) does the indirectly stimulated twitch response begin to fall.

The effects of general anesthetics and of competitive neuromuscular blockers on depolarization reinforce each other. Thus it is possible to use enflurane and tubocurarine, for example, in concentrations that by themselves have no effect on twitch response but in combination cause complete neuromuscular block. Effectively, the action of inhalation anesthetics is to decrease the margin of safety of neuromuscular blockers (Fig. 14-4). The extent of such a decrease depends on the anesthetic used. Halothane has the least effect and enflurane the greatest.

SUMMARY

The preceding list of factors influencing the action of neuromuscular blockers includes problems that vary widely in clinical significance. The effect of myasthenia gravis, for example, can be so marked that no additional relaxation is needed, whereas at the other end of the scale one encounters entities such as temperature, which is still controversial even as to the direction of the shift! When the problem is clear-cut, the solution is obvious; for example, avoid depolarizing agents in situations in which exaggerated potassium release might be expected. On the other hand, the effects of acid-base balance, temperature, and drug interaction are of the same order of magnitude as random patient to patient variation and can be approached in the same way. Thus one should not give "cookbook doses" of blocking agents but rather should titrate the drugs against the patient's response, as described further on.

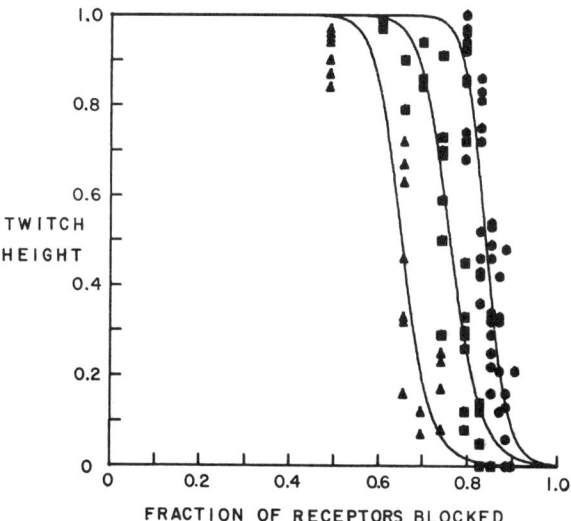

Figure 14-4. Effect of volatile anesthetics on the margin of safety of neuromuscular transmission. Plot as in Figure 14-2. Righthand curve (*circles*), no anesthetic present. Middle curve (*squares*), halothane (0.75 per cent). Lefthand curve (*triangles*), enflurane (1.68 per cent).

CLINICAL USE OF NEUROMUSCULAR BLOCKERS

Patients show marked variation in their responses to both depolarizing and nondepolarizing blockers, regardless of whether the dose is calculated in mg per kg or mg per sq m of body surface. It is wise, therefore to use a monitoring device such as a peripheral nerve stimulator (see further on) to determine the effect of the blocking agent used, and to titrate the drug against the response of the patient. R. Katz showed that 7 per cent of patients who received 0.1 mg per kg tubocurarine showed complete depression of twitch response; therefore this dose is a good place to start. Comparable doses of gallamine and pancuronium would be 0.6 mg per kg and 0.02 mg per kg, respectively. Depending on the effect of this dose, the inhalation agent used, and the kind and duration of operation, an additional dose is given. Ninety per cent twitch depression is adequate for most operations.

Succinylcholine is most commonly used for tracheal intubation. Although 0.5 mg per kg is sufficient to cause complete neuromuscular block in most individuals, the duration of block is short. The extra time gained by using 1.0 mg per kg may be useful and is far safer than repeating the original dose (see earlier).

ASSESSMENT OF DEPTH OF NEUROMUSCULAR BLOCK

There are two situations in which one needs to know the level of neuromuscular block: (1) Is the patient relaxed enough for operation? (2)

Has the patient recovered safely? A large number of indices have been used to answer one or the other of these questions. A brief list is useful.

The first group of indices involves direct measurements which, however, require specialized apparatus. The common feature is application of electric shocks to a motor nerve and observation or recording of the resultant muscular response. The simplest example is application of single shocks to the ulnar nerve every few seconds, with monitoring of the resultant flexion of the fourth and fifth digits. (The electric activity of muscle also has been used as a measure of muscle response. However, it is hard to see any advantage over the simpler twitch response.) This particular index corresponds exactly to the physiologist's standard neuromuscular preparation. Thus the response can be interpreted directly in the framework of Figure 14–2. When the twitch is completely or almost completely abolished, the degree of relaxation is suitable for the operation. Similarly, during recovery, when the simple twitch response has returned to normal, one can say that 20 per cent of the receptor pool is free. Fortunately, the diaphragm needs fewer receptors available to respond normally than do peripheral muscles. This is borne out clinically in that spontaneous respiration may be detected before an indirectly stimulated twitch response. However, a patient with 80 per cent receptor block may still be in a precarious position. Thus it is important to have a means of assessing when recovery has proceeded to a more adequate level. To this end, variants on the single shock have evolved. The simplest involves administration of a series of shocks at 30, 50, and 100 Hz. The rationale is that a tetanic response puts a greater demand on the neuromuscular synapse. As each successive stimulus arrives at the nerve ending, it depletes the local store of transmitter so that the amount of acetylcholine available for release by each succeeding stimulus falls. When the fraction of free receptors is also decreased, the tetanic response does not maintain its initial intensity; it fades. Thus the margin of safety is reduced for tetanic stimuli.

The higher the rate of stimulation, the greater the proportion of the receptor pool that must be free before a tetanic response does not fade. Unfortunately, the patient who has recovered to the level that could be examined with a tetanus is often conscious. Because production of a tetanic response can be painful, especially at the higher frequencies that yield the most information, tetanic stimulation has not proved very practical clinically. An attempt to avoid this impasse led to the introduction of the "train-of-four" approach. In this test, the ulnar nerve is stimulated with four supramaximal stimuli 0.5 seconds apart, and the ratio of the fourth twitch to the first twitch is used to determine the degree of neuromuscular block. The procedure has two advantages: it is not painful, and the first response in the train provides a built-in control for the fourth response. This is a great convenience in the clinical situation in which factors such as patient movement can change the initial tension of the muscle and hence the size of the twitch response. Unfortunately, the claim that the "train-of-four" can probe recovery much further than the single twitch does not stand up to direct measurement (see Fig. 14–5). Nevertheless, the built-in control provided by comparison of the initial and final twitches in the train makes the approach attractive.

A few comments are in order regarding determination of the nature of the block, a subject related to assessment of recovery. In this connection two phenomena may be mentioned: tetanic fade and post-tetanic facilitation (PTF). Tetanic fade has already been discussed. In the case of competitive block, the underlying mechanism is a progressive depletion of the transmitter stores. In PTF, the first twitches following a tetanus are larger than those immediately preceding it. The mechanism appears to reflect cumulation of calcium ions in the nerve terminal during the tetanus. However, this may not be the whole story or even the principal cause. The important point is that PTF itself, and in particular its relationship to neuromuscular block, is not well understood and therefore does not provide a firm basis for interpretation of mechanisms. Unfortunately, PTF is often overworked or overinterpreted. This frequently applies as well to tetanic fade. But a few words of caution are in order. Typically, the indices are used to determine the nature of a neuromuscular block. Thus one encounters claims that a tetanus is sustained during depolarizing block, whereas it fades during phase II block. However, in well-controlled experimental situations, all possible combinations of fading and sustained tetani and phase I and phase II blocks may be demonstrated. Thus the extent of fade should not be considered a reliable index of the nature of the block.

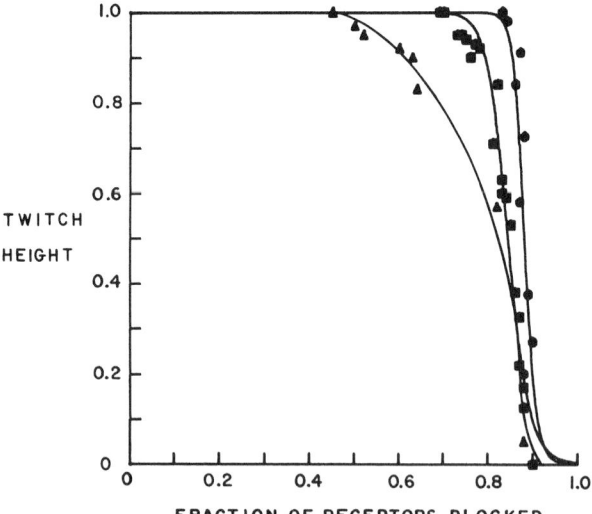

Figure 14–5. Comparison of twitch, train-of-four, and tetanus at 100 Hz as indices of receptor occlusion. Plot margin of safety as in Figure 14–2. Righthand curve (*circles*), twitch responses. Middle curve (*rectangles*), train-of-four. Lefthand curve (*triangles*), 100 Hz tetanus. Note that more receptors must be available before train-of-four response returns to normal, but that 100 Hz tetanus requires about half of the receptor pool to be free before a normal response is obtained.

The same statement applies to the extent of PTF. It is also worth mentioning that the extent of PTF is not easily translated into depth of a competitive block.

The second group of indices of depth of block requires minimal or no specialized apparatus. Aside from the obvious maneuver of noticing whether there is sufficient relaxation for operation, the components of this group are directed toward assessing the extent of recovery rather than the depth during operation. Examples may be listed in order of their appearance during recovery: (1) tidal volume (which is normal by the time the twitch response has reached control level), (2) vital capacity (which is 90 per cent of normal by the time a 50 Hz tetanus has recovered), (3) maximal inspiratory and expiratory force, and (4) head lift for five seconds. Note the relation of head lift to tetanic electric stimulation. Both allow one to probe more significant levels of recovery than can be monitored with a single twitch, but the head lift not only requires no apparatus but administers the tetanic stimulation painlessly. Eliciting a head lift does, however, require the patient's cooperation.

This brings us to another aspect of monitoring—the differential diagnosis of neuromuscular block from central mechanisms. For example, consider inadequate ventilation. Is the problem too much tubocurarine, too much morphine, or hypocarbia? A normal response to peripheral nerve stimulation and the ability to raise the head or to take a deep breath on command rule out the first explanation.

REVERSAL OF NEUROMUSCULAR BLOCK

Competitive neuromuscular blockers can be antagonized by agents such as edrophonium (Tensilon), neostigmine (Prostigmine), or pyridostigmine (Mestinon). These drugs appear to act by combining with cholinesterase, thus preventing the metabolism of acetylcholine. The acetylcholine is then available to compete more effectively with the antagonist for the receptor. Neostigmine also causes depolarization of the end plate by a direct action, but the significance of this action in the reversal of competitive antagonism is unknown.

The effect of acetylcholine is not only on the end plate of striated muscle, but also on structures innervated by the parasympathetic nervous system. Therefore in order to prevent muscarinic responses such as bradycardia, bronchospasm, or salivation, atropine 0.5 to 1.5 mg must be used before or simultaneously with the anticholinesterases.

Because of a short duration of action, edrophonium is not useful as an antagonist of competitive block. Both neostigmine and pyridostigmine may be used. Pyridostigmine has a longer duration of action and also a longer time to onset. The time from administration to maximum effect is seven to 11 minutes with neostigmine and 12 to 15 minutes with pyridostigmine. The duration of action is 37 to 58 minutes with neostigmine and 51 to 83 minutes with pyridostigmine.

The dose of neostigmine or pyridostigmine necessary to antagonize a neuromuscular block has long been debated. However, there is no basis for debate if the drug is titrated. When a peripheral monitor is used the dose may be titrated against the effect of nerve stimulation. For example, neostigmine can be given in increments of 0.5 mg either until satisfactory recovery is achieved or until succeeding doses no longer cause improvement. Because of the large margin of safety of neuromuscular transmission, an additional increment of 0.5 mg neostigmine should be given after tetanus or head lift is sustained. Pyridostigmine is used similarly, but with incremental doses of 2.5 mg.

It has been suggested that the effect of neostigmine might wear off faster than the competitive antagonist and lead to "recurarization." However, in the absence of a gross prolongation of action of the neuromuscular block, as might be produced by anuria, a single course of neostigmine will suffice if the neuromuscular block is adequately reversed in the first place.

There is no reliable antagonist of depolarizing blockers. Anticholinesterases either may cause reversal of the block or may increase it. Some authors suggest that anticholinesterases increase phase I block and reverse phase II block. Since it is difficult at present to differentiate clinically phase I from phase II block, an appropriate clinical approach is hard to determine. Some authors suggest that a test of the short-acting edrophonium be used and if the block is reversed, the longer-acting neostigmine can be given. In practice, the safest procedure is to control ventilation until spontaneous recovery occurs. Although some authors believe that phase II block can cause prolonged apnea, there is no evidence to support this view. The most likely reason for a prolonged recovery is an overdose.

APPRAISAL

In summary, neuromuscular blockers are valuable, specific, and safe drugs when carefully used. Proper use requires a background knowledge of the pertinent physiology and pharmacology plus the patience to titrate the drug accordingly rather than to give standard doses.

REFERENCES

Ali HD, Wilson RS, Savarese JJ, et al: The effect of tubocurarine on indirectly elicited train of four muscle response and respiratory measurements in humans. Br J Anaesth 47:570, 1975.

Burns BD, Paton WDM: Depolarization of the motor end-plate by decamethonium and acetylcholine. J Physiol 115:41, 1951.

Fogdall RP, Miller, RD: Antagonism of d-tubocurarine and pancuronium-induced neuromuscular blockade by pyridostigmine in man. Anesthesiology 39:504, 1973.

Gissen AJ, Katz RL: Twitch, tetanus and post-tetanic potentiation as indices of nerve-muscle block in man. Anesthesiology 30:481, 1969.

Heisterkamp DV, Skovsted P, Cohen PJ: The effects of small incremental doses of *d*-tubocurarine on neuromuscular transmission in anesthetized man. Anesthesiology 30:500, 1969.

Katz B: Nerve, Muscle and Synapse. New York, McGraw-Hill, 1966.

Katz B: The Release of Neural Transmitter Substances. Springfield, Ill, Charles C Thomas, 1969.

Katz RL: A nerve stimulator for the continuous monitoring of muscle relaxant action. Anesthesiology 26:327, 1967.

Katz, RL: Clinical neuromuscular pharmacology of pancuronium. Anesthesiology 34:550, 1971.

Katz RL (ed): Muscle Relaxants. New York, American Elsevier Publishing Co., 1975.

Miller RD: Antagonism of neuromuscular blockade. Anesthesiology 44:318, 1971.

Miller RD, Way WL: Inhibition of succinylcholine-induced increased intra-gastric pressure by nondepolarizing muscle relaxants and lidocaine. Anesthesiology 34:185, 1971.

Miller, RD, Van Nyhuis LS, Eger EI, II, et al: Comparative time to peak effect and duration of action of neostigmine and pyridostigmine. Anesthesiology 41:27, 1974.

Paton, WDM: The effects of muscle relaxants other than muscular relaxation. Anesthesiology 20:453, 1959.

Paton WDM, Waud DR: The margin of safety of neuromuscular transmission. J Physiol (Lond) 191:59, 1967.

Waud BE, Waud DR: The relation between tetanic fade and receptor occlusion in the presence of competitive neuromuscular block. Anesthesiology 35:456, 1971.

Waud BE, Waud DR: The relation between the response to "train-of-four" stimulation and receptor occlusion during competitive neuromuscular block. Anesthesiology 37:413, 1972.

Waud, BE, Waud DR: Comparison of the effects of general anesthetics on the end-plate of skeletal muscle. Anesthesiology 43:540, 1975.

Waud BE, Waud DR: Physiology and pharmacology of neuromuscular blocking agents. *In* Katz RL (ed): Muscle Relaxants. New York, American Elsevier Publishing Co, 1975, p 1.

Waud DR, Waud BE: Agents acting on the neuromuscular junction and centrally acting muscle relaxants. *In* DiPalma R (ed): Drill's Pharmacology in Medicine. New York, McGraw-Hill, 1971, p. 735.

Waud DR, Waud BE: Depolarization block and phase II block at the neuromuscular junction. Anesthesiology 43:10, 1975.

Whittaker M: Genetic aspects of succinylcholine sensitivity. Anesthesiology 32:143, 1970.

Chapter 15

INTUBATION OF THE TRACHEA

The advantages of intubation of the trachea are many: patency of the airway is reasonably assured, although not guaranteed; anatomic dead space is reduced by about half; control of respiration is facilitated; and secretions may be removed with relative ease from the tracheobronchial tree. Positive pressure can be applied to the airway with little inflation of the stomach. The patient can be placed in any position for operation with less chance of compromising the airway, while the anesthetist can be situated at some distance from the patient's head and yet maintain control of respiration.

EQUIPMENT

LARYNGOSCOPE

Laryngoscopes are of two basic types: those with straight blades, and those that are curved. Most laryngoscopes used by anesthetists offer detachable blades that can be used interchangeably on a battery-containing handle, an arrangement both economic and convenient for cleaning the instrument after use. The novice should learn to intubate the trachea using either kind, but initially proficiency with one should be developed. For the very difficult intubation, a flexible fiberoptic laryngoscope has recently been introduced. Inserted into the lumen of a tracheal tube, the flexible laryngoscope permits visualization of the larynx and the tube is threaded over it into the trachea, either orally or nasally.

TRACHEAL TUBES

Tracheal tubes are usually manufactured from natural or synthetic rubber, or plastic (Fig. 15-1). A coiled wire or heavy nylon thread may be embedded in the wall to prevent collapse and an inflatable cuff is incorporated. Natural rubber is more difficult to clean because its porosity permits ab-

Intubation of the Trachea

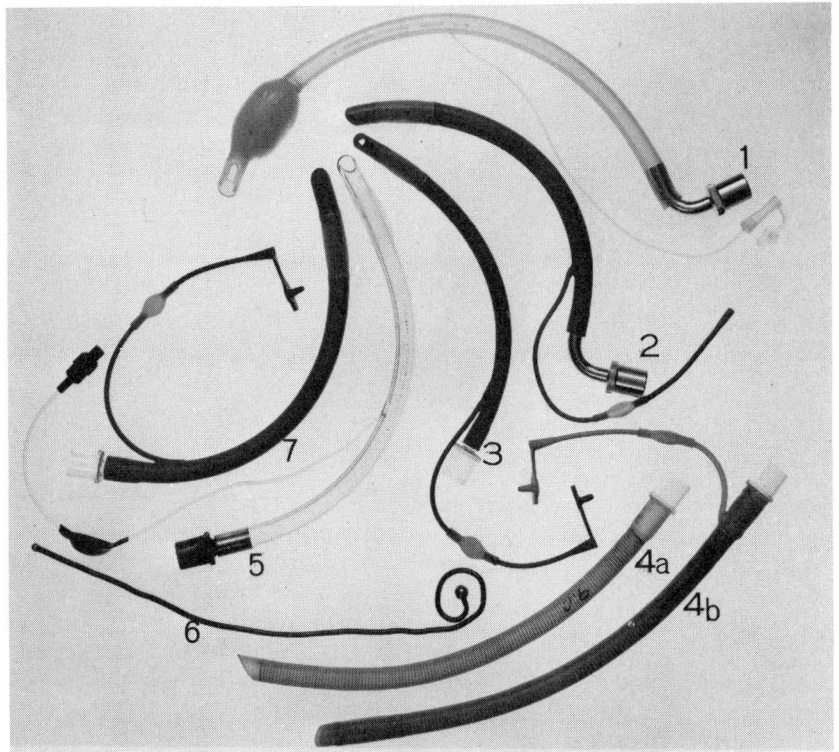

Figure 15-1. Kinds of tracheal tubes. *1*, Plastic with curved slip joint and low pressure cuff; *2*, rubber with curved slip joint; *3*, straight plastic slip joint, side opening at tip; *4a*, armored or anode tube without cuff; *4b*, with cuff; *5*, clear plastic; *6*, stylet; *7*, rubber with straight plastic slip joint, cuff, and pilot balloon.

sorption of bacteria-laden secretions, lubricants, and the chemicals used for cleaning. Although some plastic tubes stiffen with age and are thus more likely to produce trauma, others maintain flexibility and are useful because transparency facilitates cleanliness and reliability of patency. Disposable tubes are the most convenient of all.

Tubes are chosen for durability, with thin walls and maximal internal diameters to assure minimal resistance to breathing, lack of compressibility, and ease of cleaning. All but those reinforced with the coiled wire may kink or undergo compression. Noncollapsible tubes are advisable in certain kinds of operation, such as for thoracic or cervical tumors compressing the trachea, or in operations conducted in the sitting or face-down position when the head may be sharply flexed.

Endotracheal tubes are numbered according to outside diameter (Table 15-1). They are usually longer than necessary when received from the manufacturer and require cutting to lessen the possibility of bronchial intubation. Recommended lengths are also given in Table 15-1. The length

Table 15-1. Dimensions of Endotracheal Tubes

Age	Weight (lb)	Endotracheal Tube Sizes (average in boldface)			Anatomic Distances		
		Diameters		Lengths (cm) Orotracheal	Teeth to Cords (cm)	Teeth to Carina (cm)	Sagittal Diam. Trachea (mm)
		French	Magill				
Newborn	to 8	10, 12, 14	0	**11**, 12	7–8	11–12	4
1–4 mo	8–10	12, 14, 16	1	11, **12**			6
4–12 mo	10–20	14, **16**, 18	1, 1A		8.5	12–13	7
1–2 yr	20–25	16, **18**, 20	1A, 2	**12**, 13		14	7–8
2–3	25–30	18, **20**, 22	1A, **2**, 2A	**13**, 14	9		
3–4	30–35	20, 22, 24		**14**, 15		14.3	8
4–5	35–40	22, **24**, 26	2, 3, 4	14, **15**, 16			
5–6	40–45						
6–7	45–55		3, **4**, 5	15, **16**, 17	9.5	15.5	8–9
7–8	55–60	24, **26**, 28					
8–9	60–65		4, **5**, 6	15, **16**, 17, 18	9.5–10	15.5–17	9
9–10	65–70	28, **30**	5, **6**, 7				
10–11	70–80			16, **17**, 18, 19	10–11	16.3–18.5	9–11
11–12	80–90	30, 32, 34	6, **7**, 8				
12–16	90–140	34 (F)	7	17–24, **22.5**	11–15	17.5–25	11–15
Adults	130–200	36 (M)	8 (F)				
60–65		38	9 (M)	23–26	12–15	28–32	13–23
65 and over		40	10	**24**			

Intubation of the Trachea

of the tube is estimated for any patient by placing it alongside the face and neck, with the bifurcation of the trachea taken as the angle of Louis. Another method is to measure the distance from the cricoid cartilage to the tip of the xiphoid cartilage; this can be used as a rule of thumb for length of nasotracheal tubes; orotracheal tubes should be 2 cm shorter.

A connector or slip joint is placed in the proximal end of the tube, fitting snugly and preferably distending the tube; otherwise it may be dislodged. Ideally, the connector should be situated at the level of the teeth; tubes that protrude from the mouth are subject to displacement into a bronchus or may kink. The connector between the adapter and the breathing tubes of the anesthesia machine should be of large diameter, preferably curved, with smooth walls to minimize turbulence and resistance to gas flow (Fig. 15-2).

A stylet of malleable metal or plastic can be inserted to improve the curvature of an endotracheal tube. When placed within a tube the stylet is lubricated to aid in withdrawal; and it should not protrude beyond the distal end. Some use forceps to guide a flexible tube into the trachea rather than insert a stylet.

Inflatable Cuffs

An inflatable balloon or cuff allows a completely closed system, permitting easy control of respiration. When inflated, the cuff reduces the possibility but may not completely prevent passage of foreign material into the lungs. Cuffs may be of the high or low pressure kind, depending upon the

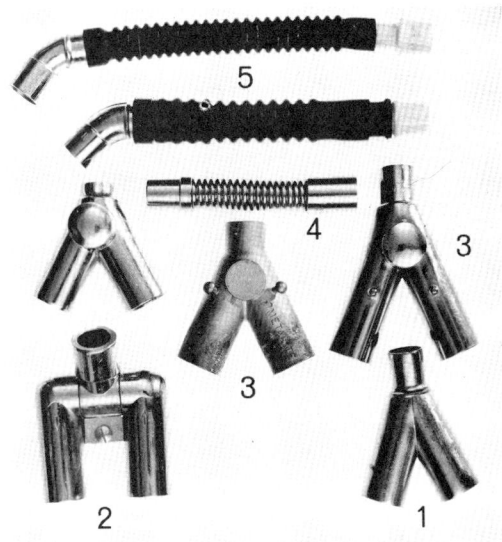

Figure 15-2. Types of endotracheal tube connectors. *1*, Y connector; *2*, Y connector with swivel neck; *3*, Y connectors with escape valve; *4*, flexible metal interconnector (rough, narrow interior walls predispose to turbulent air flow) not recommended unless respiration controlled; *5*, corrugated rubber interconnectors of two lengths and diameters, in which because of a wide lumen, turbulence is of lesser importance.

pressure used for inflation. Pressures higher than 200 torr have been measured at the interface between a high pressure cuff and the tracheal mucosa; damage to the mucous membrane should be less with the low pressure kind (see Chapter 33). The cuff should be so fixed to the endotracheal tube that it cannot become displaced and occlude the distal end. Once in place it is inflated with a measured amount of air, the extent of inflation tested by simultaneously compressing the reservoir bag while listening for escape of air at the mouth or nose. A small pilot balloon is usually incorporated to indicate inflation of the cuff. A pharyngeal pack is not recommended unless necessary because of the added irritation.

Lubricants

Uncuffed endotracheal tubes inserted under direct vision through the mouth require lubrication only if the mucous membranes are dry, but cuffed tubes are lubricated to facilitate passage through the glottis. Tap water or a water-soluble lubricant is adequate, although some believe that a lubricant containing a topical anesthetic is useful. Nasotracheal tubes require more than the usual amount of lubrication. Suction catheters are likewise lubricated for easy passage through the endotracheal tube.

Figure 15–3 illustrates some of the essential pieces of endotracheal equipment.

TECHNIQUES OF TRACHEAL INTUBATION

GENERAL PRINCIPLES

Endotracheal tubes are packaged individually in clear plastic, marked as to size. A tube of appropriate diameter and length should be selected, though it is best to have several available because the appropriate size can be determined only after viewing the glottis. The tube is examined beforehand to assure patency and the cuff inflated to detect leakage of air. The laryngoscope bulb is tested and all equipment kept clean before use. Soiled equipment—masks, tubes, and airways—should be placed in a separate container. Care and sterilization of endotracheal equipment are discussed in Chapter 7.

Before induction of anesthesia, certain observations are helpful in predicting the ease of tracheal intubation: relaxed submandibular tissues allow ready extension of the head, while tightness causes glottic exposure to be more difficult; a receding jaw causes difficulty in exposing the larynx via direct laryngoscopy; inability to open the mouth widely suggests ankylosis of the temporomandibular joint or trismus; patients with cervical arthritis often are unable to extend the head. The oral cavity is sometimes narrow and long, with minimal space between the dental arches, so that the laryngoscope tends to block a good view of the vocal cords. A large tongue

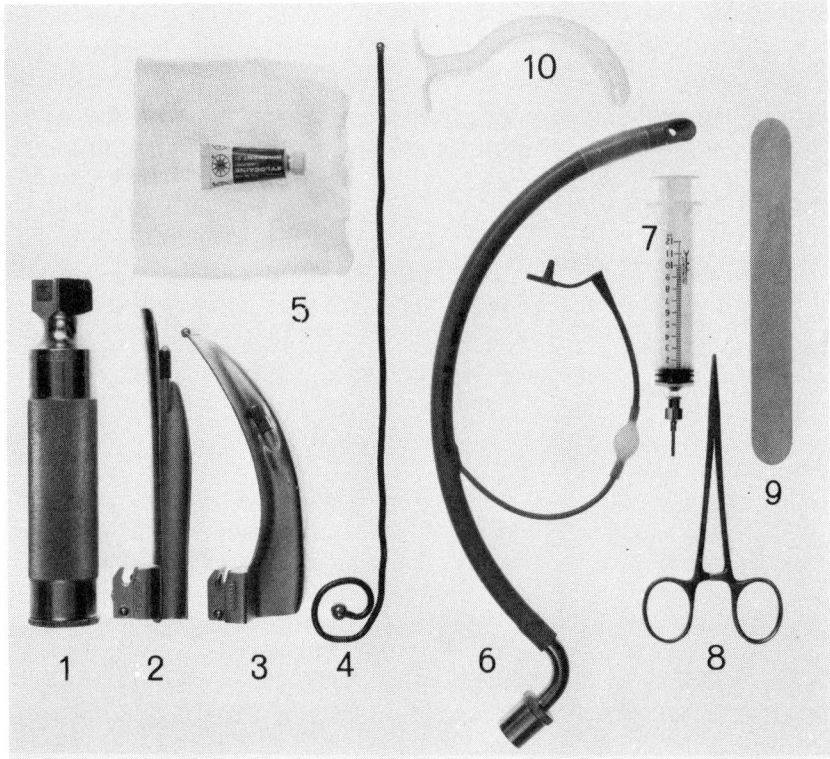

Figure 15-3. Equipment for tracheal intubation. *1*, Laryngoscope battery handle; *2*, straight blade; *3*, curved (Macintosh) blade; *4*, malleable copper stylet; *5*, sterile gauze with topical anesthetic lubricant; *6*, cuffed tube (uncut); *7*, syringe to inflate cuff; *8*, hemostat to hold cuff inflated; *9*, tongue blade for airway insertion; *10*, plastic oropharyngeal airway.

may be a hindrance, as is found in children with cretinism, mongolism, or gargoylism.

The teeth are examined. Protruding upper incisors can be damaged by the laryngoscope and cause difficulty in laryngeal exposure. Loose, chipped, capped, or diseased teeth are identified, a note made on the chart, and the patient advised of the risk of damage. If a tooth is found missing after intubation, it may be present in the mouth, pharynx, or nasopharynx. If it is not found, a chest x-ray is taken. Loose dental bridgework and partial plates are removed before intubation and care taken to avoid loss. Orthodontic appliances are removed if possible or protected against damage.

The length and angulation of the epiglottis influence the ease of intubation. The relatively narrow and flexible epiglottis of the infant or child poses problems; in the adult the long, relaxed epiglottis, which falls back over the larynx when muscular relaxation is profound, can be difficult to

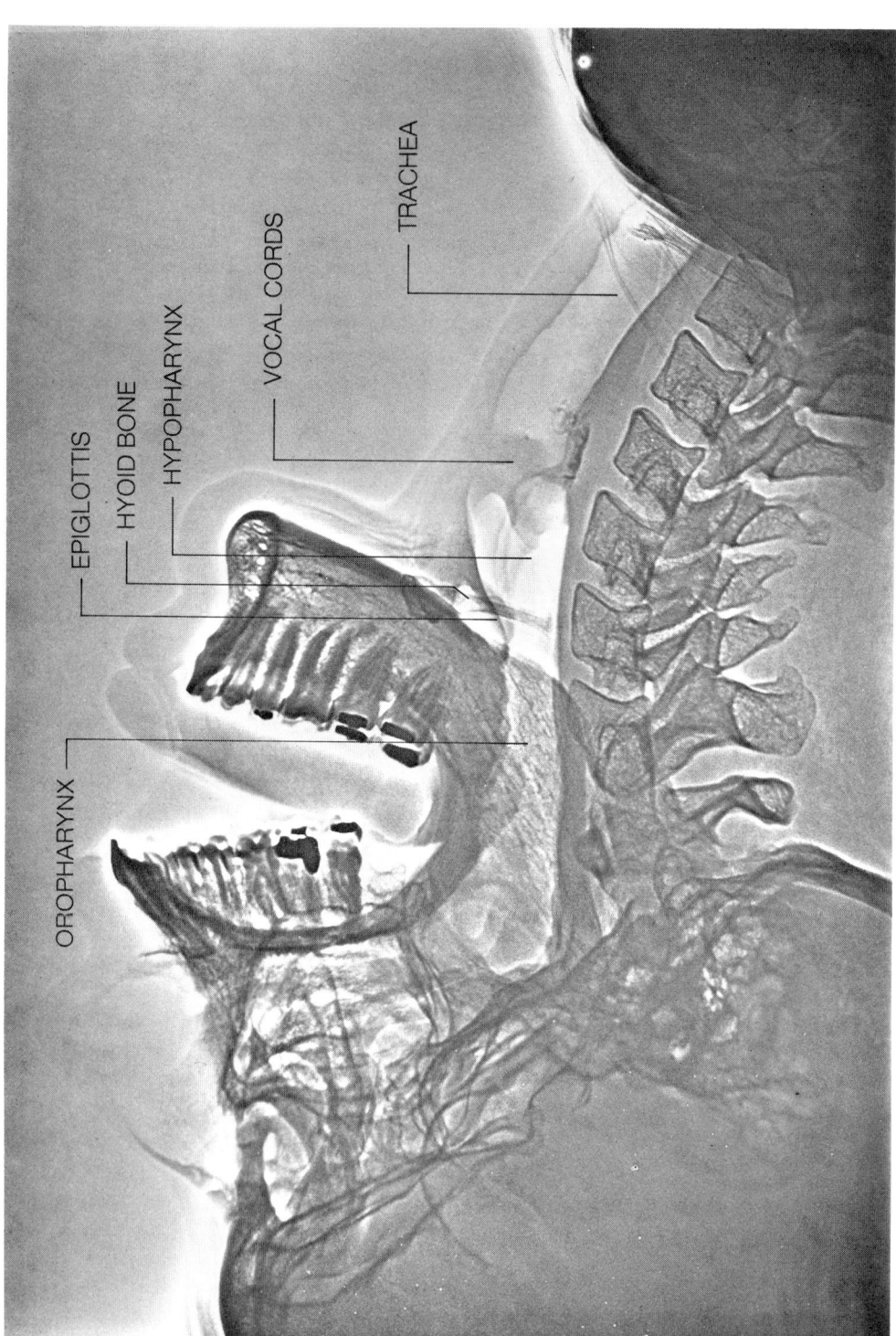

control. Anatomic features of the upper airway are shown in Figure 15–4.

With this knowledge as background, skill in intubation is more quickly attained if a predetermined plan is followed.

Technique with Straight Blade

1. The height of the operating table is adjusted so that the patient's face is approximately at the level of the standing anesthetist's xiphoid process. This allows for laryngeal suspension with the left arm flexed and the elbow held against the body at the level of the iliac crest.
2. The head, resting on a four-inch firm pillow or pad is brought into the "sniffing" position to bring the axes of the trachea, pharynx, and mouth into line (Fig. 15–5).
3. The fingers of the right hand open the jaws widely, spreading the lips to prevent bruising between laryngoscope and teeth.
4. A protective shield of lead, adhesive tape, or plastic placed over the upper incisors can prevent damage; gentleness and avoidance of pressure on teeth or gums are essential.
5. Held in the left hand, the moistened laryngoscope blade is introduced at the right side of the mouth and advanced forward and centrally along the right side of the tongue. The epiglottis is seen at the base. The wrist is held

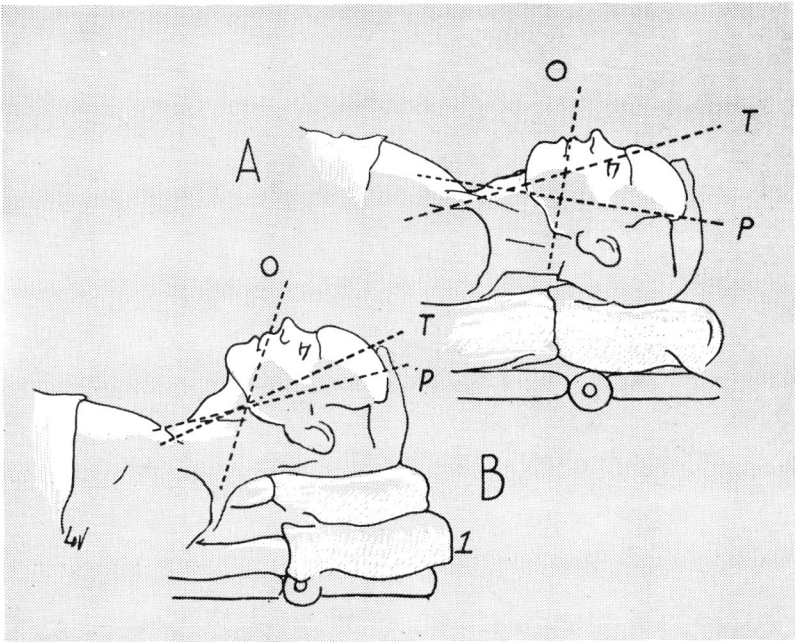

Figure 15–5. Position of the head for laryngoscopy and intubation of trachea. *A*, Ordinary position; *T*, axis of the trachea; *P*, axis of the pharynx; *O*, axis of the oral cavity. *B*, Modified position achieved with extra head rest. Flexion of cervical spine and extension at the atlantooccipital joint bring the three axes more nearly into line.

rigid to avoid using the upper teeth as a fulcrum with the blade of the laryngoscope as a lever. The right hand is placed beneath the occiput, extending the head at the atlanto-occipital joint.
6. The blade is slipped just beneath the tip of the epiglottis, and exposure of the larynx is accomplished by an upward and forward lift at a 45-degree angle, elevating mandible and head. Exposure should never be obtained by leverage on the teeth. If the glottis is not easily exposed, depression of the thyroid cartilage may help; an extra pillow or pad beneath the head is also of value. Overly deep insertion of the laryngoscope blade results in elevation of the entire larynx and exposure of the esophagus rather than the glottis.
7. The endotracheal tube with cuff deflated, concavity directed laterally, is passed to the right of the tongue and laryngoscope through the glottis, 2 to 3 cm into the trachea in the adult or until the cuff just disappears beyond the vocal cords. Occasionally, intubation is accomplished only by a 90- to 180-degree rotation of the tube with return to the forward position when in the trachea.

Rarely, the glottis is not seen but intubation is possible if the arytenoid cartilages are visible. A curved stylet or a Magill forceps helps to direct the tube anteriorly. An olive-tipped urethral bougie inserted through the endotracheal tube, permitting the tip to pass into the barely visible glottis, may allow the tube to be "threaded" into the larynx.

Common causes of failure in tracheal intubation include: inadequate muscle relaxation; insufficient depth of general anesthesia; improper position of the head, allowing the tongue to obscure the visual field; and lack of familiarity with the anatomy. On the other hand, hypoxia often occurs during intubation with the use of a neuromuscular blocker. The relaxation provided gives a false sense of security and too long a time is taken before respiration is resumed. Since the advent of succinylcholine, tracheal intubation is rarely attempted with general anesthesia alone. Better habits are developed if one learns the problems of intubation without the use of a neuromuscular blocker.

Ideal conditions for intubation are afforded the beginner by deep planes of anesthesia. Haste is not essential, since the patient continues to breathe and remains relaxed and the vocal cords move with respiration, manifestations not seen if neuromuscular block is present. If tracheal intubation is performed with a neuromuscular blocker, this is preceded by several inflations of the lung to provide a reserve of oxygen. The instructor should place a limit of one minute for intubation followed by another period of ventilation with oxygen. The interval can also be regulated if the anesthetist doesn't breathe during the intubation attempt; if the urge to breathe is felt, the patient also needs ventilation.

Technique with Curved Blade

Intubation with a curved blade involves the same maneuvers, with a few modifications.

1. The blade is passed to the right of the tongue and moved centrally, displacing the tongue to the left.
2. The epiglottis is not elevated; rather, the tip of the blade rests between the epiglottis and base of the tongue. Forward and upward lift of the laryngoscope stretches the hyo-epiglottic ligament, folding the epiglottis upward toward the blade and exposing the glottis. Failure to obtain good visualization is often caused by deep insertion of the blade, thereby fixing the epiglottis and preventing its movement. More often it is the failure to lift the blade that causes difficulty.

The theoretic advantages of the curved blade relate to the sensory innervation of the laryngeal or undersurface of the epiglottis, derived from the superior laryngeal sensory branch of the vagus. Stimulation by the straight blade is said to predispose to laryngospasm and cough. The pharyngeal surface is innervated by the glossopharyngeal nerve; stimulation of this by the curved blade is less likely to cause spasm. The curved blade allows more room for passage of the tracheal tube than the average straight blade. Occasionally exposure of the glottis is not as good as that obtained with the straight blade and a stylet may be required to insure appropriate curvature of the tube. However, when the mouth cannot be opened widely, when the teeth protrude or are in poor condition, and in thick-necked individuals and in those with a more cephalad larynx, the curved blade is more useful.

Orotracheal Intubation in the Conscious Patient

An anesthetist should be able to intubate the trachea with the patient awake when induction of general anesthesia is considered unsafe in the absence of an assured airway. Topical anesthesia is accomplished by means of a nebulizer, by application of cotton swabs to the pyriform fossae, or by transtracheal injection of local anesthetic. Topical anesthesia is done under direct vision with a laryngoscope or indirectly with reflected light and a laryngeal mirror. The structures are anesthetized in the following order: base of tongue, epiglottis, oropharynx, pyriform fossae, vocal cords, and finally, larynx and upper trachea by instillation through the glottis. A minimal amount of anesthesia is used to prevent untoward reactions, not more than 2 to 3 ml of 10 per cent cocaine, 1 per cent tetracaine, or 4 per cent lidocaine.

Orotracheal intubation with the patient awake is used to advantage in the following situations: tumors of the neck or mediastinum displacing the trachea or larynx; tumor or inflammatory swelling encroaching upon the mouth or pharynx; malformation of the jaws; and upper intestinal obstruction when aspiration of vomitus during induction of anesthesia is a threat. In the latter instance, the cuff on the tracheal tube is inflated as soon as possible after intubation prior to induction of general anesthesia. During intubation, the head of the table is elevated to minimize regurgitation.

Backward pressure on the cricoid cartilage helps to occlude the esophagus and to minimize regurgitation (the Sellick maneuver) (Chapter 28).

Blind Nasotracheal Intubation

Blind nasotracheal intubation is often the method of choice in oral and maxillofacial operations, and is useful also in emergency situations in which an airway is needed quickly, as in the obese, thick-necked person who easily becomes obstructed or the patient with hypoglossal or cervical edema. Although indicated in a patient with trismus or a fractured jaw, nasal intubation is avoided in the patient with a fractured nose or nasal obstruction; it is also contraindicated in the presence of acute sinusitis and mastoiditis, since pathogenic bacteria may be carried into the trachea. Nasotracheal intubation may be done with the patient awake and well sedated or with general anesthesia and use of a neuromuscular blocker.

A nasotracheal tube should be soft and pliable so as not to injure the nasal mucous membrane or turbinates, but of the proper consistency to resist compression and to maintain a reasonable curve. Tubes are packaged to maintain the proper curvature and well lubricated to minimize trauma. Prior topical application of cocaine or phenylephrine, 0.25 per cent, is useful in shrinking mucous membranes. A laryngoscope and Magill forceps are kept at hand in case intubation fails. Attempts are abandoned if not immediately successful and the tube is inserted under direct vision using the forceps.

When nasotracheal intubation is attempted, the occiput of the patient rests upon a firm pillow with the chin elevated. The tube is introduced with the concavity forward, hugging the floor of the nose. Advancement of the tube is slow and gentle, with rotation when resistance is encountered. Rough maneuvers, large rigid tubes, poor lubrication, and use of force against an obstruction cause epistaxis. The guides to insertion are: observing the neck for bulging produced by the tip of the tube in the hypopharynx; increase or decrease in breath sounds as the patient breathes; and resistance to passage of the tube. External, backward, or lateral movement of the larynx or rotation of the tube may be required.

Voluntary hyperpnea if the patient is awake or hyperpnea produced by hypercapnia if the patient is asleep is helpful, providing maximal abduction of the cords during inspiration. Entry into the larynx is signified by loss of breath sounds if the patient is breathing and decrease in resistance, often accompanied by cough. Success is confirmed by connecting the tube to the rebreathing system and expanding the lungs. Common errors contributing to failure of blind nasotracheal intubation are the use of a tube with poor curvature and failure to position the head properly. A fiberoptic laryngoscope inserted through a nasotracheal tube may facilitate tracheal intubation in some circumstances.

If a tracheal airway is required before induction of general anesthesia and this cannot be accomplished either by indirect or direct intubation under topical anesthesia, tracheostomy may be necessary as a first measure.

CARE AFTER TRACHEAL INTUBATION

The first steps after intubation include (1) observation of chest movement while the lungs are inflated with oxygen, and (2) listening for breath sounds bilaterally to be sure that the trachea, not the esophagus or bronchus, has been intubated. Inflation of the cuff can be detected with the fingers straddling the trachea just above the manubrium; this suggests that bronchial intubation has not occurred. After orotracheal intubation an oropharyngeal airway or soft bite block is placed between the teeth to prevent biting on the tube. The tube is secured with adhesive or umbilical tape tied around the neck. Plastic tape is useful in avoiding the need for subsequent removal of adhesive material from the tube. Suturing into place may be required for some maxillofacial operations. When there are excessive secretions, as in the face-down position, or when solutions used to prepare the operative field may loosen the adhesive, preparation of the skin with tincture of benzoin before application of the tape is helpful. Nasotracheal tubes should also be securely fixed with the connector at the level of the nares.

Cough after intubation frequently occurs when topical anesthesia is inadequate, in light planes of general anesthesia, and when the tube touches the carina. If cough is mild, transient hypertension and tachycardia result. In the more severe reaction, the spasm of thoracic muscles and bronchospasm may be difficult to overcome; ventilation may be impaired, resulting in hypoxia. Intravenous injection of a small dose of tubocurarine will relieve the chest wall spasm. If the tube is touching the carina, it should be withdrawn slightly.

After cuff inflation and fastening of the tube, the anesthetist should be sure that bronchial intubation has not occurred. A long tube may easily enter the right main stem bronchus, which comes off the trachea at a lesser angle than the left. Failure of the left side of the chest to move with ventilation or absence of breath sounds indicates bronchial intubation. If so, the tube should be withdrawn until breath sounds are equally audible bilaterally. Sometimes there is increased resistance to respiration if the bevel of the tube lies against the tracheal wall. Once the position of the tube has been confirmed, the cuff is inflated.

If the patient's position on the operating table is changed, the position of the tube should again be verified. Flexion of the head or steep Trendelenburg position may cause the tube to enter the right main stem bronchus.

On rare occasions after a difficult intubation the tracheal tube may have entered the esophagus. This is suggested by absence of distinct breath sounds and progressive development of cyanosis. Listening over the stomach with a stethoscope should detect entry of air as the reservoir bag is compressed. If doubt exists the tracheal tube should be removed immediately and ventilation carried out by means of a face mask. The stomach should be emptied of gas after tracheal intubation is accomplished.

EXTUBATION

At the conclusion of anesthesia, extubation may result in undesirable sequelae. The tube should be removed so as to avoid laryngospasm and cough, either at a relatively deep plane of anesthesia or when the patient has reacted sufficiently to have reflex control. If a neuromuscular blocker has been used, extubation is delayed until spontaneous respiration has returned. While it is essential to rid the trachea and pharynx of secretions prior to extubation, one should not persist to the point of causing continued cough and cyanosis. Secretions are aspirated from the upper airway, the catheter then passed through the tracheal tube, secretions aspirated, and the catheter withdrawn. Before and after aspiration, oxygen is administered; the cuff is deflated and the tube removed with the lungs inflated. A tube should not be removed with the aspirating catheter in place for oxygen cannot be given, and if the catheter brushes against the vocal cords, bleeding or laryngospasm may occur. After removal of the tube, the patient is again given oxygen. Laryngospasm commonly follows but is less threatening if the lungs have been oxygenated prior to extubation.

A tracheal tube should not be removed in the presence of cyanosis, when respiratory exchange is inadequate or not controllable with mask and bag, or when the operation compromises the airway. In patients with intestinal obstruction, the tube is left in place as long as possible, and the stomach is emptied via gastric tube before extubation. After maxillofacial operations resulting in a compromised airway, elective tracheostomy is performed before extubation. In the presence of inadequate respiratory exchange the tube is left in place and ventilation continued mechanically in the recovery room, a practice increasingly common in the anesthetic management of the critically ill and those who have had the combination of morphine, nitrous oxide, and a neuromuscular blocker.

COMPLICATIONS

Tracheal intubation has become a commonplace technique often used for the convenience of the anesthetist rather than for the good of the patient. Some believe there are few complications, but we have seen many.

TRAUMA DURING INTUBATION

Intubation may cause cut or bruised lips and tongue, chipped, loosened, or dislodged teeth, laceration of the pharynx, dislodged adenoid tissue, submucosal hemorrhage of the vocal cords, epistaxis, mediastinal and subcutaneous emphysema, and pneumothorax.

COMPLICATIONS WITH THE TUBE IN PLACE

Increased Resistance to Breathing. Narrow tubes and adapters or acutely angulated connectors cause turbulent air flow, increasing the work of breathing and producing respiratory fatigue. Added resistance results in hypercapnia, hypoxia, hypertension, and tachycardia, predisposing to cardiac arrest.

Obstruction of the Tube. This occurs as a result of collapse, kinking, foreign body, or secretion within the lumen; occlusion by biting; dislodged cuff overriding the distal orifice; bevel of the tube against the tracheal wall; or imperfections in the tube causing flaplike valves.

Esophageal Intubation. As noted earlier, this is sometimes difficult to detect, a complication discovered by listening for breath sounds laterally over the chest and epigastrium. Failure to recognize esophageal intubation has resulted in cardiac arrest within minutes.

Bronchial Intubation. This can be avoided by estimating the length of tube for each patient and by inserting the tube only 2 to 3 cm beyond the vocal cords. Bronchial obstruction may also result from an overinflated cuff.

Dislodgment. Failure to fasten an endotracheal tube properly may cause displacement into the pharynx or bronchus or dislodgment from nose and mouth.

Prolonged Cough and Chest Wall Spasm. If these are the result of light anesthesia, the level of anesthesia is deepened. If chest wall spasm does not respond to positive pressure with oxygen within a reasonable time, succinylcholine is given to permit expansion of the lungs.

COMPLICATIONS FOLLOWING EXTUBATION

Laryngospasm. Vocal cord spasm may follow extubation in lightly anesthetized patients; this is often alarming, particularly in infants and children, and better prevented than treated. Treatment includes administration of oxygen under pressure with reservoir bag and mask, or injection of succinylcholine.

Tracheal Collapse. Weakening of cartilaginous rings may be associated with large cervical tumors or goiter and tracheal collapse may follow extubation.

Edema or Infection of Larynx or Trachea. Improperly sterilized equipment, contaminated lubricants, insertion of an oversized tube, or an allergic response to the lubricant, rubber, or plastic may cause these reactions.

Hoarseness and Sore Throat. Some degree of denudation of respiratory tract epithelium is inevitable upon intubation. Postoperatively, patients experience sore throat and hoarseness, which invariably disappear within a day or two.

Ulceration of Tracheal Mucous Membrane. This usually occurs on the anterior wall where the tip of the tube has abraded the epithelium.

Ulceration and Granuloma of Vocal Cords. This complication is suspected when hoarseness persists for more than a few days. Contributing causes are trauma during intubation, tightly fitting tubes, protracted couth, undue movement of the head or tube, and allergic reaction to a lubricant. Most granulomas of the vocal cords seen by otolaryngologists are not attributable to anesthesia.

Aspiration of Gastrointestinal Contents. This occurs commonly in the patient with intestinal obstruction extubated before protective reflexes return, and may take place despite preventive measures in the aged and debilitated or in those with neurologic disease (see Chapter 28).

Vocal Cord Paralysis. Unilateral cord paralysis may be seen after thyroidectomy. Bilateral paralysis can occur for other reasons but we have seen this complication on several occasions after endotracheal anesthesia alone. Tubes sterilized with ethylene oxide may cause such paralysis despite presumed adequate airing; therefore it is probably a toxic effect.

This list of complications is impressive. We do not mean to dissuade anesthetists from intubation, but rather to remind them of the consequences of a careless technique. Sequelae occur more commonly during the training period of the anesthetist, becoming less frequent as skill is achieved. Critical analysis of one's technique as well as that of others does much to increase the safety and comfort for the patient when intubation is performed.

REFERENCES

Applebaum EL, Bruce DL: Tracheal Intubation. Philadelphia, WB Saunders Co, 1976.

Bannister FB, MacBeth RG: Direct laryngoscopy and tracheal intubation. Lancet 2:651, 1944.

Bowes JD, Kelly DF, Peacock JH: Intubation trauma: Effect of short-term intubation on tracheal mucous membrane of the pig. Anaesthesia 28:603, 1973.

Gillespie NA: Endotracheal Anesthesia 3rd ed, revised and edited by Bamforth BJ, Siebecker KL, Madison, University of Wisconsin Press, 1963.

Holley HS, Gildea JE: Vocal cord paralysis after tracheal intubation. JAMA 215:281, 1971.

Klainer AS, Turndorf H, Wu WH, et al: Surface alterations due to endotracheal intubation. Am J Med 58:674, 1975.

McGinnis GE, Shively JG, Patterson RL, et al: Engineering analysis of intratracheal tube cuffs. Anesth Analg 50:557, 1971.

Schellinger RR: The length of the airway to the bifurcation of the trachea. Anesthesiology 25:169, 1964.

Sellick BA: Cricoid pressure to control regurgitation of stomach contents during induction of anaesthesia. Lancet 2:404, 1961.

Stanley TH, Kawamura R, Graves C: Effects of nitrous oxide on volume and pressure of endotracheal cuffs. Anesthesiology 41:256, 1974.

Chapter 16

EVALUATION OF THE RESPONSE TO ANESTHETICS: THE SIGNS AND STAGES

The need to evaluate a patient's response to anesthetics has existed from the very beginning. John Snow recognized certain signs as guidelines for the administration of ether or chloroform. As early as January of 1847, Plomley had described three stages of anesthesia; later Snow added a fourth. To facilitate teaching during World War I, Guedel codified a system that had been used clinically for ether administration for nearly 70 years. He clearly defined the four stages of anesthesia and described the respiratory changes, pupillary alterations, eye movements, and swallowing and vomiting responses that allow estimation of depth of ether anesthesia in any one specific patient. In 1943, Gillespie added reflex responses as additional signs; that is, laryngeal and pharyngeal reactivity, lacrimation, and the respiratory response to surgical incision.

The Guedel system applied only to the unpremedicated patient allowed to breathe spontaneously during ether anesthesia, a situation that no longer exists in modern practice. Most patients receive either opioid or anticholinergic drugs as premedicants, and both alter the reliability of pupillary changes. Ether, cyclopropane, and fluroxene, which stimulate the sympathetic nervous system, cause a dose-related dilation of the pupils that is absent with halothane, enflurane, and isoflurane. The latter drugs cause a dose-related depression of blood pressure and hardly alter pulse rate, but ether, cyclopropane, and fluroxene in general demonstrate no consistent related changes in these variables. The signs proposed by Guedel and Gillespie still may be observed, but the variability among anesthetics is so great that no uniform system to evaluate depth of anesthesia is likely to evolve. Cardiovascular alterations, widely used by clinicians to evaluate the patient's response to anesthetics, are not included in Guedel's scheme. Respiratory signs, the keystone of Guedel's system, are usually invalid in today's practice of controlled ventilation and use of neuromuscular blockers. Nevertheless, evaluation of the patient's physiologic response is an important guide to anesthetic dose requirements. Guedel's system will be described first, followed by a discussion of modifications of his approach required to assess depth of anesthesia in current practice.

GUEDEL'S SIGNS AND STAGES OF ETHER ANESTHESIA

A graphic presentation of the signs and stages of ether anesthesia is given in Figure 16-1 as taken from Gillespie's chart, which emphasizes reflex alterations. The converging lines indicate progressive loss of reflex activity as anesthesia deepens.

STAGE I—AMNESIA AND ANALGESIA

Stage I is defined as lasting from the beginning of anesthesia to the loss of consciousness. Those parts of the brain of most recent phylogenetic development seem to be depressed first. This results in obtundation of intellect, memory, integrative functions, and perception of time and space. Although this is commonly called the stage of analgesia, sensation of pain is not absent and the pain threshold is apparently unchanged, but the patient's reaction to pain is altered. If warned, the patient will usually tolerate procedures that normally would not be accepted, that is, minor operations or the pain of the second stage of labor. As pointed out by Snow more than a century ago and more recently confirmed by Artusio (1954), analgesia is more profound upon emergence from ether anesthesia.

Unfortunately, an objective sign has not yet been found to indicate the transition to stage II, in which stimuli may cause the patient to react violently. Kaye states that eyelid closure in response to stroking of the eyelashes disappears at the end of stage I and this is often used as a guide.

STAGE II—DELIRIUM

Stage II, or the stage of delirium, lasts from the time of loss of consciousness to onset of a regular pattern of breathing and disappearance of the lid reflex, here meaning the normal attempt of eyelids to close when passively opened. This is the state of unconsciousness with uninhibited reaction. Patients should not undergo stimulation of any kind during this stage because the response may be injurious. This is why the prophylactic use of restraints is routine. Respiration may be irregular, and the pupils often are dilated and reactive to light. Pharyngeal and laryngeal reflexes, swallowing and laryngeal closure in response to stimulation, are obtunded at the lower limits of this stage, although vomiting can occur through plane 1 of stage III. The chief reason for rapidly increasing the inhaled concen-

Evaluation of the Response to Anesthetics

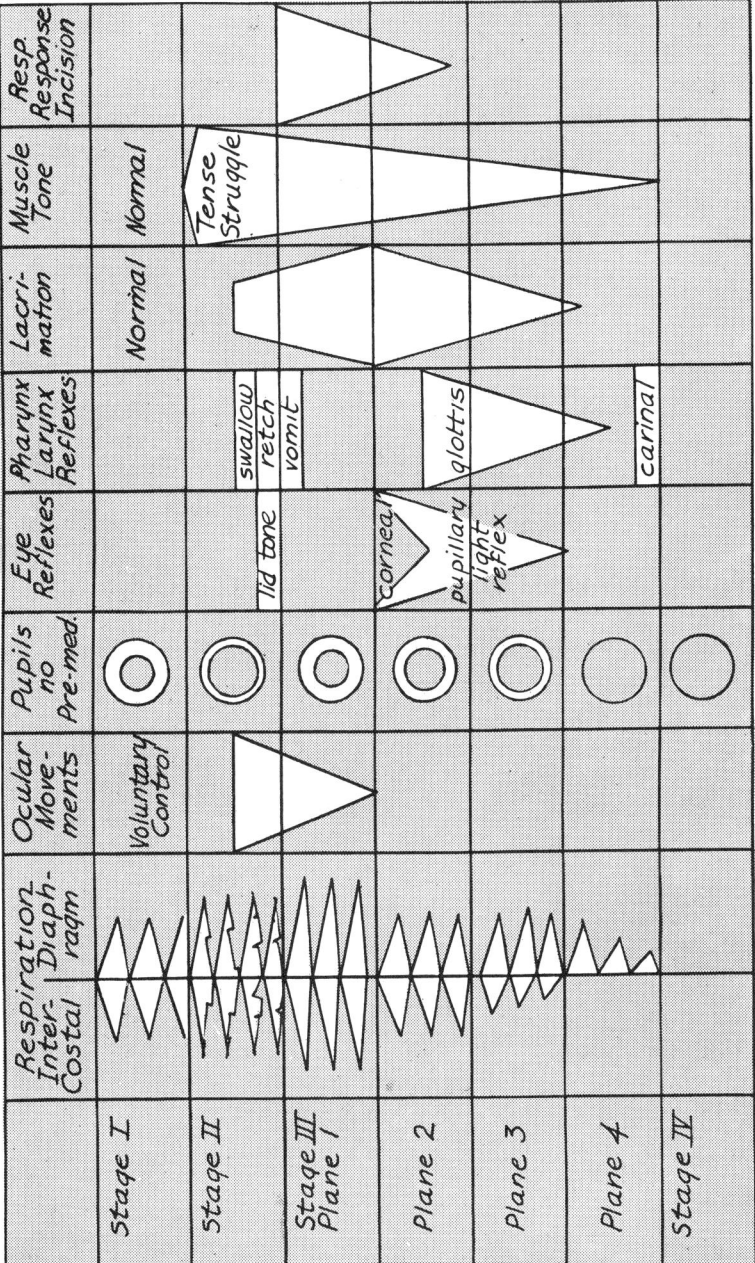

Figure 16–1. The signs and reflex reactions of the stages of anesthesia. (Reproduced with permission from Gillespie NA: Anesth Analg Curr Res 22:275, 1943.)

tration of anesthetic is to pass through this stage quickly. It is unwise to begin operation before the ensuing third stage has been reached because of the possibility of inducing movement or excitement. To paraphrase John Snow, "The surgeon wishes to know whether the patient will lie still under the knife."

STAGE III – SURGICAL ANESTHESIA

Stage III, or the stage of surgical anesthesia, lasts from the onset of a regular pattern of breathing to cessation of respiration. Most surgical procedures are performed at one of the levels of this stage. For more accurate estimation of depth of anesthesia, the third stage is arbitrarily divided into four planes.

Plane 1

Plane 1 is entered when the lid reflex is abolished and respiration becomes regular. In this plane duration of inspiration is usually longer than expiration, although this is not easily detected.

In plane 1 the eyes may oscillate and not infrequently are eccentrically fixed. Movement may not be apparent immediately when the eyelids are passively opened, especially if only one eye is inspected; it is better to examine both simultaneously. Movements may cease if the lids are kept open too long but usually return after they have been closed for a few seconds. If the extraocular muscles are tonically active, the abdominal muscles may be assumed to be in the same state. Gross ocular movement is minimal or absent during halothane anesthesia, in all planes.

Pupillary dilation may persist for a while but the pupils become distinctly smaller when well into the first plane. Reaction to light is present with ether, cyclopropane, and fluroxene and absent with halothane, enflurane, and isoflurane. The pupils tend to persist in the dilated state during cyclopropane and fluroxene anesthesia but are constricted with other agents.

During plane 1 the vomiting reflex in response to insertion of an oral airway is gradually abolished. It is interesting that swallowing, retching, and vomiting reflexes tend to disappear in that order during induction and reappear in the same order during emergence from anesthesia. The reasons for this are not clear.

Secretion of tears decreases through plane 1. The tendency for the respiratory rate and depth to increase in response to skin incision decreases. In many instances onset of peripheral venous dilation and increased cutaneous blood flow signify entry into the first plane.

Plane 2

Plane 2 lasts from the time the eyes cease to move and become concentrically fixed to the beginning of a decrease in intercostal muscle activity or thoracic respiration. Although true with ether, not infrequently with cyclopropane the eyes will not be centrally fixed, though all other signs indicate that anesthesia is in plane 2 or 3. Respirations remain regular but tidal volume is diminished, the rate tending to rise. Duration of inspiration and expiration may become equal or expiration may be slightly prolonged.

The pupils begin to dilate in plane 2 with ether, cyclopropane, and fluroxene, remaining constricted with the other agents. A rise in Pa_{CO_2} tends to produce pupillary dilation. On the whole, pupillary size is an unreliable indicator in patients given excessive amounts of premedication. Morphine tends to constrict the pupils, whereas belladonna derivatives produce dilation, with the effects of morphine generally overshadowing those of atropine or scopolamine. Whether the pupillary change is a peripheral or central influence on the autonomic nervous system has not been established. Pupillary signs are less reliable in patients over the age of 50. The best approach is to regard the dilated pupil as a sign of overdose or hypoxia until proved otherwise, except in the second stage.

Reflex closing of the vocal cords or laryngospasm begins to disappear in plane 2. The conjunctivae become lusterless and the respiratory response to skin incision disappears.

Muscle tone lessens as anesthesia deepens, but this is not always a reliable measure of depth of anesthesia. Abdominal muscle tone varies enormously among individuals, as does apparent flaccidity of the peritoneum. These phenomena are influenced by age, physical status, and the degree of intestinal or gastric distention. The tone of a flaccid muscle may be increased by a stimulus. Thus, a gentle surgeon will obtain as good abdominal exposure in the second plane as a rough surgeon in the third plane. Lack of oxygen or excess of carbon dioxide enhances muscle rigidity.

Plane 3

Plane 3 is entered when intercostal activity begins to decrease; the upper intercostals seem to become less active before the lower. Some interpret intercostal activity as secondary to diaphragmatic movement; as the diaphragm weakens, so does thoracic movement. Contraction of intercostal muscles lags behind that of the diaphragm, causing a rocking movement; to detect this lag one should observe both diaphragmatic and intercostal activity and establish the time relationship. Complete intercostal paralysis occurs in lower plane 3 while respiration is carried on solely by the diaphragm. As a consequence, tidal volume is reduced. Inspiration is now shorter than expiration and the pause between them is longer than in lighter planes of anesthesia. Some individuals, particularly men, exhibit only abdominal movement with respiration even in lighter planes of anesthesia. When the intercostals become paralyzed, passive retraction of the chest on inspiration usually occurs, giving a false impression of intercostal activity unless the time relationship is analyzed. It is unwise and unnecessary to maintain plane 3 for very long.

In mid to lower plane 3, reactivity of the pupils to light is gradually lost.

Plane 4

Plane 4 extends from the time of paralysis of the intercostal muscles to cessation of spontaneous respiration. As anesthesia deepens through this plane, diaphragmatic activity and respiratory exchange become progressively reduced until breathing stops. The pupils dilate and no longer react to light. There is little muscle tone, even in the robust person.

Tracheal tug often appears in association with deep anesthesia and intercostal paralysis. Respiratory obstruction or the actions of the accessory muscles of ventilation may produce tracheal tug, and the phenomenon is frequently observed as the diaphragm begins to regain function after use of a neuromuscular blocker. We believe that "tug" represents an unopposed action of the diaphragm, displacing the hilum of the lung and therefore increasing traction on the trachea.

STAGE IV

Stage IV lasts from the time of cessation of respiration to failure of the circulation, where respiration fails first because of a high concentration of anesthetic in the central nervous system. This is not to be confused with the apnea caused by breath-holding; nor should it be confused with the reflex breath-holding sometimes seen in lighter planes of anesthesia following manipulation of thoracic or abdominal organs, as with periosteal, pharyngeal, laryngeal, or bronchial stimulation; such breath-holding usually takes place at end inspiration and the glottis is closed. Less frequently, a prolonged expiratory effort is made or cough results.

In stage IV, which is premortem, most reflexes are absent and the circulation is about to fail, a plane of anesthesia arrived at only in error. Steps should be taken promptly to lighten anesthesia, as even brief maintenance in this plane leads to circulatory failure. The concentration of anesthetic in the blood and alveoli should be lowered by manual ventilation of the lungs with high flows of oxygen and repeated emptying of the reservoir bag.

CLINICAL ASSESSMENT OF ANESTHETIC REQUIREMENTS

Currently, anesthetists use a more logical approach than that proposed by Guedel to evaluate the effects of anesthetics. His was a static system: ether at a given dose (although then unknown) produces a given effect. He neglected the patient as a responsive organism in whom graded stimuli produce graded responses. Anesthetics alter patient reactivity, allow application of a large magnitude of stimuli, yet limit the resulting response. To evaluate fully the effect of an anesthetic, the anesthetist must evaluate both the stimulus and response. Gillespie recognized this concept when he

Evaluation of the Response to Anesthetics

added response to surgical incision to Guedel's scheme. Today's anesthetists use a stimulus-response assessment to classify adequacy of anesthetic level; it is less well defined than Guedel's scheme but more operational.

STIMULUS-RESPONSE ASSESSMENT

The stages of amnesia and analgesia and of delirium (Guedel's stages I and II) are usually not seen during induction of anesthesia at present because of the nearly routine use of intravenous induction techniques. Even during inhalation induction the two stages are not differentiated but are regarded as a single level, that of presurgical anesthesia. Excitement may occur during this stage and precautions to avoid patient stimulation during induction are still applicable. Three signs generally identify passage from the presurgical to a surgical level of anesthesia: loss of lid reflex, onset of muscle relaxation, and onset of rhythmic respiration. If these have not occurred, then the patient is at a presurgical level and stimulation must be avoided. When they are present, surgical anesthesia exists.

Three levels of anesthetic depression are recognized: presurgical anesthesia, surgical anesthesia, and overdose. Three planes of surgical anesthesia are accepted: too light, adequate, and too deep (Fig. 16-2). The thoughtful anesthetist follows a specific method in judging a patient's status. First, evaluation of afferent input to the nervous system; second, estimation of observable physiologic responses; and finally, the interaction among patient, stimulus, and anesthetic is considered and the level of surgical anesthesia deduced.

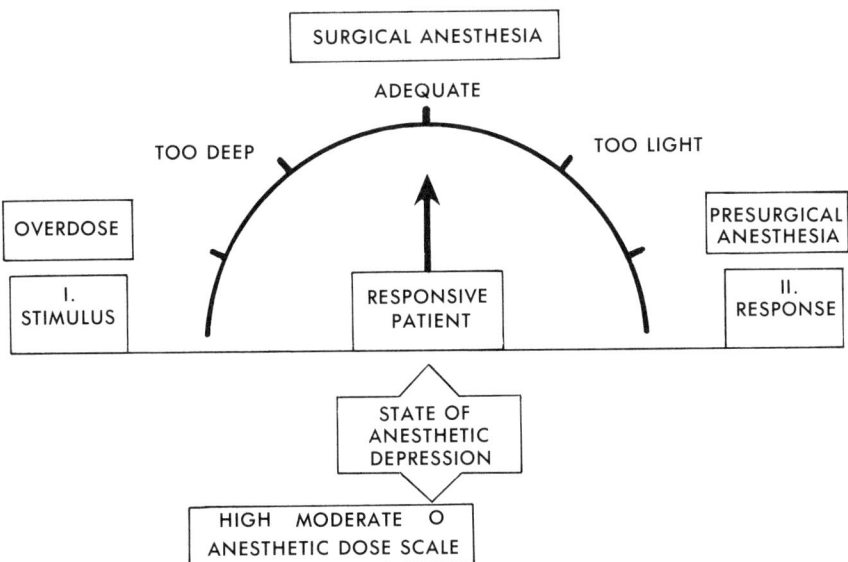

Figure 16–2. Schematic representation of evaluation of anesthetic requirements.

Stimulus Assessment

Stimulus intensity is arbitrarily classified somewhere between strong and weak. Strong stimulation results from a skin incision, anal or cervical dilation, periosteal stimulation, fracture manipulation, visceral or peritoneal traction, diaphragmatic stimulation, manipulation of the cornea, and excessive distention of the bladder. Weak stimulation results from uterine curettage, retroperitoneal dissection, wound debridement, mild distention of the bladder, and manipulation of fascia or muscle if without traction. No appreciable stimulation occurs during surgical dissection of brain, muscle, and connective tissue, bowel section and suturing, or lung resection and suturing. Inflammation usually enhances the intensity of the stimulus. Careful surgical manipulation may diminish the stimulus and the patient's age or physical status may influence the response.

Anesthetists must continuously monitor surgical activity if they are to have the information required to evaluate the anesthetized patient adequately.

Response Evaluation

Woodbridge, recognizing the large number of subtle observations the anesthetist must make, cited four components of the anesthetic state: sensory, motor, mental, and reflex functions. Table 16-1 attempts to classify the intensity of responses that may be observed in reference to Woodbridge's components. Note that observations made to evaluate depression in any one component involve nearly all body systems. Moreover, a single response may relate to several components. For example, if a patient takes a deep breath, turns the head, and develops tachycardia and hypertension when an incision is made, it is obvious that sensory depression is inadequate. Whether motor depression is inadequate depends upon the site of operation. The low intensity responses listed are undesirable in virtually every case and most anesthetists avoid drug doses that result in such responses. Utilization of this system permits logical evaluation of specific drug effects in each of Woodbridge's components.

Depth of Anesthesia and Arterial Pressure. Arterial hypotension is the chief clinical sign of depth of anesthesia with halothane and oxygen and the more common combination of halothane, nitrous oxide, and oxygen. Hypercarbia, although not to be condoned, counteracts hypotension, and with time during administration of halothane the arterial pressure rises. Both effects probably are related to increased sympathetic nervous activity. Pain perception during light anesthesia causes arterial pressure to rise. Enflurane, isoflurane, and methoxyflurane resemble halothane in their actions on blood pressure.

Evaluation of Anesthetic Requirement. A comparison of strength of surgical stimulus and observation of intensity of response allows for evaluation of specific anesthetic requirements. If the response is excessive in a

Table 16-1. EVALUATION OF RESPONSE INTENSITY

Woodbridge Component	Sensory	Motor	Mental	Reflexes		
				Circulatory	Respiratory	Gastrointestinal
High intensity response	Breath-holding Deep breathing Stiff chest Phonation Laryngospasm Tachycardia Rise or fall in BP Movement with stimulus Pupillary dilation Sweating Coughing	Fine or gross movement Abdominal tightness Muscle potentials on EKG	Movement upon stimulation Delirium Uninhibited speech or actions	Bradycardia and hypotension or Tachycardia and hypertension Arrhythmias	Spasm: laryngeal bronchiolar chest wall Salivation	Nausea Retching Vomiting Swallowing
Acceptable response	Minimal response to painful stimuli followed by accommodation Stability of cardiovascular respiratory systems	Quiet surgical field Relaxation of muscle	Amnesia Ataraxia Sleep	Absence of troublesome CV, respiratory, and gastrointestinal reflexes		
Low intensity response	No response	Muscle flaccidity Inability to reestablish normal ventilatory function at end of anesthesia	Prolonged obtundation in pre- or postanesthetic period	Bradycardia Tachycardia Hypotension Arrhythmias Intolerance to position change	Respiratory arrest*	Intestinal atony Postoperative ileus

*In the absence of neuromuscular blockers or hypocarbia.

specific area, compensatory adjustments are needed. A higher concentration of inhalation anesthetic may be administered with full recognition that this may increase depression in all areas; alternately, a specific drug, a neuromuscular blocker, may be chosen to correct the defect. Observations are repeatedly made and adjustments instituted. Occasionally, the system is disturbed by design to test the resulting response; the anesthetist may increase or reduce the inhaled concentration of anesthetic in order to observe the effect. In fact, as anesthesia progresses, the anesthetist should gradually reduce the inhaled concentration and observe the effect in order to prevent overdose as body tissues become saturated.

APPRAISAL

In many ways, this procedural assessment is a restatement of what the good clinician has always done. As powers of observation improve and experience increases, the beginner will find that a combination of signs provides a satisfactory guide to anesthetic depth. It is well known, for example, that reactivity to stimuli diminishes with age and is always less marked in the critically ill. The anesthetist must be all the more alert and observant to prevent overdose.

General anesthesia usually appears to be deeper than it actually is. It is usually easier to lighten than to deepen anesthesia. Therefore, induction should be carried a little further than seems necessary for the incision, so that the difficulties associated with inadequate anesthesia are not encountered. A middle course must be steered between light and unnecessarily deep anesthesia.

ADDITIONAL OBSERVATIONS

A correlation of the clinical signs of anesthesia with the arterial level of the anesthetic has been attempted. Although for any one individual the depth of anesthesia may correlate closely with the arterial concentration of anesthetic, the same concentration of anesthesia in a population of individuals gives wide deviations in depth. For this reason, and because arterial concentration of anesthetic is ascertained only after some delay, it is only rarely used as a clinical guide to depth.

The electroencephalogram (EEG) also has limited usefulness as a monitor of anesthetic depth. Each anesthetic differs in the EEG alterations it produces (see Chapter 11). Other factors such as tensions of oxygen or carbon dioxide and level of blood pressure can alter the EEG and thus the EEG response to anesthetics. Moreover, each anesthetic interacts differently with these modifying factors. As a result, the EEG is seldom used as a monitoring device in anesthesia.

REFERENCES

Artusio JF: Diethyl ether analgesia: A detailed description of the first stage of ether anesthesia in man. J Pharmacol Exp Ther 3:343, 1954.
Clark DL, Hosick EC, Rosner BS: Neurophysiologic effects of different anesthetics in unconscious man. J Appl Physiol 31:884, 1971.
Cullen DJ, Eger EI, II, Stevens WC, et al: Clinical signs of anesthesia. Anesthesiology 36:21, 1972.
Eger EI, II: Anesthetic Uptake and Action. Baltimore, Williams & Wilkins Co. 1974.
Gillespie NA: The signs of anesthesia. Anesth Analg 22:275, 1943.
Guedel AE: Inhalation Anesthesia. 2nd ed, New York, The Macmillan Co, 1951, pp 10–52.
Woodbridge PD: Changing concepts concerning depth of anesthesia. Anesthesiology 18:536, 1958.

Part C

REGIONAL ANESTHESIA

Chapter 17

LOCAL ANESTHETICS

The introduction of local anesthesia followed that of general anesthesia by about 40 years. Niemann, in 1860, first observed the numbing effect on the tongue of cocaine, an alkaloid obtained from the coca plant. In 1884, after Koller had produced topical anesthesia by instillation of cocaine into the conjunctival sac, the principle of local anesthesia gained quick acceptance. Perhaps this resulted from a dissatisfaction with the general anesthesia given at the time, and surgeons could now provide anesthesia for their own operations. The subsequent development of local anesthesia was assured by the synthesis of more reliable local anesthetics and the introduction of new techniques of regional anesthesia.

Local anesthesia has continued to be useful for the following reasons:

1. Simplicity: The costs are reasonable, the agents injectable, and the equipment required minimal. The need for postoperative care of the patient is lessened.

2. Most of the undesirable side effects of general anesthesia are avoided. A localized area of the body can be operated upon without loss of consciousness; hence, the term "regional" anesthesia. Modern studies support the once promulgated anociassociation theory of Crile, which held that impulses from the operative area could be noxious and lead to shock. Regional anesthesia decreases the autonomic and endocrine response to stress through interference with afferent nerve conduction.

3. The methods are ideal for ambulatory patients, for brief and superficial operations, and in situations in which recently ingested food poses the

threat of regurgitation and aspiration during general anesthesia. If the patient's cooperation is needed, as, for example, in tendon repair of the forearm, local anesthesia is a valuable technique.

Some of the reasons why regional anesthesia is not more widely used are as follows:

1. Lack of patient acceptance; patients choose to be unaware of the operation. This opposition results in part from an ineffectual approach to the patient and from anesthetists' lack of skill in the performance of nerve blocks.

2. The impracticality of anesthetizing some body areas. For example, the number of injections, the quantity of anesthetic required, and the time consumed in providing local anesthesia for a radical mastectomy are prohibitive.

3. Insufficient duration of local anesthesia: the patient fears that the anesthesia will wear off prematurely. There are, however, agents and special techniques that prolong anesthesia considerably.

4. Rapid absorption of local anesthetics into the bloodstream with untoward, rarely fatal, reactions. Although the mechanisms and the means of prevention and treatment are understood, reactions may occur because of variations in human responsiveness. These reactions, however, should be minimal if precautions are taken.

THEORIES OF ACTION

Local anesthetics applied to the body surfaces and injected about nerves are used primarily to prevent pain during surgical procedures. They are also used in the treatment of pain associated with trauma or disease. The drugs interfere with the initiation and transmission of the nerve impulse by mechanisms based on biochemical and physical changes. A good way to explain the action is to relate anesthetic activity to the transmission of the nerve impulse.

Nerve fibers, like all cells, are ensheathed in a lipoprotein membrane that separates the intracellular from the extracellular fluid. Concentration gradients between the intracellular fluid containing potassium as the major cation and the extracellular fluid containing sodium are maintained by an active metabolic process. Properties of this membrane are such that permeability to different ions alters with variations in transmembrane potential. In the resting state the membrane is relatively permeable to postassium, but much less so to sodium, and the diffusion potential produced by the concentration gradient for potassium is the major determinant of the membrane potential (-70 to -90 mv), with the exterior positive relative to the interior. Partial depolarization as the nerve impulse approaches triggers depolarization via a large increase in permeability to sodium (Fig. 17–1A). The membrane potential transiently approximates that predicted from the

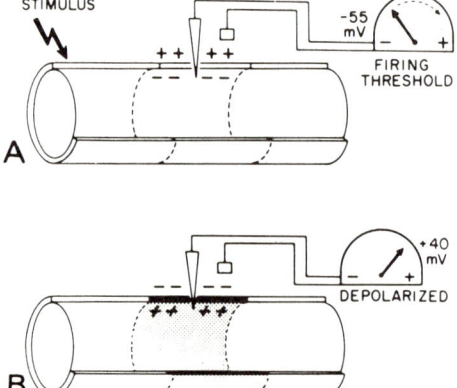

Figure 17-1. *A*, Upon stimulation, voltage across the membrane reaches −55 mv, the axon's firing threshold. *B*, Depolarization now complete, with the interior of the membrane 40 mv, positive in relation to the exterior. (Reproduced with permission from de Jong, RH: Physiology and Pharmacology of Local Anesthesia. Springfield, Ill., Charles C Thomas, 1970.)

concentration gradient of sodium (the outside becomes negative relative to the inside) and depolarization is electrically conducted to adjacent areas of the membrane (Fig. 17-1*B*). The sequence of events occurs successively as the impulse spreads along the nerve. During the latter phase of depolarization, the membrane again becomes less permeable to sodium and the nerve returns to the resting state, ready within milliseconds to repeat the response.

Local anesthetics increase the threshold for electric excitation in the nerve, slow the propagation of the impulse, reduce the rate of rise of the action potential, and eventually block conduction. These compounds act on nerve fibers by interfering with the ability of the membrane to undergo the specific change in permeability to sodium as a response to partial depolarization. The membrane is said to be stabilized at resting potential.

There are at least three theories as to how a local anesthetic may interact with the membrane. First, binding of local anesthetic molecules to the cell membrane may increase stability and prevent the opening of channels or pores for the passage of electrolytes. A conformational change in proteins associated with lipids may lead to expansion of the membrane; hence the membrane expansion theory. A second explanation involves the binding of calcium, which is displaced from the membrane, thereby allowing more ready access of sodium. Local anesthetics may increase the binding of calcium to the membrane. This is known as the surface charge theory, for which there is considerable evidence. A third possibility involves acetylcholine (ACh), which has been postulated as the transmitter substance in mediation of the nerve impulse. Released from an inactive bound form. ACh alters the permeability of the cell membrane and triggers the migration of sodium and potassium across the membrane. Once this is accomplished, ACh is rapidly hydrolyzed by cholinesterase. Local anesthetics, therefore, could interrupt conduction through competition with acetylcholine at receptor sites, but the theory is no longer tenable.

In myelinated nerve, in which the speed of conduction is facilitated by saltatory conduction, local anesthetic action takes place at the nodes of Ranvier, where the neurilemma or sheath of Schwann is present but the myelin sheath is interrupted.

DIFFERENTIAL BLOCKADE

Passage of an impulse between electrodes placed on a peripheral nerve can be displayed on an oscilloscope, with delineation of a characteristic mixed action potential. As shown by Erlanger's and Gasser's studies on electric potentials in mixed nerves, fibers of different size conduct impulses at different speeds; conduction velocity is proportional to fiber diameter. On this basis fibers may be classified as belonging to an A, B, or C group. The A fibers, from 1 μ to 22 μ in diameter, carry afferent and efferent somatic impulses at rates up to 90 m per sec. Large fibers also have the lowest excitability threshold. The smallest fibers, those carrying impulses for superficial pain, temperature, and autonomic activity, conduct slowly, and these modalities are blocked first by local anesthetics; as a corollary, weak concentrations of local anesthetics interrupt conduction in small fibers first. No theory has yet been proposed that adequately explains why the small myelinated fibers are more susceptible to block than the large. The ability to block nerve fibers differentially has been useful in diagnosis and therapy, as, for example, in differential subarachnoid block when one wishes to determine whether pain is visceral or somatic in origin. In practice, the concentration of the local anesthetic chosen should be only that needed to block the specific nerve fibers involved.

LOCAL ANESTHETIC DRUGS

More than a few reliable local anesthetics are available, but the anesthetist should understand the characteristics of a few drugs well, employ those with the greatest advantages, and use only those that have passed the test of time. The attributes of an acceptable local anesthetic are: complete reversibility of action, freedom from local irritation, high potency, effectiveness topically as well as regionally, minimal systemic toxicity, ready metabolism, stability during storage and sterilization, and a readily soluble synthetic molecule that permits chemical assay.

ESTER COMPOUNDS
Cocaine

Cocaine is still employed today in the form of the hydrochloric acid salt. It is used in 4 to 10 per cent concentrations for topical anesthesia of the nose, pharynx, and tracheobronchial tree. No more than 200 mg should be applied at a time. The local vasoconstrictive property of cocaine, unequaled by other local anesthetics, is useful in decreasing bleeding and shrinking congested mucous membranes. Vasoconstriction results from an action of cocaine that prevents reuptake of norepinephrine at nerve endings. Cocaine has been abandoned in ophthalmology because it causes opacity of the cornea and retards corneal epithelial regeneration, as do many other topical anesthetics. The high incidence of toxic reactions after injection of this drug, the liability to addiction, and the difficulty in preparing sterile solutions led to a search for a synthetic compound with fewer undesirable properties.

The clue to anesthetic activity lay in the structure of cocaine, an ester of benzoic acid, and the methylated base, ecgonine; the latter is related to tropine, the basic portion of the atropine molecule. Many local anesthetics subsequently synthesized have retained the ester structure and the chemical suffix "caine" in their nomenclature. The prototype of the esters consists of an aromatic lipophilic group, an intermediate group of several carbon atoms (ester linkage), and a hydrophilic group. The structure is as follows:

$$Ar-COO-(CH_2)_n-N\begin{matrix}R\\ \\R\end{matrix} \quad HX$$

(aromatic) (ester)   (hydrophilic) (salt)

The basic part of the ester is usually a tertiary amino alcohol which combines with acids to form soluble salts of weakly acidic reaction. The other portion of the ester is usually an aromatic acid with substituted radicals at various locations in the phenol ring. Most useful local anesthetics are secondary or tertiary amines, the compounds existing both as uncharged molecules (B) and as positively charged substituted ammonium cations (BH^+). The relative proportion of the two forms depends upon the pH of the solution and on the pK_a of the anesthetic according to the Henderson-Hasselbalch equation (see Chapter 3).

Local anesthetic solutions are marketed in the salt form, thus more stable chemically and more water soluble than the free base. There is good evidence that the salt form must be neutralized to the free base before the drug can penetrate tissues. However, it is doubtful that alkalinization of the solution prior to use is helpful in view of the excellent buffering capacity of tissues. Bromage has prepared carbonic salts of the local anesthetics, thereby providing more rapid and intense analgesia. However, the spread is wider and systemic reactions are more prone to occur. Carbon dioxide lowers tissue pH, thereby leading to ionization of the anesthetic salt.

Increased effectiveness of local anesthetic solutions when applied at a higher pH to isolated nerve fibers is the result of concentration of the charged form at the site. Again, this is of little practical concern. There is agreement that the tertiary amines penetrate the nerve membrane in the uncharged form and block the action potential from inside the membrane in charged form.

The ester compounds are hydrolyzed by esterases in plasma, of major importance in metabolism when anesthestics are absorbed into the bloodstream. The amino group bears resemblance to the quaternary amine structure of neuromuscular blockers. Since the latter compete with acetylcholine at receptor sites, some of the adverse reactions of local anesthetics may result from interference with central or peripheral synaptic transmission.

Procaine

After years of trial in the synthesis of various esters, Einhorn in 1904 prepared procaine, an ester of diethylaminoethanol and *p*-aminobenzoic acid. Procaine hydrochloride lacks topical activity but has been widely used because of minimal systemic toxicity, lack of local irritation, ease of sterilization, shorter duration of action, and low cost. The short duration and lack of cumulative toxic concentration in plasma result from the rapid hydrolysis by pseudocholinesterase. Procaine is used less and less because of competition from the amide group of anesthetics.

Chloroprocaine

Halogen substitution in the aromatic portion of the procaine molecule yields substances that are rapidly hydrolyzed in plasma and therefore less toxic than the parent compound. Chloroprocaine hydrochloride (Nesacaine), like procaine, is not topically active but is more potent and has a shorter action. It is probably the safest local anesthetic from the standpoint of systemic toxicity; hence it is advocated for use in continuous peridural anesthesia. Concentrations employed for injection range from 0.5 to 2.0 per cent in doses not exceeding 1 gm.

Tetracaine

The third drug worthy of mention in the ester series is tetracaine hydrochloride (Pontocaine, Pantocaine, Amethocaine). The potency of this compound is higher and the duration of action longer than the other anesthetics thus far mentioned, the systemic toxicity being correspondingly greater. The slow rate of hydrolysis in plasma explains in part the high incidence of reactions, but the low total dosage counteracts this disadvantage. Tetracaine is injected in 0.1 per cent concentration when the duration of anesthesia required is longer than several hours. It is the most commonly employed anesthetic for spinal anesthesia, usually combined with an equal volume of 10 per cent dextrose to increase the specific gravity and thereby control spread of the solution. As a topical anesthetic in the pharynx and tracheobronchial tree, tetracaine is employed in 1 to 2 per cent concentrations. In the conjunctival sac tetracaine retards corneal epithelial regeneration. The rapid rate of absorption from the respiratory tract mucosa accounts for the many adverse reactions reported; quantities greater than 100 mg should not be applied at one time.

AMIDES

The structure of the amide local anesthetics is essentially the same as for the esters except for the amide linkage. As a consequence, these compounds are less readily metabolized and the liability of adverse reactions is greater. On the other hand, some have significant antiarrhythmic effects on the heart.

Dibucaine

Dibucaine hydrochloride (Nupercaine, Percaine, Cinchocaine), a substituted amide, is a potent anesthetic with high systemic toxicity and long duration of action. However, because of the lesser concentration needed, the fewer the number of adverse reactions. Dibucaine is used for topical anesthesia of mucous membranes as an ointment in 0.2 per cent concentration; it is now rarely used for injection although once popular for spinal anesthesia.

Lidocaine

Lidocaine hydrochloride (Xylocaine), an acetanilid derivative, has achieved widespread acceptance since its introduction by Löfgren in 1948. Its major advantages are the rapid onset of anesthesia and the freedom from local irritation. Potency and duration of action are moderately greater than for procaine, and topical activity, although good, is not as effective as that of cocaine. Lidocaine lacks the vasoconstrictive property of cocaine, and because of the amide structure is slowly detoxified in circulating plasma. Some of the drug is metabolized in liver microsomes and part is excreted unchanged in urine. For these reasons the drug is considered twice as toxic as procaine, and doses greater than 0.5 gm should not be used when the recommended 0.5 to 2.0 per cent concentrations are employed for injection. Concentrations of 4 per cent are employed for topical anesthesia; 80 mg seems to be a safe dose. Lidocaine is remarkably free from allergic reactions and therefore a good substitute for the ester compounds when reactions to the latter have occurred.

Mepivacaine

Mepivacaine hydrochloride (Carbocaine) contains an amide radical linked to a saturated heterocyclic ring of the piperidine group. In comparison to lidocaine, mepivacaine acts equally quickly but increases duration of anesthesia by approximately 20 per cent. For this reason the addition of epinephrine is not required for nerve block of ordinary duration. Concentrations suggested range from 1 to 4 per cent for injection and topical anesthesia, with the maximal dosage no higher than 500 mg. Adverse reactions are few, and studies on its metabolism are not extensive. Although tissue irritation is minimal, the drug has not been used in spinal anesthesia to any extent.

Prilocaine

In order to overcome the disadvantage of the slow metabolism of lidocaine, prilocaine (2-propylamino-*o*-propionotoluidide) (Citanest), an amide, was synthesized. Prilocaine is at least as effective as lidocaine in terms of concentration, latency, and duration of action. A major disadvantage of prilocaine is the development of methemoglobinemia, approaching 10 per cent of hemoglobin concentration in some cases. Furthermore, the oxygen dissociation curve for hemoglobin is shifted to the left with less ready release of oxygen. Cyanosis has been observed, and the treatment suggested is intravenous injection of methylene blue. This is not an overwhelming disadvantage in normal individuals, but the consequent decrease in oxygen-carrying capacity in patients with anemia and in the fetus when placental transfer occurs is a major disadvantage.

Bupivacaine

Bupivacaine hydrochloride (Marcaine) was synthesized in 1957 by Ekenstam, and has since been extensively used. The compound, an anilide derivative, differs from mepivacaine in that a butyl group is substituted for the methyl. More potent and with a markedly longer action than lidocaine or mepivacaine, probably as a result of increased tissue protein-binding, the drug is used in concentrations ranging from 0.25 to 0.75 per cent for the complete span of regional nerve blocks. Epinephrine in 1:200,000 concentration is added to the solution when indicated; the total amount of drug injected at a time should not exceed 200 to 500 mg, since its toxicity approximates that of tetracaine. With weaker concentrations, motor fiber block is inadequate, 0.75 per cent being necessary for that purpose in abdominal operations. While onset of anesthesia may be somewhat slower than with lidocaine or mepivacaine, the duration is two to three times longer. With repeated injection the drug accumulates in the bloodstream, with arterial concentrations 20 to 40 per cent higher than the venous; the placental barrier is readily crossed.

Etidocaine

Etidocaine (Duranest), the most recently introduced of the local anesthetics, is an amide structurally similar to lidocaine but of greater potency and longer duration of action. Its properties in relation to the others are shown in Table 17-1, while its general pharmacologic and toxicologic actions differ little from the group characteristics.

Table 17-1 lists the local anesthetics discussed in this chapter (with the exception of prilocaine, and their structure-activity relationships, while Table 17-2 lists some data of practical use in regional anesthesia.

LONG-ACTING LOCAL ANESTHESIA

In the treatment of postoperative and intractable pain, there has been a need for a local anesthetic with a duration of action longer than six to eight hours. Hence bupivacaine and etidocaine have been useful additions to the existing local anesthetics. One must bear in mind that local anesthesia by definition is a reversible process. In this respect, the long-lasting effects of certain proprietary compounds do not represent true anesthesia; careful histologic examination after experimental injection of these compounds often reveals destruction of nerve fibers.

Solutions of local anesthetics in oil were once thought to act as repositories from which the anesthetic was gradually released, thereby extending the action. Prolongation of anesthesia has not been demonstrated by this means. In some instances the oily base remains at the site, causing abscess or granuloma formation. Proprietary long-acting anesthetic mixtures often contained benzyl alcohol, eugenol, bromosaligenin (Bromsalizol), salicyl alcohol (Saligenin), or phenol. These agents are not local anesthetics and are destructive to nerve fibers. Fortunately, the mixtures were employed only to provide relief from pain after anorectal surgery or episiotomy, areas of the body in which neurologic deficit is of little consequence. One must be certain never to inject these solutions near the larger peripheral nerves or in the vicinity of the spinal cord, for the resulting neuritis may lead to pain more severe than that originally experienced or cause transverse myelitis. However, in the treatment of the intractable pain of terminal malignancy or to relieve the muscle spasm of paraplegia, weak solutions of ethyl alcohol or phenol, 6 per cent, have been injected into the subarachnoid space. In these situations the resulting neurologic deficit is overbalanced by the therapeutic effect.

INTRAVENOUS USE OF LOCAL ANESTHETICS

Although high blood levels of local anesthetic are responsible for most adverse systemic effects, several of the local anesthetics have been given intravenously either as adjuncts to general anesthesia or in the treatment of a miscellaneous group of ailments. Intravenous injection of procaine was once considered the best means of treating ventricular arrhythmias during general anesthesia. Procaine was also given as a continuous infusion in 0.1 per cent concentration to add to the effect of general anesthesia. Although central nervous system stimulation was not observed if the drug was given carefully, the frequent appearance of hypotension led to abandonment. Probably, rapid hydrolysis of procaine given only to the point of tolerance in the conscious patient prevented more serious side effects than would have been otherwise anticipated.

Intravenous injection of lidocaine has been advocated for the same reasons that led to the use of procaine. Lidocaine appears to depress laryngeal and tracheal reflexes, thereby permitting maintenance of pharyngeal and tracheal airways in light planes of general anesthesia. Patients thus treated are said to require less analgetics for pain and to vomit less postoperatively than when given general anesthetics alone. Because of its antiarrhythmic properties, lidocaine is effective during cardiac surgery, in resuscitation after cardiac arrest, and for treatment of irritability in myocardial infarction. Many of the effects noted following the intravenous injection of local anesthetics were predictable from their pharmacologic actions. General anesthesia seems to obtund several of the more undesirable actions, but not all.

TOPICAL ANESTHESIA

Topical anesthesia is often inexpertly done, and the incidence of adverse reactions is therefore high. Preliminary topical anesthesia of the respiratory passages is useful in eliminating pharyngeal and tracheal reflexes and cough when airways are inserted before induction or during light planes of general anesthesia. The drugs used for this purpose have already been described and the safe dosage limits are listed in Table 17–2. Preferably only one drug should be used for a procedure. Blood levels of local anesthetic during topical anesthesia may equal those obtained after intravenous injection, and primary myocardial depression is the probable cause of sudden collapse; therefore, preparation should be made for resuscitation should such a reaction occur.

Because topical anesthetization is an uncomfortable procedure requiring cooperation, the appropriate preanesthetic sedation should be provided and atropine given for the drying effect. Salivary secretions interfere with anesthesia by diluting the anesthetic and preventing sufficient contact with mucous membranes.

Anesthetic ointments should be water soluble and sterile. Ointments are often applied to airways before insertion, but unless this is preceded by topical anesthesia they do not immediately prevent cough. At least one minute is required for onset of anesthesia with most topical drugs, the duration of anesthesia being no longer than 20 to 30 minutes. Either a water-solu-

Table 17–1. Structure-Activity Relationships of Local Anesthetics

Agent	Chemical Configuration			Physico-Chemical Properties		Biological Properties		
	Aromatic Lipophilic	Intermediate Chain	Amine Hydrophilic	Partition Coefficient	% Protein Binding	Equi-Effective* Anesthetic Conc.	Approx. Anesthetic* Duration (min)	Site of Metabolism
A. Esters								
PROCAINE	$H_2N-\phi-$	$COOCH_2CH_2$	$-N(C_2H_5)_2$	0.6†	5.8§	2	50	Plasma
TETRACAINE	$H_9C_4-N(H)-\phi-$	$COOCH_2CH_2$	$-N(CH_3)_2$	80†	75.6§	0.25	175	Plasma
B. Amides								
MEPIVACAINE	(2,6-dimethylphenyl)	NHCO	N-pyrrolidinyl-CH$_3$	0.8‡	77.5‖	1	100	Liver

BUPIVACAINE	![2,6-dimethylphenyl with CH₃ groups]	NHCO	N(C₄H₉)(pyrrolidine ring)	27.5‡	95.6‖	0.25	175	Liver
LIDOCAINE	![2,6-dimethylphenyl with CH₃ groups]	NHCOCH₂	N(C₂H₅)(C₂H₅)	2.9‡	64.3‖	1	100	Liver
ETIDOCAINE	![2,6-dimethylphenyl with CH₃ groups]	NHCOCH(C₂H₅)	N(C₂H₅)(C₃H₇)	141‡	94‖	0.25	200	Liver

*Data derived from rat sciatic nerve blocking procedure
†Oleylalcohol/pH 7.2 buffer
‡n-Heptane/pH 7.4 buffer
§Nerve homogenate binding
‖Plasma protein binding—2 μg/ml
¶(Reproduced with permission from Covino, BG, Vassallo, HG: Local Anesthetics. Mechanisms of Action and Clinical Use. New York, Grune & Stratton, 1976.)

Table 17-2. Suggested Uses, Concentrations, and Maximal Dosage of the Local Anesthetics*

Drugs	Topical	Dose (mg)	Injection	Dose (mg)
Esters:				
Cocaine hydrochloride	Respiratory tract 5-10% (4-2 ml)	200	Not employed	
Procaine hydrochloride Novocain Ethocaine	Ineffective		Infiltration 0.5% (200 ml) Peripheral nerves 1-2% (100-50 ml)	1000
Chloroprocaine hydrochloride Nesacaine	Ineffective		Infiltration 0.5% (200 ml) Peripheral nerves 2% (50 ml)	1000
Tetracaine hydrochloride Pontocaine Pantocaine	Respiratory tract 1-2% (8-4 ml)	80	Infrequently used for infiltration and nerve injection, 0.1 to 0.25%	100
Amides:				
Dibucaine hydrochloride Nupercaine Percaine Cinchocaine	Infrequently used 0.2% (15 ml)	30	Infrequently used	
Lidocaine hydrochloride Xylocaine lignocaine	Respiratory tract 2-4% (10-5 ml)	200	Infiltration 0.5% (100 ml) Peripheral nerves 1-2% (50-25 ml)	500
Mepivacaine hydrochloride Carbocaine	No data		Infiltration 0.5-1.0% (100-50 ml) Peripheral nerves 1-2%	500
Bupivacaine hydrochloride Marcaine	No data		Infiltration and peripheral nerves 0.25-0.75%	500
Etidocaine hydrochloride Duranest	No data		Infiltration and peripheral nerves 0.25-0.75%	500

*Use of local anesthetics for specialized techniques is not shown.

ble jelly or solution may be introduced into the pharynx so that gargling will result in anesthesia. Pledgets of cotton soaked in anesthetic solution and wrung out before application can be applied to the mucous membranes with the aid of a head lamp and laryngeal mirror. Once anesthesia of the pharynx has been obtained, a small amount of anesthetic can be instilled into the trachea under direct vision. Spraying or atomization is commonly employed, but is ineptly done as a rule because the droplets vary so much in size. Large droplets from an ordinary spray cause cough and lead to overdose, while small droplets from a nebulizer pass through finer bronchioles and are rapidly absorbed, producing toxic effects. The most efficient atomizers supply droplets ranging in size from 30 to 100 μ; these devices should incorporate a reservoir so that the quantity of drug used can be readily observed.

A safe concentration and volume of anesthetic (tetracaine 1 per cent, or lidocaine 4 per cent, 2 ml total) can be injected into the trachea percutaneously through the cricothyroid membrane; the resulting cough helps to spread the anesthetic. This is done aseptically and used only in situations where anatomic relationships are clearly defined and there is no local disease. Vigorous cough is hazardous in certain types of valvular heart disease in which the hypoxia and Valsalva effect can lead to circulatory collapse.

ADVERSE EFFECTS OF LOCAL ANESTHETICS

Untoward reactions to local anesthetics are often erroneously ascribed to sensitivity or idiosyncrasy, whereas they can be explained on known pharmacologic grounds even though exceedingly small doses may have been responsible for the effects observed.

SYSTEMIC REACTIONS

Cause

Systemic reactions are encountered with symptoms referable to the central nervous, respiratory, and cardiovascular systems. These reactions result from absorption into the bloodstream of toxic amounts of the drug, causing convulsions, drowsiness, or unconsciousness. Whether a depressive or excitatory response occurs seems to depend upon a balance of effect of the local anesthetic on inhibitory and excitatory centers in the brain. The excitatory response is enhanced by respiratory and metabolic acidosis. The depressant effect on the medullary centers may lead to apnea and vascular collapse. Local anesthetics depress the myocardium directly by a quinidinelike effect on conduction, contractility, and irritability. For this reason, procaine and lidocaine have been employed as antiarrhythmic agents. The hypotension resulting from the action on the myocardium is compounded by a peripheral vasodilatory action. Part of the depressive action may be countered by reactive sympathetic activity. Some or all of these effects occur rapidly in response to injection of much less than the expected toxic doses. The most feared outcome is simultaneous respiratory and cardiac arrest.

Because the circulating blood level of anesthetic is a prime factor in systemic reactions, the site of injection is of paramount importance. The intravenous route is most dangerous, but absorption from the pharyngeal, tracheal, and bronchial mucosa yields high blood concentrations almost as rapidly because of the vascularity of these areas, rapid absorption of anesthetic from the lungs, and direct circulation of the drug to the myocardium. It is not surprising that most instances of sudden cardiovascular collapse involve topical anesthesia of the respiratory tract. Other hazardous injection sites include tissues about the head and neck and the paravertebral region; least dangerous are the subcutaneous areas of the trunk and limbs. Hyaluronidase, because of its spreading action, is sometimes added to local anesthetic solutions to increase the percentage of successful nerve blocks, but systemic reactions are more likely to occur because of rapid absorption. Anesthetic solutions taken by mouth result in few reactions, probably because of absorption into the portal venous system and rapid metabolism in the liver.

A second factor in the causation of reactions is the rapidity of hydrolysis once an anesthetic reaches the circulation. The enzymes involved are cholinesterases formed in the liver. Hydrolysis of the ester compounds proceeds at varying rates, toxicity being related quantitatively to this factor alone. The generalization may be made, therefore, that the esters are likely to be less toxic than the amides.

Prevention

Total Amount of Anesthetic. The least possible amount of anesthetic should be used. The total amount of drug injected over a period of time is more significant than the initial concentration or volume. It is essential to employ the minimal effective concentration and the smallest volume, bearing in mind that sensory nerve impulses are blocked by lesser concentrations.

Use of Epinephrine. The rate of absorption of anesthetic should be slowed in every way possible; this is accomplished by slow injection and repeated aspiration for blood, particularly in vascular areas, to avoid intravenous injection. The vasoconstrictive property of epinephrine retards absorption; additional benefits are prolongation of anesthesia and decreased bleeding. Near maximal prolongation of anesthesia and probably maximal protection are obtained with 1:200,000 concentrations of epinephrine, 0.5 mg per 100 ml of solution. Epinephrine should be measured with a syringe rather than added to the anesthetic solution according to the number of drops. Only minimal effective concentrations should be employed, because epinephrine carries a toxicity of its own. Many so-called reactions to local anesthetics represent the pharmacologic effects of epinephrine: apprehension, tremor, pallor, sweating, tachycardia, and palpitation. Epinephrine is dangerous in the patient with myocardial disease or coronary arteriosclerosis because of the increased work of the heart resulting from the positive chronotropic and inotropic actions as well as arrhythmogenic properties. Local injection of anesthetic solutions containing epinephrine may result in gangrene when injected into closed spaces such as the finger. Little benefit derives from adding epinephrine to topical anesthetics.

Barbiturates and Diazepam. Preanesthetic administration of a short-acting barbiturate, secobarbital, or pentobarbital in sedative doses, once believed to protect against the central stimulating properties of local anesthesics, provides little more than relief from apprehension. Narcotic rather than sedative doses of the barbiturate are necessary to prevent convulsions. Diazepam is much more effective in prevention and therapy. deJong has shown in the cat that the median convulsant dose of lidocaine (8.4 mg per kg) is approximately doubled by the prior use of 0.25 mg per kg diazepam, the equivalent of 15 mg in a 60-kg adult.

Treatment

Rapid intravenous injection of pentobarbital or thiopental has been the initial treatment of choice for incipient or fully developed convulsions, but the barbiturates may add to the circulatory and respiratory depression already present. Recently diazepam has been employed intravenously in 5 mg doses for the treatment of convulsions. The dangers of a convulsion dervive from cerebral hypoxia, bodily injury, the possibility of the aspiration of vomitus, postictal depression, and respiratory and circulatory arrest attendant upon the hypoxia. Consequently, oxygen should be given by inhalation simultaneously with injection of the barbiturate. It has been suggested that the short-acting neuromuscular blocker, succinylcholine, be used to stop convulsive movements. Although this may minimize oxygen demands secondary to muscle contractions, some believe it does not prevent the cerebral hypoxia contingent upon cortical hyperactivity. We believe that the production of apnea by succinylcholine in inexperienced hands may lead to more problems in the way of pulmonary ventilation. Furthermore, succinylcholine is seldom available in the place where reactions are most likely to occur—the physician's office.

Circulatory depression as indicated by hypotension or a weak pulse should be treated with a vasopressor drug given intravenously or intramuscularly. Single dose ampules of ephedrine or phenylephrine should be at hand. It matters little which vasopressor is given in an emergency so long as myocardial depression and peripheral vasodilation are reversed before cardiac standstill occurs. Cardiac arrest should be managed according to the plan suggested in Chapter 30.

LOCAL IRRITATION AND TISSUE DESTRUCTION

A number of new local anesthetic substances were introduced to practice before tests were made of tissue destruction (see Long-acting Local Anesthesia). It is not enough merely to report absence of an inflammatory response in the test animal; new anesthetics should also be injected about nerves to detect neuron destruction. The anesthetics described here are safe from this standpoint. A technique used to detect tissue damage involves injection of a local anesthetic into the anterior chamber of the rabbit's eye; irritation or destruction is indicated by development of corneal opacity. Still another method has been observation of the effect of local anesthetics on ciliary activity in human bronchial ciliated epithelium removed by biopsy. Toxic properties are suggested if the paralyzing effect on ciliary movement is not reversible.

ALLERGIC REACTIONS

True allergic reactions to the local anesthetics are infrequent. We have observed an anaphylactic reaction in a patient with multiple allergies who developed bronchospasm and cardiac standstill following topical application of cocaine for tonsillectomy. It has not been possible to predict allergic reactions reliably either by skin patch tests or by conjunctival instillation. Dermatitis following repeated exposure to local anesthetics, particularly procaine, occurs not infrequently in professional personnel, and cross-sensitivity has been demonstrated; further use of local anesthetics calls for substitution of a compound of a different chemical nature.

PRACTICAL SUGGESTIONS FOR THE USE OF LOCAL ANESTHETICS

A patient scheduled for nerve block should refrain from eating or merely eat an easily digested meal not less than four hours before the procedure. Vomiting may occur as a psychogenic response or accompany a systemic reaction to the local anesthetic. A sedative dose of one of the short-acting barbiturates or diazepam can be prescribed to allay apprehension. If ambulatory, the patient should be accompanied by a relative or friend and not be permitted to drive an automobile after a sedative. Patients should be questioned for untoward reactions to the local anesthetics, and the general physical condition should be known.

When possible a patient should be recumbent at the time of injection and the skin prepared with an antiseptic that will not stain clothing or bed linen. Although freshly prepared solutions of local anesthetics may be reliable, it is simpler to employ the sterile, single dose ampules of the drug. One calculates in advance the quantity of anesthetic to be injected, keeping well below the toxic dose. This is done by choosing the minimal effective concentration, understanding the anatomic course of nerves, and injecting at a point at which maximal effect is obtained with the least amount of solution. Use of epinephrine has already been discussed. A common mistake is not to wait long enough for the anesthetic to take effect or to inject only into the subcutaneous tissues, thereby missing intracutaneous nerve fibers. Injection should be unhurried, with frequent aspiration for blood and constant observation. Observation of the face may disclose muscle twitches that precede a more generalized reaction. Continuous conversation serves to reassure the patient and to allow detection of garrulousness, excitement, or loss of consciousness.

Upon completion of a procedure using local anesthetic, particularly a complicated one, the patient should be watched for some time to detect delayed complications. If an untoward reaction to the anesthetic has occurred, the patient should be fully informed so that repetition is avoided. Lastly, a record must be kept of the procedure as a protection for both patient and physician.

REFERENCES

Covino BG, Vassallo HG: Local Anesthetics. Mechanisms of Action and Clinical Use. New York, Grune & Stratton, 1976.

deJong RH: Physiology and Pharmacology of Local Anesthesia. Springfield, Ill, Charles C Thomas, 1970.

de Jong RH, Heavner JE: Diazepam prevents local anesthetic seizures. Anesthesiology 34:523, 1971.

Munson EA, Wagman IH: Diazepam treatment of local anesthetic-induced seizures. Anesthesiology 37:523, 1972.

Symposium on local anaesthetics. Br J Anaesth 47:Suppl, 1975.

Chapter 18

SPINAL ANESTHESIA

Spinal anesthesia entails the injection of a local anesthetic into the subarachnoid space. Introduction of the method followed invention of the hollow needle and syringe in the middle of the 19th century, the discovery by Koller of the local anesthetic properties of cocaine in 1884, and the initial performance of lumbar puncture by Quincke in 1891. Administration of the first spinal anesthesia has been attributed to Corning, who in 1885 attempted to anesthetize the lower half of the body of a patient by injecting cocaine into the region of the spinal column. The anesthesia, which reached completion after a lapse of about 20 minutes, possibly resulted from diffusion of cocaine into the peridural space. Three surgeons—Bier in Germany, Matas in America, and Tuffier in France—independently in 1898 and 1899, were among the first to administer spinal anesthesia in the true sense of the term.

ACTION AND FATE OF ANESTHETICS IN THE SUBARACHNOID SPACE

When a local anesthetic is injected into the subarachnoid space there is almost immediate onset of anesthesia. Spinal nerve roots, dorsal root ganglia, and the periphery of the cord to some extent are the loci of action. The main effects probably result from anesthetization of the anterior and posterior nerve roots. Because of the high initial concentration gradient and lipoid solubility of the local anesthetic, absorption takes place rapidly into nerve fibers. Fibers of smallest diameter are affected first, possibly because of more rapid diffusion through the myelin sheath, possibly because of the large surface area and the lesser distance in penetration. Disappearance of neural function occurs more or less in the following order: autonomic activity, superficial pain, temperature sensation, vibratory and position sense, motor power, and finally, touch.

As the anesthetic spreads from the lumbar region, more and more fibers are affected, with gradually decreasing concentration in the cerebrospinal fluid (CSF), until at the upper reaches conduction is interrupted only in autonomic fibers and those mediating pinprick. The concentration of procaine in CSF necessary for block of superficial sensation is approximately 0.2 mg per ml and for tetracaine, 0.02 mg per ml. A span of several dermatomes is present between complete motor block and the highest point of sensory or autonomic interruption. Thus, it is possible to produce abdominal muscle relaxation without paralyzing the upper intercostal muscles or diaphragm. On the other hand, mere sensory blockade does not guarantee sufficient muscle relaxation for performance of operation.

Anesthesia wanes as the anesthetic is absorbed into the systemic circulation from nerves and CSF, via lymphatics and capillaries. Ultimately the anesthetic is metabolized in the liver and excreted in urine. For ester compounds, hydrolysis takes place in the circulation and liver; the concentration of esterases in CSF is negligible. Thus, duration of spinal anesthesia depends upon the vascular and lymphatic supply of the spinal cord and the rapidity of absorption. Duration of anesthesia also relates to the amount of anesthetic injected. A small amount injected into the subarachnoid space and then permitted to spread widely results in incomplete anesthesia of short duration, whereas a larger quantity concentrated in one area produces more complete and longer-lasting effects. The local anesthetic used, physical, metabolic, and physiologic factors explain the variable duration of spinal anesthesia.

PHYSIOLOGIC EFFECTS

CIRCULATION

Appearance of marked degrees of arterial hypotension after administration of spinal anesthesia was an early concern and is still considered a relative disadvantage despite use of vasopressor drugs and intravenous fluids to support the pressure. The hypotension of spinal anesthesia results from interruption of sympathetic nerve impulses to systemic blood vessels and interruption of baroreceptor reflexes that control blood pressure. The higher the level of sympathetic block, the more consistent and profound is the fall in pressure and the less chance for compensatory vasoconstriction in unanesthetized areas of the body. Blood pressure tends to decline more if the initial level of pressure is high. Postural effects are marked as in any type of neurologic hypotension, and the lowering of pressure is further aggravated in the presence of hypovolemia.

Circulatory studies indicate that a decrease in total peripheral vascular resistance accounts for the drop in pressure in some individuals; in others, a decrease in cardiac output is found. The latter probably results from venous dilation and pooling of blood, with decreased venous return to the heart. Accessory factors include bradycardia resulting from block of accelerator impulses to the heart or decrease in endogenous release of norepinephrine from sympathetic nerve endings, thereby reducing myocardial contractility. Vasoconstriction in unanesthetized areas of the body may compensate partially for the hypotension. With total autonomic block, the reflex vasoconstrictive response to hypotension initiated from the baroreceptors is interrupted.

RESPIRATION

Under ordinary circumstances paralysis of intercostal muscles does not cause respiratory insufficiency if the cervical origin of the phrenic nerves is not reached by the anesthetic; diaphragmatic action alone should provide adequate ventilation. During abdominal operation, however, movement of the diaphragm may be limited by retractors or packs; thus, respiratory assistance with oxygen should be provided. When diaphragm and intercostal muscles both are paralyzed, this emergency is treated as is any other instance of respiratory failure. Patients often complain of difficulty in breathing during spinal anesthesia because of lack of perception of abdominal and thoracic movements.

BOWEL AND URINARY TRACT

Because of sympathetic block the effect of spinal anesthesia on the bowel is that of unopposed parasympathetic activity, the intestines being contracted and hyperactive, the sphincters relaxed. However, opioids oppose this action, and high doses of atropine tend to minimize vagal influence. Spillage of feces during intestinal anastomosis or defecation may occur, although uncommonly. The ureters show peristalsis with relaxation of the ureterovesical orifice; this may aid in removal or elimination of ureteral calculi. Renal blood flow tends to decrease unless the arterial blood pressure is maintained. The usual adrenocortical response to stress is lacking during spinal anesthesia because of the block of afferent impulses from the operative field.

FACTORS INFLUENCING SPINAL ANESTHESIA

The composition of the solution injected into the subarachnoid space and the technique of injection are influenced by: duration, intensity, and level of anesthesia desired; body height or length of the vertebral column; intra-abdominal pressure and obesity: and anticipated position of the patient during operation. One can combine the measures listed further on to influence duration, intensity, and level of block.

DURATION OF ACTION

The average duration of anesthesia with the commonly used drugs is 60 minutes for procaine and lidocaine and 120 minutes for tetracaine. For

Spinal Anesthesia

operations of indeterminate duration, a continuous technique may be chosen.

The duration of the anesthetic action may be increased by addition of epinephrine to the anesthetic mixture, 0.5 mg being the optimal amount. An average increase in duration of approximately 30 to 100 per cent can be expected, depending upon the concentration of epinephrine. Phenylephrine, usually 2 mg, also increases the duration but to a lesser extent. Extension of anesthesia is thought to result from prolonged exposure of nerve fibers to the anesthetic, possibly with more thorough penetration and fixation.

When epinephrine is given with tetracaine, the onset of anesthesia is slower; whether as a result of the vasoconstriction and slow penetration of nerve fibers or change in the physical characteristics of the solution has not been determined. The slow onset often prompts the anesthetist to lower the head of the operating table in an effort to spread the block with a hyperbaric solution, but this usually leads to a level higher than wanted. Since a high level results, the anesthetist is tempted beforehand to reduce the total dose of anesthetic and this, in turn, leads to inadequate anesthesia. A disadvantage of long-acting anesthesia is that the patient is left with numbness and paralysis for a long time postoperatively. It is better, therefore, to resort to a continous technique if anesthesia of long duration is required, especially in the elderly.

SERIAL INJECTION

A plastic catheter is placed in the subarachnoid space, permitting additional doses of anesthetic to be injected as needed. This technique provides almost unlimited duration of anesthesia, affording better control of dosage particularly in the very ill or elderly patient for whom selection of a proper dose as a single injection may be a problem. Injection of anesthetic in small increments also lessens the rapidity of onset and the degree of hypotension. Although this is a cumbersome technique with a higher potential for neurologic sequelae, the advantages outweigh the disadvantages.

DOSAGE

The average anesthetic dose of tetracaine for individuals of varying height and for expected levels of sensory anesthesia is shown in Table 18–1 and Figure 18–1. Sacral levels permit performance of operations on the perineum; levels at the groin allow for operation on the legs and thighs; xiphoid levels permit lower abdominal procedures; and a sensory level to the nipples is necessary for upper abdominal operations. It must be remembered that the upper level of anesthesia as tested by pinprick is merely a sensory level and that motor nerves to muscle are blocked several dermatomes below.

Table 18-1. DOSE OF TETRACAINE FOR SPINAL ANESTHESIA*

Operation	Tetracaine (mg) Height (cm)		
	152	167	184
	mg		
Upper abdomen	14	16	18
Lower abdomen	12	14	16
Inguinal—bladder	10	12	14
Extremities	8	10	12
Rectal	4	6	8

*Tetracaine is injected as 0.5 per cent, in 5 per cent dextrose in water; for a 12 mg dose, mix 1.2 ml of 1 per cent tetracaine with 1.2 ml of 10 per cent dextrose in water. With procaine, the dose is 10 times that of tetracaine, injected as 5 per cent procaine in CSF. *These doses are approximate,* chosen to make memorization easy. Dose and body height are not the only factors influencing anesthetic level. Position before and after injection, volume and baricity of the solution, inclusion of vasoconstrictors, rate of injection, cough and straining, and pressure and volume of the CSF affect the level (see text).

CONCENTRATION OF LOCAL ANESTHETIC

If sensory block alone is sought, a lesser concentration of anesthetic is needed than if conduction in the larger motor fibers is to be interrupted. For example, a 0.2 per cent solution of procaine is employed for differen-

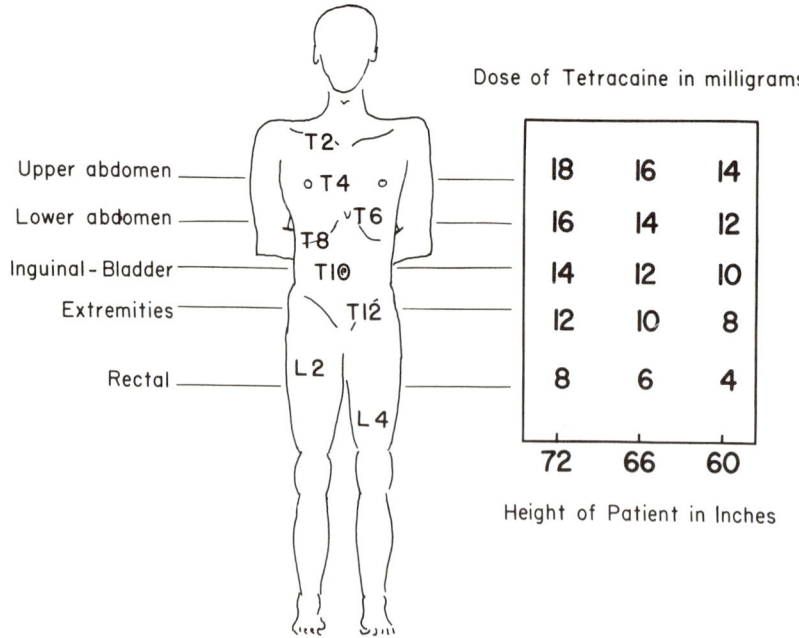

Figure 18-1. Approximate sensory levels of anesthesia required for the operative site indicated.

tial block of sympathetic nerves when spinal anesthesia is used as a diagnostic or prognostic test. Therefore, if muscle relaxation is not essential, a weak solution is used.

SPECIFIC GRAVITY OF SOLUTION

The specific gravity of CSF varies, depending upon temperature and solute content (average 37°C, 1.005 ± 0.003). By dissolving the local anesthetic in distilled water, a solution with a specific gravity less than CSF results (hypobaric); with CSF or 10 per cent dextrose as the diluent, a hyperbaric solution is obtained. Differences in specific gravity when combined with position, during and after injection, are used to influence the spread of anesthetic. If, for example, a hyperbaric solution is selected and the patient is seated during and after injection, a low block is obtained; injection of a hypobaric solution would result in a higher level of anesthesia. When a heavy solution is injected slowly into the subarachnoid space it remains more or less as a bolus acted upon by gravity. In none of these maneuvers is the anesthetic confined to the site, for the difference in specific gravity is equalized as the anesthetic solution spreads. However, the area exposed to the higher concentration remains anesthetized for a longer time. Dextrose solution mixed with tetracaine seems to shorten the time of onset and to prolong anesthesia as well as insure uniform block. Unilateral anesthesia is often attempted in an effort to diminish some of the undesirable physiologic effects of spinal anesthesia, but it is hardly successful unless the original position is maintained for about 40 minutes.

Because of the spinal curvatures (Fig. 18-2) a hyperbaric solution tends to reach the third to sixth thoracic segments if the patient lies supine with legs extended. The curves may be altered by flexing the thighs on the abdomen; the reduction in lumbar lordosis limits cephalad spread of a hyperbaric solution.

INTRA-ABDOMINAL PRESSURE AND OBESITY

Increased intra-abdominal pressure dictates a reduction in volume and dose of local anesthetic used. Elevated pressures compress the vena cava

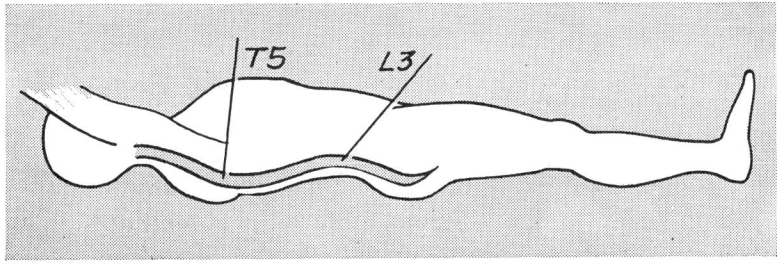

Figure 18-2. Spinal column curvatures that influence spread of anesthetic.

and increase pressure in the peridural plexus of veins, the resulting dilation encroaching upon the subarachnoid space, thereby lessening capacity. The solution therefore, is injected into a lesser volume of CSF and spreads over a wider area. Pregnancy, ascites, large abdominal tumors, intestinal obstruction, and marked obesity are situations in which abdominal pressure may be elevated.

POSITION

Subsequent moving of the patient into position for operation is another factor in choice of anesthetic solution. Hypobaric solutions are of value for operations carried out in the lateral or prone position, since injection can be made with the operative site uppermost. If the Trendelenburg position is elected, as for a vaginal procedure, use of a hypobaric solution minimizes the likelihood of high block. If cholecystectomy is the procedure, a high, solid block is needed, and in our opinion a hyperbaric solution is best. Once spinal anesthesia is fully developed, a change in body position may be followed by hypotension (supine to lateral, or to prone position).

EQUIPMENT AND STERILIZATION

Appropriate choice of equipment and drugs and attention to asepsis are essential in spinal anesthesia because of the threat of neurologic complications. Everything required for the administration of spinal anesthesia should be packaged in one tray. If a choice of local anesthetic is desired, ampules can be packaged, sterilized separately, and added to the tray as needed. The tray should contain:
1. Drape with central opening
2. One 5-ml plain tip syringe for the local anesthetic, a 10-ml syringe for hypobaric solutions
3. One blunt tip, 18-gauge needle for mixing the anesthetic solution
4. One 2-ml Luer-Lok syringe for superficial anesthesia
5. One 25-gauge hypodermic needle for skin infiltration
6. One 22- and one 26-gauge lumbar puncture needle, $3^{1}/_{2}$ inches long, each with stylet, and a 21-gauge introducer for the smaller needle
7. One 2-inch 22-gauge needle for intramuscular injection
8. Forceps and sponges
9. Ampule file
10. Spinal anesthetics, skin anesthetic, and vasopressor drug
11. A medicine glass or metal cup

The local anesthetics should be reputable products. A variety of disposable spinal anesthesia trays containing all the materials necessary and sterilized in ethylene oxide are now commercially available and are quite satisfactory (Fig. 18–3). When ampules of local anesthetic are wrapped

Spinal Anesthesia

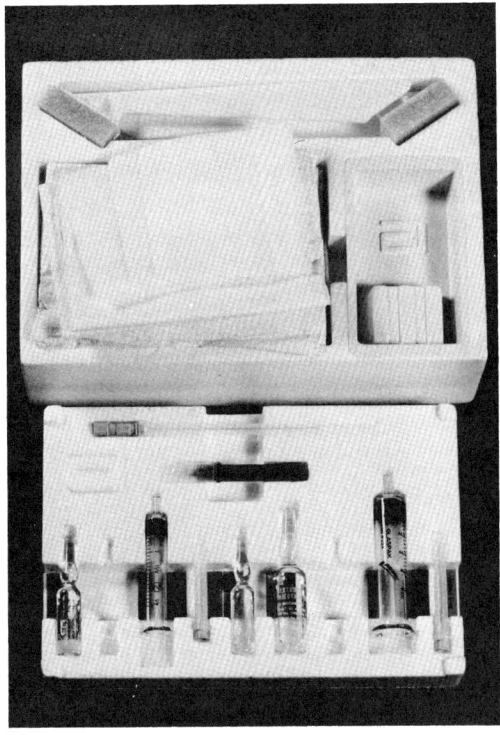

Figure 18-3. Disposable spinal tray. (Courtesy of Abbott Laboratories.)

separately, they are sterilized at 260 C and 27 pounds pressure for 10 minutes, as in ethylene oxide. As a rule, drugs are not resterilized even though little deterioration takes place with autoclaving; this includes epinephrine, whose potency is not reduced by such treatment. Sterilization of ampules by immersion in antiseptic solutions is no longer practiced as the antiseptic can penetrate a cracked ampule. Detection of contamination is difficult and neurologic damage has followed injection.

CHOICE OF SPINAL ANESTHESIA

In the majority of cases, spinal anesthesia is given for operations on the lower abdomen, inguinal regions or lower extremities, although in some clinics it is used for upper abdominal operations as well. The conditions provided for intra-abdominal operation are unrivaled because of the excellent muscle relaxation, contracted bowel, quiet breathing, and relative decrease in bleeding owing to the hypotension usually present. Some of the conditions for which spinal anesthesia is the method of choice are as follows: in husky muscular patients, when food has recently been ingested, in cesarean section for prematurity, alcoholism or barbiturate addiction, a difficult airway problem, use of controlled hypotension, and hepatic, renal, or metabolic disease. Spinal anesthesia cannot be elected without consideration for the patient's emotional and physical make-up and the needs of the surgeon. Among the contraindications are prior difficulty with spinal anesthesia, residual neurologic deficit, backache, unhappy emotional experience with spinal anesthesia, the presence of neurologic disease, and concurrent use of anticoagulants. Other deterrents are the prospects of difficult lumbar puncture or the possibility of introducing infection. The patient's back is examined to predict these things and to determine the best position for puncture. Lesser contraindications include very young patients, mental aberration, morbid fear of this kind of anesthesia, decreased blood volume, severe anemia, and a marked increase in intra-abdominal pressure.

Common reasons for dislike of spinal anesthesia are the patient's fear of being conscious during the operation, apprehension that anesthesia may wear off prematurely, and worry about complications such as headache, or residual paralysis. It is unwise to force spinal anesthesia upon an unwilling patient.

PREPARATION FOR ANESTHESIA

Premedication is given to allay apprehension. A drying agent is not used unless supplementation with general anesthesia is planned, although some believe that atropine decreases nausea and vomiting and diminishes the parasympathetic effect of spinal anesthesia on the bowel. Before anesthesia, a blood pressure cuff is applied, vital signs are recorded, and an anesthesia machine is readied for use. An intravenous infusion is started for administration of fluids or injection of drugs, should hypotension or pain develop.

LUMBAR PUNCTURE AND INJECTION

The lateral decubitus is the routine position for lumbar puncture; however, if difficulty is expected, puncture is often easier in the sitting position. A prone position is used when anesthesia in the lumbar and sacral dermatomes is induced with hypobaric solutions. If a hyperbaric solution is given, the side to be operated upon should be lowermost, and uppermost if a hypobaric technique is chosen. An assistant should flex the back, support the patient, and prevent exposure. At this time the skin of the back may be shaved. The anesthetist palpates the vertebral spines, selecting the appropriate interspace; an imaginary line between the iliac crests (Tuffier's line) intersects the spine at the third or fourth lumbar space, both below the level of the estimated termination of the spinal cord at the second lumbar space.

After washing the hands, the anesthetist dons sterile gloves and opens the spinal tray. Equipment is approached with a "no touch" technique; that is, the barrels of syringes and tips of needles are not handled. Ampules are identified, inspected for imperfections, and the questionable ones discarded.

The patient is forewarned before each maneuver. The skin is prepared with a colored antiseptic, avoiding contamination of needles and syringes. Beginning at the lumbar puncture site and working concentrically, the back is painted over a wide area. The sponge stick is set aside and the back covered with a sterile drape. The anesthetist is seated with the spine at eye level (Fig. 18-4) and the skin is not touched until dry. A skin wheal is raised, using the 25-gauge needle and small syringe with infiltration to the supraspinous ligament. Then an intramuscular injection of a pressor drug may be given to avoid or minimize the expected fall in blood pressure; preferably a 22-gauge intramuscular needle and 2-ml syringe are used for injection into the sacrospinalis muscle. Pressor drug and dose used are matters of individual preference. (See Chapter 27.)

Lumbar puncture is done carefully to avoid injury to soft tissues, ligaments, or periosteum. Trauma is probably responsible for many complaints after spinal anesthesia, including backache and sciatic radiation of pain. The lumbar puncture needle is grasped in the manner in which a pencil is held, between thumb and forefinger. With stylet in place, the needle is advanced perpendicularly to the plane of the back, but slightly cephalad. Tissues penetrated are the supraspinous and interspinous ligaments, the ligamentum flavum, and lastly the dura. After some experience one learns to distinguish these structures by a sense of touch. If bone is met, the needle is withdrawn subcutaneously and redirected. Usual causes of failure include poor positioning of the patient, selection of the wrong interspace (too low), or failure to advance the needle in the midline. If the midline structures are calcified, the needle is directed toward the interlaminar space via a lateral approach.

Rotation of the needle places the bevel well within the subarachnoid space at an average depth of 6 cm from the surface. Blood-tinged CSF or lack of free flow contraindicates injection of the anesthetic; blood-tinged fluid which clears is not a contraindication. One should not inject the anesthetic in the presence of a paresthesia, as the needle tip may lie within or against a nerve root; permanent neurologic damage will follow intraneural injection. However, another interspace can be tried.

The anesthetist then stands, and with the needle supported to prevent dislodgment, the syringe is firmly attached to the needle hub. If CSF can be aspirated easily, the anesthetic is injected at a slow rate, mixing being avoided during injection. Syringe and needle are removed after final demonstration of a free flow of CSF.

SACRAL OR TAYLOR APPROACH

A longer needle is inserted at the second sacral foramen and directed medially and cephalad toward the midline of the lumbosacral space, a tech-

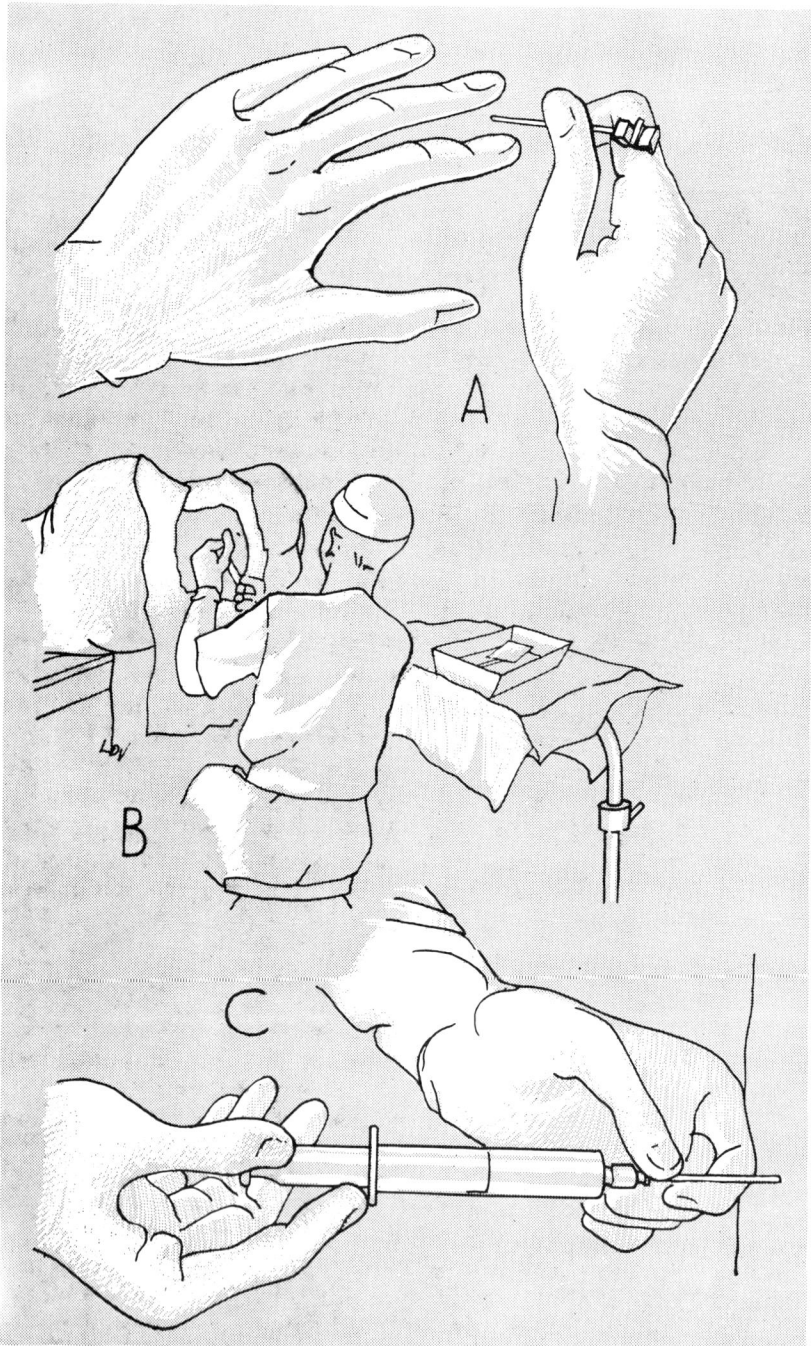

Figure 18-4. Details of spinal anesthesia technique. *A*, Insertion of lumbar puncture needle. Left hand fixes skin over chosen lumbar intervertebral space. *B*, Position for lumbar puncture. Anesthetist sits with eyes at level of lumbar spine. Spinal tray on separate table to right. *C*, Position of hands to aspirate and inject fluid.

nique useful with the prone patient, also helpful in surmounting calcific or bony obstruction at higher sites.

CONTINUOUS SPINAL ANESTHESIA

First described by Lemmon in 1940 and subsequently modified by Tuohy, this technique permits intermittent injection to provide anesthesia of unlimited duration. The method is chosen when the length of operation is indeterminate, when procedures longer than several hours are anticipated, or when better control of anesthesia is essential.

After lumbar puncture with a Tuohy-Huber point needle, a previously marked plastic catheter with stylet is passed, the tip wedged in the needle tip. The stylet is withdrawn a centimeter or so, the catheter further advanced and when it is certain that the catheter has passed the needle tip, the stylet is removed. Without the stylet it is hardly possible to pass the catheter beyond the needle tip because the warm CSF softens the plastic. The catheter is not inserted more than a centimeter or two because it may coil and interfere with spread of the anesthetic. Care is taken to avoid withdrawal of the catheter with the introducing needle in place, lest the tip be sheared: the catheter is advanced little by little as the needle is extracted while the markings on the catheter indicate the distance from the tip. A needle adapter is inserted in the free end of the catheter and the catheter fixed to the skin to prevent dislodgment. After aspiration of CSF, the anesthetic is injected. The anesthesia syringe is protected by a sterile towel and fixed to a small armboard to protect it and avoid accidental pressure on the plunger.

The most controllable solution for continuous spinal anesthesia consists of 3 to 5 per cent procaine in CSF. CSF is withdrawn after lumbar puncture and mixed with the local anesthetic before insertion of the catheter. Withdrawal of 10 ml of CSF causes a reduction in CSF pressure and dilation of vessels in the subarachnoid space; this diminishes the capacity and lessens the ease of introduction of the catheter. It is more practical, therefore, to use tetracaine in a 0.2 to 0.4 per cent concentration in dextrose. Baricity of the solution also leads to better control of anesthesia. With either anesthetic, however, initial injection should be no more than 0.5 to 1.0 ml as a larger volume may result in a high level of anesthesia. When continuation of analgesia or blockade may be helpful, as follows vascular surgery, the catheter is left in place for several hours, with intermittent injection to maintain sympathetic blockade. It is probably unsafe to allow the catheter to remain in the subarachnoid space for a longer period.

MANAGEMENT OF SPINAL ANESTHESIA

The time immediately following injection is critical. The position may be maintained for five to ten minutes if localization of anesthesia is desired, as in the sacral region or leg. During positioning for operation the patient is cautioned to relax and to permit passive turning. Straining, or breath-holding may raise the level of anesthesia to unwanted heights, blood pressure may decline. For these reasons the anesthetist must devote full attention to the patient, alternately testing the level of anesthesia with pinprick and determining the blood pressure. An assistant can help to arrange the drapes, the protective screen, and the arm rest. Levels are tested and recorded over at least the first half hour after injection. Motor power is tested by asking the patient to dorsiflex the feet (S1, S2), flex toes (L4, L5), raise knees (L2, L3), or tense the rectus muscles (T6 to T12) by lifting the head. Intercostal paralysis is detected by palpation in the intercostal spaces.

Onset of anesthesia is usually evident within one to two minutes of injection. Occasionally onset is delayed for five to ten minutes, perhaps because of slow diffusion or penetration of the anesthetic. Failure to obtain anesthesia, however, most commonly results from injection into the space between the dura and arachnoid. The term "rachi-resistance" was coined to describe spinal anesthetic failure, but even while admitting that in some individuals a slow onset of anesthesia occurs, we believe that technical errors are responsible in the majority of instances. Surgical incision should not be made unless it is certain that anesthesia is adequate. If anesthesia does not appear, the injection may be repeated if there is time, or general anesthesia substituted.

During spinal anesthesia the same careful observation is required as during general anesthesia. Respiratory insufficiency is not easily detected. If the slightest suspicion is aroused, however, oxygen is given by mask. High intercostal paralysis may be accompanied by a feeling of suffocation and signs of sensory and motor paralysis in the arms. If phrenic nerve roots are blocked, accessory muscles of respiration may be called into action, although these too will be weakened. The patient is unable to speak for lack of ability to move air and may lose consciousness. Paralysis of respiration is treated with positive pressure oxygen via mask or endotracheal tube and is carried out until the high level of anesthesia recedes.

Arterial hypotension is considered to be present with significant lowering below preoperative values or when systolic blood pressure declines below 80 torr. Hypotension is potentially more hazardous if coronary and cerebral insufficiency have been diagnosed preoperatively. Treatment consists of oxygen by mask, rapid administration of fluids, and intravenous injection of a pressor drug (see Chapter 27). Small doses are given intravenously to avoid excessive elevation of pressure, while a larger amount is given intramuscularly for sustained effect. If repeated injection of a pressor drug is necessary, continuous infusion is preferable to sustain the pressure.

The anesthetist should remain at the head of the table, encouraging the patient, monitoring vital signs, and supplementing with general anesthesia when needed. Nausea and vomiting are not uncommon. Opioids used for premedication, cerebral ischemia, psychologic factors or traction on viscera may be responsible for the gastrointestinal symptoms. Supplementation with general anesthesia is necessary when analgesia or muscle relaxation is inadequate, when nausea and vomiting are protracted, or when the patient chooses to be unconscious. As a rule, only a light plane of general anesthesia is needed, obtainable with nitrous oxide and intravenous injection of a short-acting barbiturate. Circulatory depressant properties of most general anesthetics are magnified during spinal anesthesia because of lack of compensating sympathetic activity.

DELAYED SEQUELAE OF SPINAL ANESTHESIA

SEQUELAE OF LUMBAR PUNCTURE

Headache

The syndrome of decreased intracranial pressure, consisting primarily of headache but occasionally accompanied by difficulty in hearing and vision, is the most common complication of lumbar puncture. The opening in the dura made by the lumbar puncture may persist for days or weeks (Fig. 18–5). With escape of CSF, pressure falls. Headache is postural, ap-

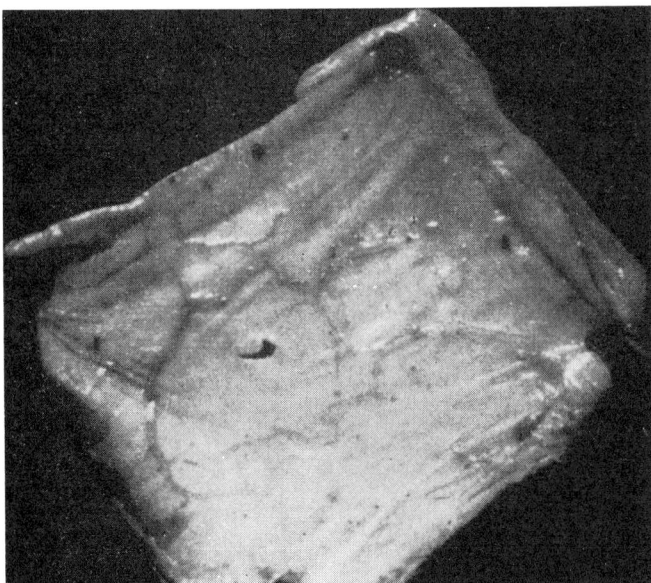

Figure 18–5. Puncture opening in dura, two days old. Diameter of needle 0.8 mm. Magnification 4×. (Reproduced with permission from Franksson C and Gordh T: Acta Chir Scand 94:443, 1946.)

pearing in the head-up position and suggesting that loss of CSF permits traction on intracranial pain-sensitive structures.

In a series of 9277 administrations of spinal anesthesia studied by the authors, the overall incidence of headache was 11 per cent. Headache occurred in highest frequency in patients in the third and fourth decades of life (Table 18–2). Frequency of headache was also higher in females, a result in part of inclusion of obstetric cases in the group, for headache followed vaginal delivery in 22 per cent of patients. Even if obstetric cases are not included, however, headache was still more frequent in women.

The incidence of headache diminished with decreasing diameter of needle used (Table 18–3); not only were there fewer headaches, but severity and duration were less. In this series of cases a 16-gauge needle was employed for continuous spinal anesthesia. Technical difficulties were more common, and the incidence and severity of headache and ocular complaints was high.

Treatment of headache consists of keeping the patient flat in bed, using analgetics, or attempting to increase cerebrospinal fluid pressure. Body hydration or application of a tight abdominal binder, thereby raising pressure in the peridural venous plexus, sometimes relieves milder headaches.

Table 18–2. RELATION OF AGE TO INCIDENCE OF SPINAL HEADACHE

Age (yr)	Number of Anesthetics	Headache	
		No.	Per Cent
10–19	537	51	10
20–29	1994	321	16
30–39	1883	261	14
40–49	1759	192	11
50–59	1736	133	8
60–69	1094	45	4
70–79	297	7	2
80–89	27	1	3
Total	9277	1011	

Table 18–3. RELATION OF GAUGE OF NEEDLE USED FOR LUMBAR PUNCTURE AND INCIDENCE OF HEADACHE

Gauge	Number of Anesthetics	Headache	
		No.	Per Cent
16	839	151	18
19	154	16	10
20	2698	377	14
22	4952	430	9
24	634	37	6
Total	9277	1011	

The mechanism of relief of headache after peridural placement of fluid has not been established. When headache is protracted and severe, the symptoms may be completely relieved in a high percentage of cases by application of an autologous "blood patch." An epidural injection of 10 to 15 ml of blood serves to seal the dural fistula. However, back pain and signs of meningeal irritation have been noted in more than a few instances after this therapy.

Ocular and Auditory Complications

Auditory complaints were noted in 0.4 per cent of 9277 anesthetized patients and consisted of buzzing, popping, clogging of the ears, humming, roaring, or loss of hearing altogether, with few exceptions associated with a postural headache. Auditory difficulties may relate to alterations in fluid pressure in the cochlea. Difficulty with vision occurred in 0.4 per cent of the patients; double vision, blurring, trouble in focusing, and spots before the eyes were the complaints. In all but eight of the 34 patients visual problems arose in association with postural headache. We found three cases of abducens palsy or lateral rectus muscle paralysis, and the symptom of prolonged double vision in three others suggested that paralysis might also have been present. The six cases followed use of a 16-gauge needle for continuous spinal anesthesia. One theory holds that with brain displacement or traction, the abducens nerve with a long intracranial course is paralyzed by stretch.

Traumatic Puncture or Infection

Traumatic lumbar puncture without injection of the anesthetic has led both to transient or permanent neurologic deficit. This occurs usually after repeated attempts, with production of paresthesias and recovery of blood or blood-tinged CSF. Epidural abscess and bacterial meningitis have followed lumbar puncture and spinal anesthesia. In the vast majority of instances, such complications must be ascribed to faulty technique.

SEQUELAE OF ANESTHETIC INJECTION

Adhesive Arachnoiditis and Cauda Equina Syndrome

The complication most feared is chronic progressive adhesive arachnoiditis, which, we believe, is a nonspecific pathologic response to an intrathecal irritant. The ultimate effects of arachnoiditis relate to ischemia of the spinal cord. Transverse myelitis has also been described and perhaps is related to destruction of neural tissue by the injected substance, or to intraspinal or intraneural injection. Either of these two processes may result in paralysis of the lower limbs and intestinal and bladder dysfunction, as well as involvement of the spinal cord and roots at higher levels. Sensory changes alone may occur. In our study of spinal anesthesia, accurate information concerning 86 per cent of the patients was obtained over a period of at least six months after discharge from the hospital. There were no instances of adhesive arachnoiditis, cauda equina syndrome, or transverse myelitis. We believe that these good results relate to proper selection of the patient for this technique and its careful application.

Minor Neurologic Sequelae

Residual signs or symptoms of numbness following spinal anesthesia occurred in 0.8 per cent of the patients, in the majority restricted to the lumbar and sacral dermatomes. None of the patients had other neurologic signs and most complaints disappeared within six months. Subjective complaints consisted of numbness, tingling, heaviness, or burning. Sensory deficit was not always found. These sequelae must relate to anesthetic injection.

Exacerbation of Pre-existing Neurologic Disease

Although a cause and effect relation between spinal anesthesia and exacerbation of neurologic disease can rarely be proved, we believe that spinal anesthesia should not be given to patients with certain neurologic diseases. This reservation applies to congenital, active, or inactive disease, it embraces trauma, bacterial, and viral infection, neoplasms, and systemic disease with neurologic concomitants. Exceptions to the rule are made only when a technique other than spinal anesthesia is potentially more hazardous or less safe in the hands of the administrator.

Detection of neurologic disease after spinal anesthesia calls for repeated postanesthetic visits. Patients are questioned for difficulty in voiding or defecation, residual numbness, or paralysis. Any deviation from normal is investigated even at the expense of suggesting a relation to anesthesia. It is important to detect symptoms early, for we believe that progression of disease can be halted, perhaps by surgical exploration or in some cases by administration of corticosteroids. In many instances unrelated neurologic disease has been found.

In any instance of neurologic complaint, and this point cannot be emphasized enough, it is essential to seek other causes rather than to ascribe all to spinal anesthesia. The majority of serious neurologic symptoms appearing after spinal anesthesia as administered today can be attributed to coincident or previously unrecognized disease. Thorough neurologic examination must be performed, appropriate diagnostic methods used, and consultation sought.

APPRAISAL

It is not an easy matter to assess the role of spinal anesthesia in modern anesthetic practice. With the widespread use of balanced anesthesia techniques and the resurgence of interest in peridural anesthesia, one might expect decreased interest in the subarachnoid technique. Nevertheless, the manufacturers sell millions of spinal sets annually. Because the method is more predictable in its results and the onset of anesthesia more rapid, these advantages still prevail in the choice over peridural anesthesia. General practitioners, surgeons, and obstetricians find the method useful when an anesthetist is not available. However, headache after lumbar puncture remains a major problem, particularly in obstetrics, and neurologic sequelae still are reported; the latter commonly are reasons for legal action against the physician concerned.

REFERENCES

Converse JG, Landmesser CM, Harmel MH: The concentration of pontocaine hydrochloride in the cerebrospinal fluid during spinal anesthesia and the influence of epinephrine in prolonging the sensory anesthetic effect. Anesthesiology 15:1, 1954.

DiGiovanni AJ, Galbert MW, Wahle WM: Epidural injection of autologous blood for post lumbar-puncture headache. Anesth Analg 51:226, 1972.

Dripps RD, Vandam LD: Long-term follow-up of patients who received 10,098 spinal anesthetics: I. Failure to discover major neurological sequelae. JAMA 156:1486, 1954.

Egbert LD, Deas TC: Effect of epinephrine upon the duration of spinal anesthesia. Anesthesiology 21:345, 1960.

Ernst EA: *In vitro* changes of osmolality and density of spinal anesthetic solutions. Anesthesiology 29:104, 1968.

Freund FG, Bonica JJ, Ward RJ, et al: Ventilatory reserve and level of motor block during high spinal and epidural anesthesia. Anesthesiology 28:834, 1967.

Gibbons RB: Chemical meningitis following spinal anesthesia. JAMA 210:900, 1969.

Greene NM: Physiology of Spinal Anesthesia. 2nd ed, Baltimore, The Williams & Wilkins Co, 1970.

Helrich M, Papper EM, Brodie BB, et al: The fate of intrathecal procaine and the spinal fluid level required for surgical anesthesia. J Pharmacol Exp Ther 100:78, 1950.

Lund PC: Principles and Practice of Spinal Anesthesia. Springfield, Ill, Charles C Thomas, 1971.

Phillips OC, Ebner H, Nelson AT, et al: Neurological complications following spinal anesthesia with lidocaine. A prospective review of 10,440 cases. Anesthesiology 30:284, 1969.

Smith TC: The lumbar spine and subarachnoid block. Anesthesiology 29:60, 1968.

Vandam LD, Dripps RD: Long-term follow-up of patients who received 10,098 spinal anesthetics: II. Incidence and analysis of minor sensory neurological defects. Surgery 38:463, 1955.

Vandam LD, Dripps RD: Exacerbation of pre-existing neurologic disease after spinal anesthesia. N Eng J Med 255:843, 1956.

Vandam LD, Dripps RD: Long-term follow-up of patients who received 10,098 spinal anesthetics: III. Syndrome of decreased intracranial pressure (headache and ocular and auditory difficulties). JAMA 161:586, 1956.

Vandam LD, Dripps RD: Long-term follow-up of patients who received 10,098 spinal anesthetics: IV. Neurological disease incident to traumatic lumbar puncture during spinal anesthesia. JAMA 172:1483, 1960.

Chapter 19

PERIDURAL AND CAUDAL ANESTHESIA

We have first presented the subject of spinal anesthesia because we believe that the beginner should learn this technique before going on to peridural (epidural) anesthesia. In addition, the two methods are similar except for certain technical differences; that is to say, choice and application to the patient are almost the same for both, action and fate of the local anesthetics are similar, the physiologic consequences are almost identical, and management of anesthesia differs little. Throughout the discussion comparisons between the two methods will be made.

Peridural anesthesia results upon injection of a local anesthetic into the space surrounding the dura mater, within the spinal canal. Note was made earlier that Corning in 1885 was possibly the first to do this, although it was done unsuspectingly. In 1901 Sicard and Cathelin independently introduced local anesthetics into the peridural space via the sacrococcygeal hiatus. Subsequently, sporadic attempts were made to approach the space at higher levels, but the method did not take hold until Pages in 1921 and Dogliotti in 1927 achieved anesthesia with greater consistency via a lumbar approach. Peridural anesthesia via the caudal route is used today for procedures performed in the sacral region—anorectal operations, vaginal procedures, and obstetric delivery. However, because of uncertainty in achieving the level of anesthesia via the caudal approach, the need for large volumes of local anesthetic solution, and a failure rate in the vicinity of 5 to 10 per cent, the lumbar approach to the peridural space is more commonly used for obstetrics. The latter has gained popularity not only because of fear of development of neurologic complications of spinal anesthesia, but for its usefulness in obstetrics.

ANATOMY

The anatomic features of the peridural space explain in part the action of the local anesthetics injected into it as well as the requirements for concentration and volume. In essence, the peridural space extends from the base of the skull to the coccyx. The spinal cord present within it is enveloped by the meninges, the dura being outermost, with the cord terminating at or just above the second lumbar vertebra and the subarachnoid space at the second sacral foramen. The outer limits of the space are formed by the ligamentum flavum and the periosteum lining the vertebral canal; traversing the space via the intervertebral and sacral foramina are the spinal nerves, enveloped by the dura to the point of exit at the foramina. Other structures within the peridural space are the peridural plexus of veins, loose areolar tissue, and fibrous connections between the dura and the spinal column, most prominent anteriorly and more extensive in the elderly.

The volume of the peridural space varies from region to region, depending upon the configuration of the vertebral canal and the contents of the dural sac. The most prominent enlargements of the spinal cord are the lower cervical, the upper thoracic, the lumbar, and the upper sacral segments, corresponding to the brachial and lumbosacral plexuses, respectively. Areas of larger capacity in the peridural space are the caudal canal and the lumbar region. The peridural space varies in capacity, with alterations in volume of the dural sac owing to changes in position and to the volume of blood in the peridural plexus of veins, again influenced by position and intra-abdominal pressure.

NEGATIVE PRESSURE IN THE PERIDURAL SPACE

An important aspect of the peridural space is the negative pressure demonstrable upon initial entry with a needle, a useful sign. Although some claim this is an extension of the negative pressure developed within the thorax, negative pressure can also be demonstrated in the cadaver. Thus, it is thought that flexion and lengthening of the spine increase the volume of the relatively closed peridural space, creating a true vacuum. However, in the living subject the pressure in the thoracic region is subatmospheric, less negative in the lumbar region, and not demonstrable in the caudal canal. Probably the most likely explanation relates to the pressure in the peridural plexus of veins. Pressure in the space is negative as long as a body position favors a negative pressure in the veins. Perhaps pertinent is the explanation that needle entry into the space "tents" the dura ahead of it, causing local expansion of the space with development of negative pressure; this is confirmed by a simultaneous rise in pressure within the subarachnoid space.

RESULTS OF PERIDURAL INJECTION
SITE OF ACTION OF THE LOCAL ANESTHETIC

The action of local anesthetics deposited within the peridural space is believed to occur in several ways. Perhaps the major action takes place at the nerve roots and dorsal root ganglia beyond the point of meningeal covering, the result of outward diffusion of anesthetic through the intervertebral foramina. On the other hand, the anesthetic is found in the subarachnoid space, access being gained either by diffusion across the meninges or by retrograde diffusion through the intervertebral foramina via the perineural spaces and lymphatics. The periphery of the spinal cord is also affected so that block of ascending and descending pathways may be observed. At any time during peridural anesthesia a concentration of local anesthetic sufficient for sensory blockade is present in CSF.

SPREAD, ONSET, AND DURATION OF ANESTHESIA

The volume of fluid injected into the peridural space is the major influence in the spread of a local anesthetic. Unlike spinal anesthesia, position and gravity influence distribution to a lesser extent while the baricity of the anesthetic solution is of no importance. Spread is influenced more by the structures within the space and the changing volume of the space in the sitting or lateral positions owing to the volume of the dural sac and venous plexus. Some believe rapidity of injection is another variable, for it may influence the escape of fluid through the intervertebral foramina and the extent of spread cephalad or caudad. Finally, concentration of the anesthetic solution determines the completeness of the block insofar as nerve fiber size and the number of fibers are concerned.

In summary, then, it is the mass of local anesthetic, concentration times volume, that determines the spread and the solidity of the block. Differential block of nerve fibers can also be had by altering the concentration of the anesthetic. Latency and duration of anesthesia are affected by the aforementioned factors as well as by specific properties of the local anesthetic. Epinephrine slows vascular absorption and decreases peak concentrations of anesthetic in the bloodstream by approximately one half to one third. Termination of anesthesia depends upon absorption of the anesthetic from the nerves and peridural space via vascular and lymphatic channels.

IMPORTANCE OF VASCULARITY

Because the peridural area is highly vascularized and the concentration and volume of anesthetic injected are relatively large, a significant incidence of systemic reactions to the local anesthetic may be expected. For this reason, epinephrine is added to the anesthetic solution unless there is some contraindication to its use. Epinephrine increases duration of anesthesia; a concentration of 1:200,000 is usually employed. Under conditions of increased vascularity, as in pregnancy at term, the likelihood of absorption is increased.

PHYSIOLOGIC EFFECTS

Although the physiologic results of spinal and peridural anesthesia are almost the same, there is a difference in that absorption of the local anesthetic from the peridural space may give rise to systemic effects, a possibility already mentioned. Likewise, the systemic actions of epinephrine may be evident. Depending upon the concentration of anesthetic employed, motor block may be less intense and is slower to appear than in spinal anesthesia, while some sensory input may continue via large fibers.

Hypotension can follow peridural anesthesia for most if not all the reasons listed under spinal anesthesia. In comparisons of spinal and peridural anesthesia of equal degree, the hypotension encountered with the latter tends to be less profound. The concomitant use of epinephrine in peridural anesthesia does not prevent hypotension. Despite an increase in heart rate and stroke volume, peripheral resistance declines to a greater degree. In addition to the neurogenic effects on circulation, some of the changes noted may result from absorption of the local anesthetic into the bloodstream. It should also be emphasized that pressor drugs are rarely used prophylactically before peridural anesthesia.

TECHNICAL ASPECTS

EQUIPMENT

Basic equipment and principles of sterilization are the same as for the spinal technique. In peridural anesthesia the anesthetic should be added to the prepared tray in a single dose ampule rather than risk injection of a contaminated solution from a multiple dose vial. Additional equipment required is as follows:

1. For single dose anesthesia, a well-designed needle is required. The essentials are: a sizable hub that can be grasped firmly as the needle is advanced, a rigid shaft, and a short bevel point with rounded edges to minimize inadvertent dural puncture. We prefer a 19-gauge, thin-walled needle, about 9 cm in length.
2. For continuous anesthesia we use a 17- or 18-gauge, 7.6 cm, thin-walled Tuohy needle with a Huber point. In conjunction, a disposable vinyl plastic catheter is used which receives a 23-gauge Luer-Lok needle. The tubing is marked at 10, 11, and 15 cm, the leading edge beveled, and a fairly rigid stylet inserted. With a Teflon catheter, a stylet is not necessary.
3. A 10-ml Luer-Lok syringe for attachment to the catheter and serial injection.
4. An 18-gauge short-bevel needle for puncturing the skin and ligaments to permit entry of the Tuohy needle.
5. A 10-ml plain-tipped syringe is used for the "loss of resistance" test, while a 20-ml syringe may be used for initial injection.

All the equipment is commercially available in presterilized, packaged form.

AGENTS AND TECHNIQUE

Currently used local anesthetics, concentrations employed, approximate latency of onset, and duration of anesthesia are shown in Table 19-1. We employ 1.5 and 2.0 per cent lidocaine or mepivacaine and from 0.25 to 0.75 per cent bupivacaine. A few clinicians employ dichloroprocaine for the continuous method, in order to avoid cumulative concentrations in plasma.

Single Dose Technique

The routine position of the patient is the lateral decubitus, with the anesthetist seated as for lumbar puncture. The spine need not be flexed as much as in spinal anesthesia, for some believe that inadvertent dural puncture is less likely with minimal flexion. The skin of the back is prepared and draped, and the skin and deeper tissues then are anesthetized. Entry is made at a spinal interspace corresponding as closely as possible to the dermatomes at the center of the area to be anesthetized. More uniform results can be expected from a standard midline insertion at L2 to L3.

Several techniques have been suggested to detect entry into the peridural space; the loss of resistance method is perhaps most commonly used. We prefer this when a smaller needle is employed for single injection. A syringe containing air, distilled water, or preferably saline is attached to the needle as it is advanced, maintaining steady gentle pressure on the plunger. After the ligamentum flavum has been pierced a sudden loss of resistance is experienced, fluid or air entering the peridural space and displacing the dura. If distilled water is used, pain may be experienced as it enters the space. When the hanging drop method of Gutierrez is selected, a drop of local anesthetic placed in the needle hub is sucked inward as negative pressure is encountered.

Once entry has been gained, aspiration is tried by rotating the needle to several quadrants to detect blood or CSF; if either is recovered the

Table 19-1. ACTION OF LOCAL ANESTHETICS IN SINGLE DOSE PERIDURAL ANESTHESIA*

Agent	Usual Conc. (%)	Volumes (ml)	Total Dose (mg)	Onset (min)	Duration (min)
Esters:					
Chloroprocaine	1-3	15-30	150-900	–	30-45
Procaine	1-2	15-30	150-600	–	45-60
Tetracaine	0.25-0.5	15-30	37.5-150	–	180-360
Amides:					
Lidocaine	1-2	15-30	150-500	15	60-180
Mepivacaine	1-2	15-30	150-500	15	60-180
Bupivacaine	0.25-0.75	15-30	37.5-225	16.5	180-360
Etidocaine	1-1.5	15-30	150-300	10.85	180-360

*Data compiled from reports in the literature.

needle is removed and inserted at another space. A trial injection of 3 ml of anesthetic is then made. Although not infallible, this measure should reveal subarachnoid puncture; if not demonstrable, the anesthetizing dose of local anesthetic is injected. Usually 1.5 to 2.0 ml of anesthetic are required for each spinal segment anesthetized in the younger age group, with injection performed at a rate of 1 ml per second. A faster injection may produce paresthesias, a higher level of anesthesia, and a higher blood concentration; slow injection should result in more localized anesthesia. However, there is little agreement on the role of the rapidity of injection other than that a protracted injection provides better quality of block. The anesthetic diffuses in both directions, usually more cephalad than caudad, particularly in the elderly. The patient's position at the time and soon after injection has relatively little influence on spread, in contrast to spinal anesthesia. We do not recommend the use of thoracic peridural anesthesia by the beginner because of the greater hazards entailed.

Serial Technique

After performance of peridural puncture and injection of the test dose, the first anesthetizing dose is injected. Then a catheter is passed through the needle, the tip wedged at the needle point. The wire stylet is then withdrawn a millimeter or two, and the catheter further advanced; when it is certain that the catheter has passed the tip of the needle into the peridural space, the stylet is removed. Without the stylet, it is sometimes difficult to pass the catheter beyond the needle point. The catheter should be inserted into the peridural space not more than a centimeter or two because it may coil and interfere with spread of the anesthetic or may traumatize nerves or blood vessels. Furthermore, paresthesias are almost uniform if the catheter is advanced 4 to 5 cm. Care is taken to avoid withdrawal of the catheter with the introducing needle still in place lest the tip of the catheter be sheared. An attempt is made to maintain the catheter in its initial position or to advance it slightly as the needle is extracted. The markings on the catheter indicating distance from the tip help in determining appropriate depth of insertion. A needle adapter is then inserted in the free end of the catheter and the catheter fixed to the skin to prevent accidental withdrawal or kinking. Subsequent injections of one half to one third of the initial dose are made every 45 to 60 minutes. However, repeated injection may result in tolerance or tachyphylaxis, which may relate to local changes in hydrogen ion concentration. In the use of lidocaine, a slowly metabolized drug, the cumulative dose may reach toxic levels; as a rule, such concentrations are not attained during the course of an operation of average duration.

In using this technique precautions with regard to asepsis and avoidance of trauma must be taken. The anesthesia syringe should be protected in a sterile towel and fixed to an armboard such as that used to protect intravenous infusions, to avoid detachment of the syringe from the catheter or accidental pressure on the plunger.

MANAGEMENT AND SEQUELAE

Subsequent management of peridural anesthesia is the same as for spinal anesthesia, with attention paid to maintenance of circulation, and respiration, and supplementation with general anesthesia when called for. There has been no thorough study undertaken to detect development of neurologic sequelae after peridural anesthesia. However, isolated instances of neurologic complications have been infrequently reported. Major problems may be summarized as follows:

1. Inadvertent subarachnoid injection, with the resultant high spinal anesthesia requiring immediate treatment for respiratory paralysis and circulatory depression. Postural headache usually follows introduction of the large needle.

2. Systemic reactions to the local anesthetic in the form of convulsions, hypotension, and loss of consciousness, requiring specific treatment. The systemic effects of epinephrine are hazardous in the presence of arteriosclerotic heart disease, but the smaller total doses used in the elderly counteract this tendency. Furthermore, epinephrine may intensify the block.

3. Inability to obtain anesthesia or recovery of blood dictates use of another technique. Failure may be the result of catheter entry into a peridural vein. The onset of anesthesia may be absent or slow; the patient may manifest an unusual circulatory reaction owing to the epinephrine injected and drowsiness or a convulsion may ensue.

CAUDAL ANESTHESIA

While the first planned approach to the peridural space was made via the sacral canal and subsequently called caudal anesthesia, the method has been used largely in obstetrics, gaining popularity in the 1940s as a means of producing painless childbirth. Misapplication of the technique led to failures, complications, and a subsequent decline in its popularity in obstetrics. However, the method is safe and useful, particularly for operations performed in the anal and sacral regions and for culdoscopy.

ANATOMY

The sacrum comprises the fused five sacral vertebrae. This triangular bone articulates with the lumbar spine above, the iliac bones laterally, and the coccyx below. The posterior midline crest represents the vertebral spines, while the sacral cornua below are the remnants of the articular processes. Lack of fusion or absence of the laminae of the fifth or fourth and fifth vertebrae gives rise to the sacral hiatus between the cornua. This site is covered posteriorly by the dense sacrococcygeal ligament formed from the supraspinous and interspinous ligaments as well as the ligamentum flavum. The posterior sacral foramina give passage to the posterior primary divisions of the sacral nerves. Osseous anomalies in the sacrum are frequent.

The sacral canal contains the following structures: the dural sac, which terminates approximately at the level of the second sacral foramen; the anterior and posterior divisions and dorsal root ganglia of the sacral nerves enveloped by the dura to their exits at the anterior and posterior foramina; a rich network of peridural veins; and some loose fat and areolar tissue. The capacity of the sacral canal varies according to body habitus and is more capacious in the female.

Because of the variable anatomy of the sacrum, the presence or absence of obesity, and the presence or absence of local contraindications, the sacrum should be examined during the preoperative visit to determine the feasibility of injection.

TECHNIQUES AND COMPLICATIONS

The patient lies in the prone position with the table flexed at the hips, the sacrum horizontal, and the heels turned outward to separate the buttocks and expose the hiatus. In the pregnant woman the lateral decubitus position is elected. Important landmarks are: the posterior superior iliac spines; the second sacral foramen, 1 cm below and medial to the spines; and the hiatus between the sacral cornua, about 4 cm above the tip of the coccyx (Fig. 19-1). The hiatus can be felt as a distinct depression.

The sacral area is thoroughly prepared with antiseptic and draped, a gauze sponge having first been placed between the buttocks to prevent leakage of irritating solutions onto the genitalia. Anesthetic infiltration of the skin and underlying ligaments is made with a hypodermic needle. A 20-gauge, 4-cm needle with stylet or a Tuohy needle is used for injection; this is inserted almost perpendicular to the skin until a distinct feeling of penetration of the sacrococcygeal ligament is experienced. The needle is then advanced a centimeter or two somewhat parallel to the sacrum, with the bevel downward. The stylet is withdrawn and used to measure the distance inserted, certainly not as far as the S2 level. With a dry syringe, aspiration is gently done in four quadrants to detect the appearance of CSF or blood; recovery of either necessitates repositioning the needle. Five ml of air are then injected, with the fingers held over the site of the needle tip; a sensation of crepitus indicates that the needle lies on the dorsum of the sacrum, requiring reinsertion. If the needle is well positioned, an initial injection of 5 ml is made to be sure that subarachnoid entry has not occurred; the

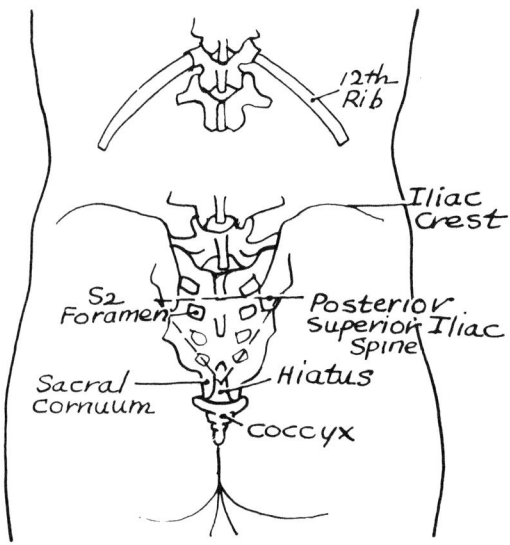

Figure 19-1. Landmarks for caudal anesthesia.

remainder of the anesthetic solution is then placed. Usually about 10 to 15 ml of 1.5 to 2.0 per cent lidocaine, mepivacaine, or procaine, with 1:200,000 epinephrine, are required for sacral anesthesia. Onset with lidocaine or mepivacaine is apparent in two to five minutes; with procaine, in five to ten minutes; complete anesthesia is obtained in 20 to 30 minutes with any of the drugs. Because of the variation in capacity of the sacral canal as well as obstacles to diffusion of the drug, the resultant level of anesthesia may vary widely. The most controllable technique is to inject the drug serially with the needle still in place or to resort to a continuous technique with the use of a plastic catheter. Inadequate anesthesia can be corrected by transsacral injection, which is a paravertebral approach to the sacral canal. In 5 to 15 per cent of individuals the presence of ligamentous and osseous abnormalities precludes the attainment of satisfactory anesthesia.

Complications resulting from caudal anesthesia include systemic reactions to the local anesthetic and, in obstetrics, high levels of anesthesia with arterial hypotension and interference with the forces of labor. Injury to the fetal head has been reported when injection was made during the second stage of labor. Infection is a serious delayed complication.

APPRAISAL

Peridural anesthesia is a useful technique not only for surgical and obstetric procedures but in the diagnosis and treatment of pain and autonomic nervous system dysfunction, wherein prolonged neural blockade may be beneficial. The technical problems inherent in the method can be largely overcome through practice, but in every series reported there has been a higher failure rate than with spinal anesthesia. The chief reason for selection of peridural rather than spinal anesthesia is to avoid lumbar puncture headache and the potential for neurologic complications. If the beginner masters spinal anesthesia first because it is the easier method, the approach to problems of peridural anesthesia will be better understood.

REFERENCES

Bromage PR: Mechanism of action of extradural anaesthesia. Br J Anaesth 47 (Suppl):199, 1975.

Cohen EN, Levine DA, Colliss JE, et al: Role of pH in development of tachyphylaxis to local anesthetic agents. Anesthesiology 29:994, 1968.

Covino BG, Vassallo HG: Clinical aspects of local anesthesia. *In* Covino, BG and Vassallo, HG: Local Anesthetics. Mechanisms of Action and Clinical Use. New York, Grune & Stratton, 1976.

Gunther RE, Bauman J: Obstetrical caudal anesthesia. I. A randomized study comparing 1 per cent mepivacaine with 1 per cent lidocaine plus epinephrine. Anesthesiology 31:5, 1969.

Stanton-Hicks M d'A: Cardiovascular effects of extradural anaesthesia. Br J Anaesth 47 (Suppl): 253, 1975.

Wilkinson GR, Lund PC: Bupivacaine levels in plasma and CSF following peridural administration. Anesthesiology 33:482, 1970.

Chapter 20

REGIONAL NERVE BLOCKS

Although this is an introductory text, we believe it important for the beginner in anesthesia to think at the outset in terms of regional anesthesia. Consequently, in this chapter we describe the techniques of nerve block most commonly employed for operation and, in the instance of sympathetic nerve block, some commonly used therapeutic measures. There are other nerve blocks that anesthetists will wish to master as they achieve experience. The descriptions given here are more or less in outline form, but using this as a background, in addition to reading and experience, proficiency ultimately will be attained.

In order to succeed with nerve block, one should understand the anatomy of a typical spinal nerve (Fig. 20-1). Anterior and posterior nerve roots of a somatic nerve join at the intervertebral foramen to form the nerve trunk. In the immediate vicinity of the foramen the dorsal root ganglion is present, the spinal dura blends with the perineurium, and the anterior and posterior primary divisions of the nerve are formed. Thereafter, the rami communicantes connect with the sympathetic chain and a recurrent sympathetic branch enters the spinal canal. In general, the posterior primary divisions supply the skin and muscles posterior to the transverse processes of the vertebrae, comprising the axial skeleton. The anterior divisions supply structures of the appendicular skeleton anterior to the transverse processes, as well as the chest and abdomen. In the midline anteriorly the nerves overlap for a short distance, while any one area of skin has a sensory contribution from at least three nerves, an overlapping of three dermatomes. The approach to spinal nerves for blocking purposes is dictated by the anatomy of the region involved, obviously differing for neck, thorax, and abdomen, and the extent of anesthesia sought. For the chest and abdomen, nerve blocks are done paravertebrally for the most part, while for the neck to some extent and for the extremities, regional blocks involve the major somatic nerve plexuses and peripheral nerves.

Regional Nerve Blocks

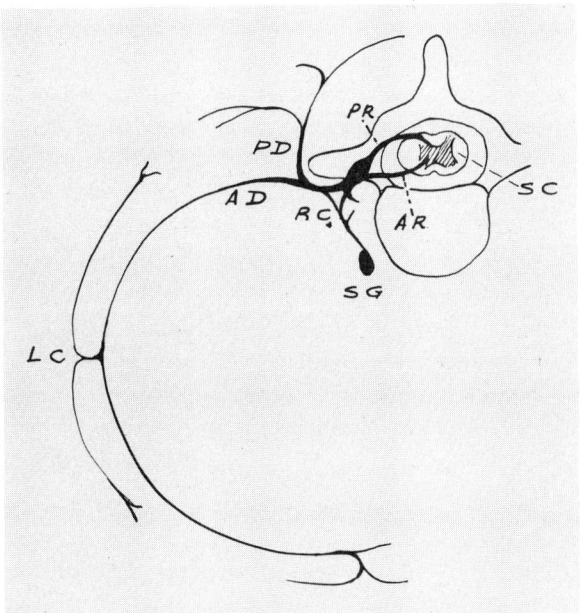

Figure 20–1. Diagram of a typical spinal nerve. SC = spinal cord; AD = anterior division; PD = posterior division; RC = rami communicantes; SG = sympathetic ganglion; LC = lateral cutaneous nerve.

PARAVERTEBRAL NERVE BLOCK

CERVICAL PLEXUS BLOCK

The cervical plexus is formed from the anterior primary divisions of the first four cervical nerves. These nerves are interconnected, communicate with the last four cranial nerves, and receive gray rami communicantes from the cervical sympathetic chain. The most important contributions of the plexus are those to the ansa hypoglossi that supplies the infrahyoid muscles, and to the roots of the phrenic nerve derived from the third and fourth nerves. The first cervical nerve has no sensory component, but the others carry sensation from the head and neck via the superficial cervical plexus. The deep cervical plexus segmentally innervates those muscles that arise and insert on the corresponding cervical vertebrae and transverse processes.

The cervical plexus may be blocked from either a posterior or a lateral approach, the former being more painful and having less precise landmarks. For the lateral approach the patient's head is turned away to permit palpation of the transverse processes and to displace the sternomastoid muscle and carotid sheath anteriorly. After raising a skin wheal, injection of 10 to 20 ml of a 0.5 to 1.0 per cent solution of procaine or lidocaine is made at the midpoint of the posterior border of the sternomastoid muscle; this should anesthetize the superficial cervical plexus which carries sensation from head and neck (Fig. 20-2). The injection should "fan out" both superficial to and beneath the deep fascia, to reach all nerve filaments. Then the second, third, and fourth nerves are blocked at the transverse processes. A landmark for the fourth transverse process is just above the midpoint of the posterior border of the sternomastoid muscle, where the external jugular vein crosses the muscle. The upper border of the thyroid cartilage suggests the space between the third and fourth cervical vertebrae. After the transverse processes are identified, injection with 5 ml of 1.0 to 1.5 per cent procaine or lidocaine is made successively with the needle point against bone at either the anterior or posterior tubercle.

Possible complications of deep cervical nerve block include bleeding from the vertebral artery, subarachnoid or peridural injection, phrenic nerve paralysis, and laryngeal nerve block as indicated by hoarseness. It should not surprise one if Horner's syndrome develops or if anesthesia spreads to involve the upper divisions of the brachial plexus.

With superficial plexus block, operations can be performed in the region between the jaw and the clavicle, in the anterior and posterior cervical triangles. Deep cervical block provides relaxation of the strap muscles, but analgesia is not complete because afferent sympathetic fibers may remain unblocked. The surgeon should manipulate tissues gently and infiltrate with local anesthetic if necessary as the dissection proceeds.

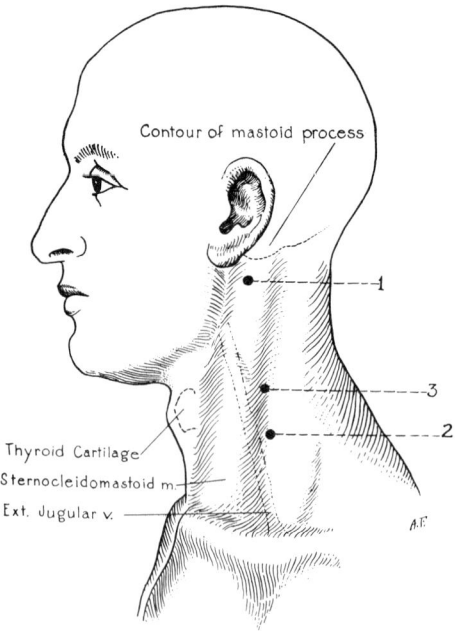

Figure 20-2. Landmarks for the cervical plexus: *1* is one fingerbreadth below the mastoid process, corresponding to C2; *3* is opposite the superior cornu of the thyroid cartilage corresponding to C5 – also the midpoint of the posterior border of the sternocleidomastoid muscle where block of the superficial cervical plexus is done; *2* is at the level of Chassaignac's tubercle, or the sixth transverse process – also used as a landmark in stellate ganglion block and the interscalene approach to the brachial plexus. (Reproduced with permission from Labat GL: Regional Anesthesia. 2nd ed, Philadelphia, WB Saunders Co, 1928.)

INTERCOSTAL BLOCK

The 12 thoracic nerves forming the intercostals present a peculiar anatomy of their own. In the intercostal space, vein, artery, and nerve relate to each other in that order from above downward. From the intervertebral foramen outward, the intercostal nerve lies between the external intercostal muscle and the internal intercostal membrane. Beyond the angle of the rib the nerve courses between intercostal muscles and then forward, splitting the internal intercostal muscle so that the latter forms an internal and a medial muscle. At the costal cartilages the external intercostal muscle is no longer present. Thus, the nerves have varying relationships, depending upon the presence or absence of the intercostal muscles. The lower six intercostals pass posterior to the costal cartilages between the origins of the diaphragm and the tranversus abdominis muscles, entering the abdominal wall; there they lie between the transversus abdominis and the internal oblique muscles. A lateral cutaneous branch leaves the intercostal nerve anterior to the posterior axillary line, then splitting into anterior and posterior divisions. Thus, the intercostal nerve should be blocked posterior to this point to obtain satisfactory superficial anesthesia of the abdominal wall. Furthermore, block of at least three somatic nerves is necessary for complete anesthesia in any one dermatome.

Intercostal nerve block provides satisfactory anesthesia of the abdominal wall, permitting relatively superficial intra-abdominal procedures such as liver biopsy, cholecystostomy, gastrostomy, or loop colostomy. In these instances the parietal peritoneum requires infiltration with anesthetic. More extensive intra-abdominal operations necessitate celiac and mesenteric plexus block to interrupt afferent visceral sympathetic impulses.

For unilateral intercostal block the patient is positioned with that side uppermost; for bilateral block the prone position, if tolerated by the patient, is more convenient. The ribs are identified with the injection made posterior to the posterior axillary line, using needles of the shortest possible length to avoid entering the pleura. We prefer to contact the rib below, perpendicularly, and to "walk off" the rib into the space above; the external intercostal fascia is sensed as the needle enters the space. A skin wheal is hardly necessary, and injection is made as the needle is advanced to the rib. No more than 3 to 4 ml of 0.5 to 1.0 per cent procaine or lidocaine are required for each space. As already noted, several nerves must be blocked above and below the proposed abdominal incision for complete anesthesia. Thus, for the upper abdomen, thoracic nerves five through eleven should be injected. One should calculate in advance the total amount of local anesthetic needed to avoid injection of toxic amounts.

Multiple injection of the intercostal nerves is painful, often requiring premedication with opioids if the condition of the patient allows. Subsequently, operation is made more comfortable if 20 to 40 per cent nitrous oxide is given by mask.

PARAVERTEBRAL SOMATIC NERVE BLOCK

The landmark for any one of the spinal nerves is usually the corresponding vertebral spine; however, it is not easy to identify the spines. The most prominent is not always the seventh cervical, as stated (the vertebra prominens). Spines also vary in shape and slope, depending upon segmental location. Thus, the cervicals are bifid and more or less perpendicular to the long axis, the thoracic spines are round at the tips, sloping downward acutely in the midthoracic region, and the lumbar spines are oblong at the ends and perpendicular to the long axis of the back.

For the dorsal approach to a somatic nerve, a point 4 cm from the midline is selected. The needle is guided perpendicularly onto the rib or transverse process. Then the needle is redirected inferiorly and inward at a 45-degree angle in both planes. If the needle is redirected upward after initial insertion, more paresthesias are encountered, and there is more chance of subarachnoid injection through the intervertebral foramen. In the thoracic region the needle is advanced only 2 cm beyond the lower border of the rib or transverse process. Markers on the needle are helpful. The tip of the needle then lies between the external intercostal muscle and the internal intercostal membrane; deeper insertion carries the hazard of pleural entry. Five ml of 1 per cent procaine or lidocaine are sufficient to anesthetize not only the intercostal nerve but the sympathetic ganglion as well. Paresthesias in the lumbar region are not unusual; here, depth of penetration to the transverse process is greater than in the thoracic region and paravertebral injection, also at a greater depth, carries less hazard.

BLOCKS OF THE UPPER EXTREMITY

BRACHIAL PLEXUS

Soon after the introduction of local anesthesia in 1884, Halsted, a surgeon, injected cocaine under direct vision into the brachial plexus in order to perform radical mastectomy. After 1900 and the synthesis of procaine, the plexus was anesthetized percutaneously—first via an axillary approach whereby the needle was advanced above the clavicle, then more or less directly via a supraclavicular insertion. Supraclavicular block remained the method of choice until Adriani resurrected axillary block, this time with perivascular injection about the axillary artery into the median, radial, and ulnar nerves. Finally Winnie proposed the interscalene approach to the plexus, with insertion of the needle at the level of the sixth cervical transverse process. At present both the axillary and interscalene methods have supplanted the supraclavicular technique because of an appreciable incidence of pneumothorax with the latter. The success of all these techniques rests upon a common anatomy.

Anatomy

Composed of the anterior divisions of the last four cervical and first thoracic nerves, the plexus can be envisioned as extending from the transverse processes to the apex of the axilla, where the terminal nerves are formed. All components are contained in a sheath of cervical fascia so that injection of a sufficient volume of anesthetic at any of the sites mentioned previously results in anesthetization of the plexus. The plexus itself is concentrated within a circumscribed area, just above the first rib; in relation to the cupula of the pleura between the anterior and middle scalene muscles. Here the plexus is joined by the third portion of the subclavian artery, to form a neurovascular bundle continuing into the axilla. The prominent pulsation of the artery as it lies in the subclavian groove on the first rib can be used as a guide to the plexus in supraclavicular injection (Fig. 20-4). Landmarks such as the midpoint of the clavicle or the external jugular vein as it crosses the sternocleidomastoid muscle are also employed.

Finally it should be noted that other nerves may be anesthetized as the large volumes needed for complete brachial block are injected: phrenic nerve with resulting diaphragmatic paralysis; inferior laryngeal nerve with vocal cord paralysis; the ascending nerves to the head in the paravertebral sympathetic chain causing Horner's syndrome; postganglionic autonomic fibers arising in the stellate ganglion; and the upper cervical nerves which carry sensation from the back of the head, the anterior and posterior cervical triangles, and the cutaneous areas over the upper thorax and shoulder.

In all varieties of brachial plexus block the plexus should be approached with a clear concept of its location, the point of crossing the first rib, the relation to the pleural cupula immediately beneath, and a knowledge of other landmarks such as the scalenus muscles and the anterior tubercle of the sixth vertebral transverse cervical process. The anesthetist usually stands at the side of the recumbent patient, whose head may or may not be turned away, with the shoulder girdle drawn down or the arm abducted. The area is prepared and draped so that all landmarks are visible. Depending upon the dexterity of the anesthetist, either hand may be employed for needle insertion. The needle should be the shortest possible compatible with reaching the plexus; a 2 cm, 23 gauge needle is usually satisfactory.

Axillary Block of the Brachial Plexus

Because of the ease and accuracy of placement of the needle as well as the minimal incidence of complications, axillary approach to the brachial plexus has largely replaced the original supraclavicular approach. Additional advantages are that the axillary block may be repeated if necessary during the course of a lengthy operation, and it is a technique easily applied to a child or to a somewhat uncooperative patient.

The skin of the axilla should be shaved and the arm abducted to 90 degrees, with the forearm flexed at a right angle and lying flat on a table (Fig. 20-3). A tourniquet is placed just below the axilla to direct the local anesthetic toward the supraclavicular region. The operator stands at the patient's side, with the axillary artery isolated and fixed between the index and middle fingers of one hand. A skin wheal is raised as high in the axilla as possible, usually 1 to 3 cm above the insertion of the pectoralis major muscle on the humerus. At this point the terminal nerves of the plexus have not yet begun to diverge from the artery. A 2-cm, 23-gauge needle is inserted at a 45-degree angle in the direction of the artery, to enter the neurovascular sheath. A distinct impression of penetration of fascia may be experienced as well as production of paresthesias or perforation of the artery. The latter is of little moment when a small needle is used and immediately withdrawn. Pulsations transmitted to the needle are a good sign. In the original technique, injection of local anesthetic in concentrations from 1.5 to 2.0 per cent was made as follows: superior and lateral to the artery to anesthetize the musculocutaneous and median nerves; superior and medial for the ulnar nerve; and inferior and lateral for the radial nerve. From 5 to 10 ml of anesthetic are injected at each site for a total volume of 30 to 40 ml, depending upon the girth of the arm and the accessibility of structures. Recent observations suggest that mere injection into the neurovascular sheath without repositioning the needle results in successful block. De Jong has described a technique for injection of the musculocutaneous nerve in the arm because this is frequently missed during axillary block. Block of the intercostal brachial nerve is accomplished merely by extending the initial skin wheal around the arm. This does not prevent tourniquet pain.

Complications of axillary block are limited essentially to minimal extravasation of blood in a small percentage of cases. If properly performed, the solidity and extent of the nerve block are as good as in supraclavicular block, the anesthetic apparently diffusing upward to reach the supraclavicular branches of the plexus as demonstrated by injection of radiopaque solutions.

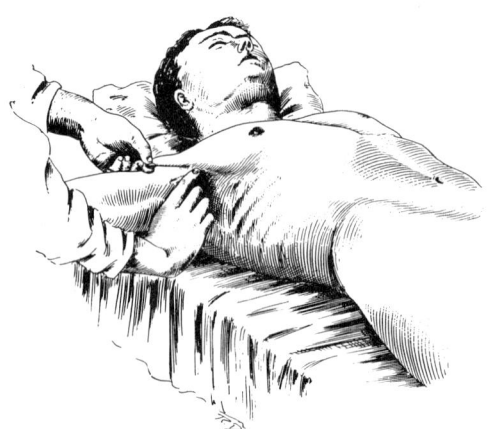

Figure 20-3. Perivascular axillary block of the brachial plexus. (Reproduced with permission from Labat GL: Regional Anesthesia. 2nd ed, Philadelphia, WB Saunders Co, 1928.)

Interscalene Brachial Plexus Block

Winnie has described several perivascular techniques for block of the brachial plexus based on the concept that the plexus is enveloped in a fascial compartment extending from the cervical vertebrae to the distal axilla. In the interscalene approach, the head is lifted to accentuate the clavicular head of the sternomastoid muscle. Starting at the lateral border above the clavicle, the finger is rolled across the belly of the anterior scalene muscle to the groove between the anterior and middle scalenes. At the level of the sixth cervical transverse process or Chassaignac's tubercle, a 2.5- to 4-cm, 22-gauge needle is inserted into the groove perpendicular to the skin (thus slightly caudad, dorsal, and mesial). Penetration of fascia may be felt, a paresthesia elicited, or a transverse process touched. With the needle thus placed in the fascial compartment, 20 to 40 ml of procaine or lidocaine, 1.0 to 1.5 per cent, are injected into the space; volume is considered important here. With large volumes both cervical and brachial plexuses are blocked. Although pneumothorax is avoided, Horner's syndrome and phrenic nerve palsy appear frequently.

Supraclavicular Block

A skin wheal is raised at a point 1 cm above the clavicle midway between the acromial tip and the sternoclavicular articulation, thus approximately at the lateral border of the first rib (Figure 20–4). To avoid puncturing the subclavian artery, the artery is depressed with the index finger of one hand while inserting the needle just above the fingertip with the other.

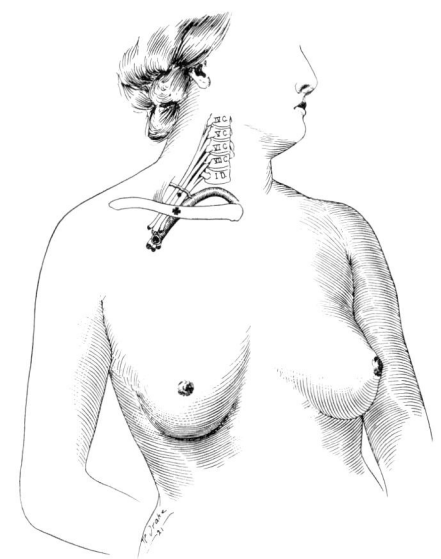

Figure 20–4. Landmarks for the supraclavicular block of the brachial plexus. (Reproduced with permission from Labat GL: Regional Anesthesia. 2nd ed, Philadelphia, WB Saunders Co, 1928.)

Although some prefer to use a capped needle to prevent pneumothorax, we do not believe that entrainment of air is responsible for this complication. Direction of the needle is backward, inward, and downward. When paresthesias are elicited in the fingers, the anesthetic is slowly injected; usually 20 to 25 ml of 1.5 to 2.0 per cent procaine or lidocaine are adequate.

One of the important details of this technique is instruction of the patient in the accurate reporting of paresthesias; these are described as sensations resembling those of "electric shock" or striking the "funny bone." Patient cooperation calls for just the right amount of sedation. After the anesthetic is injected, it is unlikely that further paresthesias will be elicited, probably because of anesthetization of sensory nerves. If the rib is not reached at the expected depth, anywhere from 0.5 to 5 cm beneath the skin depending upon the habitus of the patient, the needle is withdrawn to avoid entering the pleura and the direction altered. Once the rib is touched, the plexus has already been by-passed.

An intracutaneous and subcutaneous wheal is then made in bracelet fashion about the upper arm to interrupt sensory fibers of the second and third thoracic nerves carried in the intercostobrachial nerve. While this may be necessary for operation performed on the upper arm, it does not, as alleged, prevent tourniquet pain. Tourniquet pain represents ischemic pain transmitted by small autonomic fibers that travel perivascularly to enter the spinal cord through unblocked pathways.

The most serious complication of supraclavicular nerve block is development of tension pneumothorax, reported as occurring in 1 to 3 per cent of blocks. That pneumothorax develops gradually suggests slow escape of air from the lung rather than entrainment of air during injection. Phrenic nerve paralysis is found in approximately 25 per cent of patients, though it causes little difficulty. Horner's syndrome, recurrent laryngeal nerve paralysis, and hematoma may develop. In a small number of patients persistent subjective paresthesias and sensory deficit have been noted. These are inherent in the technique, probably resulting from the deliberate elicitation of paresthesias and intraneural injection of the anesthetic.

NERVE BLOCK AT THE ELBOW

There is usually little need to block the radial, median, or ulnar nerve at the elbow because of the ease of performance of axillary block, but occasionally elbow block may be necessary. Block at the elbow does not prevent pain when a forearm tourniquet is used. The techniques of Labat described here are those commonly employed.

Median Nerve

Both median and radial nerves are approached at the arm, where a crease is formed when the supinated forearm is held at a right angle; the

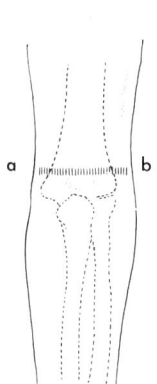
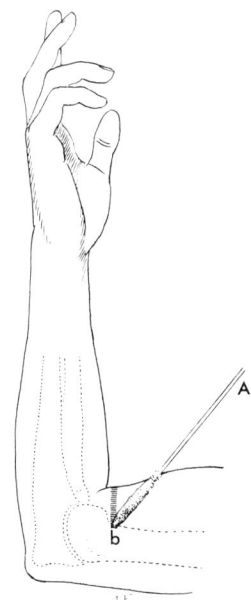

Figure 20-5. *A* is an applicator to show the level of injection of the median and radial nerves at the elbow. (Reproduced with permission from Labat GL: Regional Anesthesia. 2nd ed. Philadelphia, WB Saunders Co, 1928.)

forearm is then extended (Fig. 20-5). The tendon of the biceps is palpated, the pulsation of the brachial artery identified, and a skin wheal is raised just medial to the artery for block of the median nerve. The point is about midway between the medial condyle of the humerus and the medial border of the biceps. Occasionally the median nerve can be rolled beneath the finger. A 4-cm, 23-gauge needle is inserted perpendicular to the skin through deep fascia, where a paresthesia may be produced. From 2 to 3 ml of 2 per cent procaine or lidocaine are injected, or 5 ml are introduced fanwise in the absence of a paresthesia.

Radial Nerve

At the same level as for the median nerve, the needle is inserted 1 cm lateral to the biceps tendon through deep fascia, in a direction toward the operator's index finger as it is held against the posterior surface of the lateral condyle of the humerus. The intermuscular septum is thereby penetrated between the brachioradialis and brachialis muscles, about 10 cm above the lateral condyle in the axis of the humerus. The needle is advanced to bone, where 10 ml of a 2 per cent procaine or lidocaine solution are injected fanwise over a distance of 6 to 7 cm. It should be recalled that once the radial nerve has supplied the muscles arising from the lateral condyle—the extensors, external rotators, and supinators—it is purely sensory to forearm and hand.

Ulnar Nerve

Block of the ulnar nerve at the elbow is easily performed because the nerve can be rolled beneath the fingers as it lies in the groove between the medial condyle of the humerus and the olecranon process of the ulna. The patient is positioned to lie on the opposite side with the forearm extended, or supine with the forearm flexed and the arm held across the chest. Injection is made directly into the nerve with 2-cm, 25-gauge needle inserted from above downward into the groove, the nerve held immobile between two fingers. Paresthesias are easily produced, whereupon 1 to 2 ml of 2 per cent procaine or lidocaine are injected.

Block of the nerves at the elbow can be performed in rapid succession to produce anesthesia in the hand. For operations on the forearm, a bracelet injection of local anesthetic is made at the elbow to anesthetize the descending cutaneous nerves of the forearm.

NERVE BLOCK AT THE WRIST

Median Nerve

Satisfactory anesthesia for operation on the hand is obtained by block of the nerves at the wrist. Block of the median nerve is made at a level corresponding to the tip of the styloid process of the ulna at a point between the tendons of the palmaris longus and flexor carpi radialis muscles (Fig. 20-6). The main part of the nerve lies beneath the volar fascia, either beneath or just to the radial side of the palmaris longus tendon. To identify the latter, the patient flexes the wrist against counterpressure with the fingers and thumb held straight. A 2-cm, 25-gauge needle is directed perpendicularly to a depth of 0.5 cm below deep fascia and 1 to 2 ml of a 2 per cent solution of procaine or lidocaine are injected if a paresthesia is elicited; if not, an additional 2 ml are injected fanwise.

Ulnar Nerve

Ulnar nerve block at the wrist is performed at the same level as for the median nerve (Fig. 20-6). With the hand supine and the tendon of the flexor carpi ulnaris held between the fingers, the needle is inserted perpendicularly, tangential to the tendon, beneath deep fascia where injection is made as for the median nerve. A good landmark is the ulnar artery, with injection beneath fascia just lateral to it, then dorsally and subcutaneously to reach the smaller branches of the nerve. One to 2 ml of 2 per cent procaine or lidocaine are used.

Radial Nerve

At the wrist the radial nerve, now purely sensory, has diverged from the radial artery at the lower third of the forearm, turned dorsally, and

Regional Nerve Blocks

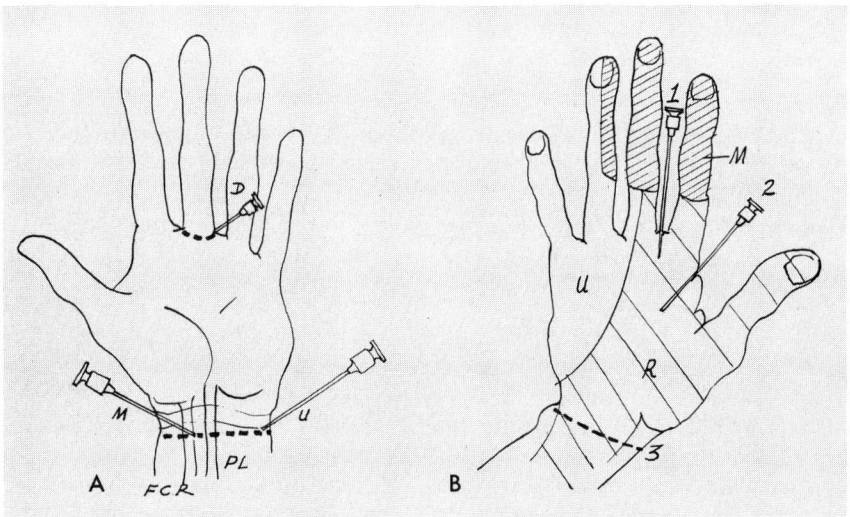

Figure 20-6. *A.* Palmar surface of the hand. Needles at *M* and *U* show points of injection for median and ulnar nerves, respectively. The dotted line is at the level of the styloid process of the ulna. Needle at *D* shows site of injection for field block of finger. *FCR* = flexor carpi radialis tendon; *PL* = palmaris longus tendon. *B.* Dorsum of the hand showing cutaneous distribution of radical (*R*), ulnar (*U*), and median (*M*), nerves. Needles *1* and *2* indicate approaches to the interosseous spaces. The dotted line indicates bracelet injection for cutaneous nerves. (Reproduced with permission from Vandam LD: Anesthesia for hand surgery. *In* Flynn JE (ed): Hand Surgery. Baltimore, The Williams & Wilkins Co, 1966.)

pierced the deep fascia to supply cutaneous branches to the wrist, the dorsum of the hand, and the dorsum of the first, second, and third fingers (Fig. 20-6). Here, at the same level as for block of median and ulnar nerves, a subcutaneous and intracutaneous bracelet will anesthetize not only the radial branches but other cutaneous nerves of the forearm extending into the proximal part of the palm. Specifically, for the radial nerve fibers, the radial artery is identified, the skin over it penetrated, and the needle then angled dorsally and parallel to skin, with injection subcutaneously for the length of the needle. Again, about 2 ml of a 2 per cent solution of procaine or lidocaine are used.

HAND AND DIGITAL BLOCK

Commonly employed nerve blocks of the hand are largely of the field and infiltrative variety. As a rule, it is best to inject via the dorsum of the hand rather than through the skin of the palm (Fig. 20-6). Injection should not be made into an infected area. In all instances it is important to avoid excessive distention of tissues and the use of epinephrine, both of which may comprise circulation to the fingers.

The digits are anesthetized by subcutaneous infiltration bilaterally at the base of the finger (Fig. 20-6). Operations on the fifth finger involving palm and metacarpal bone can be performed with ulnar nerve block at the elbow or at the wrist. Extensive operations on the thumb require both median and ulnar nerve block as well as block of the radial and other cutaneous nerves. The other fingers and their respective metacarpals are anesthetized by infiltration into the interosseous spaces. Injection is made from the dorsum, infiltrating the space down to the palm: about 5 ml of 1 per cent procaine or lidocaine are required. In interosseous injection, additional field block of the cutaneous nerves is necessary.

BLOCKS OF THE LOWER EXTREMITY

ANATOMY

The lower extremity is supplied by the anterior primary divisions of the five lumbar and upper three or four sacral nerves. In the pelvis these nerves form a deep-seated, widely spaced plexus that is not so readily accessible to block as is the brachial plexus. The peripheral nerves formed from the plexus emerge at several points. The femoral nerve derived from the upper four lumbar nerves crosses over the brim of the pelvis beneath the inguinal ligament to supply the extensors of the knee as well as the skin of the anterior thigh and part of the leg in the distribution of the saphenous nerve. The obturator nerve formed from the first four lumbar nerves leaves the pelvis through the obturator canal to supply the adductors of the thigh and the skin on the medial surface. The remainder of the lower extremity is supplied by the great sciatic nerve, the largest in the body. With contributions from L4, L5, S1, S2, and S3, the sciatic nerve exists from the pelvis posteriorly through the greater sciatic notch. On the posterior surface of the thigh, nerves to the hamstrings or flexors of the knee are given off; at the midpoint, division into the two terminal branches occurs—the common peroneal and the tibial. In general, the peroneal nerve (L4, L5, S1, S2) supplies all structures on the front of the leg and the dorsum of the foot: the tibial nerve supplies the posterior portion of the leg and the plantar surface of the foot. A number of cutaneous and motor nerves to the muscles of the buttocks and pelvis are given off directly from the plexus.

FEMORAL NERVE BLOCK

The femoral nerve is blocked just below the inguinal ligament at the lateral border of the fossa ovalis. Three structures—femoral vein, artery, and nerve, in medial to lateral relation—lie in the fossa. With a finger on the pulsating femoral artery, paresthesias of the femoral nerve are easily elicited, since it lies laterally. Five to 10 ml of 1 per cent procaine or lidocaine are injected. Block of the nerve is not sufficient for operation on the anterior surface of the thigh unless combined with a lateral femoral cutaneous nerve block. The femoral nerve is sensory to the medial surface of the thigh by way of the intermediate and medial cutaneous nerves.

LATERAL FEMORAL CUTANEOUS NERVE BLOCK

The lateral femoral cutaenous nerve (L2, L3) is easily blocked just medial to the anterior superior spine of the ilium. Infiltration is performed fanwise down to the iliac spine and beneath the inguinal ligament with 5 to 10 ml of 1 per cent procaine or lidocaine. This block alone is sometimes sufficient for superficial operation on the lateral surface of the thigh. Rarely, the nerve is involved in the syndrome of meralgia paresthetica (Roth), characterized by numbness and paresthesias in the distribution of the nerve.

OBTURATOR NERVE BLOCK

Block of the obturator nerve is seldom performed and is less easily done than the others. The block is utilized mostly therapeutically or for prognosis in painful conditions involving the hip. The patient is positioned with the thigh abducted and externally rotated. With the pubic tubercle as a landmark, the needle is inserted below and perpendicularly until the body of the pubis is met. Redirection of the hub of the needle downward and medially is done to guide the needle upward and laterally into the obturator canal. In performing this block continued reference to the skeleton is helpful. Paresthesias are rarely produced, and the criterion of successful block may be merely weakness of adduction of the thigh or relief of pain.

SCIATIC NERVE BLOCK

Sciatic nerve block results in anesthesia on the back of the thigh and leg. With many other types of anesthesia available for the patient in a poor physical state, sciatic block is seldom used; however, as a means of relieving pain it is occasionally valuable. One hazard of sciatic block is intraneural injection; because the perineural sheath is dense, development of pressure may cause ischemia with resulting paralysis. Labat advises bisection of a line drawn between the posterior superior spine of the ilium and the posterior tip of the greater trochanter of the femur. The needle is introduced perpendicular to the skin 2 cm below, on a line drawn perpendicular to the first, where paresthesias are sought. Since the sciatic nerve is large, 10 to 20 ml of 2 per cent procaine or lidocaine are required. The sciatic nerve can also be blocked via an anterior approach, but the percentage of successful blocks with this method is much lower.

PERONEAL NERVE BLOCK

The peroneal nerve is easily blocked at the point at which it encircles the fibula, just beneath the head. Some difficulty may be encountered in palpating the nerve, since it is flattened at this point. In this location the nerve is easily injured by pressure or stretch, thus accounting for postoperative foot drop. There is little need to block the nerve in the popliteal space.

TIBIAL NERVE BLOCK

If necessary, the tibial nerve can be blocked at the medial margin of the popliteal space just lateral to the tendons of the semimembranosus and semitendinosus muscles. As in sciatic block, 2 per cent concentrations of anesthetic should be employed.

ANKLE BLOCK

Anterior and posterior tibial nerves are both blocked at a level on the ankle corresponding to the uppermost ends of the malleoli of tibia and fibula (Fig. 20-7). The leg is positioned so that the knee is flexed, with the sole of the foot flat on the table. For anterior tibial nerve block the operator stands on the lateral side, introducing the needle between the prominent tendons of the tibialis anticus and extensor hallucis longus muscles. When the needle touches bone, it is withdrawn slightly and liberal infiltration made. For the posterior tibial nerve, the operator stands on the medial side and the needle is inserted medial to the calcaneous tendon until bone is touched. Again, slight withdrawal and infiltration are done. Paresthesias are sought in both instances and elicited relatively easily. Ankle block is completed with a superficial cutaneous bracelet infiltration and deep infiltration at the posterolateral compartment to block the sural nerve. Toe block is similar to that for the fingers.

SYMPATHETIC NERVE BLOCKS

STELLATE GANGLION BLOCK

Stellate ganglion block with interruption of sympathetic nervous impulses to the arm is beneficial in the treatment of peripheral vascular disease, sympathetic dystrophy, and perhaps as an adjunct to operation on the hand when vessel, nerve, or bone healing is in jeopardy. As noted earlier, brachial plexus and peripheral nerve block are also accompanied by sympathetic nervous interruption.

Anatomy

The sympathetic fibers that course through the ganglion supply blood vessels, sweat glands, and pilomotor fibers to the skin of the head, arm, and upper chest wall, as well as deeper blood vessels, pupils, salivary glands, and the heart and lungs. Preganglionic fibers to the ganglion originate from the first through the eighth thoracic spinal segments and synapse either in the ganglion or in the upper cervical ganglia, thereafter accompanying blood vessels and nerves in a peripheral distribution. Deep pain sensation may be transmitted via perivascular autonomic fibers; these enter the cord via the posterior nerve roots and white rami communicantes, where the cell bodies are located in the dorsal sensory ganglia.

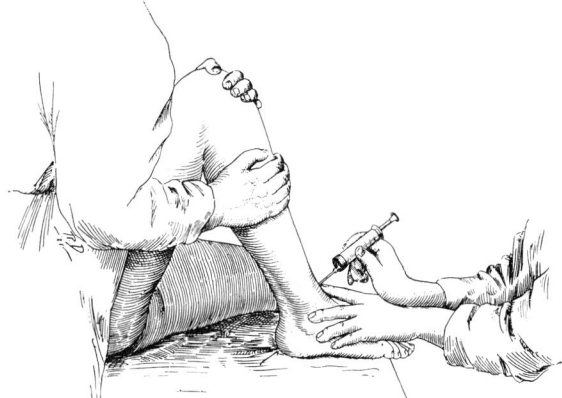

Figure 20-7. Approach to anterior tibial nerve block, same level as posterior tibial injection. (Reproduced with permission from Labat GL: Regional Anesthesia. 2nd ed, Philadelphia, WB Saunders Co, 1928.)

The stellate ganglion usually is composed of the conjoined ganglia of the inferior cervical and first thoracic sympathetic ganglia. It is a discrete, more or less encapsulated structure with its own blood supply, lying upon the seventh cervical vertebral transverse process and the neck of the first rib. Posteromedially situated is the longus colli muscle; posterolaterally, the scalenus muscles; and anteriorly, the cupula of the pleura. Adjacent structures include the carotid sheath, the first portion of the subclavian artery, the thyrocervical and vertebral arteries, the phrenic and recurrent laryngeal nerves, the esophagus, the vertebrae, and the spinal nerves.

Technique

Many approaches to stellate ganglion block have been described. These are classified according to point of entry in the neck and the relation to the sternocleidomastoid muscle—anterior, anterolateral, lateral, or posterior paravertebral.

A safe technique is that described by de Sousa Pereira, utilizing the anterior tubercle of the sixth cervical transverse process (Chassaignac's, or the carotid tubercle—Figure 20-2) as a landmark. With the patient semierect and the sternomastoid muscle and carotid sheath displaced medially, the tubercle may be felt just beneath the skin, easily reached with a short, small-gauge needle. Infiltration of 15 to 20 ml of 0.5 per cent procaine or lidocaine and downward diffusion produce effective block with little likelihood of major complications.

The simplest of all approaches in our experience is a median paratracheal injection performed just beside the cricoid cartilage, corresponding to the level of the sixth cervical vertebra (Fig. 20-8). With the patient supine in a semierect position, the sternomastoid muscle is displaced lat-

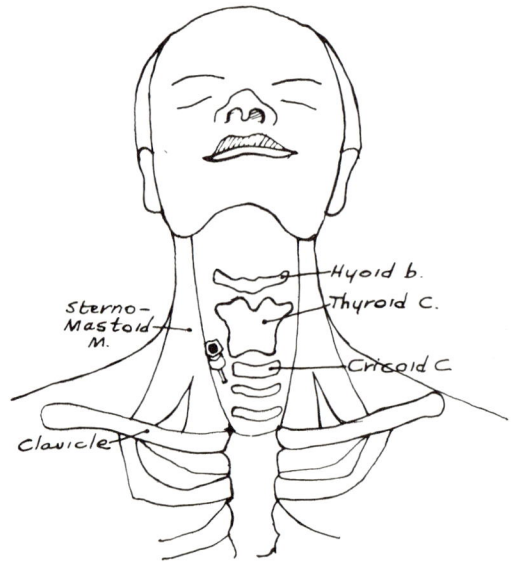

Figure 20-8. Median paratracheal injection of the stellate ganglion.

erally. A pillow placed beneath the shoulders so that the neck is hyperextended accentuates the anatomic relations. A 4-cm, 23-gauge uncapped needle is inserted perpendicular to the skin and tangential to the trachea until bone is met at a depth of from 2.5 to 4 cm. This may be either the sixth vertebral body or the base of the transverse process. The cervical sympathetic chain lies laterally at a distance no greater than 1.5 cm from the point of contact. After slight withdrawal of the needle to avoid injection into the longus colli muscle, 10 to 20 ml of 0.5 per cent procaine or lidocaine are injected slowly, with intermittent aspiration. At termination the patient is tilted upright to facilitate downward diffusion to the ganglion.

The first sign of successful stellate ganglion block is usually ptosis of the eyelid on the blocked side, followed by miosis. Enophthalmos is an illusion seemingly produced by paralysis of the sympathetic component to the levator palpebrae superioris muscle. Scleral injection, warmth, and dryness of the face follow. These are the signs of Horner's syndrome and indicate interruption of the cervical sympathetic impulses to the head. To be certain of satisfactory effect in arm and hand, warmth, anhidrosis, and vasodilation should be apparent.

Complications

As already noted, phrenic, recurrent laryngeal, or brachial nerve block may ensue. The patient should be warned beforehand of these occurrences, particularly of the ocular changes, the dryness of the face, nasal congestion, and possible hoarseness. Major complications resulting from stellate ganglion injection are pneumothorax, perforation of blood vessels, and subarachnoid injection. Block of the ganglion should not be attempted in the presence of a decreased clotting tendency.

For sustained block of six to eight hours' duration, tetracaine in 0.1 per cent concentration is added to 0.5 per cent procaine or lidocaine containing, in addition, epinephrine in 1:200,000 concentration. Bupivacaine or etidocaine in 0.25 per cent concentration with epinephrine will produce block lasting up to 12 hours. Continuous ganglion block by injection through an indwelling catheter seems too traumatic a procedure. Prolonged block with injection of 6 per cent phenol has been advocated to relieve chronic refractory pain, reputedly with little resultant neuritis. In this procedure, experience and placement of the needle under radiographic guidance are necessary to lessen complications.

PARAVERTEBRAL LUMBAR BLOCK

Apart from block of the stellate ganglion, paravertebral lumbar block is the most commonly performed sympathetic nerve block. The block is done as a diagnostic, prognostic, or therapeutic measure for vasospasm in the lower extremity or for sympathetic dystrophy.

Anatomy

The approach to the sympathetic chain is based upon its location on the anterolateral surface of the lumbar vertebral body in the retroperitoneal space, in close association with the celiac, semilunar, and mesenteric plexuses. Injection is made into the area of the first and second lumbar sympathetic ganglia—the lowermost portion of the thoracolumbar division of the autonomic nervous system, the site of maximal sympathetic outflow to the legs.

Technique

For unilateral block the patient may be positioned in the lateral decubitus position, but for bilateral block the prone position is more convenient. The trunk is bowed either by flexing the operating table or by placing a pillow beneath the abdomen to open the space between rib cage and iliac crest. Long, marked needles, 10 to 12 cm in length, 21- to 22-gauge, are required because of the depth entailed.

A line about 7 cm long is drawn from a vertebral spine to the point of intersection with the last rib. Insertion at this level should take the needle to the first or second lumbar vertebra. The needle is inserted either 4 or 7 cm from the midline at a 45-degree angle, inward. At the shorter distance the transverse process of the lumbar vertebra is met approximately 5 cm below the surface. The needle is then redirected downward at a 45-degree angle until the vertebral body is touched from 7.5 to 10 cm below the surface; in so doing, a paresthesia may be produced in the lumbar nerve. After setting the marker as an indication of depth, the needle is progressively redirected until it just slides off the vertebral body.

When insertion is made 7 cm from the midline, contact with the vertebral transverse process is missed, paresthesias are less likely, and the procedure is less painful. With either point of entry, a second needle is placed about 3 to 4 cm below, in the same plane. From 5 to 10 ml of 0.5 to 1 per cent procaine or lidocaine are then injected. Signs of successful block include increase in skin temperature, anhidrosis, and vasodilation in the leg. Recording of skin temperature or skin conductivity should be done as an index of therapeutic result. Complications are few: blood vessel perforation, arterial hypotension, and rarely inadvertent subarachnoid block.

CELIAC BLOCK

Celiac block is merely an extension of lumbar paravertebral sympathetic block, the needle being advanced into the retroperitoneal space 1 to 2 cm beyond the anterolateral surface of the vertebral body. Care is taken to avoid penetration of the aorta on the left or the inferior vena cava on the right. Since the capacity of the retroperitoneal space is large, and the celiac and mesenteric plexuses are diffuse, a large volume of anesthetic is required—from 30 to 40 ml of 0.5 per cent procaine or lidocaine.

Celiac block is usually performed for the relief of abdominal pain in acute or chronic pancreatitis or carcinoma of the pancreas, or in sympathetic imbalance involving the bowel such as acquired megacolon. Signs of a successful block include relief of pain and, sometimes, signs of sympathetic paralysis in the legs. Arterial hypotension is not infrequent because of widespread sympathetic blockade involving the splanchnic circulation and lower extremities. In situations in which prolonged block for a day or two might be beneficial, continuous lumbar peridural anesthesia is a more manageable technique.

INTRAVENOUS REGIONAL ANESTHESIA

Intravenous injection of a local anesthetic between two tourniquets to produce anesthesia in the arm was introduced by Bier in 1908. After sporadic application, the method fell into disuse until it was reintroduced by Holmes in 1963. The method entails bloodless exsanguination of the extremity and subsequent injection of a measured quantity of local anesthetic, which is confined to the area by use of a tourniquet. Onset of anesthesia is fairly prompt, probably relating to diffusion of the anesthetic to sensory nerve endings and in part to the pressure of the tourniquet on larger nerve fibers. Release of the tourniquet at the termination results in rapid disappearance of anesthesia, but with the possibility of central nervous and cardiovascular symptoms relating to the entry of a bolus of local anesthetic into the systemic circulation. However, the concentration of local anesthetic in plasma is less than that following brachial plexus or caudal block. Three peak concentrations are observed, relating respectively to release of local anesthetic from the vascular space, the extravascular space, and then from tissue compartments.

TECHNIQUE

For operations on the foot a pneumatic tourniquet is applied to the calf; for operations on the hand or wrist, to the forearm; and for operations above this level, to the arm. Initially the tourniquet is inflated just above venous pressure to permit venipuncture close to the site of operation with a temporarily maintained small scalp vein needle or a catheter with a small fluid-filled syringe attached. The tourniquet is then released to permit exsanguination of the part by elevation above venous pressure, and an Esmarch bandage or a pneumatic splint is applied. The tourniquet is then inflated about 100 torr above the level of systolic blood pressure. With the part positioned for operation, injection of the local anesthetic is made, usually 0.5 per cent lidocaine after prior flushing of the plastic tubing and needle with saline. The dose of lidocaine ranges from 1.5 to 3.0 mg per kg; for a subject weighing 60 kg the volume would be from 20 to 40 ml, the amount adjusted for muscle mass. After injection, the needle is removed and the operation proceeds.

In the ordinary course of events tourniquet pain is apt to appear after 40 to 45 minutes. Consequently, when a procedure approaching this length is anticipated, two pneumatic tourniquets are utilized, the proximal deflated and the distal inflated with the onset of pain. Pain may also be relieved by use of an opioid intravenously or by administration of subanesthetic concentrations of nitrous oxide by mask.

Intravenous regional anesthesia is employed largely for minor operations on the arm, less so in the foot or leg, and in either case when the procedure lasts less than an hour or so. Examples include incision and drainage; reduction of phalangeal or wrist fracture; excision of tumors or ganglia; removal of foreign bodies; repair of lacerations; and tendolysis and synovectomy. The time limitation is imposed by onset of tourniquet pain. Although toxic reactions to the local anesthetic are now rare, the anesthetist must be prepared to treat such occurrences by the recommended means (see Chapter 17).

APPRAISAL

There are distinct advantages in avoiding general anesthesia if a regional technique will suffice. Regional methods, however, require much of the anesthetist, patient, and the surgeon. Anesthetists must prepare patients carefully through informative discussion and adequate premedication. A detailed knowledge of anatomy is required as is a skilled, gentle technique. One must know the characteristics of the local anesthetic used, its potential for harm, and the treatment required should a toxic reaction develop. Finally, psychological support must be provided during the operation and appropriate supplemental drugs given when needed. The surgeon must be delicate in all manipulations and aware that the patient is awake. These admonitions are particularly important during intra-abdominal procedures. Some anesthetists and surgeons are unwilling to undertake these responsibilities, turning instead to general anesthesia as an easier but not necessarily better alternative.

REFERENCES

Adriani J: Labat's Regional Anesthesia. Philadelphia, W B Saunders Co, 1967.
Bonica JJ: Clinical Applications of Diagnostic and Therapeutic Nerve Blocks. Springfield, Charles C Thomas, 1959.
Burnham PJ: Regional block at the wrist of the great nerves of the hand. JAMA 167:847, 1958.
Erickson E (ed): Illustrated Handbook in Local Anaesthesia. Chicago, Year Book Publishers, 1969.
Harris WH, Slater EM: Regional anesthesia by the intravenous route. JAMA 194:1273, 1965.
Moore DC: Regional Block. 4th Edition. Springfield, Charles C Thomas, 1975.
Thorn-Alquist AM: Intravenous regional anaesthesia: A seven year survey. Acta Anaesth Scand 15:23, 1971.
Winnie AP, Collins VJ: The subclavian perivascular technique of brachial plexus anesthesia. Anesthesiology 25:353, 1964.

Part D

INTRAVENOUS SUPPORTIVE THERAPY

Chapter 21

INTRAVENOUS FLUIDS AND ACID-BASE BALANCE

The intravenous administration of drugs, electrolyte solutions, plasma, albumin, and blood components is an integral part of anesthetic management. In conjunction with principles of parenteral fluid therapy, this chapter is devoted to a discussion of the basic physiology of fluid, electrolyte, and acid-base balance. A subsequent chapter deals with blood transfusion and the technical aspects of intravenous administration.

THE BODY FLUID COMPARTMENTS

In practice the anesthetist is primarily concerned with monitoring the intravascular volume. Routine measurements such as blood pressure, pulse, central venous pressure (CVP), and ECG readings are all related to the adequacy or inadequacy of the circulating volume. The validity of these observations depends upon an understanding of the relationship between total body water and the various subcompartments: the two major subcompartments—intracellular and extracellular—and the subdivisions of the latter, the intravascular and interstitial compartments; these are all in equilibrium.

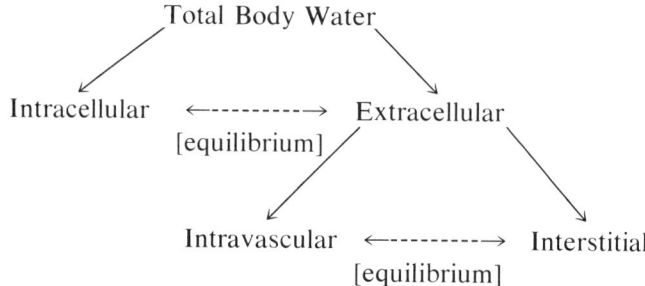

Total body water refers to the total amount of water in the organism, expressed as a per cent of the total body weight. The lean body mass is defined as the functional tissues consisting of bone, essential fat, and all vital tissues. Studies have shown that approximately 70 per cent of the adult mammalian functional mass consists of water, but the human organism contains a variable amount of fat, which has a much lower water content per gram than any other tissue. Therefore, a wide range of total body water exists in both women and men, with men having a greater body water content than women.

Representative total body water measurements are as follows:

	Range %	*Mean %*
Men	40–68	60
Women	30–53	50

The measurement of body fluid volumes depends upon the dilution principle. A known quantity of a measurable substance is injected into the fluid compartment and the concentration is determined once the substance is in equilibrium throughout.

$$\text{Fluid volume} = \frac{Q \text{ (known quantity of test substance)}}{\text{concentration}}$$

Estimation of total body water is made using substances which theoretically have equal distribution both inside and outside cells. Various substances, such as deuterium oxide (heavy water), urea, sulfanilamide, antipyrine, and creatinine have been used. Potential errors in measurement can be related to metabolism, protein binding, or inability of the substances to assume homogeneous distribution. Using deuterium oxide, a mean total body water of approximately 60 per cent for men and 50 per cent for women has been estimated.

RELATIONSHIP OF EXTRACELLULAR VOLUME TO BLOOD VOLUME

Extracellular fluid volume comprises approximately 20 per cent of ideal body weight or about one third of the total body water. As previously stated, there are two major components: the intravascular or plasma volume, and the interstitial fluid. The proportion of extracellular fluid present intravascularly is determined largely by the oncotic pressure of protein. Approximately one fifth of the extracellular fluid volume is plasma, while four fifths constitute interstitial fluid.

The organism utilizes several mechanisms to maintain an appropriate balance between the size of the intravascular space and the intravascular volume, in order to insure adequate venous return to the heart. Homeostatic mechanisms include mobilization of protein via the lymphatics and vasoconstriction, primarily in the capacitance vessels. Ultimately, changes in extracellular fluid are reflected by proportional changes in both interstitial volume and the plasma component of the intravascular space. Therefore, maintenance of a normal extracellular fluid volume is essential in the maintenance of blood volume.

Measurements of extracellular fluid compartments have employed sucrose, inulin, or mannitol, all of which are excluded from the cell interior. However, because these substances fail to enter all the extracellular fluid compartments uniformly, the measurements are not quite accurate. Plasma volume is determined by intravenous injection of a dye such as Evans blue, or of radioactive iodinated human serum albumin (RIHSA). The whole blood volume is computed by adding the red blood cell volume as determined by injection of chromium-tagged cells. Average figures for the fluid compartments are given in Table 21–1.

RELATIONSHIP OF EXTRACELLULAR TO INTRACELLULAR FLUID VOLUME

The distribution of water is not limited to any particular compartment, since it is a freely movable solvent for all the body solutes. Solute distribution, on the other hand, has several limitations. The size of molecules

Table 21–1. AVERAGE FLUID VOLUMES

Measurement	Absolute Value		Relative Value (% Body Weight)	
	Male	Female	Male	Female
Weight (kg)	70	60	—	—
Hematocrit, large vessels (per cent)	44	40	—	—
Plasma volume (ml)	3150	2700	4.5	4.5
Red blood cell volume (ml)	2100	1500	3.0	2.5
Blood volume (ml)	5250	4200	7.5	7.0
Hematocrit, whole body (per cent)	40	36	—	—
Total body water (L)	42.0	30.0	60	50
Extracellular water (L)	16.4	14.2	23.4	23.7

such as the plasma proteins limit their movement from one compartment to another. Certain electrolytes, like sodium, do not readily traverse cell membranes. The result is that water diffuses across the barriers to maintain osmotic equilibrium.

In order to understand this solute-solvent relationship the concept of osmolarity is basic. One gm molecular weight (one mole) of a substance contains 6.06×10^{23} (Avogadro's number) molecules. One osmole is defined as one mole (Avogadro's number) of a nondissociating substance in 1 L of solution. The term milliosmol (mOsm) is defined as one thousandth of an osmole of the substance in solution. Osmolarity is equal to the number of osmoles per liter of solution, while osmolality is defined as the number of osmoles per 1000 gm of solvent. In dilute solutions such as exist in the human organism, osmolality is approximately equal to osmolarity. Conventionally, these values are expressed in terms of mOsm with the normal osmolality of extracellular fluid equal to 285 to 295 mOsm per liter.

The major extracellular cation is sodium; each cation is accompanied by an anion. Beside sodium, other osmotically active particles found in small amounts are urea and glucose. In patients with uremia or severe hyperglycemia, these molecules add significantly to the total osmolality. Other substances such as ethanol or mannitol can also increase the total osmolality. Both urea and ethanol readily cross cellular membranes and therefore do not cause acute shifts in water between the extracellular and intracellular compartments. However, substances such as sodium, glucose, and mannitol do not readily cross cell membranes, therefore potentially causing loss of intracellular fluid. In clinical conditions such as heat stroke, water is selectively lost without solute. When this occurs a hyperosmolar state exists. The hyperosmolar state corresponds to a serum osmolality greater than 340 mOsm, or a serum sodium greater than 160 mEq/L, or both. Some drugs, for example bicarbonate, given intravenously markedly raise osmolarity. A 50-ml ampule of sodium bicarbonate contains 50 mEq of $NaHCO_3$ (100 mOsm) per 50 ml or 2000 mOsm per liter.

Excessive administration of salt-free water to a patient not on oral intake is associated with the hypo-osmolar state. Hypo-osmolarity corresponds to a serum osmolality less than 240 mOsm or a serum sodium less than 110 mEq/L. Rapidity of change of serum osmolality or serum sodium is another factor affecting a patient's tolerance to osmolar changes.

Administration of fluid containing 140 mEq of sodium expands extracellular volume without producing appreciable change in serum sodium concentration, as the solution is isotonic. Hypotonic salt solution increases the size of the extracellular space while decreasing serum sodium concentration. Clearly, serum sodium concentrations alone should not be used to estimate the size of extracellular fluid volume.

The volume of intracellular water is approximately twice that of extracellular water. Consequently, about two thirds of sodium-free water given a patient and not excreted in urine enters the intracellular compartment in response to osmotic equilibrium. Only one third of the water remains extracellularly, and in the absence of vasodilatation or protein shift only about one fifth of extracellular water is intravascular once osmotic equilibrium is established.

CHEMICAL STRUCTURE OF FLUID COMPARTMENTS

A diagram of the chemical structure of the body compartments expressed in mEq/L is shown in Figure 21-1. In the extracellular fluid compartment the important cations are sodium, between 135 to 140 mEq, calcium, 4.5 to 5.5 mEq, and magnesium, 1.5 to 2.5 mEq. Changes in serum potassium levels induce cardiac effects such as arrhythmias long before any abnormalities cause fluid shifts secondary to osmotic effects. Similarly, changes in serum calcium and magnesium produce neurologic and cardiac signs before osmotic effects are observed. The clinical problems produced by the most common extracellular cation abnormalities and their treatment are summarized in Table 21-2.

The major extracellular anions are chloride, between 100 to 106 mEq/L, and bicarbonate, between 24 to 28 mEq/L. These anions are frequently referred to as the exchangeable anions. When renal reabsorption of one anion is increased, renal excretion of the other is enhanced. A common example is found in the patient with chronic obstructive lung disease with carbon dioxide retention. Values for bicarbonate between 35 and 40 are associated with those for chloride between 85 and 95.

Recently, the importance of serum inorganic phosphorus has been appreciated. An essential clinical effect of inadequate amounts of inorganic phosphorus can be traced to reduced adenosine triphosphate (ATP) and 2,3-diphosphoglycerate levels, both of which shift the oxygen dissociation curve to the left, with diminished release of oxygen to the tissues. This kind of abnormality is found in the chronically ill patient in negative nitrogen balance through lack of oral intake, and in some patients on a hyperalimentation regimen without inorganic phosphorus supplementation.

Normally the total sodium and potassium in mEq/L should not exceed the sum of chloride and bicarbonate by more than 15 mEq. Should a larger difference arise, the presence of some other anion such as lactate, ketone, or salicylate should be suspected. This phenomenon is defined as an anion gap, as follows:

$$\textit{Anion Gap } [<15 \text{ mEq}]$$
$$[(\text{mEq Na}^+ + \text{mEq K}^+) - (\text{mEq HCO}_3^- + \text{mEq Cl}^-)]$$

The diagnosis and therapy of acid-base abnormalities are discussed later.

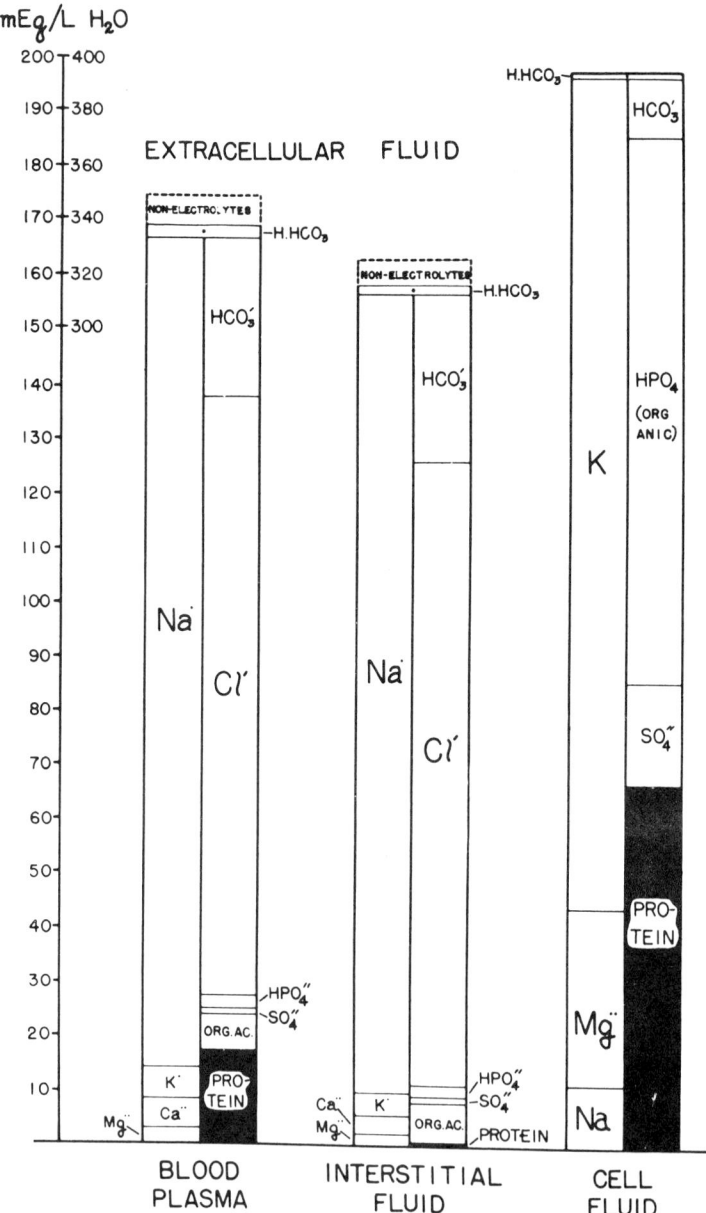

Figure 21-1. Chemical structure of the body compartments. (Reproduced with permission from Gamble JL: Extracellular Fluid. Cambridge, Harvard University Press, 1947.)

Intravenous Fluids and Acid-Base Balance

Table 21-2. Extracellular Cation Abnormalities and Their Treatment

	$\uparrow K^+$	$\downarrow K^+$	$\downarrow Ca^{++}$	$\downarrow Mg^{++}$
Major clinical problems	Cardiac arrhythmias: ultimately sinus arrest	Cardiac arrhythmias: ultimately ventricular fibrillation	Inotropic cardiac failure	Hyperreflexia and tetany
		Muscle weakness or loss of reflexes	Hyperreflexia and tetany	Psychiatric symptoms
				Increased arrhythmias with digitalis
Most common causes	Renal failure	Diuretic therapy	Alkalosis	Alcoholism
	Acidosis	Treatment of acidosis	Hypoparathyroidism	Diuretic therapy
	Iatrogenic	Alkalosis	Massive transfusion (RARE)	Chronic renal disease
		Dehydration		GI losses
Laboratory values	>5 mEq/L	<3 mEq/L	<4.5 mEq/L <9 mg per 100 ml	<1.5 mEq/L <1.8 mg per 100 ml
ECG changes	Peaked T wave	ST depression	Prolonged Q-T interval	No distinctive abnormalities
	Loss of P wave	T wave inversion		
	Loss of peaked T wave	U wave (may be a positive or negative wave)		
	Bradycardia			
	Spread of QRS			
Acute therapy in 70-kg adult (life-threatening situations only)	100 mEq NaHCO₃ IV over 2 minutes	K⁺ IV at 1 mEq per minute	CaCl 250 mg IV every 5 minutes until symptoms reverse; if calcium gluconate is used, multiply dose by 3	MgSO₄ 5 gm per hour IM or IV
	50 gm glucose, 20 U regular insulin IV			

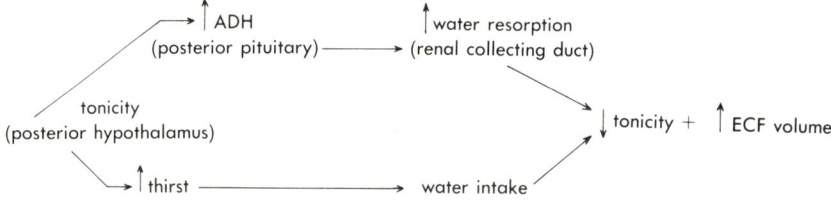

Figure 21-2. The tonicity maintenance system.

PHYSIOLOGIC CONTROL OF EXTRACELLULAR TONICITY AND VOLUME

The homeostatic systems for maintenance of extracellular tonicity are diagrammed in Figure 21-2. Sensors present in the posterior hypothalamus induce two compensatory responses when tonicity rises: (1) thirst develops, increasing water intake; and (2) more antidiuretic hormone (ADH) is produced and water is resorbed from the renal tubules. Restoration of normal tonicity occurs at the expense of increasing extracellular fluid volume. The volume maintenance system then returns the extracellular fluid volume toward normal.

The mechanism for maintenance of extracellular fluid volume is shown in Figure 21-3, reacting to increased extracellular fluid volume by decreasing renin release from the renal juxtaglomerular apparatus. Renin cleaves a hepatic-produced plasma polypeptide to yield angiotensin II. A decreased level of angiotensin II leads to less release of aldosterone from the adrenal cortex, in turn resulting in less sodium resorption from the proximal renal tubules. Other poorly understood mechanisms reduce salt intake. Decreased sodium resorption and decreased sodium intake lower extracellular fluid tonicity. The decrease in tonicity causes shifts of water intracellularly, decreased thirst, and less ADH release, changes that return extracellular volume toward normal.

Homeostatic mechanisms may be upset by a number of factors, the most important being: (1) restriction of oral intake; (2) fluid and electrolyte deficits or excesses related to the primary disease; (3) fluid and electrolyte deficits or iatrogenically produced excesses; (4) inappropriate ADH secretion; and (5) increased adrenocortical steroid secretion.

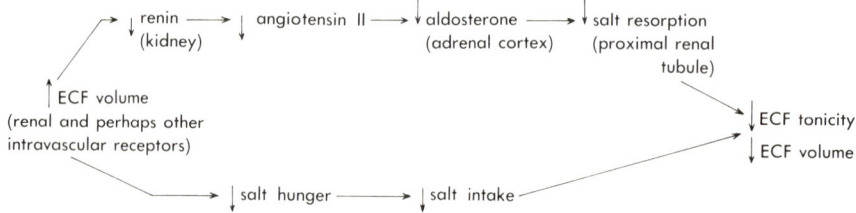

Figure 21-3. The extracellular volume maintenance system.

INTRAVENOUS FLUID THERAPY

ROUTINE PARENTERAL FLUID THERAPY IN ELECTIVE SURGERY

Most patients facing elective operation have their oral intake withheld during the 12 immediately preoperative hours, resulting in unreplaced solute and water loss. Water is lost from the body primarily via the kidneys, lungs, skin, and a small amount through the gastrointestinal tract. That portion lost from the lungs and skin constitutes the insensible loss, ranging from 800 to 1000 ml daily in the normal adult. In addition, a minimal obligatory 500 ml of urinary water are required for excretion of waste products. The optimal urine volume is expressed as 1 ml/kg of body weight per hour, approximately 1700 ml in a 70-kg adult. This potential water-conserving capability of the kidney provides a margin of safety, the chief means of adjustment when water must be conserved. It should be remembered that the normal glomerular filtrate is approximately 180 L daily, equal to approximately 60 times the plasma volume. Obviously, most of this is reabsorbed in the renal tubules and returned to the circulation. Although renal function in adults can limit losses in the fluid-restricted patient, infants are less able to deal with unreplaced losses, in part owing to the increased ratio of surface area to weight. In adults not operated on until afternoon, some anesthetists order an early clear liquid breakfast before oral intake is discontinued. An alternative approach is to give an intravenous infusion of a crystalloid solution preoperatively.

In view of the loss of fluid preoperatively, it is logical to administer one third to one half of the estimated 24-hour fluid requirement parenterally during the course of a major operation in the adult. Thus, an average 70-kg adult would receive approximately 600 to 1000 ml of fluid during the course of a one- to two-hour operation. This presumes no significant fluid or blood loss. To minimize the hazard of excess free water administration, at least one third of the fluid should be a solute-containing solution, either as saline or lactated Ringer's solution. Since most of these patients have had no caloric intake over the past 12 to 16 hours, it is good practice to include 25 to 30 gm of dextrose in the fluid administered. Obviously modifications of this approach are required for the dehydrated or previously salt-restricted patient. Intravenous fluids can often be omitted in healthy patients undergoing minor procedures.

FLUID THERAPY IN THE DEHYDRATED PATIENT

Patients with a history of vomiting, diarrhea, gastric suction, or intestinal fistulas may have suffered massive fluid losses from the gastrointestinal tract. In addition, those with peritonitis or bowel obstruction may lose large volumes of protein-rich fluid into the lumen of the gut or abdominal cavity. In the diabetic with hyperglycemia and acetonuria, or in some kinds of renal failure, impressive deficits arise as a result of renal salt and water losses. Extensive second- and third-degree burns result in massive losses of fluid, salt, and protein into the involved areas. Febrile patients or those exposed to tropical conditions can lose large amounts of fluid by sweating or through the respiratory tract. Finally, chronically ill or psychotic patients frequently fail to maintain adequate oral nourishment over prolonged periods.

The condition of this kind of chronically ill, malnourished patient falls into the category of the "depletion syndrome" because of several characteristics: depletion of essential substrates, amino acids, glycogen, fats, and caloric reserves necessary for vital system function; and a significant decrease in intracellular water with a corresponding slight increase in the extracellular component. The increase in extracellular water occurs primarily in the interstitial compartment, with a concomitant fall in the intravascular compartment or plasma volume. These patients have a deficiency in total body potassium, phosphate, and sodium, and decreased serum proteins and a tendency toward a decreased serum osmolality. Frequently such patients appear stable until subjected to the combined physiologic stress of anesthesia and operation. Under these circumstances the circulation often rapidly decompensates and does not respond readily to treatment.

Useful signs in evaluating a patient with these problems include the state of consciousness or sensorium and the degree of cardiovascular change in response to postural stress. Significant dehydration is generally accompanied by mental changes and obvious signs of hypovolemia. A fully conscious patient with an intact sensorium who can sit upright for at least a minute without a significant increase in pulse rate or fall in mean arterial pressure is unlikely to have more than a 10 per cent deficit in extracellular fluid volume. On the other hand, an obtunded patient with an obstruction or perforated small bowel causing peritonitis, with associated hypotension and tachycardia while lying supine, is obviously deficient in extracellular fluid volume. Since morphine is a vasodilator of the capacitance vessels, intravenous injection of small doses often unmasks a pre-existing deficit in intravascular volume. Thus it is essential to restore the extracellular fluid volume toward normal before operation to achieve adequate cardiovascular, cerebral, and renal function.

Other common signs of dehydration are: furrowing of the tongue, dry oral mucosa, and loss of skin or tissue turgor. However, a dry oral mucosa is occasionally observed when a patient breathes largely through the mouth.

The approach to a patient with dehydration certainly depends upon the evolving physical findings and the initial response to fluid therapy. In a patient with normal cerebral function, cardiovascular stability, and an adequate urine output, only documented losses and insensible loss are replaced. Alternatively, in the hypotensive, dehydrated patient, the extracellular space is repleted with isotonic saline or lactated Ringer's solution. It may be necessary to give up to 1 L of crystalloid every 15 minutes, up to 3 to 4 L, bearing in mind the nature of cardiopulmonary reserves. When more careful replacement is suggested, it is better to try a fluid challenge of 200 ml of crystalloid over a period of 10 minutes with observation of CVP or pulmonary wedge pressure. Fluids are continued until vital signs stabilize, urine output reaches 50 ml per hour, CVP rises excessively, or rales develop, as detected by auscultation. If signs of intravascular fluid overload appear before cardiovascular stability or adequate urine output occurs, fluid administration is slowed. Under these circumstances it is likely that the primary fault is inadequate myocardial function, and administration of a positive inotropic drug such as dopamine or isoproterenol should be considered, with simultaneous injection of the diuretic furosemide. In any case it is vital to restore cardiovascular stability before induction of anesthesia because vasodilation further comprises circulatory integrity. If circulatory stability cannot be achieved before operation, minimal general or local anesthesia may be the only acceptable solution.

For the reasons discussed, the serum sodium level cannot be used as an index of the amount of salt solution required. Misuse of the serum sodium level results in replacement errors both in magnitude and direction. A high hemoglobin or even a normal hemoglobin level in a chronically ill patient should heighten suspicion of severe dehydration. Modest decreases in hemoglobin or hematocrit are useful indices that the extracellular deficit has been effectively treated.

Some anesthetists and surgeons select blood or colloid over saline for treatment of dehydrated patients with peritonitis, bowel obstruction, or severe burns. Such patients can indeed suffer large internal losses of protein-rich fluid. Provided that sufficient amounts are administered, saline alone is almost always effective in restoring circulatory stability. However, an excess of saline may be required, thus involving the risks discussed later on. Hence there is a reason to use colloid for at least part of the fluid replacement in these patients.

Some prefer a balanced salt solution to isotonic saline. The composition of the several available parenteral fluid solutions is given in Table 21–3. When using isotonic saline in large amounts, 30 mEq of bicarbonate are

Table 21–3. COMPARISON OF EXTRACELLULAR FLUID AND VARIOUS REPLACEMENT SOLUTIONS

Solution	Na (mEq/L)	K	Cl (mEq/L)	Total Base	pH	Ca^{++} (mEq/L)	Mg^{++}	Calories per L
ECF	138	5	108	27	7.4	5	3	12
D_5W	0	0	0	0	4.5	0	0	200
Normal saline	154	0	154	0	6.0	0	0	0
Lactated Ringer's	130	4	109	28	6.5	3	0	9
Normosol	140	5	98	50	7.4	0	3	24

often added to each liter of solution administered. Provided that acid-base abnormalities are diagnosed by appropriate blood gas measurements and corrected with sodium bicarbonate, there is little proved advantage or disadvantage in using more expensive and complex salt solutions. Acid-base evaluation is, of course, mandatory in patients receiving massive replacement therapy regardless of solution chosen.

It is unwise to administer potassium routinely to the dehydrated patient without knowing the electrolyte status. The possibility of either hypokalemia or hyperkalemia exists, since severe dehydration can result in renal failure with resultant hyperkalemia. When hypokalemia is present, commercially balanced salt solutions usually fail to supply sufficient potassium to correct the deficit. We add up to 40 mEq of potassium to replacement solutions given to the hypokalemic patient. Potassium should not be given more rapidly than 1 mEq per minute per 70 kg. Should the dose exceed 0.5 mEq per minute per 70 kg, the electrocardiogram must be monitored continuously and serum potassium measured before the start and at no less than two-hour intervals.

Ill-advised treatment frequently causes severe salt and water depletion. The effects of administering too little or too much water and certain solutes are shown in Table 21-4. Iatrogenic dehydration most often occurs in patients who are salt restricted and receiving diuretics for treatment of hypertension or congestive heart failure. Depletion may become evident only after a vasodilating anesthetic is administered. It is preferable to establish CVP monitoring before beginning anesthesia for such patients. If both hypotension and a decrease in CVP follow induction of anesthesia, administration of isotonic saline or colloid is indicated. At times the intravascular volume needed to maintain cardiovascular stability during anesthesia proves to be too great at the termination of anesthesia. Nevertheless, anesthetists and their colleagues should realize that circulatory stability during the vasodilation of anesthesia may at times require administration of more volume than is best for the patient, once anesthesia is gone and remobilization of excess fluid occurs. Occasionally patients can only be managed by large volume administration intraoperatively, followed by vigorous fluid restriction and diuresis after operation.

HAZARDS OF EXCESS FLUID AND ELECTROLYTE ADMINISTRATION

In addition to using parenteral fluids to treat dehydration, many anesthetists give them for other purposes: as a substitute for blood transfusion, to treat shock, and to protect the kidney during major operations. Before discussion of the possible advantages of administering parenteral fluids to patients in excess of probable loss, we shall first examine the hazards.

Table 21-4. Effects of Administering Too Little or Too Much Water and Certain Solutes

Substance	Amount Administered	
	Too Little	Too Much
Water	Serum solute and sodium concentration increased Highly concentrated urine Thirst Oliguria Fever Circulatory failure	Serum solute and sodium concentration decreased Very dilute urine Polyuria Intracranial hypertension Headache, confusion, nausea, and vomiting Weakness Muscle twitchings and cramps Convulsions Coma
Sodium	Extracellular fluid volume decreased Hemoconcentration Lost tissue elasticity Microcardia Hypotension Circulatory failure Uremia	Extracellular fluid volume increased Edema formation and congestive heart failure Tendency to potassium deficiency
Potassium	Apathy Lethargy Muscle weakness Electrocardiographic changes Ileus or diarrhea Hypopotassemia Metabolic alkalosis	Hyperpotassemia Electrocardiographic changes Muscle weakness Cardiac arrest
Phosphorus	Hypophosphatemia ?Other effects	Hyperphosphatemia Hypocalcemia Tetany
Carbohydrate	Ketosis Protoplasmic catabolism augmented Tendency to greater water and electrolyte losses	Hyperglycemia Glycosuria Hepatic failure

(Reproduced with permission from Talbot NB et al: N Engl J Med 252:856, 1955.)

HAZARDS OF EXCESS FREE WATER ADMINISTRATION

Water Intoxication

Release of ADH occurs in response to stress, general anesthesia, opioids, pain, blood loss, and positive pressure ventilation. Thus postoperatively patients often develop elevated ADH levels despite normal or decreased extracellular fluid tonicity. When the extracellular fluid is already hypotonic, continued secretion of ADH is considered inappropriate.

Unlike a patient whose tonicity maintenance system is intact, a patient with inappropriate ADH secretion fails to excrete excess free water. The results of administering excess solute-free water to this patient are dilutional hyponatremia, intracellular water shift with cell swelling, and cerebral symptoms ranging from mild lethargy and disorientation to delirium, coma, and convulsions. The condition can be made worse by administration of opioids in a misdirected effort to treat delirium. Symptoms of water intoxication usually begin on the first to third postoperative day, and if convulsions occur, the fatality rate is high. The syndrome is rarely seen in adults given less than 2 L of free water on any postoperative day, including water absorbed from irrigating solutions or during transurethral resection. Water intoxication is more common in patients over 60 years of age. Serum sodium levels at the onset of symptoms are usually in the 118 to 131 mEq range, with 122 mEq an average value. Urine osmolality is higher than serum osmolality, with a typical value of 500 mOsm per L. Treatment includes fluid restriction to less than 1 L of isotonic saline per day with no free water intake. Oral intake of water by the uncooperative or confused patient must be prevented. Serum osmolality can be raised more quickly by the use of mannitol or diuretics, or by 2.5 per cent sodium chloride given intravenously. However, in the absence of serious symptoms, fluid restriction alone is effective. Symptoms may persist for days despite return of serum sodium levels to normal. Because of the hazards of water intoxication, administration of sodium-free water should be limited to replacement of demonstrated or probable losses, including those caused by overnight fluid restriction.

HAZARDS OF EXCESS SALT ADMINISTRATION

Just as ADH levels may be elevated postoperatively despite decreased extracellular tonicity, so, too, are adrenocorticoid levels raised despite increased extracellular fluid volume. As with ADH, elevations in circulating glucocorticoids and aldosterone are in part related to stress. However, part of the rise in aldosterone level may be a homeostatic response to a functional decrease in extracellular fluid volume when fluid is lost to sites from which it cannot be rapidly remobilized. Extracellular fluid in such locations comes more slowly into equilibrium with radioisotopic tracers; that fluid which is sequestered presumably is not readily available for purposes of circulatory homeostasis. Many investigators have documented such functional losses of extracellular fluid following major operation or trauma. Moreover, the postoperative tendency toward renal salt conservation can be overcome by saline overloading, in contradistinction to postoperative renal free water conservation, which is not overcome by free water loading.

Nevertheless, large saline excesses are not without hazard. Previously healthy individuals given large amounts of isotonic salt solution (3000 ml or more) in the treatment of shock have developed fetal pulmonary edema.

Smaller volumes may cause difficulty in pulmonary oxygen diffusion even in the absence of overt edema. Pulmonary problems may not occur until several days postoperatively, when the functionally lost fluid becomes available. Most patients tolerate excess saline better than excess free water; however, indiscriminate use of salt solution without demonstrable indication is poor practice.

INDICATIONS FOR ISOTONIC SALT SOLUTION OTHER THAN AS REPLACEMENT THERAPY

Several situations exist in which modest use of isotonic salt solution is justified in amounts exceeding probable losses. In a patient requiring intravascular volume replacement of less than 20 per cent of blood volume, or for whom colloid or volume expander is not available, blood volume can be maintained with saline given in amounts two to three times the blood lost. Saline is substituted for much of the blood formerly used to prime heart-lung oxygenating devices (see Chapter 26). Such hemodilution has reduced the amount of hemolysis seen as a consequence of cardiopulmonary bypass and conserves limited blood supplies.

A second use of salt solution lies in rapid expansion of the intravascular volume prior to anesthetic techniques that result in vasodilation. Thus, rapid administration of approximately 500 to 1000 ml prior to spinal anesthesia decreases the magnitude of hypotension and the need for vasopressors. Fluid necessary for overnight replacement therapy can be administered in this manner.

Finally, fluid administration beyond replacement of measured loss is commonly used to protect the kidneys. Both animal and clinical studies suggest that an intraoperative diuresis of 50 ml per hour or more decreases the risk of postoperative renal failure, especially in patients with major trauma or those undergoing resection of an aortic aneurysm. Diuresis should be attempted in these patients by volume administration alone. However, excessive fluid often leads to interstitial pulmonary edema and all of the undesirable consequences. In these cases, it is preferable to induce diuresis with mannitol or furosemide rather than with large volumes of fluid. It is not possible to give exact figures on the limits of fluid administration above measured losses because of associated factors. Other factors to consider in making a decision are the duration of operation, the operation per se, whether on the abdomen, chest, or the extremities, and both postoperative fluid and myocardial status.

ACID-BASE BALANCE

An understanding of appropriate fluid and electrolyte therapy is not complete without an appreciation of basic acid-base balance. This subject is further considered in Chapter 33.

In simplified acid-base terminology, an acid is defined as a chemical substance that donates H^+ ions (proton donor), and a base as a substance that accepts H^+ ions (proton acceptor). In the body economy several different acids are found, such as hydrochloric acid in the stomach, lactic acid, organic acids, and carbonic acid, the end product of aerobic metabolism. Conversely, the several bases present include ammonia and the bicarbonate ion. A typical acid-base reaction occurring *in vivo* is:

$$H_2CO_3 \rightleftharpoons H^+ + HCO_3^-$$
$$\text{Acid} \qquad\qquad\qquad \text{Base}$$

The acidity of a solution is determined by the concentration of H^+ ions, or more specifically, by H^+ ion activity. Acidosis implies an excess of H^+ ions in tissues and acidemia is defined as H^+ ion concentration above normal. Conversely, alkalosis refers to a deficit of H^+ ions at the cellular level, whereas alkalemia is a less than normal H^+ ion concentration. Acidosis and alkalosis are clinical diagnoses, whereas acidemia and alkalemia are values obtained directly by analysis of arterial blood. Acidity is conveniently expressed by the symbol pH, which relates to H^+ activity, in dilute solutions approximated by H^+ ion concentration.

Mathematically, pH is defined as the negative logarithm of the H^+ ion concentration. The pH scale is derived from the ionization constant of water, water representing the basic solvent. Water dissociates weakly into 1×10^{-7} H^+ ions and an equal number of OH^- (hydroxal) ions. When the negative logarithm of H^+ ion concentration is calculated, it is equal to a pH of 7.

$$pH = -\log_{10}[H^+]$$
$$= -\log_{10} 10^{-7}$$
$$pH = (-)(-7) = 7$$

At a pH of 7 it is apparent that the number both of H^+ and OH^- ions is equal; therefore a chemically neutral solution exists. Blood normally has a pH slightly on the alkalotic side of neutrality, with 4×10^{-8} mEq H^+ ion per liter. In order to convert an H^+ ion concentration of 4×10^{-8} mEq/L into pH, one takes the logarithm of 4, which equals 0.60, and to this adds the logarithm of 10^{-8}, which is -8.0. The resultant figure is -7.40, in pH terminology equaling $+7.40$.

Carbon dioxide and water constitute the major products of aerobic metabolism, and their combination into carbonic acid is unique in that it represents the only volatile acid produced by the organism. Elimination by the lungs of this potential source of H^+ ion via carbon dioxide and water enables the carbonic acid-bicarbonate system to be an effective buffering system. All other acids, both organic and inorganic, produced by metabolic processes are handled only by the kidney. It is important for the body to maintain a stable and narrow range of H^+ ion concentration in order for cellular enzymes to function properly. This is the reason for the elaborate buffering systems. A buffer system is defined as a weak acid and its conjugate base, or conversely as a weak base and its conjugate acid. A substance functioning in this manner is said to be amphoteric. Buffer systems are important in that they minimize changes in free H^+ ion concentration in spite of relatively large additions to or removal of H^+ ions from the system. Four major buffer systems function in the body: carbonic acid–bicarbonate system, reduced hemoglobin-oxyhemoglobin, serum proteins (carbamino compounds), and phosphates (major intracellular buffer).

Many expressions of the state of acid-base balance are used. One commonly employed is the Henderson-Hasselbalch equation, depicting the dependency of pH of blood on the bicarbonate-carbonic acid relationship.

$$pH = pK + \log \frac{[HCO_3^-]}{[H_2CO_3]}$$

Intravenous Fluids and Acid-Base Balance

In practice the carbonic acid term in the denominator is replaced by a term which is the solubility coefficient of dissolved carbon dioxide (s = .03) times the partial pressure of carbon dioxide (P_{CO_2}). From arterial blood gas measurements, pH and Pa_{CO_2} are measured directly, allowing for calculation of plasma bicarbonate.

$$pH = pK + \log \frac{[HCO_3^-]}{s \times P_{CO_2}}$$

[Value of pK = 6.1]

Thus the pH of blood depends upon the ratio of bicarbonate to dissolved carbon dioxide, the normal ratio being 20:1.

STATE OF ACIDOSIS OR ALKALOSIS

The pH of arterial blood ranges between 7.35 and 7.45. Values below 7.35 represent acidemia, potentially harmful, whether of respiratory or metabolic origin, because cellular acidosis must be assumed until proved otherwise. More importantly, absence of acidemia does not unequivocally rule out cellular acidosis or at least localized acidosis. At the cellular level acidosis increases myocardial irritability, decreases myocardial contractility, and decreases the responsiveness of the cardiovascular system to catecholamines, even though in response excess catecholamine secretion occurs. Measurements of pH values alone are poor predictors of circulatory stability. For example, the heart of a young, vigorous, diabetic patient may withstand a pH value of 7.0 to 7.1, whereas an older patient with myocardial ischemia may be unable to tolerate a pH of 7.25. Also on clinical grounds a state of alkalemia (pH above 7.45), once considered innocuous, can no longer be viewed so. Pa_{CO_2} normally ranges between 35 and 45 torr. Pa_{CO_2} levels above 45 represent hypercarbia or alveolar hypoventilation. On the other hand, Pa_{CO_2} levels below 35 represent hypocarbia or alveolar hyperventilation.

Clinical assessment of acid-base balance has been made easier by analysis of arterial blood gases. The interpretation is simple if the two directly measured variables, Pa_{CO_2} and pH_a, are used as the basis for analysis (Table 21-5). Incorporating this information into the clinical picture and then using the information derived from blood gas measurements and bicarbonate and base deficits, suggest the appropriate therapy. Once the figures are assembled, the next step is to place them in the clinical context. For example, respiratory acidosis and metabolic acidosis may coexist. How can one decide whether the Pa_{CO_2} and pH_a abnormalities result entirely from the respiratory circumstances and if the pH change is appropriate to the change in Pa_{CO_2}? As a basic approximation for each increase of 10 torr in Pa_{CO_2} above 40, the corresponding pH change is 0.05 units in the opposite direction. This oversimplification is sufficiently accurate for diagnosis and treatment of acute or combined acid-base disorders in the majority of situations. Table 21-6 lists approximate values of pH_a which can be expected at different levels of Pa_{CO_2} assuming no metabolic component.

Table 21-5. Blood Gas Analysis

	Pa_{CO_2}	pH_a
Normal respiratory state	35–45	7.45–7.35
Primary Pulmonary Dysfunction		
Acute resp. acidosis	>45	<7.35
Chronic resp. acidosis	>45	Norm. range
Acute resp. alkalosis	<35	>7.45
Chronic resp. alkalosis	<35	Norm. range
Primary Metabolic Dysfunction		
Uncompensated metabolic acidosis	Norm. range	<7.35
Partially compensated metabolic acidosis	<35	<7.35
Completely compensated metabolic acidosis	<35	Norm. range
Uncompensated metabolic alkalosis	Norm. range	>7.45
Partial compensated metabolic alkalosis	>45	>7.45
Completely compensated metabolic alkalosis	>45	Norm. range

Acute Respiratory Acidosis

Acute respiratory acidosis can be corrected only by improving the alveolar ventilation, either spontaneously by the patient or by mechanical means. The intravenous administration of bicarbonate may result in transient improvement of pH at best and is to be avoided, unless measures are taken simultaneously to insure adequate alveolar ventilation.

Table 21-6. Predicted pH at Different Pa_{CO_2} Levels in Absence of Metabolic Acid-Base Abnormality

Respiratory acidosis — Pa_{CO_2}, torr	Predicted pH (approximate)
70	7.25
60	7.30
50	7.35
Respiratory alkalosis — Pa_{CO_2}, torr	Predicted pH (approximate)
30	7.5
20	7.6
10	7.7

NOTE: Each change in Pa_{CO_2} of 10 torr when Pa_{CO_2} is greater than 40 torr produces a pH change of about 0.05 unit in the opposite direction.
Each change in Pa_{CO_2} of 10 torr when Pa_{CO_2} is less than 40 torr produces a pH change of about 0.10 unit in the opposite direction.

Chronic Respiratory Acidosis

In chronic respiratory acidosis, the net fall in pH is minimized by renal compensation via reabsorption of bicarbonate. Thus, a patient in chronic CO_2 retention, a state of chronic respiratory acidosis, would be expected to have a pH only slightly lower than normal or at best, in the low or normal range, if one subscribes to the principle that the body usually does not overcompensate. Frequently, however, these patients show pH values slightly on the high side of normal, explainable on the basis of a superimposed metabolic alkalosis, since diuretic therapy may lead to hypokalemia and hypochloremia. Hypochloremia in moderately severe CO_2 retention should be expected as the kidneys augment excretion of chloride in order to enhance bicarbonate reabsorption. When these patients receive mechanical ventilatory assistance, care should be taken to avoid normalizing Pa_{CO_2} too rapidly, since this will result in acute alkalosis, the hazards of which are discussed later.

Metabolic Acidosis

In metabolic acidosis, pH_a is less than normal in spite of a reduction in Pa_{CO_2}. If the blood is tonometered to a normal Pa_{CO_2} of 40 torr, a further reduction in pH occurs. The resulting bicarbonate value is far less than expected from the pH-Pa_{CO_2} relationship if the change is related solely to changes in Pa_{CO_2}. The discrepancy in bicarbonate values is referred to as base deficit and the source of excess H^+ ions is obviously the nonvolatile acids. The H^+ ions in turn combine with available bicarbonate and are eliminated through the lungs as CO_2 and H_2O. Approximate values for base deficit or excess when the Pa_{CO_2} is kept constant at 40 torr are listed in Table 21-7.

The common causes of metabolic acidosis are: diabetic ketoacidosis,

Table 21-7. Predicted pH_a at Different Levels of Acid or Base Excess When Pa_{CO_2} Is Kept Constant at 40 Torr

Acid excess, mEq/L (Reported as base deficit)	Predicted pH (approximate)
−21	7.1
−14	7.2
− 7	7.3
Base excess, mEq/L	Predicted pH (approximate)
+ 7	7.5
+14	7.6
+21	7.7

NOTE: For each 7 mEq of acid or base excess, pH changes about 0.10 unit in the appropriate direction. Acid excess is more commonly reported as base deficit or as negative base excess; hence it is reported with a minus sign.

lactic acidosis, renal failure, alcoholic ketoacidosis, and drug ingestion (salicylates and methanol).

When metabolic acidosis is present, the primary cause must be eliminated. However, in the interim, the cardiovascular system is supported with appropriate amounts of sodium bicarbonate intravenously, as follows:

1. Assume that the extracellular fluid volume is 20 per cent of ideal body weight and that bicarbonate is confined to the extracellular space.
2. The base deficit expressed in mEq is multiplied by the extracellular fluid volume: [(mEq/L) × (L)].
3. One half the calculated dose of sodium bicarbonate is given intravenously and after a short interval, arterial blood gases are measured for pH.

Several alternative ways are available to quantitate metabolic acidosis. Base excess or deficit can be calculated from a more exact nomogram or slide rule, available in most hospitals. Other methods include measurement of standard bicarbonate and of CO_2 combining power.

Standard bicarbonate represents an estimate of blood bicarbonate concentration on the basis of titrating Pa_{CO_2} down to 40 torr. Standard bicarbonate is measured in an anaerobically drawn blood sample or equivalently corrected by a nomogram. Measurement is reported as bicarbonate level rather than deviation from normal.

CO_2 combining power differs from the standard bicarbonate primarily in that the sample is not handled anaerobically. Thus, blood drawn for CO_2 combining power is not useful in providing data for Pa_{CO_2} or pH. In addition, CO_2 combining power is usually reported in volumes per cent, which must then be converted to mEq/L.

Respiratory Alkalosis

Respiratory alkalosis is most often secondary to hypoxemia; it is also related to central nervous system disorders or iatrogenic-induced hyperventilation. If the primary cause is not corrected, the kidneys, in time, should augment excretion of bicarbonate, resulting in a measured base deficit not to be confused with metabolic acidosis. In this situation, with Pa_{CO_2} below normal, the pH is on the high side of normal rather than below.

Metabolic Alkalosis

Metabolic alkalosis correlates clinically with deficits of chloride or potassium or a combination thereof. Hypokalemia exerts several deleterious effects on the organism beside causing metabolic alkalosis; namely, increased myocardial irritability and generalized muscle weakness. In order to correct metabolic alkalosis it is important to supply not only potassium but chloride ion as well. This allows the kidneys to excrete the excess bicarbonate and to reabsorb chloride.

Additional adverse effects of metabolic alkalosis include deficient oxygen delivery to tissues owing to shift of the oxygen dissociation curve to the left, and interference with the central control of respiration. These are discussed in Chapter 33.

Common causes of metabolic alkalosis are loss of gastric secretions in vomiting or nasogastric suction, diuretic therapy, chronic hypercarbia, inadequate dietary intake, chronic steroid administration, and excessive exogenous administration of bicarbonate as employed in cardiac resuscitation.

APPRAISAL

Today's anesthetist is called upon to administer anesthesia to older patients who have considerable limitations of cardiopulmonary reserves for major operations, conditions that would have been unthinkable two decades ago. This challenge cannot be met by improved intraoperative anesthesia and operative technique alone. An appreciation is required of fluid, electrolyte, and acid-base physiology, and a working knowledge of the various fluid therapy modalities available for treatment. The assessment of these problems and institution of therapy are often required far in advance of operation for a successful outcome.

REFERENCES

Davenport HW: The ABC of Acid Base Chemistry. 6th ed, Chicago, University of Chicago Press, 1974.
Hayes, MA: Water and electrolyte therapy after operation. N Engl J Med 278:1054, 1968.
Kassirer JP: Serious acid base disorders. N Engl J Med 291:773, 1974.
Leaf A: Regulation of intracellular fluid volume in disease. Am J Med 49:291, 1970.
Loeb JN: The hyperosmolar state. N Engl J Med 290:1184, 1974.
Morgan HG: Acid-base balance in blood. Br J Anaesth 41:196, 1969.
Rastegar A, Thier SO: Physiologic consequences and bodily adaptations to hyper- and hypocapnia. Chest (Suppl) 62:28S, 1972.
Roth E, Lax LC, Maloney JV, Jr: Ringer's lactate solution and extracellular fluid volume in the surgical patient. A critical analysis. Ann Surg 169:149, 1969.
Schrier R: Symposium on water metabolism. Kidney Int 10:1, 1976.
Vidt DG: Use and abuse of intravenous solutions. JAMA 232:533, 1975.

Chapter 22

BLOOD COMPONENT THERAPY

Well-documented differences in blood volume exist between adult men and women and between adults and newborn infants and children, but the average percentages of body weight are as follows:

Men	7.5 (75 ml/kg)
Women	6.5 (65 ml/kg)
Newborn infants	8.5 (85 ml/kg)

Muscularity and physical activity tend to increase the blood volume, whereas obesity, inactivity, and chronic disease tend to decrease it.

When blood is lost, replacement with whole blood, its components, colloids, or crystalloids is necessary when: insufficient volume is present to fill the intravascular space, oxygen-carrying capacity per unit volume is inadequate to meet tissue oxygen needs at a reasonable cardiac output, or coagulation factors such as fibrinogen and platelets are insufficient to permit effective blood coagulation. The percentage of blood volume lost before these requirements can no longer be met differs among patients. Normal subjects suffer little functional impairment after a 10 per cent loss in total blood volume, 20 per cent of oxygen carrying capacity, or 40 per cent of coagulation factors. Losses twice this amount may be compatible with survival, but place extreme demands on the patient's reserves.

MAINTENANCE OF INTRAVASCULAR VOLUME

Cessation of blood loss is dependent upon protective local reactions at the bleeding site, vascular smooth muscle contraction in severed vessels secondary to both mechanical and reflex sympathetic stimulation, and formation of a fibrin clot, which depends upon the integrity of clotting mechanisms.

An immediate compensation for loss of intravascular volume is a reduction in the size of the intravascular bed via vasoconstriction in the splanchnic system, the kidneys, and the venous capacitance vessels, the latter containing 60 to 70 per cent of the total blood volume. Vasoconstriction conceals the symptoms and signs of hypovolemia in healthy volunteers after an acute 20 per cent volume loss in the supine position, or after a 10 per cent loss when upright. A good example of a 10 per cent blood loss is when a donor gives one unit of blood, approximately 400 ml, without the appearance of tachycardia or postural hypotension. However, when losses exceed this amount or when anesthetics, drugs, or an adverse physiologic circumstance such as acidemia interfere with vasoconstriction, smaller blood losses may result in hypotension.

A second compensation for acute blood loss consists of transfer of interstitial fluid and extravascular protein to the intravascular space, thus restoring plasma volume. Acute blood loss of 10 per cent is largely replaced by this mechanism over approximately 24 hours. The process is facilitated in the microcirculation by a lowered transcapillary pressure secondary to increased precapillary constriction, and mobilization of interstitial fluid. At the same time lymph returned to the circulation, largely via the thoracic duct, is rich in plasma proteins.

Immediate treatment of blood loss maintains the intravascular volume and tissue perfusion without the need for activation of the normal homeostatic mechanisms. When the volume is not immediately replaced, little change in hemoglobin or hematocrit can be detected until interstitial fluid is mobilized. Since the process takes many hours, a change in hemoglobin concentration or hematocrit is a poor way to assess the magnitude of acute untreated blood loss. When volume expanders such as saline or dextran are used, the hematocrit decreases in proportion to replacement volume.

VOLUME EXPANDERS

Albumin or plasma protein solutions are useful for limited volume expansion because they are more readily available than whole blood and do not transmit hepatitis or result in hemolytic transfusion reactions. When simple volume expansion is the sole therapeutic goal, they are preferred over blood. On a logistic basis high molecular weight dextran-70 is more available than albumin, but the main deterrent to its use is a prolongation of clotting time when amounts in excess of 15 ml per kg are administered, approximately 1000 ml in a 70-kg individual.

Crystalloids, such as 0.9 per cent sodium chloride and lactated Ringer's solution, are widely used as volume expanders, both in emergencies and for definitive replacement. Compared with dextran, saline carries the disadvantage of redistribution between the extravascular and intravascular space in a ratio of approximately 4:1. Therefore, the amount of saline required to maintain intravascular volume is three to four times larger than the amount of blood lost. As saline is inexpensive and readily available, the need for larger amounts is not a disadvantage *per se*. However, in vulnerable patients the interstitial distribution of saline involves the pulmonary extravascular space, resulting in a barrier to pulmonary gas exchange. Also, once large quantities of saline are administered, the addition of plasma protein fraction to the circulation may cause mobilization of fluid from the extracellular space. This can lead to left-sided heart failure in patients with limited cardiac reserves. Thus, crystalloids should be used as blood substitutes primarily for replacement of modest blood losses or in an emergency when oncotically active expanders are not immediately available.

Large volumes of salt-free solution such as dextrose and water are poor volume expanders because they simply represent excess free water as the glucose is metabolized, and they pose the hazard of water intoxication.

MAINTENANCE OF OXYGEN-CARRYING CAPACITY

Since most oxygen in arterial blood is carried by hemoglobin, a reduction in hemoglobin causes a decrease in arterial oxygen content. The amount of oxygen supplied to tissues depends upon the arterial oxygen content and the cardiac output. If hemoglobin content is reduced, oxygen delivery to tissues must be maintained by a hyperdynamic circulation. This subject is covered in detail in Chapter 33.

WHOLE BLOOD THERAPY

The selective administration of blood components is preferable to routine use of whole blood, since most patients require only specific components (Table 22-1). This approach has been made possible by improvements in techniques of collection, processing, and storage of blood. Blood component therapy for the most part avoids the major adverse effects of whole blood administration, which include serum hepatitis, hemolytic reactions, and sensitization to minor erythrocyte antigens.

The once commonly used blood anticoagulant, ACD, a mixture of citric acid, sodium citrate, and dextrose, has largely been replaced by CPD, a mixture of sodium citrate, citric acid, a phosphate buffer, and dextrose. CPD offers several advantages over ACD in the decreased degradation of 2, 3-diphosphoglycerate, a higher pH at equilibration, increased red blood cell survival, and lower potassium levels in storage.

Whole blood is best used only when blood loss is severe enough to cause hypovolemic shock. Under this circumstance there is a distinct advantage in the blood being as fresh as possible. In aging, the effectiveness of stored blood is diminished by reduced erythrocyte viability and a decreased oxygen availability secondary to changes in 2, 3-diphosphoglycerate with leftward displacement of the oxyhemoglobin dissociation curve, both significant in blood replacement.

TABLE 22-1. BLOOD COMPONENT THERAPY

Blood Therapy Type	Indications
A. Whole blood (Type Specific)	A. Acute hemorrhage
B. Packed red blood cells	B. Severe chronic anemia Patient history — congestive heart failure Anemia in elderly debilitated patient Anemia in hepatic failure (cirrhosis) Anemia in renal failure (anuria, uremia)
C. Leukocyte-deficient red blood cells (washed RBC's)	C. Patient history — multiple transfusions Organ transplantation
D. Frozen red blood cells	D. Rare blood types Autotransfusion Organ transplantation

E. Platelet concentrates	E. Thrombocytopenic patient for:
	  major surgery
	  cancer (acute leukemia)
	  postchemotherapy, radiation therapy
	Bleeding thrombocytopenic patient
	Intraoperative massive blood replacement with stored bank blood

F. Fresh frozen plasma	F. Intraoperative massive blood replacement with stored bank blood Specific coagulation factor deficiencies

Reactions to Blood Administration

Hemolytic Reactions. Administration of incompatible blood leads to agglutination of the donor's red cells with resultant hemolysis. The signs and symptoms noted immediately or shortly after the start of transfusion may include any or all of the following: hives, chills, palpitations, fever, chest or flank pain, dyspnea, headache, and flushing of the skin. In severe reactions these symptoms may be accompanied by cardiovascular collapse, hemoglobinuria, and incoagulability of blood. Such reactions may be observed following transfusion of as little as 75 ml of incompatible blood. During general anesthesia the only signs of a hemolytic reaction may be hypotension, poor peripheral perfusion as evidenced by cyanosis, or diffuse bleeding at the operative site. A hemolytic transfusion reaction must be considered an emergency, varying directly with the amount of blood given. Therefore, the transfusion should be stopped immediately. Short of a fatality, the major long-term complication is development of anuria secondary to acute tubular necrosis (ATN). This lesion seems to result from renal cortical vasoconstriction induced by release of renin and formation of the potent vasoconstrictor angiotensin.

The treatment of circulatory collapse requires careful cardiovascular monitoring and often additional administration of fluids. At the earliest possible moment a urine specimen should be examined for the presence of free hemoglobin, which is often grossly apparent. There may be value in alkalinizing the urine, especially if done early in order to prevent precipitation of acid hematin in the tubules. Mannitol, 25 gm in 10 per cent solution, and furosemide, 40 mg, are administered intravenously to induce diuresis. Subsequently, if ATN develops, the patient is started on an anuric regimen to forestall overhydration and potassium intoxication, and consideration is given either to peritoneal or hemodialysis if a diuretic phase fails to appear or potassium intoxication is imminent.

The commonest cause of transfusion reactions owing to serologic incompatibility is misidentification of donor or recipient. Figures show that only 5 per cent of blood reactions result from serologic incompatibility detectable before transfusion. Because of the many minor blood groups one can never hope to give completely compatible blood, but major reactions are preventable by meticulous crossmatching and identification of donor and recipient.

The ordinary saline technique of crossmatching may fail to detect all antibodies capable of causing hemolysis. The end point of the normal crossmatch is agglutination of the erythrocytes incompatible with the serum of a prospective recipient. However, recipient serum may contain incompatible antibodies that attach to the surface of donor cells, causing hemolysis *in vivo* without agglutination *in vitro*. These "incomplete" antibodies on the red cell surface can be detected by the Coombs test, which employs the serum of rabbits previously immunized against human globulin causing agglutination of erythrocytes coated with the globulin.

Allergic Reactions. These result from the transfer of allergens from donor to recipient and are manifested as pruritus, urticaria, asthma, angioneurotic edema, and, rarely, frank anaphylaxis. By and large these symptoms are not severe during general anesthesia, when antigen-antibody reactions and liberation of histamine seem to be depressed. Blood administration is not discontinued because of mild urticaria, but the rate of flow is slowed while appraisal is made; nor do we always give antihistamines for mild urticaria. For more severe manifestations such as wheezing, an antihistamine such as diphenhydramine (Benadryl) is given, followed by epinephrine, aminophylline, and hydrocortisone if indicated. If an anaphylactic reaction occurs, aggressive therapy is instituted consisting of ventilatory support with oxygen, epinephrine 0.5 mg intramuscularly, aminophylline, hydrocortisone, blood volume expansion, and peripheral vasoconstrictors to support the pressure.

Transmission of Disease

Hepatitis. The disease most frequently transmitted by blood transfusion is type B viral hepatitis. It is not easy to determine the incidence of this complication because of nonicteric forms of the disease, but the incidence is lower when blood donor selection excludes high risk hepatitis carriers, drug addicts, and professional donors. The risk increases linearly with the number of units of blood transfused. The disease may also follow use of plasma, pooled plasma, and some products of protein fractionation, and the incubation period may range from 14 to 60 days. A fatality rate of 12 per cent has been reported but mortality is lower below the age of 40. According to recent reports, there is some hope of preventing or modifying the disease by the use of high titer immune globulins.

The discovery of a hepatitis-associated antigen—hepatitis type B surface antigen (HB_sAg)—found in the blood of a high percentage of patients who develop serum hepatitis has proved helpful in studying the disease. Routine screening of blood donors for the presence of the antigen should reduce the incidence of serum hepatitis and is now mandatory in Red Cross blood banks and most hospital laboratories. However, screening does not detect a large percentage of carriers. Another approach that has reduced infection is limiting blood donors to volunteers rather than paid producers. It is important to know that infectious hepatitis can also be transmitted by blood or blood products, and that low levels of type B surface antigen may go undetected in blood capable of causing the disease.

Bacterial Contamination. Patient reaction to massive bacterial contamination of bank blood is a rare complication, manifested by chills and hyperpyrexia and, in the severe case by cardiovascular collapse and death within a short time. The severe reactions apparently result from contamination of blood with gram-negative bacteria and their endotoxins. Vigorous treatment must be initiated with broad-spectrum antibiotics, myocardial inotropic agents, corticosteroids, and appropriate blood volume expansion. Careful bacteriologic control of bank blood, adequate refrigeration, and discarding blood containers that are opened and unused are the preventive measures.

Similar reactions have occurred in patients receiving contaminated intravenous crystalloids or colloids. Therefore, all fluids to be infused must be routinely examined before starting and cloudy fluid or fluid in cracked bottles should be cultured and then discarded. Contaminated parenteral fluid supplies with low bacterial counts have gone undetected for long periods as the sources of infection in recipients.

PACKED RED BLOOD CELLS

Packed red blood cells are prepared by removing two thirds of the plasma and anticoagulant solution from a unit of whole blood by either centrifugation or undisturbed sedimentation, resulting in a hematocrit between 65 to 70 per cent. There are several advantages in using packed red blood cells as opposed to whole blood.

A unit of packed cells has an oxygen carrying capacity equal to that of a unit of whole blood with approximately one third the volume of plasma, thereby reducing the possibility of circulatory overload while achieving the desired improvement in oxygen carrying capacity. This is of value in transfusions in patients with the potential for congestive heart failure, in the chronically anemic patient whose plasma volume is usually expanded, in the anuric patient, in those in chronic renal failure to reduce the acid and potassium load of a whole blood transfusion, and in the patient with severe hepatic dysfunction to minimize the ammonia and citrate load. Elderly debilitated patients with anemia, although hypovolemic, should be given packed cells because they are often unable to tolerate major increases in blood volume.

LEUKOCYTE-DEFICIENT RED BLOOD CELLS

Often an allergic reaction to blood is caused by incompatible leukocytes. Leukocyte antibodies can be found in patients who have had multiple transfusions, in some multiparous women, and in those who have had tissue or organ transplantation. Lymphocytes and granulocytes also carry tissue antigens. The reaction is characterized by chills, fever, headache, nausea, and malaise. Prior sensitization of organ transplant recipients to incompatible antigens may jeopardize survival of the transplanted organ. Several methods are available to remove 70 to 90 per cent of the leukocytes normally found in the blood, including centrifugation, nylon filtration, dextran sedimentation, red blood cells washed in saline, and reconstitution of frozen red blood cells. Washing red blood cells in saline requires that the cells be exposed to the environment, therefore the cell pack should be used within 24 hours to minimize bacterial contamination.

Reconstituted Frozen Red Blood Cells

Red blood cells with an added cryoprotective agent such as glycerol can be frozen and stored for years, the freezing completely inhibiting cellular metabolism. Prior to transfusion the cells are thawed and the glycerol removed by washing, which removes the plasma and most of the nonerythrocytic formed elements, such as leukocytes. The advantages of freezing include storing red blood cells of rare types, accumulating blood for autotransfusion, stockpiling blood of various kinds without plasma proteins and few leukocytes, and building reserves in case routine blood bank supplies run short. The primary disadvantage is the higher costs of blood preparation.

MAINTENANCE OF COAGULATION FACTORS

Of the three independent problems resulting from blood loss, coagulation difficulties occur least frequently. Fortunately, only 10 to 20 per cent of the labile coagulation factors are needed for effective coagulation. The labile coagulation factors (V and VIII) are found only in fresh blood or fresh frozen plasma—factor V or proaccelerin and factor VIII or antihemophiliac globulin. Deficiencies of factor V or factor VIII result in prolonged clotting times. With meticulous technique (constant temperature block and predetermined tilt pattern), the one-tube clotting time is a useful and reproducible test, the normal clotting time being less than four minutes. Administration of 250 ml of fresh frozen plasma every time half the estimated blood volume is replaced should prevent bleeding owing to insufficient factor V or VIII.

Reduced platelet levels are another source of coagulopathy, not easily diagnosed and difficult to treat. Blood with insufficient platelets has an essentially normal clotting time but the clot fails to retract normally. Viable platelets can be obtained only from fresh blood or from platelet concentrates. The normal platelet count ranges from 200,000 to 400,000 per mm^3 and can fall to 50,000 per mm^3 without impairment of the coagulation mechanism, provided the platelets are functionally normal.

Patients with advanced liver disease and those receiving oral anticoagulants may show hypoprothrombinemia. However, decreased levels of prothrombin are usually not a problem in replacement therapy, since adequate amounts of prothrombin are present in bank blood; the level must decrease to below 40 per cent of normal before bleeding occurs. Hypoprothrombinemic patients usually have relatively normal clotting times but prolonged prothrombin times. If the problem is caused by oral anticoagulants and liver function is not impaired, intravenous vitamin K can correct the deficiency within four to six hours.

The third most common kind of intraoperative coagulopathy, increased fibrinolysis, occurs during massive transfusion with deficiency of labile clotting factors and thrombocytopenia. This is usually associated with intravenous release of thromboplastins, causing widespread inappropriate intravascular microclotting and depletion of clotting factors, especially fibrinogen and platelets. This entity, called consumption coagulopathy or disseminated intravascular coagulopathy (DIC), is observed after hemorrhage secondary to placenta previa, during prostatic surgery, cardiopulmonary bypass, and following hemolytic transfusion reaction and heat stroke or malignant hyperthermia. DIC is not easily diagnosed rapidly because the clot may not lyse at room temperature for many hours. Lysis does not occur with normal blood in 24 hours. In severe cases a poor quality clot forms or clotting does not take place at all. Specialized laboratory tests are available for diagnosis, but results may not be available for hours. The treatment of choice when diagnosis is certain is administration of heparin intravenously, a potentially dangerous therapy. Thus hematologic consultation should be obtained whenever DIC is suspected. The use of antifibrinolytic agents such as ε-aminocaproic acid (EACA) is inappropriate and more dangerous than heparin.

PLATELET CONCENTRATES

Indications for platelet transfusion include: patients scheduled for major operations in whom the platelet count is below 50,000 per mm^3, and for the treatment of patients with thrombocytopenia with pronounced bleeding. Usually thrombocytopenia in the nonsurgical patient is not severe enough to increase the risk of bleeding significantly until the platelet count falls below 10,000 mm^3. Cancer patients, the acute leukemic, or those who have had chemotherapy or radiation therapy often have moderate thrombocytopenia with platelet counts between 10,000 and 30,000 mm^3. When they are scheduled for operation, prophylactic treatment of the thrombocytopenia is necessary. Patients with thrombocytopenia secondary to increased platelet destruction derive minimal benefit from platelet transfusion because donor platelets are destroyed nearly as rapidly as the recipients' autologous platelets. Repeated platelet transfusion increases the risk of formation of antibodies to platelets thus diminishing the response to subsequent platelet transfusions. Platelet concentrates should be given the donor within hours, so that the platelets remain viable. Other sources of platelets include fresh whole blood, platelet-rich packed red blood cells, and platelet-rich plasma.

Platelet concentrates are prepared by plasmapheresis, a process by which whole blood is drawn into a special collecting system and plasma containing the platelets is separated from red cells by centrifugation. The remaining packed red blood cells can be reinfused into the donor or placed in the blood bank.

FRESH FROZEN PLASMA

To qualify as fresh, plasma must be separated from whole blood within four to six hours after collection, not used immediately, and frozen and stored at −18°C. When frozen it is used within two hours of thawing. Fresh frozen plasma contains all the plasma clotting factors except platelets and the labile factors V and VIII, which disappear upon storage if unfrozen. Fresh frozen plasma is given only after proof of compatibility by typing and crossmatching. The prime indication for its use is the treatment of major clotting factor deficiencies (V, XI, and XIII) and the treatment of other specific clotting factor deficiencies (VII, VIII, IX, and X) when specific concentrates are unavailable. Fresh frozen plasma can be effectively used to treat the hemophiliac with factor VIII deficiency, but cryoprecipitated plasma is a preferred source, since its factor VIII is thereby concentrated. Cryoprecipitate enriched with factor VIII is obtained by centrifugation at 4°C when fresh frozen plasma is thawed. The preparation is also indicated when multiple clotting factor deficiencies exist, as in severe liver disease, defibrination states, and during massive blood replacement with stored bank blood.

OVERLOAD OF THE CIRCULATION

In massive blood loss, whether replacement is with blood, colloid, or crystalloid, volume overload of the circulation can easily occur. It is possible to pass from a state of an inadequate blood volume to one of gross overload without receiving an unusually large volume. This occurs more readily in the elderly, in those with a history of congestive heart failure, and in debilitated patients. However, inadequate volume replacement with the consequent arterial hypotension can produce irreversible cardiac or cerebral damage before adequate perfusion is restored. The only approach is careful observation of all patients and use of the appropriate monitoring devices.

PRINCIPLES OF RAPID VOLUME REPLACEMENT

The need to give blood rapidly is modified by the state of the patient's cardiovascular system. The problem of what volume to give is simplified by determining the adequacy of venous return to the ventricles, hemodynamically referred to as assessing "preload function." Factors involved in preload function are the inotropic state of the myocardium and the relationship of intravascular space to intravascular volume.

Central venous pressure (CVP) is used to assess the return of blood to the right ventricle, and pulmonary wedge pressure (PWP, measured by a Swan-Ganz catheter) permits assessment of blood returned to the left ventricle. The application and use of these monitoring devices are discussed in Chapter 8. This discussion is confined to the use of these monitors as guides to rapid fluid replacement.

In most situations the right and left ventricles are considered to have equal functional capabilities; therefore, measurement of CVP is an adequate estimate of overall myocardial function. CVP can be considered as a measure of the compliance characteristics of the venous system relative to the volume in the capacitance vessels. The system can be assessed via sequential measurement called the "delta factor," or change in pressure from a previous baseline with intravenous administration of a finite volume of fluid. This is correlated with improvement observed in the systemic arterial circulation, increase in blood pressure, elevated urine output, and other evidence of improved peripheral circulation.

There are several techniques of applying a fluid challenge to monitor augmentation of intravascular volumes. Using the CVP monitor, one approach is a so-called 2 to 5 cm rule, as follows:

1. Give 50 to 200 ml of crystalloid over a ten minute period; the exact amount depends upon the patient's condition.

2. Observe the systemic circulation for improvement in blood pressure, peripheral circulation, and urinary output. Assess the pulmonary circulation by auscultation of the chest.

3. Evaluate changes in CVP. If the increase is less than 2 cm H_2O, administer more fluid. An increase of more than 5 cm H_2O suggests that continued volume expansion is unlikely to cause further improvement. If the increase is between 2 and 5 cm H_2O, wait 10 minutes, then re-evaluate CVP and the clinical situation. If CVP returns to less than 2 cm H_2O

increase, continue to give fluid. If CVP remains between 2 and 5 cm H_2O, give a smaller quantity of fluid and repeat the evaluation.

PWP is a better guide to rapid fluid therapy in patients with a disparity between left and right ventricular function. An approach as outlined previously using PWP can be followed by a 3 to 7 torr limit. The probability of such elevations exists in patients with a history of recent myocardial infarction (especially if pulmonary edema was present), in septic shock, following massive trauma, and in chronic obstructive pulmonary disease with cor pulmonale. If pulmonary wedge pressure rises 7 torr or more above baseline values, volume expansion should be withheld pending therapy directed at improving left ventricular function.

Certain measures increase the safety of rapid blood transfusion: warming blood to body temperature and monitoring body temperature; continuous, direct monitoring of arterial blood pressure; measuring arterial and mixed venous blood gases (pulmonary artery) to assess alveolar ventilation, arterial oxygenation, and acid-base balance; monitoring breath sounds via an esophageal stethoscope to detect pulmonary edema and evaluate heart sounds; and monitoring urine output, CVP, and PWP.

In spite of this approach some patients develop heart failure, often immediately postoperatively. This necessitates appropriate ventilatory support with oxygen, use of positive inotropic drugs, and diuretic therapy. In the awake patient, morphine given intravenously in repeated 1 to 5 mg doses is helpful, causing a decrease in venous tone as well as providing sedation and analgesia.

The need for positive inotropic drugs and diuretics is urgent. Furosemide, 10 to 40 mg intravenously, has an immediate onset of action through a direct vasodilating effect and a potent diuretic effect on the kidney. Since vasopressors are discussed in Chapter 27, the remarks here are confined to those appropriate to the situation at hand. Dopamine has a positive inotropic effect, thereby increasing cardiac output, but has less arrhythmogenic tendency than isoproterenol. It is the drug of choice following rapid transfusion resulting in a high PWP or CVP. At low doses (1 to 2 mEq/kg body weight) dilation of the renal vessels occurs via the so-called dopaminergic receptors. As the dose is increased to (5 to 15 mEq/kg body weight), the action becomes more predominantly one of beta-adrenergic stimulation, and with greater increase in dose (> 20 mEq/kg body weight), an alpha-adrenergic stimulation. Isoproterenol is effective as treatment in myocardial failure, especially when secondary to propranolol therapy.

Calcium chloride or calcium gluconate is reserved for those patients with hypocalcemia secondary to pre-existing disease or after massive blood transfusion in patients with myocardial dysfunction. Digitalis is not routinely recommended for acute myocardial failure during or immediately following anesthesia; however, if necessary, digoxin may be used. Other supportive measures for acute heart failure include utilization of PEEP (see Chapter 33) and phlebotomy.

INTRAVENOUS TECHNIQUE

APPARATUS

Disposable equipment, now universally used for intravenous fluid therapy, is both safer for the patient and economical. Occasionally, anesthesia for short procedures can be accomplished without an intravenous infusion, but most operations require an intravenous route for blood, fluid replacement, or medication. There are two categories of intravenous devices: one is the so-called "butterfly needle," and the other is the plastic catheter. In the critically ill and in those who are given large volumes of fluid, the preferred device is a plastic catheter threaded well into the vein and stabilized externally.

The butterfly needle, available in various gauges, was devised for infusion into the scalp veins of infants; hence it is also called a scalp vein needle. The needle is thin walled, with a plastic catheter extension terminating in a female adapter for the infusion set. Plastic wings on the needle fold to form a grip for the fingers during insertion and then are flattened against the skin and taped in position. While simple to use, the butterfly needle is not as reliable as a catheter threaded into a vein.

Two kinds of plastic catheter are available: the "intracath," introduced through a needle, and the "extracath," introduced over a needle. Once introduced into a vein the intracath is more flexible, more easily advanced often deliberately into the central venous circulation. For routine peripheral use the extracath is preferred because it offers a larger bore for a given catheter size, causes less bleeding at the venipuncture site, and eliminates the possibility of catheter transection by the introducing needle. The latter results from improper technique.

The major disadvantages of the plastic catheter include high cost, an increased incidence of thrombophlebitis, and an increased potential for shearing and loss of the catheter to the circulation. Thrombophlebitis is usually of the aseptic variety, increasing with the duration of maintenance, and may be, in part, a consequence of rigid fixation in a small vein. Catheters are changed, or discontinued if possible, within 72 hours. In the event of transection the fatality rate may be high if the loose catheter migrates to the lungs and heart; the catheter must be retrieved surgically during fluoroscopic localization.

When infusion of large amounts of fluid is anticipated, a minimum of two 16-gauge peripheral intravenous catheters should be placed exclusive of one to measure CVP. The smallest catheter or needle permitting rapid blood administration is of 20 gauge, but this requires a high pressure head. A linear relationship exists between hydrostatic pressure and laminar flow rate and a fourth power relationship between the cross-sectional area of the catheter and flow; doubling the height of the infusion bottle doubles the flow rate, while doubling the internal diameter of the catheter increases flow rate 16 times (Poiseuille's law). A unit of blood can be infused through a 14-gauge catheter in about five minutes using an elastic cylindric in-line bulb with check valves, or by applying external pressure via a hand-inflated air bladder surrounding a plastic blood container. The once common method of introducing air under pressure into a blood container above the fluid level has been abandoned because of the hazard of air embolism.

TECHNIQUE OF CATHETER INSERTION

The skin is routinely prepared for venipuncture with 70 to 90 per cent isopropyl alcohol. Mechanical cleansing is probably as important as the bactericidal action of the antiseptic, which is allowed to dry before venipuncture. Betadine solution may be preferred as an antiseptic. When using an 18-gauge or larger catheter, a skin wheal is made first with a 25-gauge needle and 0.5 per cent lidocaine or procaine is given to minimize discomfort. The largest, straightest, and most visible vein that will remain accessible during operation is chosen for puncture. The veins on the dorsum of the hand are often excellent from the standpoint of size, visibility, and minimal chance of inadvertent arterial cannulation (Fig. 22-1), but it is sometimes difficult to maintain immobilization in the immediate postoperative period. Veins of the midforearm are more suitable for immobilization over long periods. Leg veins are avoided if possible because of the hazard of thrombosis. Spasm of veins can be overcome by dependent drainage, by application of moist heat, or by rubbing or tapping the puncture site. A tourniquet is applied as close as possible to the site without pinching the skin or pulling hair, best accomplished with a wide tourniquet; a blood pressure cuff inflated to 40 torr is good.

The intravenous needle may be inserted attached to the adaptor of the infusion tubing or to a syringe. With anticipated easy venipuncture the intravenous tubing is attached and pinched to produce a negative pressure. Use of a syringe is preferable in difficult venipuncture, as it makes both handling the needle and aspiration of blood easier. Extracaths are best inserted attached to a syringe. With the vein fixed proximally by the tourniquet and held distally by stretching the skin, the needle is inserted through the skin to one side of the vein and advanced steadily and directly over the vein, with the bevel upward until penetration occurs (Fig. 22-2). The needle is threaded into the vein with a slight rotary movement and the tourniquet removed before infusion is started. If an extracath is used, the entire unit is advanced into the vein a few millimeters before sliding the catheter off the introducing needle. Catheters are not advanced past a venous valve lest a perforation occur. If a vein is torn or penetrated through and through, the needle should be removed, pressure applied, and the arm elevated above venous pressure to lessen hematoma formation.

The catheter is fixed with adhesive tape to maintain connection between the needle and the intravenous adaptor and to prevent accidental dislodgement; nonallergenic tape is used if there is sensitivity to adhesive tape. The wrist or elbow is held immobile on a padded board if the catheter site lies over those areas, care being taken to avoid applying the tape to

Blood Component Therapy

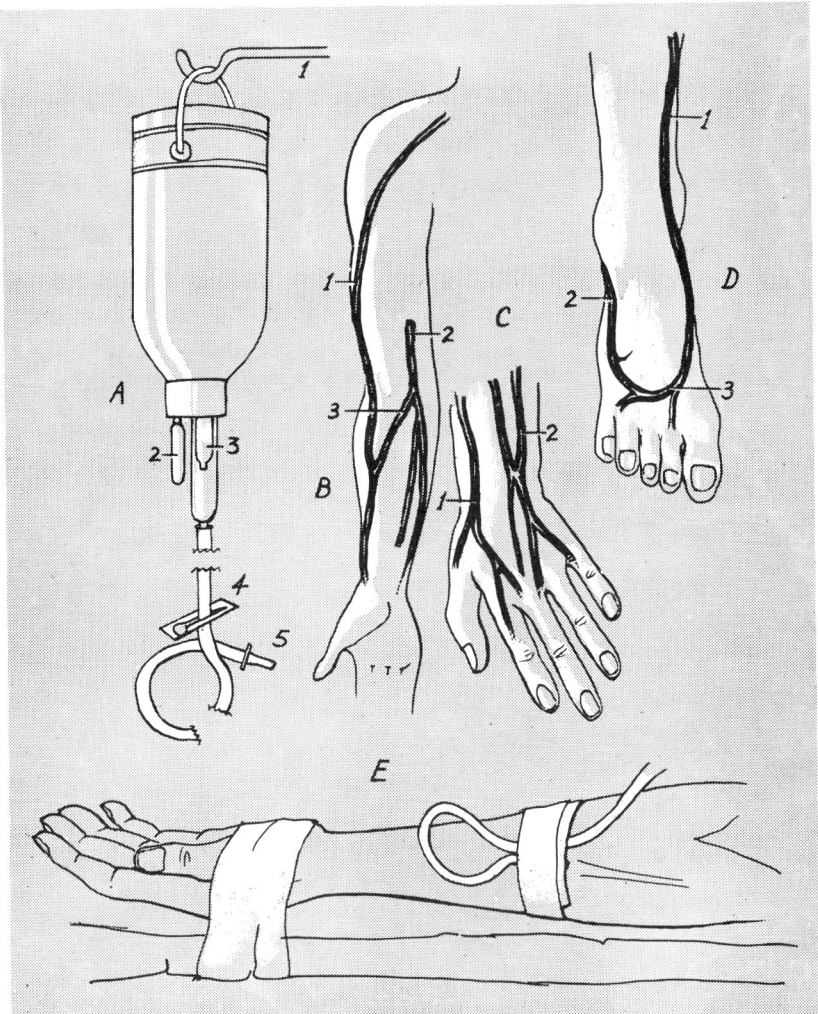

Figure 22-1. *A*, Components of intravenous apparatus: *1*, Hook on pole of adjustable height; *2*, air inlet; *3*, drip bulb; *4*, pinch clamp for controlling flow of fluid; *5*, adapter for insertion into needle or catheter. *B*, Veins of arm: *1*, cephalic; *2*, basilic; *3*, antecubital. *C*, Veins of dorsum of hand: *1*, cephalic; *2*, basilic. *D*, Veins of dorsum of foot: *1*, great saphenous vein; *2*, small saphenous vein; *3*, dorsal venous arch. *E*, Fixation of intravenous needle and tubing to arm.

hairy skin or placing it circumferentially in such a way as to increase venous pressure (Fig. 22-1). After insertion, the system is checked to make sure that infiltration has not occurred. Blood should flow back into the tubing if the container is lowered below heart level. The infusion site is re-examined for infiltration at intervals.

Some anxious, vasoconstricted patients benefit from having venipuncture done after inhalation anesthesia has produced vasodilation. When

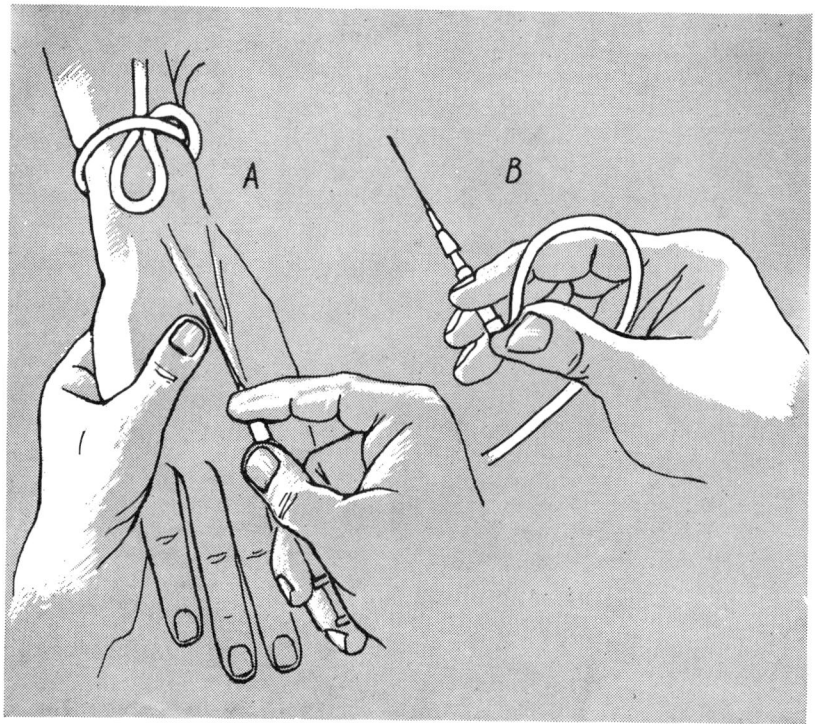

Figure 22-2. Technique of venipuncture. See text for explanation.

comfort alone is the issue, this is more pleasant for the patient than repeated and unsuccessful attempts at venipuncture. However, if vasoconstriction is the result of hypovolemia or if the patient has a full stomach, an intravenous route is mandatory before attempting anesthesia induction, even if a cutdown is necessary.

The following complications from intravenous therapy have been observed: localized cellulitis and lymphangitis, venous thrombosis or thrombophlebitis, air embolism, extravasation with tissue slough or neuritis, accidental injection of the wrong drug, and accidental intra-arterial infusion.

REFERENCES

Carey JS, Scharschmidt BF, Culliford AT, et al: Hemodynamic effectiveness of colloid and electrolyte solutions for replacement of simulated operative blood loss. Surg Gynecol Obstet 131:679, 1970.

Chaplin H, Jr: Packed red blood cells. N Engl J Med 281:364, 1969.

Gollub S, Svigals R, Bailey CP, et al: Electrolyte solution in surgical patients refusing transfusion. JAMA 215:2077, 1971.

Jesch F, Webber LM, Dalton JW, et al: Oxygen dissociation after transfusion of blood stored in ACD or CPD solution. J Thorac Cardiovasc Surg 70:35, 1975.

Mollison PL: Blood Transfusion in Clinical Medicine. 5th ed, Philadelphia, F.A. Davis Company, 1972.
Moss GS, Salletta JD: Traumatic shock in man. N Engl J Med 290:724, 1974.
Robertson HD, Polk HC: Blood transfusions in elective operations: Comparison of whole blood versus packed red cells. Ann Surg 181:778, 1975.
Rosenblum R: Physiologic basis for the therapeutic use of catecholamines. Am Heart J 87:527, 1974.
Sutnick AI, London WT, Millman I, et al: Viral hepatitis: Revised concepts as a result of the study of Australian antigen. Med Clin North Am 54:805, 1970.
Umlas J: Washed, hyperpacked, frozen and shelf red blood cells. Transfusion 15:111, 1975.

Part E

THE SPECIALTIES

Chapter 23

OBSTETRIC ANESTHESIA AND PERINATOLOGY

The history and practice of obstetric anesthesia have long been influenced by the biblical quotation from Genesis, "In sorrow ye shall bring forth children." Until modern times, attempts to relieve the pain of childbirth were looked upon as sinful, meeting with reactions varying from mere disapproval to persecution. It was not until 1852, when John Snow administered chloroform to Queen Victoria during the birth of her eighth child, that any acceptance was gained toward making childbirth a tolerable experience.

Since then great strides have been made in providing comfort and safety for the parturient; however, in many areas obstetric anesthesia remains outside the pale of anesthetic practice. Fewer than one fourth of all vaginal deliveries in this country are attended by physician anesthetists. This situation probably relates to a shortage of anesthetists interested in obstetrics, inadequate residency training in obstetric anesthesia, and the unpredictability of delivery, thus preventing prior scheduling. While maternal deaths from the traditional hazards of hemorrhage, infection, and toxemia have markedly decreased, deaths from anesthesia remain one of the leading causes of maternal mortality. Aspiration of gastric contents accounts for over half of maternal deaths, while profound hypotension following regional anesthesia is the cause of many others. Nearly all are preventable.

Obstetric anesthesia is further complicated in that in no other aspect of practice does the anesthetic so influence the course of the procedure and therefore the actions taken by the obstetrician. And, as noted, the manner of pain relief may drastically affect the course of labor and delivery. Therefore, anesthetist and obstetrician must remain in constant communication to provide optimal conditions for the parturient and the infant. Further, the woman in labor must be consulted as to her wishes with regard to pain relief.

This chapter attempts to place in perspective the approach to the woman in labor and to present information to upgrade obstetric anesthetic care to the level of that given surgical patients.

PHYSIOLOGIC CHANGES IN PREGNANCY

To provide optimal care for the parturient, one must have a basic knowledge of the physiologic changes that occur during pregnancy. All organ systems are affected, to a greater or lesser extent, influencing anesthetic management.

RESPIRATION

The respiratory system undergoes significant changes throughout pregnancy. As the gravid uterus enlarges, it encroaches upon the diaphragm, compressing the lungs and decreasing functional residual capacity. This deficit is balanced by a flaring outward of the ribs, so that vital capacity is essentially unchanged. Therefore, total lung capacity is only slightly decreased as a result of reduction in residual volume.

The gravid patient tends to hyperventilate, for reasons not entirely clear but probably related to the central stimulating effect of estrogens. Near term, respiratory rate increases by 10 to 15 per cent and tidal volume by 20 to 30 per cent. Thus there is a marked increase in minute volume and an even greater increase in alveolar ventilation, demonstrated by a Pa_{CO_2} in the low 30s. To maintain a normal pH, base is excreted resulting near term in a base deficit ranging from 5 to 8. The implications of these alterations for anesthetic management will be discussed.

CIRCULATION

The cardiovascular system undergoes multiple changes. Blood volume increases early, reaching a peak at approximately 32 to 34 weeks of gestation. At term the increase is approximately 25 per cent, with a 10 per cent increase in red cell mass and 30 to 40 per cent expansion of plasma volume. These disproportionate changes in blood components result in the so-called physiologic anemia of pregnancy, that is, the hematocrit is usually in the low 30s while the actual red cell mass is increased.

Changes in cardiac output have been extensively studied and are the subject of some controversy. It is agreed that cardiac output increases early in pregnancy, reaching a level 20 to 30 per cent above normal at 24 to 28 weeks. Earlier data had indicated that cardiac output falls during the third trimester and at term is actually lower than normal. However, these measurements were made with the patient in a supine position; cardiac output in the third trimester falls in the supine position owing to compression of the vena cava by the gravid uterus, decreasing venous return to the heart. When cardiac output is measured with the patient in the lateral position, the decrease in the third trimester is not nearly as great as once thought, so that even at term, cardiac output may be increased.

During labor further alterations in cardiac output occur, primarily owing to uterine contractions. Each time the gravid uterus contracts, approximately 300 ml of blood are ejected into the central circulation, resulting in an additional 15 to 20 per cent increase in output. In the unanesthetized parturient this increase is augmented by another 10 to 15 per cent as a result of catecholamine stimulation in response to pain.

The highest cardiac output is found in the immediate postpartum period. Compression of the vena cava no longer obtains, while a large portion of the blood volume previously sequestered in the uterus is now autotransfused into the central circulation. At this time the cardiac patient is at greatest risk.

What are the implications of these changes for anesthesia? One of the most important phenomena is the supine hypotensive syndrome. As noted, when the pregnant woman lies on her back the gravid uterus compresses the vena cava, interfering with venous return to the heart, thereby causing a decrease in cardiac output and hypotension. Also in the supine position the gravid uterus compresses the aorta above the level of the uterine arteries, simultaneously decreasing both uterine and placental blood flow. If the sympathetic blockade of regional anesthesia is added, hypotension is a common consequence. While the hypotension may not reach a dangerous level for the mother, it may be dangerous for the fetus. Therefore, particularly during regional anesthesia, the supine position is avoided either by resorting to the lateral position or by elevating the right hip with a wedge.

Changes in both cardiac output and ventilation markedly influence the course of inhalation anesthesia. The decrease in functional residual capacity with more rapid lung washout means that the anesthetic concentration rises in arterial blood more rapidly. Alveolar hyperventilation also adds to this effect. However, the increase in cardiac output tends to slow induction with the more soluble agents. The net effect, nonetheless, is one of more rapid induction with inhalation agents.

The decrease in functional residual capacity also implies that the pregnant woman will become hypoxic more rapidly if respiratory depression occurs. Further, the compensatory metabolic acidosis in response to hyperventilation also implies that respiratory obstruction or depression may rapidly lead to acidosis. Both factors dictate that one must guard assiduously against respiratory depression or obstruction in the parturient.

GASTROINTESTINAL TRACT

In the gastrointestinal tract the cardioesophageal sphincter tends to dilate both indirectly as a response to compression of the stomach by the uterus, and directly as a response to estrogens. Thus the pregnant woman is prone to gastroesophageal reflux, as evidenced by the common complaint of heartburn. During labor, gastric motility is decreased so that gastric emptying is markedly prolonged, extending several hours postpartum. Prolonged gastric emptying time, coupled with an incompetent esophageal sphincter, implies that the woman in labor is prone to aspiration of gastric contents. For this reason all woman in labor are considered to have a full stomach; thus the airway must be protected if general anesthesia is administered.

PAIN PATHWAYS IN LABOR

Discomfort through most of the first stage of labor is caused by uterine contractions and cervical dilation. Sensation from the uterus is carried in sympathetic fibers of thoracic spinal nerves 10 through 12. Therefore, sympathetic blockade of those fibers will relieve the pain of uterine contraction and cervical dilation (Fig. 23-1).

Late in the first stage and in the second, as the fetal head descends into the pelvis and pain is caused by distention of pelvic structures and perineum, sensation is carried by somatic fibers originating in sacral roots 2 to 4. Therefore, block of these sensory fibers is necessary to relieve the discomfort of this stage of labor.

At delivery, since perineal relaxation as well as pain relief are required, it is necessary to block sacral motor fibers as well, particularly for forceps delivery.

METHODS OF PAIN RELIEF

As in any kind of pain, the distress of labor is greatly affected by both anxiety and expectation. This should be kept in mind when providing analgesia for labor and delivery. Pain can be approached either centrally with some form of sedation or general anesthesia, or peripherally via regional anesthesia. Many deliveries are carried out without anesthesia, employing suggestion, hypnosis, or the Lamaze technique.

PHARMACOLOGIC AGENTS IN THE FIRST STAGE

Parenteral agents used during the first stage of labor include the opioids, tranquilizers, and barbiturates. Opioids offer the most logical approach to relief of pain, since they are pain specific. While opioids cause respiratory depression in both mother and newborn, moderate doses

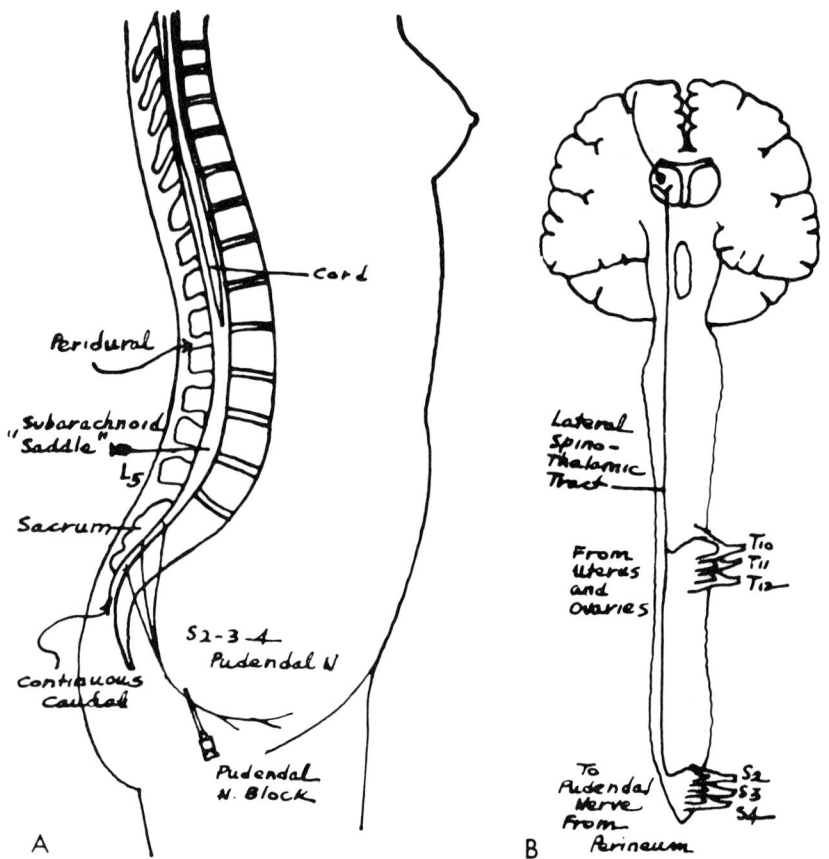

Figure 23-1. Sites of injection and sensory pathways in obstetric regional anesthesia: *A*, Peridural, subarachnoid, caudal, and pudendal block; *B*, block of afferent input to T10–T12 via lumbar peridural block relieves pain of first stage. Block of the pudendal nerve, saddle block, caudal block, or extension of lumbar peridural block relieve pain of the second stage. (After JJ Bonica.)

provide reasonable pain relief with an acceptable degree of depression. Although morphine sulfate is the standard by which all opioids are judged, its usefulness in obstetrics is somewhat limited by a rather long duration of action. Occasionally moderate doses such as 0.1 mg per kg are used early in labor. Shorter-acting opioids such as meperidine 1 mg per kg or fentanyl 1 μg/kg are used. Intravenous injection is preferable to the intramuscular route because absorption is more reliable and onset of action more rapid. The analgetics are not given at intervals of less than four hours for meperidine or one hour for fentanyl and are not given at all if delivery is expected within an hour. In using opioids it should be kept in mind that respiratory depression lasts far longer than the analgetic effect; this is especially true with the longer-acting agents such as morphine or meperidine.

Tranquilizers are also useful in the conduct of labor. While having no specific analgetic effect of their own, they do potentiate the action of opioids. Further, they relieve that aspect of pain resulting from anxiety. Generally speaking, all tranquilizers cross the placental barrier but the effect on the fetus is minimal. Therefore, almost any of the common tranquilizers may be used if the dose is kept low. Hydroxyzine 1 mg per kg provides excellent tranquilization with minimal depression. Diazepam is an exception: while this useful tranquilizer causes little respiratory depression in the mother, it leads to inordinate flaccidity of both skeletal and smooth muscle in the newborn. Temperature control is therefore affected and bowel and bladder hypotonia may ensue. Further, the solvent in diazepam, a glycol, competes with bilirubin for albumin binding sites so that the physiologic jaundice of infancy may be enhanced.

Barbiturates now play only a small role in the conduct of labor, not only failing to relieve pain but possibly accentuating the pain response. Further, the depression produced by the high doses needed to control pain is not readily reversed in either mother or infant. The only current use for a barbiturate is for the patient in desultory labor who needs a good night's sleep in order to institute a satisfactory labor pattern. Should active labor begin during the period of action of the barbiturate, the infant may be depressed upon delivery.

Inhalation agents are useful for analgesia in low concentrations during labor or delivery, thereby minimizing the risk of aspiration. Volatile agents such as trichloroethylene or methoxyflurane may be self-administered, inhaled from simple drawover vaporizers during contractions. If the patient falls asleep, the vaporizer falls away from the face and the anesthetic is no longer inhaled. The concentration of methoxyflurane achieved by this method does not exceed 0.5 per cent. However, this method should not be used without supervision and patients are warned against propping the vaporizer against the face in order to breathe the anesthetic continuously. Nitrous oxide is a safe analgetic; however, administration is generally limited to the delivery room because of the need to administer a safe combination with oxygen via an anesthesia machine. Concentrations of nitrous oxide in oxygen from 20 to 60 per cent provide excellent analgesia for delivery with the patient awake and maintaining a satisfactory airway. However, not all patients accept these regimens.

REGIONAL ANESTHESIA

Basically, any of five regional techniques can be used to provide analgesia during the first stage: paracervical, paravertebral lumbar sympathetic, lumbar epidural, caudal, or subarachnoid block (Fig. 23–1). Lumbar epidural and caudal anesthesia are most commonly used, providing analgesia for delivery with relative safety for mother and fetus. Lumbar paravertebral sympathetic block, technically difficult and not often used, provides excellent analgesia for the first stage of labor, but is inadequate for delivery. Paracervical block is also inadequate for delivery and is associated with a high incidence of fetal bradycardia owing to absorption of epinephrine in the local anesthetic solution. Spinal anesthesia confined to the sacral area, obtained by intrathecal injection of 4 or 5 mg of tetracaine or 40 to 50 mg lidocaine, provides good pain relief for both labor and delivery. Subarachnoid anesthesia is generally reserved for the second stage because of limited duration of the single injection and the high incidence of headache, even with the small-gauge lumbar puncture needles employed.

Continuous caudal anesthesia was popular for vaginal delivery in the 1940s and 1950s because of its relative safety and a low incidence of inadvertent dural puncture. The technique is suitable by either single injection or intermittently via catheter, with 20 ml of 1 per cent lidocaine or 2 per cent chloroprocaine providing excellent relief from the pain of uterine contractions and perineal pressure. As anesthetists have begun to specialize in obstetric anesthesia, this technique has become less popular. Disadvantages include the high dose of local anesthetic required during labor, the high incidence of sacral anatomic variations, and difficulty in positioning the parturient for insertion of the needle. Should cesarean section become necessary, the level of anesthesia of a caudal block cannot reliably be raised to that required.

Lumbar epidural anesthesia is the method of choice in many institutions where continuous anesthesia supervision prevails in delivery areas. The catheter technique (see Chapter 19) requires only 6 to 10 ml of 1 per cent lidocaine, 0.25 per cent bupivacaine, or 2 per cent chloroprocaine to provide satisfactory analgesia for the first stage of labor. As the fetal head descends and pressure is applied to pelvic structures, the dose is increased to provide sacral anesthesia. Generally from 10 to 15 ml of 1.5 per cent lidocaine or 3 per cent chloroprocaine are required for delivery. The technique offers the advantage of suitability for cesarean section if that procedure becomes necessary. As in caudal anesthesia, lumbar epidural block is not without complications, the most common being inadvertent dural puncture and a high incidence of lumbar puncture headache. A second major problem, common to all forms of regional anesthesia, is maternal hypotension. The sympathetic blockade resulting with these techniques causes peripheral vasodilation, decreased venous return, and a fall in blood pressure, hazardous for both mother and fetus. Hypotension can be minimized by adequate hydration, infusion of 500 to 1000 ml of a balanced salt solution prior to institution of the block, and avoidance of the supine hypotensive syndrome. Should hypotension occur, treatment entails intravenous injection of 10 to 20 mg ephedrine. A vasopressor with a predominantly alpha-adrenergic stimulant action, neosynephrine or methoxamine, causes uterine artery constriction and fetal acidosis. Furthermore, alpha-adrenergic stimulators in conjunction with oxytocics may cause threatening degress of hypertension.

Finally, a major complication of the regional techniques relates to local anesthetic overdose. Local anesthetics cross the placental barrier; thus a high maternal blood level results in high fetal levels with ensuing circulatory and central nervous system depression. Local anesthetic overdose may result from inadvertent intravenous injection or repeated injection of the slowly metabolized amide compounds. The usual signs of local anesthetic overdose are seen in the mother (see Chapter 17), and in the fetus bradycardia occurs.

Pudendal nerve block performed by the obstetrician provides adequate pain relief and perineal relaxation for normal vaginal delivery, including application of outlet forceps. When combined with inhalation analgesia, more extensive procedures such as midforceps rotation may be performed. Many vaginal deliveries, especially in multipara, can be satisfactorily accomplished with only perineal infiltration of a local anesthetic for episiotomy and repair.

GENERAL ANESTHESIA FOR DELIVERY

Delivery can also be performed with general anesthesia, a technique gradually abandoned because of the increased risk for both mother and baby. As noted earlier, women in labor are suspect for a full stomach and at risk for aspiration of gastric contents during general anesthesia. If general anesthesia is necessary, rapid tracheal intubation with a cuffed tube is mandatory. Further, the duration of anesthesia prior to delivery should be minimal because general anesthetics cross the placenta, and given time, reach concentrations that cause depression of the fetus. The primary indication for general anesthesia in vaginal delivery is the need for relaxation during intrauterine manipulation such as version and extraction of a second twin or extraction of a breech delivery. For these problems halothane in a concentration of 1.5 to 2 per cent or enflurane 1 to 3 per cent are the agents of choice. Be forewarned, however, that placental bleeding is controlled only when the uterus is contracted; halothane and enflurane cause uterine muscle relaxation and oppose the action of oxytocics. To minimize postpartum hemorrhage, the lungs should be hyperventilated with oxygen to eliminate the anesthetic immediately after intrauterine manipulation is completed.

If general anesthesia for vaginal delivery is necessary for any other reason, primarily for psychiatric problems, the preferred technique is to place the patient's legs in stirrups for delivery prior to anesthetic administration. Thiopental, 3 to 4 mg per kg, is administered followed by 1 mg per kg of succinylcholine intravenously for tracheal intubation, then maintenance with 70 per cent nitrous oxide until the baby is born. After delivery, anesthesia is maintained with additional doses of thiopental or intravenous opioids. The endotracheal tube is not removed until the mother is fully awake, to avoid vomiting and aspiration.

EFFECTS OF ANESTHESIA ON LABOR

By plotting centimeters of cervical dilation versus time, a standard curve for progress of labor can be depicted (Fig. 23-2). As a rule any anesthetic or analgetic given during the latent stage of labor tends to prolong that stage, while that given in the active phase will have little effect on progression of labor. Regional anesthesia is often implicated in slowing or cessation of labor. However, appropriate timing minimizes the problem. When regional anesthesia such as lumbar epidural is administered during the active phase transient slowing of contractions is observed, but once anesthesia is established the contractions accelerate. Another effect of epidural or spinal anesthesia entails the matter of rotation of the fetal head to the occiput anterior position. This depends in large part on perineal tone, so that early perineal relaxation results in a higher incidence of transverse arrest and persistent posterior presentations. Additionally, anesthesia of the perineum abolishes the reflex urge to bear down. Although the ability to cooperate remains, obtundation of this reflex increases the number of forceps deliveries, not a problem in modern obstetric practice.

CESAREAN SECTION

In centers with a large proportion of high risk patients, a cesarean section rate of over 15 per cent is common. One reason for the propensity to perform cesarean section is the availability of safe anesthesia. Choice of regional or general anesthesia for cesarean section hinges upon many factors. As the parturient is considered to have a full stomach, regional anes-

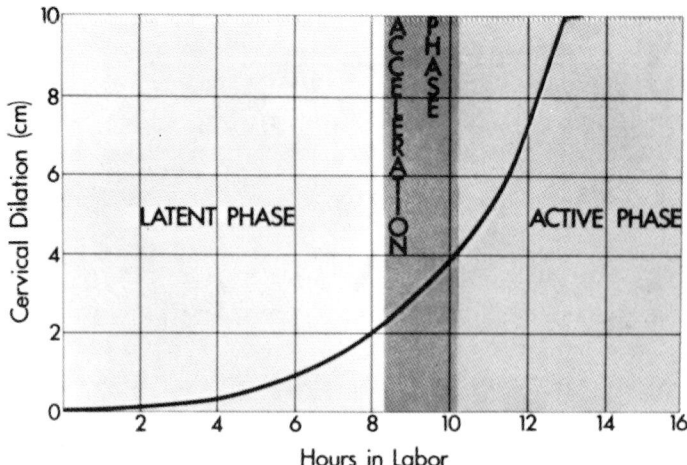

Figure 23-2. Labor progress curve.

thesia is advantageous. However, if the indication for section is fetal distress or maternal hemorrhage, the necessity for rapid delivery overrides all other considerations. For elective cesarean section the choice of anesthesia largely relates to patient or physician preference, although the somewhat longer time required for delivery in a second or third cesarean section may recommend regional rather than general anesthesia.

If general anesthesia is elected, the operating table is tilted to the left or a wedge placed under the patient's right hip to displace the uterus from the vena cava. Oxygen is administered through a face mask while prepping and draping are accomplished. When the obstetrician is ready to make the incision, anesthesia is induced. A sleep dose of 3 to 4 mg per kg of thiopental is followed immediately by 1 mg per kg of succinylcholine intravenously; cricoid pressure is applied and a cuffed endotracheal tube inserted. The surgeon then proceeds. Anesthesia is maintained either with 70 per cent nitrous oxide in oxygen or 50 per cent nitrous oxide in oxygen and 0.5 per cent halothane, or 0.2 per cent methoxyflurane. Relaxation is obtained with an infusion of 0.1 per cent succinylcholine. If the infant is delivered within ten minutes, minimal neonatal depression occurs.

At one time delivery of the infant was delayed for ten minutes after presumed placental transfer of the injected thiopental, to allow redistribution of the drug from the fetal brain, a practice now believed unwise. The amount of thiopental reaching the fetal brain after a 4 mg per kg maternal dose is hardly depressant and delay only prolongs anesthesia time prior to delivery with the possibility of neonatal depression from the inhalation agent. An infant should be delivered as quickly as possible consistent with safe surgical practice.

If regional anesthesia is selected, the choice lies between subarachnoid and epidural block. Spinal anesthesia is more reliable and rapid in onset, but dural puncture results in a high incidence of headache. Lumbar epidural block only occasionally results in dural puncture, but the procedure is technically more difficult, and requires a higher dose of local anesthetic. In either case a sensory level of T4 is necessary for patient comfort. The dose of drug required to achieve this level ranges from 7 to 10 mg of tetracaine in the subarachnoid space to 15 to 25 ml of 2 per cent lidocaine, 3 per cent chloroprocaine, or 0.75 per cent bupivacaine in the peridural compartment.

APPROACH OF THE ANESTHETIST TO THE PREGNANT PATIENT

Traditionally the obstetric patient has received little attention from anesthetists. While the surgical patient can receive reassurance and ask questions preoperatively, the parturient is often not seen until delivery is imminent. The supposition is that obstetric delivery represents an emergency situation and the patient must accept whatever anesthetic care is available. Actually, this premise is untrue, as the obstetric patient knows of the forthcoming delivery for many months while under the care of an obstetrician. Therefore, good practice demands that the obstetric patient be given the same opportunity to be interviewed by an anesthetist as the surgical patient; this is best managed by an appointment during the third trimester. Some anesthetists maintain regularly scheduled office hours, and during visits procedures can be explained and questions answered.

Whether or not the obstetric patient has been seen prior to entering the hospital, she should be visited by an anesthetist as soon as she is admitted to the labor floor. An interview early in labor allays anxiety considerably and permits the more pleasant administration of the anesthetic elected.

In preparation for delivery, certain basic principles need to be followed. Blood should be drawn for a complete blood count and a second tube labeled and refrigerated for typing and crossmatching should the need for transfusion arise. A 16- or 18-gauge plastic catheter is inserted intravenously for administration of fluids, medications, and blood when necessary. A blood pressure cuff is applied and left in place throughout labor and delivery. Monitoring of heart rate, by either precordial stethoscope or electrocardioscope, is appropriate for vaginal delivery and mandatory for cesarean section. Invasive forms of monitoring such as central venous pressure or an intra-arterial line are rarely needed but may be indicated in the event of complications.

Routine administration of oral antacids has been recommended for the parturient whose stomach contains highly acid fluid (see Chapter 28). It is the aspiration of this acid fluid that leads to the high morbidity and mortality; hence, the contention that an antacid such as magnesium trisilicate will raise gastric pH to a safer level. This measure is purportedly effective in preventing the aspiration syndrome only if the antacid has been ingested at least 30 minutes beforehand. More data are required and investigations are underway.

FETAL MONITORING

It has been said that the perinatal period is the most dangerous in the life span of a human being. This means that the care of the fetus should approach that available in an intensive care unit. Until recently the extent of knowledge of fetal physiology was limited. The obvious difficulty in caring for the fetus *in utero* is accessibility, an excuse once employed to limit fetal monitoring to manual palpation of uterine contractions and intermittent abdominal auscultation for fetal heart rate. This approach resulted in many depressed infants without forewarning, frequently leading to emergency cesarean sections because of fetal bradycardia. Several decades ago, therefore, physicians began to look for methods of continuously monitoring fetal heart rate and uterine contractions.

Fetal monitoring during labor has taken two forms—the bioelectronic and the biochemical. Bioelectronic monitoring has reached an advanced state. The prototype instrument permits detection of fetal heart rate by direct electrocardiography with a fetal scalp electrode, indirect electrocardiography via a maternal abdominal electrode, or ultrasonic detection utilizing the Doppler phenomenon. The signal is fed into a cardiotachometer and converted to heart rate. A second receiver records uterine contractions either directly via a catheter inserted transcervically or indirectly by means of a tocodynamometer on the abdomen. Signals from both fetal heart and uterus are recorded on a two-channel hot stylus paper. A continuous record of fetal heart rate and uterine contraction is made (Fig. 23-3A), the correlation between the two providing useful information. In general, a stable fetal heart rate at 120 to 160 beats per minute is normal. However, the heart does not always beat regularly, considered to be a sign of a mature fetal autonomic nervous system and a normal heart. Lack of variability is considered ominous and is frequently a sign of fetal acidosis, although some drugs including general and local anesthetics and sedatives tend to minimize beat-to-beat variability.

Occasionally fetal heart rate is unstable with contractions, and the relation between contraction and heart rate is examined for abnormality. The changes of concern are those involving transient slowing of rate, known as periodic decelerations. These are of two kinds. In the first variety, heart rate slows as uterine pressure increases, beginning and ending simultaneously with contraction (Fig. 23-3B); the rate is a mirror image of the contraction. This is called *early deceleration* and usually results from compression of the fetal head on the perineum, not associated with acidosis and not considered a sign of fetal distress.

A second kind of deceleration (Fig. 23-3C) resembles early deceleration but is out of phase with the contraction, beginning late and not terminating until the contraction has subsided. This pattern is referred to as *late deceleration,* an ominous sign occurring with uteroplacental insufficiency or any disturbance that causes fetal hypoxia. Late decelerations are also associated with fetal acidosis, many times an indication for expeditious delivery.

The most common kind of deceleration resembles neither of the previously mentioned patterns (Fig. 23-3D). Changes in fetal heart rate that are unrelated to contractions and quite irregular in contour are called *variable decelerations,* seen at times in almost all labors. Variable decelerations are believed to signify umbilical cord compression and are vagally mediated. Unless the changes in fetal heart rate are extreme, below 70, and prolonged beyond 30 seconds, they are usually benign.

Fetal monitoring has been used as as a prognostic means of evaluating high risk pregnancies prior to labor. The oxytocin challenge test applied to the pregnant woman before onset of labor entails fetal monitoring while instituting an intravenous infusion of pitocin to simulate labor. The response of the fetal heart to three consecutive contractions over a ten-minute

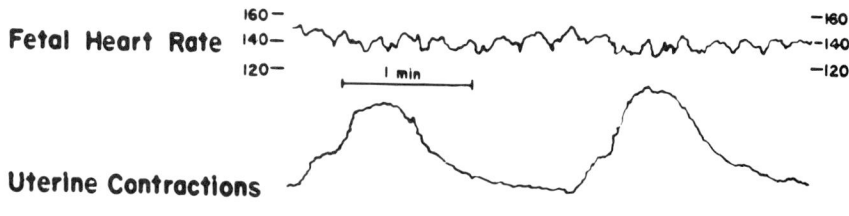

FIGURE 3A. NORMAL TRACING

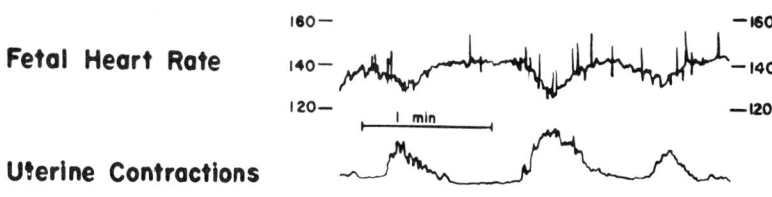

FIGURE 3B. EARLY DECELERATIONS

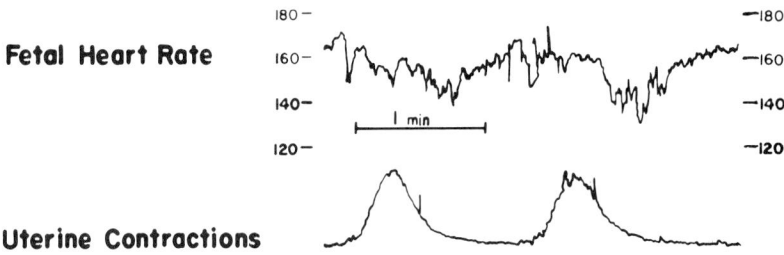

FIGURE 3C. LATE DECELERATIONS

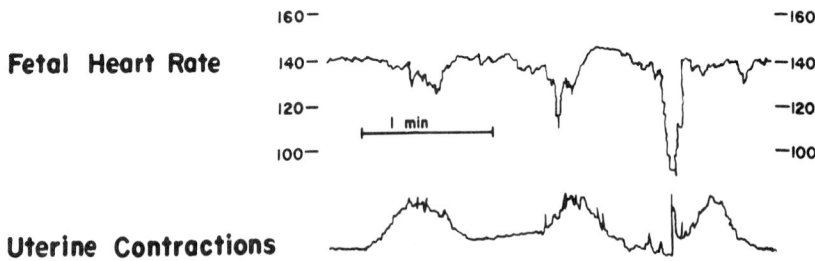

FIGURE 3D. VARIABLE DECELERATIONS

Figure 23-3. Bioelectronic monitoring of fetal heart rate and uterine contractions.

period is noted; the presence of late decelerations constitutes a positive test, generally an indication for planned early delivery by expeditious means. Recently a nonstress test has been utilized, involving attachment of the monitor to a pregnant woman before labor and observing and recording fetal movements *in utero*. A healthy fetus responds to movement with acceleration of heart rate while an endangered fetus may show no change in rate or deceleration.

Bioelectronic monitoring provides only part of the picture. As in any intensive care patient, one wishes to detail biochemical changes, especially arterial blood gases. Fetal blood can be obtained from the scalp. Fortunately, with regard to pH the capillary blood thus obtained is for all clinical purposes equivalent to arterial blood. Further, the pH of capillary blood correlates well with the condition of the fetus. Combined with bioelectronic monitoring, scalp capillary pH provides the best possible index of fetal condition.

EVALUATION AND CARE OF THE NEONATE

The goal of all obstetric anesthetic management is the birth of a vigorous newborn, and that of fetal monitoring to detect depression of the fetus before irreversible damage occurs. Despite all measures, some babies are physiologically depressed at birth and require resuscitation. The anesthetist as an expert in management of the unconscious patient is the logical person to supervise neonatal resuscitation.

Neonatal depression can be ascribed to several causes. One category of anesthetic concern is drug depression. For all practical purposes, all drugs used in anesthesia cross the placental barrier. As a rough rule of thumb if the mother is narcotized, so is the fetus. The extent of passage of a drug across the placenta depends upon several factors, including molecular weight, degree of ionization, and lipid solubility (see Chapter 3). Neuromuscular blockers are exceptions to the rule in that they cross the placenta in such small amounts in the ordinary doses given the mother that little or no impairment of fetal neuromuscular transmission occurs.

Birth trauma also causes neonatal depression. Prolonged or precipitant labor may result in a concussionlike syndrome. Manipulative procedures, particularly mid- and high forceps delivery, also tend to traumatize the fetus.

The most important cause of neonatal depression is asphyxia, a combination of hypoxia and acidosis. Asphyxia may result from maternal respiratory deficiency or hypotension, increased intrauterine pressure as observed in tetanic contractions, umbilical cord compression, or, most commonly, from inherent placental defects, as found in toxemia or diabetes.

Resuscitation of the newborn, as of the adult, has its ABC's (see Chapter 30). Establishing an *A*irway and assuring *B*reathing are the first steps. Support of the *C*irculation is also essential, but there is an additional

C in newborn resuscitation, that is, avoidance of Cold. The newborn does not shiver, and when the temperature falls heat is generated from brown fat, an oxidative process that increases oxygen consumption to such a degree that hypoxia can ensue.

In order to determine whether or not a baby is depressed, a method of evaluation is necessary. The most commonly used is the score devised by Virginia Apgar in 1953 (Table 23-1). This system provides a simple means of assessing the vitality of the newborn: a high Apgar score indicates a vigorous baby and a low score the opposite. The five indices of the Apgar score should be assessed exactly at one and five minutes after delivery, defined as that instant when both the head and feet of the infant are seen. Simply looking at an infant and stating that the Apgar score is 10 or 7 or 5 is meaningless.

All infants, whether depressed or not, must have the airway cleared. Nose and mouth are gently suctioned, and the head extended and positioned below the trunk while the infant is in a bassinet maintained at 32 to 34°C with infrared or radiant heating. The lungs *in utero* are fluid filled. The infant must generate enough pressure to open collapsed alveoli; in addition, the fluid filling the trachea and bronchi must be drained. Once this is accomplished and the Apgar score derived, treatment of the infant can proceed. Neonates with Apgar scores at one minute of 7 to 10 (a score of 10 is rare) require only observation, warmth, and perhaps further pharyngeal suctioning.

Newborns scoring 5 or 6 are mildly depressed, often as a result of opioids or anesthetic depression. In general, the mildly depressed can be resuscitated by external stimulation, preferably by gently slapping the soles of the feet, and by mask oxygen applied to the face. Assisted ventilation is usually not necessary.

Table 23-1. THE APGAR SCORE*

Sign	0	1	2
Heart rate	Absent	Less than 100 beats per minute	Over 100 beats per minute
Respiratory effort	Absent	Irregular, slow, gasping	Regular, rhythmic
Muscle tone	Limp	Some flexion of extremities	Active motion
Reflex response to stimulation	None	Grimace	Vigorous cry
Color	Pale, completely cyanotic	Body pink, extremities blue	Completely pink

*The Apgar method of scoring: 60 seconds after complete delivery of infant (disregarding cord and placenta), the five objective signs are evaluated and each given a score of 0, 1, or 2. A score of 10 characterizes an infant in the best possible condition.

An infant not responding to these measures or one with an Apgar score of 3 or 4 is moderately depressed. Once the airway has been cleared, positive pressure ventilation by mask, 30 to 40 breaths per minute, is applied. Along with suctioning and stimulation, this is usually adequate.

A newborn with an Apgar score of 0, 1, or 2 is severely depressed, requiring heroic measures. The airway is cleared by suction using a laryngoscope and direct vision. Positive pressure ventilation, preferably with 100 per cent oxygen, is given via an endotracheal tube. If intubation is not feasible, time is not wasted and mask ventilation or mouth to mouth ventilation is employed. Babies thus depressed in most instances have suffered brainstem hypoxia and the lungs must be ventilated before breathing resumes. Additionally, these infants are quite acidotic, the acidosis causing pulmonary artery vasoconstriction. Acidosis is corrected via administration of sodium bicarbonate, 2 to 4 mEq/kg into umbilical vein or artery. The bicarbonate is prepared by diluting 5 mEq with an equal volume of 5 per cent dextrose in water and injecting the appropriate volume. Improvement of the infant is monitored both clinically and by measurement of the pH of umbilical artery blood. While there is controversy concerning the use of sodium bicarbonate in the newborn because of the hypertonicity of the solution, the drug is lifesaving in the severely depressed. Because these babies also have cardiovascular depression, it is necessary to support the circulation. If heart rate is below 100 or absent, external cardiac massage is initiated at least at a rate of 100, remembering that the newborn has a large liver and spleen. Thus chest compression via the fingers only should be applied to the midpoint of the sternum (see Chapter 30).

Few drugs are of value in resuscitation of the newborn. The use of analeptics has been abandoned; they are not effective in the presence of acidosis and may further exacerbate an already depressed myocardium. Calcium in a dose of 10 mEq and epinephrine 50 to 100 μg intravenously may be used for the infant *in extremis*, but those requiring this kind of therapy rarely survive.

Opioid antagonists are useful in resuscitation. The antagonists that initially were available also exerted narcotic effects of their own, and if given to the neonate depressed from a cause other than maternal opioids might worsen the depression. With the new antagonist naloxone this is no longer a problem, as the drug itself does not produce depression and completely reverses opioid-induced depression. A dose of 5 μg per kg may be given either intramuscularly or intravenously to any newborn in whom opioid depression is suspected. Lack of response to the antagonist is evidence of depression from other causes. A newborn suffering opioid depression reversed by naloxone may become renarcotized owing to the short action of the antagonist. Obviously these babies need close observation.

In resuscitation, meconium aspiration merits special notice. Aspiration of meconium into the lungs can result in severe pneumonitis, often fatal. To minimize this problem all neonates with evidence of thick meconium should undergo tracheal aspiration using a laryngoscope and endotracheal tube. Small suction catheters are inadequate for this procedure because of the viscosity of the meconium. Suction is applied directly to the endotracheal tube by mouth as the tube is withdrawn. Saline lavage of the tracheobroncheal tree is still a controversial measure.

RESPIRATORY DISTRESS SYNDROME OF THE NEWBORN

The respiratory distress syndrome (RDS) of the newborn (hyaline membrane disease) remains a major cause of death in premature infants, although recent advances in treatment have reduced immediate mortality and long-term morbidity. Perhaps the most effective treatment is the application of continuous positive airway pressure (CPAP), which allows the infant to breathe spontaneously and prevents alveolar collapse during expiration. Once the enzymes needed to form surfactant become effective, CPAP is no longer necessary. A test is available for disclosing those infants likely to develop RDS. As the disease is caused by lack of surfactant, and amniotic fluid inevitably contains fetal tracheal fluid, analysis of amniotic fluid should detect the presence or absence of the mature surfactant principle. The ratio of lecithin, a major component of surfactant, to sphingomyelin in amniotic fluid provides an index of fetal lung maturity; a ratio greater than 2:1 correlates significantly with an incidence of RDS lower than 10 per cent.

APPRAISAL

It is a truism that the future of any country rests upon its children. As birth rates decline, a higher premium is placed on life and the tenet becomes even more important. Only through provision of the best possible care for mother and newborn will each individual be able to achieve a true life potential. The anesthetist plays a major role in this kind of care. Too long have we abrogated our responsibilities with the excuse that there are too few to provide obstetric care or that we are not sufficiently trained to do the job. Standards of care for obstetrics must be upgraded to equal or surpass those provided the surgical patient.

REFERENCES

Apgar V: A proposal for a new method of evaluation of the newborn infant. Anesth Analg 32:260, 1953.
Beard RW: The detection of fetal asphyxia in labor. Pediatrics 53:157, 1974.
Covino BJ: Local anesthesia. N Engl J Med 286:1035, 1972.
DeVore JS: Resuscitation of the newborn. Clin Obstet Gynecol 19:3, 1976.
Finster M, Poppers PJ, Sinclair JC, et al: Accidental intoxication of the fetus with local anesthetic drug during caudal anesthesia. Am J Obstet Gynecol 92:922, 1965.

Gluck L, Kulovish MV, Borer RC, et al: Diagnosis of the respiratory distress syndrome by amniocentesis. Am J Obstet Gynecol 111:440, 1971.

Gordon HR: Fetal bradycardia after paracervical block; correlation with fetal and maternal blood levels of local anesthetic (mepivacaine). N Engl. J Med 279:910, 1968.

Gregory GA, Gooding CA, Phibbs RH, et al: Meconium aspiration in infants—a prospective study. J Pediatr 85:848, 1974.

Gregory GA, Kitterman JA, Phibbs RH, et al: Treatment of the idiopathic respiratory distress syndrome with continuous positive airway pressure. N Engl J Med 284:1333, 1971.

Hon EH, Quilligan EJ: Electronic evaluation of fetal heart rate. Clin. Obstet Gynecol 11:145, 1968.

James LS, Adamsons, K Jr: Respiratory physiology of the fetus and newborn. N Engl. J Med 271:1353; 271:1403, 1964.

Marx GF: Aortocaval compression incidence and prevention. Bull NY Acad Med 50:443, 1974.

Mandelli M, Morselli PL, Nordid G, et al: Placental transfer of diazepam and its disposition in the newborn. Clin. Pharmacol Ther 17:564, 1975.

Paul RH: Clinical fetal monitoring; experience on a large clinical service. Am J Obstet Gynecol 113:573, 1972.

Roberts RB, Shirley MA: Reducing the risk of acid aspiration during cesarean section. Anesth Analg 53:859, 1974.

Scanlon JW, Brown WU, Weiss J, et al: Neurobehavioral responses of newborn infants after maternal epidural anesthesia. Anesthesiology 40:121, 1974.

Schiff D, Chan G, Stern L: Fixed drug combinations and the displacement of bilirubin from albumin. Pediatrics 48:139, 1971.

Texts and Symposia

Bonica JJ: Principles and Practice of Obstetric Analgesia and Anesthesia. Philadelphia, F. A. Davis, vol 1, 1967.

Shnider SM, Moya F (eds): The Anesthesiologist, Mother, and Newborn. Baltimore, The Williams & Wilkins Company, 1974.

Chapter 24

PEDIATRIC ANESTHESIA

GENERAL CONSIDERATIONS

As compared with an adult the child, especially the neonate, has unique anatomic, physiologic, and biochemical characteristics. Those responsible for the anesthetic care of infants and children should be familiar with these differences.

RESPIRATORY SYSTEM

The infant's upper airway is prone to obstruction because of small nares, a large tongue in relation to the size of the mandible, and abundant lymphoid tissue. The diameter of the trachea is quite small so that edema causes disproportionate narrowing of the airway. The horizontally placed ribs result in a cylindrical thorax and limit its expansion almost entirely to movement of the diaphragm. The sternum and anterior rib cage are compliant, intercostal and accessory muscles of respiration are poorly developed, and the highly placed diaphragm is easily restricted by any increase in volume of the abdominal contents. Although thoracic volume is enlarged mostly by diaphragmatic excursion, the flexible thoracic cage is readily expanded when positive pressure is applied to the airway. Except for the susceptibility to upper airway obstruction, which persists throughout childhood, these anatomic features become less important with age.

Lung development is not sufficiently complete for adequate gas exchange until 28 weeks of gestation, when the fetus weighs approximately 1 kg. Alveoli containing a film of surfactant as well as adjacent pulmonary capillary networks begin to mature after this time. At birth the terminal air sacs are shallow and wide-necked, and the alveoli are lined with cuboidal epithelium. As the alveoli mature, the epithelium becomes flattened and more permeable to gas exchange. The alveolar surface area is approximately one third that of the adult, and since metabolic rate is roughly twice that of the adult, lung reserves are limited. The number of alveoli increases tenfold from birth to adulthood.

Alveolar ventilation (V_A) of the newborn is proportionately about twice that of the adult. The high metabolic demand is met by increasing respiratory rate (f) rather than volume (Table 24-1). Dead space volume (V_D) is roughly the same in both the infant and adult per kg of body weight and the ratio of dead space to tidal volume (V_D/V_T) remains constant (Table 24-1). However, when administering anesthesia it should be realized that the volume of dead space in anesthetic apparatus is more significant in the infant than in the adult owing to the smaller airway volumes of the infant.

Functional residual capacity (FRC) is rapidly established at birth and is large enough to provide adequate buffering of inspired gases. The increased ratios of FRC and residual volume (RV) to total lung capacity (TLC) found in infants as compared with adults indicate the presence of a greater volume of air in the lungs after exhalation (Table 24-1).

The absolute value for total respiratory compliance in the neonate is

Table 24-1. RESPIRATORY DATA IN THE ADULT AND NEONATE

Alveolar Ventilation	Adult	Neonate
$\dot{V}_A$ (ml/kg/min)	60	100-150
V_T (ml/kg)	7	6
V_D (ml/kg)	2.2	2.2
V_D/V_T	0.3	0.3
f (min)	20	40
Lung Volumes	**Adult**	**Neonate**
FRC (ml/kg)	34	30
RV (ml/kg)	17	20
FRC/TLC	0.40	0.48
RV/TLC	0.20	0.33
Respiratory Mechanics	**Adult**	**Neonate**
Total respiratory compliance	20	1
Specific respiratory compliance (compliance/L lung volume)	1	1
Total flow resistance	1	12
Specific resistance	1	1
Acid-Base Status	**Adult**	**Neonate**
Pa_{CO_2} (torr)	38-40	32-35
Plasma HCO_3 (mEq/L)	24-28	17-22
pH	7.38	7.38
Alveolar-Arterial Oxygen Differences (AaD_{O_2})	**Adult**	**Neonate**
Pa_{O_2} (torr)	80-100	60-80
AaD_{O_2} (torr)	10 (105-95)	25 (105-80)

(From Nelson, NM: Neonatal pulmonary function. Pediatr Clin North Am 13:769, 1966.)

quite small; however, the specific compliance (compliance related to total lung volume) is about the same for infant and adult. Similarly, although resistance to air flow through the smaller airways of the newborn is increased, when measurements are related to lung volume, newborn and adult values are comparable (Table 24-1). This means that during artificial ventilation approximately the same airway pressure is required to ventilate adequately both neonatal and adult lungs.

Arterial blood in the neonate reveals the presence of a mild respiratory alkalosis and metabolic acidosis. The low plasma (and CSF) bicarbonate level reflects that of the mother, who chronically hyperventilates in the last trimester. This central acidosis apparently stimulates the newborn's respiratory center, producing mild hyperventilation. The low plasma bicarbonate level is also indicative of the neonate's compromised ability to compensate for acidosis (Table 24-1). The lower normal range for Pa_{O_2} of 60 to 80 torr commonly found in this age group is the result of shunting 20 to 30 per cent of the cardiac output at birth through the still patent foramen ovale and ductus arteriosus (Table 24-1).

CIRCULATORY SYSTEM

Following the first several breaths and expansion of the lungs after birth, pulmonary vascular resistance decreases and there is functional closure of the foramen ovale and ductus arteriosus. Should hypoxemia be prolonged at birth, pulmonary vascular resistance increases, thus retarding ductus closure with consequent venoarterial shunting, persistent hypoxemia, and systemic arterial hypotension.

The heart of the neonate has to pump approximately 80 per cent of the blood volume present in fetal life, since the placental circulation is eliminated after birth. For the same reason, the vascular bed of the neonate is decreased by 25 per cent. This leads to a reduction in cardiac work and a diminishing heart size in the first year of life. The stroke volume of the neonatal heart is roughly proportionate to that of the adult (a mere 4 to 5 ml in the neonate), but heart rate is doubled, resulting in a cardiac output about twice that of the adult. This elevated output is required to meet the relatively greater metabolic rate of the infant (Table 24-2).

Normal neonatal systolic blood pressure is in the range of 60 to 80 torr and pulse varies between 120 and 140 per min. Systolic blood pressure normally rises to 100 torr and pulse rate falls to 100 per min at about six years of age (Table 24-2). Accurate measurement of blood pressure in the infant and child is only possible if the proper equipment is used. Wide cuffs result in falsely low readings, while narrow cuffs give high values. The proper cuff covers approximately two thirds of the length of the upper arm. More sophisticated blood pressure monitoring equipment than the usual sphygmomanometer (such as the Doppler device or the intra-arterial catheter-transducer) is both useful and practical for complex operations in infants and children.

Table 24-2. Cardiovascular Data in Infant and Child

Cardiovascular Data	
Stroke volume (ml)	4–5
Heart rate (min)	120
Cardiac output (ml/min)	500–600
Metabolic rate (cal/kg/hr)	
Neonate and infant	2
Adult	1

	Blood Pressure and Pulse	
Age	Approximate Systolic BP (torr)	Approximate Pulse (min)
2 hr	60	120–160
5 days	80	120–160
6 mo	90	110–130
6 yr	100	100
10 yr	110	90
15 yr	120	80

Estimated Blood Volume	
	ml/kg
Newborn	85
Infant	80
Child	75
Adult	65

Heart rate is labile in infants and blood pressure at times difficult to measure. Continuous monitoring of heart and respiratory sounds with a precordial or esophageal stethoscope is essential during pediatric anesthesia. The experienced anesthetist can determine changes in depth of anesthesia by detecting alterations in heart sounds. Auscultatory changes can warn of inadequate blood replacement and impending shock.

TEMPERATURE CONTROL

The newborn has an incompletely developed thermoregulatory mechanism, causing it to be dependent upon the environment for maintenance of body temperature. Body surface area, especially in the premature infant, is relatively large. Neonates lack subcutaneous fat insulation, have poor peripheral vasomotor control, and inadequate sweating and shivering responses. Their main source of heat-producing energy is the brown fat (nonshivering thermogenesis) which is located largely between the shoulder blades, around the neck, and behind the sternum. Prematures lack this brown fat.

Oxygen consumption is reduced if body temperature is kept relatively constant. Exposure of the neonate to a cold environment (less than 27° C) leads to nonshivering thermogenesis, increases oxygen consumption, and induces metabolic acidosis. If body temperature falls the cardiorespiratory system becomes depressed, especially when hypothermia occurs during anesthesia. Conservation of body heat through use of thermoregulatory blankets and other devices is important in the operative management of neonates.

Development of hyperthermia with a body temperature higher than 40° C is a dangerous complication during pediatric anesthesia. Predisposing factors are fever, dehydration, elevated ambient temperature, drugs that diminish sweating (atropine, scopolamine) or disturb temperature regulation (barbiturates, phenothiazines, general anesthetics), and excessive surgical drapes. Fever increases oxygen consumption and carbon dioxide production, stimulates the cardiorespiratory system, and causes metabolic and respiratory acidosis. If uncorrected, convulsions, hypoxic brain damage, arterial hypotension, and cardiac arrest may occur.

If the child is febrile, operation should be delayed to allow time for fluid replacement and other efforts directed at reducing body temperature. If fever persists despite these measures, and the child requires immediate operation, anesthesia is induced and prompt measures such as external cooling are instituted to restore normothermia (see Management of Anesthesia further on).

FLUID BALANCE AND METABOLISM

Maintenance of fluid balance in infants and children is a special matter. The size of the body water compartments and the relative volume of circulating blood vary considerably from birth to adulthood (Fig. 24–1). Renal immaturity and a high basal metabolic rate result in a greater turnover of body water and a higher daily fluid requirement in infants as com-

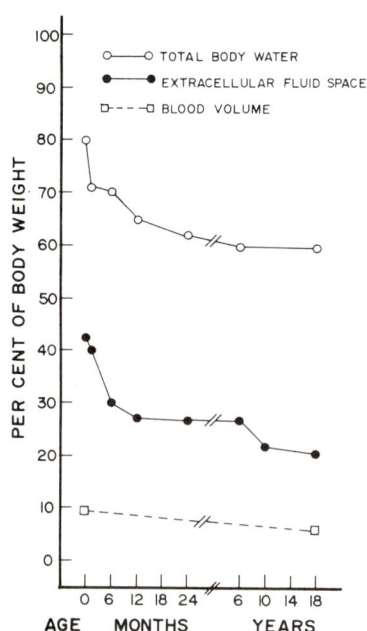

Figure 24–1. Body water and blood volume in the pediatric age group.

pared with adults (Table 24-3). Losses of fluid are less well tolerated and result in rapid dehydration if not replaced (see Preoperative Evaluation and Preparation). Investigations of operative fluid requirements in the newborn have shown that the neonatal kidney lacks the ability to retain sodium and water and that shifts of fluid and electrolytes during operation are similar to those seen in adults. The higher percentage of body mass in the form of water also necessitates a relatively higher dose of drugs such as succinylcholine and digoxin per kg of body weight, owing to a larger distributional space (see Table 24-8).

Carbohydrate and fat rather than amino acids are the principal sources of metabolic fuel in the first days of life. It is therefore important to maintain glycogen stores and an adequate blood glucose level, by providing liberal quantities of glucose in intravenous fluids given during operation (10 per cent glucose is recommended for premature infants).

In general, the capacity for metabolism of drugs in the neonatal period is less well established than in the infant and child. Furthermore, renal clearance rates for almost all drugs are decreased in the neonate, especially in the premature infant. Therefore, all drugs given the neonate should be administered with strict attention to dose and response.

Table 24-3. MAINTENANCE FLUIDS IN PEDIATRIC PATIENTS AND NORMAL URINE OUTPUT

Electrolytes	*Daily Dose*
Na	3 mEq/kg
K	2 mEq/kg
Cl	2 mEq/kg

Body Weight and Age	*24-Hour Fluid Requirement*
Premature and full term newborn less than 5 days of age	50-70 ml/kg
Premature and full term newborn over 5 days of age (5 days to 1 month of age)	150 ml/kg
3-10 kg (over 1 month of age)	100 ml/kg
10-20 kg	1000 ml plus 50 ml/kg over 10 kg
20 kg to adult	1500 ml plus 20 ml/kg over 20 kg

Normal Urine Output	
1 to 4 days old (ml/kg/hr)	0.3-0.7
4 to 7 days old (ml/kg/hr)	1.0-2.7
Over 7 days old (ml/kg/hr)	3
Over 2 years old (ml/kg/hr)	2
5 years old to adult (ml/kg/hr)	1
Insensible loss (ml/kg/day)	28

PREOPERATIVE EVALUATION AND PREPARATION

PSYCHOLOGICAL CONSIDERATIONS

The infant and child do not understand the reasons for hospitalization and separation from the family. The parents' apparent concern may complicate the picture, and the child often senses and reflects the parental attitude. It is not easy to establish rapport with a young child. Poor or inept preparation for operation can result in psychic trauma that may last for years. The child from one to three years of age is most vulnerable, while problems lessen and gradually level off at seven to eight years of age. Appropriate preoperative sedation is usually relied upon to provide the necessary tranquility.

GENERAL EVALUATION

During the preoperative visit it is important, as with all patients, to inquire into any history of familial difficulty with anesthesia. Evidence of respiratory infection, so prevalent in children, should lead to cancellation of elective operation for the following reasons: rhinorrhea, often a sign of early infection deeper in the respiratory tract, can produce airway obstruction by way of secretions, hyperactive laryngeal reflexes, and laryngospasm, also predisposing to laryngeal edema following tracheal intubation. Symptoms of upper respiratory infection in the child are also often premonitory signs of an impending systemic infection.

The normal variation in hemoglobin levels in infancy should be known to those involved in the care of these patients (Fig. 24–2). The criteria for diagnosis of anemia in various age groups are listed in Table 24–4. Note that

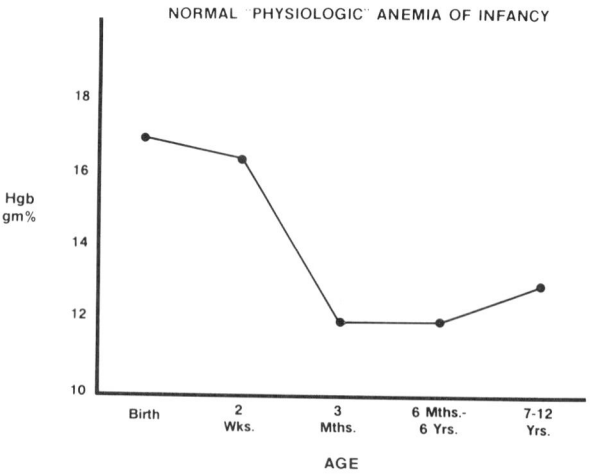

Figure 24–2. Normal "physiologic" anemia of infancy.

Table 24-4. CRITERIA FOR DIAGNOSIS OF ANEMIA

Age	(Hgb gm per 100 ml)
Cord blood	13.5
2 weeks	13.0
2 to 3 months	9.5
6 months to adult	10.0

while a hemoglobin level below 13 gm per 100 ml may be considered as anemia at two weeks of age, a level below 9.5 gm per 100 ml signifies anemia at two to three months. In addition to a hemoglobin level, a urinalysis should be done routinely as part of the minimal laboratory evaluation in all children preoperatively.

Congenital anomalies must be anticipated in children presenting for operation, especially in the neonate. Coexistent cardiac anomalies are frequently found and may have serious implications.

ASSESSMENT OF THE CARDIOPULMONARY SYSTEM

Assessment of pulmonary function in the infant is not easily done. The ventilometers in use today are not sufficiently sensitive to measure the small inherent volumes. Arterial puncture for blood gas analysis may result in arterial thrombosis and thus should be done only if necessary. Capillary blood sampling unfortunately approximates true arterial blood only in the healthy infant. The pattern of respiration is unreliable. In particular, the premature neonate tends to breathe irregularly, so a change in respiratory rhythm must persist to be significant. Color is often of little diagnostic value because of the normal presence of peripheral cyanosis. Breath sounds may be difficult to hear because of noisy respirations and retracting intercostal spaces. Radiographs of the chest are easily misinterpreted because they are often unavoidably obtained during exhalation.

For these reasons, assessment of impaired pulmonary function in the infant must center around detection of classic clinical signs of respiratory distress, such as sternal and intercostal retraction, flaring nostrils, and grunting respirations. With these signs of respiratory distress, a neonate with diaphragmatic hernia or major bowel obstruction will frequently need respiratory assistance preoperatively. This usually requires tracheal intubation and positive pressure ventilation before operation is begun.

STATE OF HYDRATION

Fever, tachycardia, and high urine specific gravity point to the presence of dehydration. The estimated per cent of dehydration in infants is evaluated clinically by the criteria listed in Table 24-5. Although the amount of fluid replacement depends upon the extent of dehydration, ad-

Table 24-5. ESTIMATED STATE OF HYDRATION IN THE INFANT

Signs and Symptoms	% Dehydration
Tissue turgor poor	5
Sunken fontanelle	10
Sunken eyes	10-20
Acute weight loss	% loss of original weight before illness (must be reliable information)

ministration of a balanced electrolyte solution such as lactated Ringer's solution is usually adequate for electrolyte needs. Replacement volume is 10 ml per kg per estimated per cent dehydration (Table 24-5). The dehydrated patient is usually hypovolemic. Albumin (5 per cent) or plasma protein fraction should be given in a dose of 10 ml per kg to the dehydrated patient as part of the fluid replacement. Potassium deficits have been estimated to be as large as 8 to 12 mEq per kg in severe dehydration and should be replaced with potassium chloride or phosphate when adequate urine volume is established.

Dehydration in infants is accompanied by moderate to severe metabolic acidosis requiring correction preoperatively. Anderson's formula is appropriate even in infants as an estimation of bicarbonate dosage for partial correction of metabolic acidosis [$0.3 \times$ wt kg $\times$ base deficit $=$ mEq $NaHCO_3$]. The metabolic alkalosis of pyloric stenosis should be treated preoperatively with a kind and volume of electrolyte solution and potassium similar to that recommended previously for dehydration, to prevent compensatory hypoventilation in the postoperative period.

PREMEDICATION AND PREOPERATIVE FEEDING

Atropine in relatively high doses (0.03 mg per kg intramuscularly, maximum 0.6 mg) helps to prevent the vagal reflexes, especially cardiac reflexes, which are readily elicited in pediatric patients. Atropine is a better premedicant than scopolamine in children because of its greater cardiotonic effect. The antisialogogue action is sufficient for the commonly used anesthetics. With this dose of atropine, bradycardia is rarely seen following administration of succinylcholine or traction on either the extraocular muscles or the viscera. Atropine should be withheld preoperatively if the patient has an elevated body temperature, but may be given intravenously before induction of anesthesia (0.02 mg per kg, maximum 0.4 mg).

Premedication for patients under one year of age is limited to atropine alone. For patients over one year, sedation may be added according to individual preference and adjusted for dosage, depending upon the patient's clinical status. For example, morphine (0.1 to 0.2 mg per kg intramuscularly) or meperidine (1.5 mg per kg intramuscularly) is commonly employed as preoperative sedatives for patients in good physical condition.

Pentobarbital (2 to 3 mg per kg) may be given when the patient is apprehensive. As an alternative, pentazocine or diazepam, in doses of 1 mg per kg and 0.2 mg per kg respectively, have been found to provide good preoperative sedation in children. Since the level of sedation may be inadequate before 30 minutes and the effect of atropine on heart rate and reflexes diminishes after 75 minutes, induction of anesthesia should begin from 30 to 75 minutes following premedication.

Another alternative for premedication is available if a well-staffed preoperative holding room is at hand. Under these circumstances, a suspension of thiopental (15 to 25 mg per kg) may be given rectally in the presence of the parents before transporting the child to the operating room, to create the least possible psychic trauma.

It is best to omit giving opioids and sedatives in children who are restless as a result of respiratory depression and hypoxia. However, patients with cyanotic congenital heart disease are an exception to this rule. These children become unconscious from hypoxia induced by crying and excitement and may improve their state of consciousness and oxygenation after receiving morphine (see Table 24-8). This is attributed not only to the depressant effect of morphine on metabolism, but also to a dilation of the pulmonary outflow tract and vasculature, thus decreasing the right to left intracardiac shunt.

Operations on infants should be given priority on the schedule in order to avoid dehydration. A safe preoperative feeding schedule for pediatric patients is outlined in Table 24-6. For afternoon procedures, patients are seldom allowed oral intake after 6 A.M., as the schedule may be altered to bring them to the operating room earlier.

EQUIPMENT

Adult circle systems are not satisfactory for children younger than seven or eight years of age because they are more cumbersome, have excessive dead space, and present more resistance to respiration than the more commonly used pediatric systems. A Revell circulator overcomes these disadvantages but is not commonly used. The Columbia pediatric valve has proved useful for conversion of the adult circle system to pediatric use. Circle carbon dioxide–absorbing systems specifically designed for

Table 24-6. PREOPERATIVE FEEDING IN CHILDREN

Age	Feeding Schedule
<6 mo	Clear fluids after midnight up to 4 hours preoperatively
<4 to 5 yr	Clear fluids after midnight up to 6 hours preoperatively
>4 to 5 yr	NPO after midnight

pediatric patients with minimal dead space and low resistance valves (Bloomquist system) have achieved limited popularity, probably because less complicated devices are available. The prevailing system in anesthesia for neonates and infants is the Jackson-Rees modification of Ayre's T-piece. A variety of nonrebreathing valves may be incorporated into a Magill circuit for children over two to three years of age. These systems are simple and lightweight, with low resistance, and are easily gas sterilized. They require high flows of dry gases which must be humidified to prevent drying of respiratory mucosa in the infant and for operations exceeding one hour in older children.

The Ayre T-piece system is shown in Figure 24-3. Required gas flows are two-and-a-half to three times predicted minute volume, to prevent rebreathing. The small 500-ml reservoir bag is easy to manipulate and gives a good "feel" for the infant's pulmonary resistive forces and adequacy of ventilation. The humidifier provides adequate humidification of gases.

The Sierra valve pictured in Figure 24-4 is one of many nonrebreathing valves available. This valve is excellent for children over three years of age because of its light weight and minimal dead space. It allows spontaneous or controlled respiration without manipulation. Again, humidification of gases is easily accomplished. Both Ayre's T-piece and the Magill-Sierra valve system are readily adapted for scavenging exhaled anesthetics (Figs. 24-3, 24-4).

Masks of the Rendell-Baker Soucek type that minimize dead space are best for the neonate and infant under one year of age (Fig. 24-5). For the child over one year, a mask with an inflatable rim provides a good fit.

The number one straight laryngoscope blade is best for neonates and

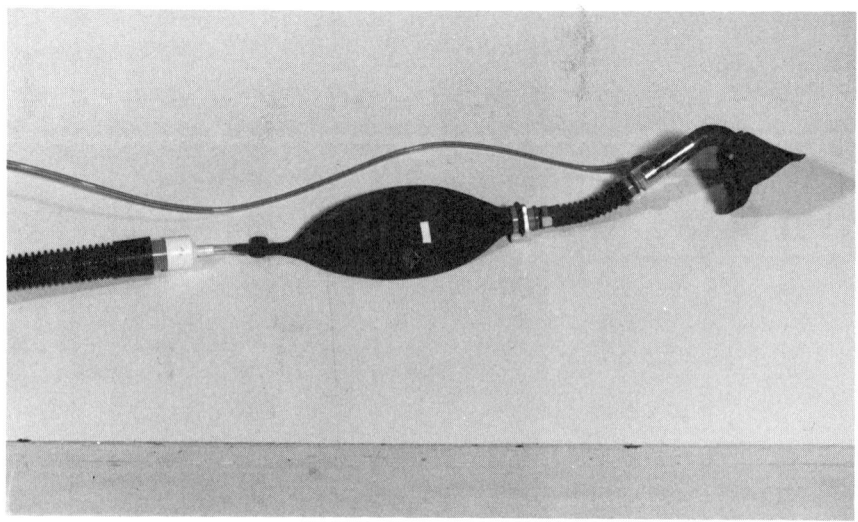

Figure 24-3. Jackson-Rees modification of Ayre's T-piece. Humidifier should be used in system as seen in Figure 24-4. Note connection at tail of bag for anesthetic exhaust.

Pediatric Anesthesia

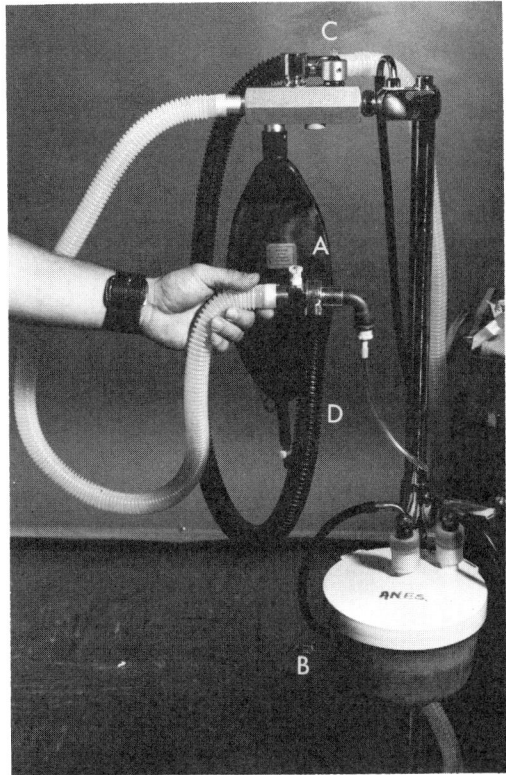

Figure 24-4. Sierra nonrebreathing valve A, in Magill circuit, B, cascade humidifier incorporated in system, C, Georgia valve provides "leak" for surplus anesthetics, D, exhaust tubing attached to exhalation port of both Sierra and Georgia valves (C).

infants, although number 0 blades are available for the premature newborn. Curved blades are less effective in exposing the infant glottis because insertion of the blade tip in the vallecula utilizing the usual upward, forward pull only serves to push the high, anterior larynx out of view. The Cole endotracheal tube (Fig. 24-5), designed to provide decreased resistance and

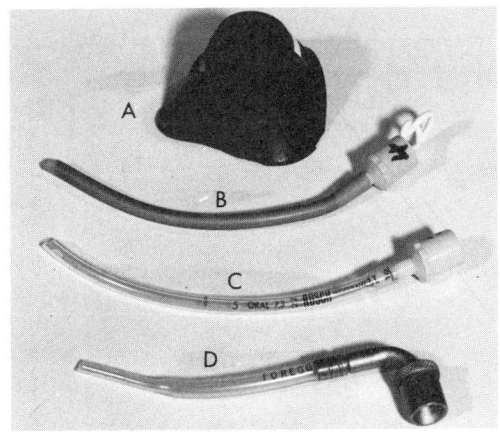

Figure 24-5. A, Rendell-Baker Soucek mask. B, Armored, C, Rusch plastic, and D, Cole endotracheal tubes.

improve laminar flow, is excellent for the neonate and small infant, but it kinks easily and should only be used when access to the airway is easy. Clear plastic tubes must be thin-walled and soft but should resist kinking. Armored tubes are useful in operations on the head and neck in which reliability of patency is a necessity, but they are easily flipped out of the trachea when the operation involves the oropharynx. Approximate sizes and lengths of endotracheal tubes for children are listed in Table 24–7. A good rule of thumb for the average French size for children over one year of age is "18 plus the age" (a six-year-old requires 18 plus 6 or a size 24 French tube). If tube size is in millimeters, convert to French size by multiplying by four and adding two; e.g., a 3.5-ml tube $(3.5 \times 4) + 2 =$ size 16 French tube.

All of this equipment is gas sterilizable, following which particular attention should be given to adequate aeration (a minimum of 72 hours without aerator and 12 hours with aerator), especially for equipment that comes into direct contact with the patient. All plastic tubes marked for single use only should not be resterilized with ethylene oxide in order to avoid formation of toxic substances that can damage tissues.

MONITORING

For the purposes of this chapter we shall emphasize only the minimal number of monitoring devices required for safe anesthetic procedure in infants and children.

Body temperature should be monitored continuously in all anesthe-

Table 24–7. ENDOTRACHEAL TUBE SIZES FOR PEDIATRIC ANESTHESIA

Age of Patient	Approximate French Size	Approximate Internal Diameter (mm)	Length (cm)
Newborn (under 2.3 kg)	11–12	2.5	10
Newborn (2.3–3 kg)	13–14	3.0	11
Newborn to 6 mo	15–16	3.5	11
5 to 12 mo	17–18	4.0	12
12 to 20 mo	19–20	4.5	13
18 months to 3 yr	21–22	5.0	14
3 to 4 yr	23–24	5.5	16
5 to 6 yr	25–26	6.0	18
6 to 7 yr	27–28	6.5	18
8 to 9 yr	29–30	7.0	20
10 to 11 yr	31–32	7.5	22
12 to 13 yr	31–32	7.5	23
14 yr	33–34	8.0	24

tized pediatric patients. Telethermometers are available to measure rectal, esophageal, or tympanic membrane temperature. The thermometer can be connected to a servocontrolled system and water mattress, to maintain a reasonably constant body temperature. Less complicated equipment such as insulated heating pads may be sufficient, since the primary problem of concern here is loss of body heat. While it is best to use temperature-controlled equipment on all anesthetized children, this is a necessity in patients under five years of age and in older children when the operation may last longer than two hours. This equipment should be readily available in all cases to treat large deviations ($\pm 2°$C) in body temperature. Other methods of maintaining body temperature in small infants include a radiant heating lamp that can be used before and after operation and an orthopedic wrap for the extremities. Exposed viscera should be protected by dressings soaked in warm solution.

Other useful monitoring devices routinely applied are a properly fitting blood pressure cuff and a precordial or esophageal stethoscope. ECG monitoring is advisable, especially in major operations (consider the patient with tracheoesophageal fistula requiring posterolateral thoracotomy, for whom a precordial or esophageal stethoscope is impractical). The newer stable ECG monitors and disposable surface electrodes provide reliable readings. It must be emphasized, however, that blood pressure readings and heart sounds are the reliable guides to adequacy of cardiac output, not the ECG tracing. Intra-arterial blood pressure monitoring is used in open heart operations on children of all ages and in other procedures in which continuous recording of arterial pressure is desirable (e.g., hypotensive anesthesia).

Finally, simple visual and tactile monitoring are indispensable: pulmonary resistive forces can be continuously evaluated with the anesthetic reservoir bag, the color of blood in the wound and the color of the nail beds observed, and muscular tone checked in an exposed arm. Many clinicians use a nerve stimulator to determine the level of neuromuscular blockade in patients given neuromuscular blockers.

MANAGEMENT OF ANESTHESIA

INDUCTION

The child requires quiet, constant reassurance and gentle physical contact during induction of anesthesia. In general, for an elective operation in a healthy child under seven to eight years of age, a halothane, nitrous oxide-oxygen induction is satisfactory. A good technique is to cup the mask at the chin, off the face, and to use high flows (no greater than 70 per cent nitrous oxide), increasing the halothane concentration at 0.5 per cent increments until 3 per cent is reached (Fig. 24–6). The mask is gradually lowered as consciousness is lost, placed firmly on the face, and the gas

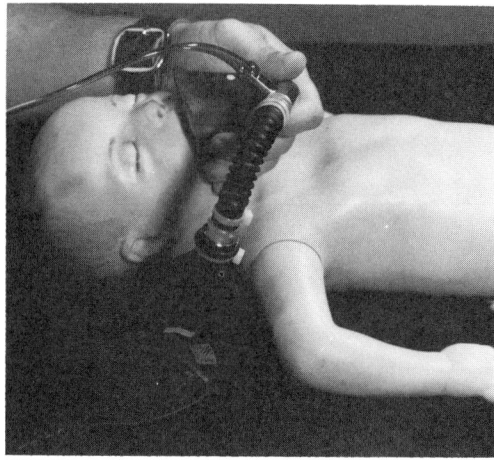

Figure 24-6. Inhalation induction with mask cupped at chin. See text.

flows, concentration of oxygen, and anesthetics are changed to appropriate levels. In the basically healthy child over seven to eight years of age the option of an intravenous thiopental induction (5 mg per kg) should be considered.

Ketamine is a safe, effective induction agent, especially in the one- to ten-year age group. At present we use this drug (5 to 7 mg per kg intramuscularly) for induction of anesthesia in cardiac operations. The prolonged crying and struggling sometimes seen with mask induction are avoided with this technique and the cardiocirculatory system remains stable throughout induction. Ketamine should not be used for induction of anesthesia in short operations because of its prolonged effect.

Airway obstruction commonly seen during induction can be readily overcome by the insertion of an oral airway. One of the major advantages of halothane is its ability to depress laryngeal reflexes, permitting early airway insertion. Once an airway is guaranteed, gently assisted respirations with 3 to 5 cm of water positive end-expiratory pressure will discourage the tendency toward laryngospasm. The mask should be held firmly in place as suggested in Figure 24-6, and, especially in the neonate and small infant, the fingers should support the mandible, not compress the soft tissue against the floor of the mouth.

A good intravenous route should be established in all but the simplest surgical procedures for administration of drugs, fluid, and blood products when needed. With experience, a 20-gauge short plastic catheter can usually be inserted percutaneously in the neonate but if a cutdown is required, the catheter should be no smaller than size 18 French to facilitate blood administration. If the catheter can be inserted into the superior or inferior vena cava, valuable venous pressure measurements can be obtained.

Fluid infusion in neonates and infants should be arranged to allow for administration of drugs through a side channel containing a minimum of

Pediatric Anesthesia

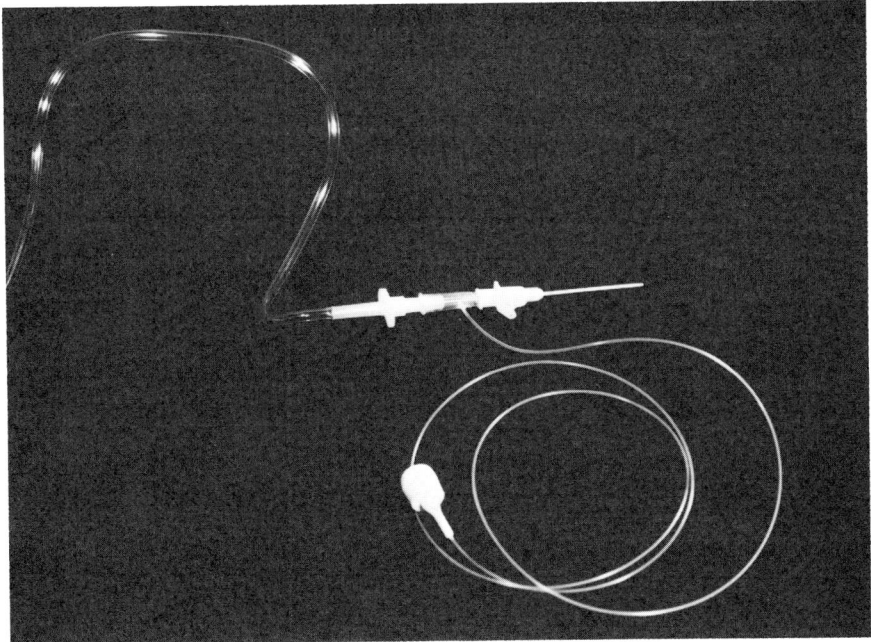

Figure 24-7. Intravenous side channel volume less than 0.1 ml for administration of drugs to neonate.

dead space (Fig. 24-7). Small bubbles of air in tubing may add up to a significant volume in the neonate and must be meticulously removed before connection to the patient is made.

TRACHEAL INTUBATION

Tracheal intubation is required in intrathoracic, intra-abdominal, and neurosurgical operations, in most head and neck procedures, and in all cases in which a neuromuscular blocker is used. The length of operation and age of the patient do not necessarily affect the decision for or against intubation. For example, a newborn having a bilateral inguinal herniorrhaphy, a procedure occasionally lasting up to two hours, may be managed safely by mask.

Knowledge of the anatomic differences between the infant and adult larynx is important for safe, rapid tracheal intubation.

1. The vocal cords in the infant are situated between the C2 and C4 vertebral bodies rather than at the C5 to C6 location as in the adult. The high location of the glottis therefore may cause difficulty in visualization.
2. The angle formed by epiglottis and vocal cords is more acute in the infant than in the adult. Exposure of the glottis is therefore better accomplished with a straight blade directly lifting the epiglottis, rather than with a curved blade inserted between the base of the tongue and the epiglottis.

Table 24-8. DRUGS USEFUL IN PEDIATRIC ANESTHESIA

Drug	Dose	Remarks
Alphaprodine	0.5–1.0 mg/kg IV	Initial dose
	0.5 mg/kg/hr	Maintenance dose
Atropine	0.02 mg/kg IV	
Dexamethasone	*Under 1 year old:*	For decreasing edema
	4 mg IV	
	Over 1 year old:	
	8 mg IV	
Diazepam	0.2 mg/kg IM*	Sedative dose or IM*
	0.1 mg/kg IV	Premedication dose
Digoxin	*Premature:*	
	0.55–0.66 mg/kg	Oral, digitalizing dose
	Full-term newborn and infant:	
	0.66 mg/kg	2/3 dose parenterally
		1/2 dose initially
		1/4 dose q 6–12 hr
	Over 2 year old:	
	0.44 mg/kg	Maintenance dose
		1/8 digitalizing dose
		q 12 hr
Droperidol	0.1 mg/kg IM or IV	Sedative or premedication dose
d-Tubocurare	*Newborn:*	
	0.25–0.50 mg IV	Initial dose. *Not* per kg
	1/4 initial dose	Maintenance dose
	Infant:	
	0.4 mg/kg IV	Initial dose
	1/5 initial dose	Maintenance dose
	Child:	
	0.2 mg/kg IV	Initial dose
	1/4 initial dose	Maintenance dose
Fentanyl	1–2 µg/kg IV	Anesthetic dose
	(.001–.002 mg/kg)	
Ketamine	5–10 mg/kg IM	Induction dose
	1–2 mg/kg IV	Maintenance dose
Furosemide	1 mg/kg/dose	

*Poorly absorbed, IM

3. In the infant, unlike the adult, the anterior attachment of the vocal cords to the larynx is below the posterior attachment. For this reason a curved tube may become impeded at the anterior commissure. Gentle rotation of the tube overcomes this problem.
4. In the infant, the larynx is funnel-shaped owing to narrowing at the cricoid cartilage; the diameter of the airway at this point is therefore less than at the vocal cords. Hence, the tube accommodated by the glottis may not pass readily through the cricoid ring. Forcing the tube into the trachea may result in ischemia and edema of the mucous membrane with complications such as respiratory obstruction following extubation.

The appropriate kind and size of endotracheal tube have been discussed under Equipment in this chapter. One size larger and one smaller

Table 24-8. DRUGS USEFUL IN PEDIATRIC ANESTHESIA (Continued)

Drug	Dose	Remarks
Lidocaine	1 mg/kg IV	Antiarrhythmic dose
	2-3 mg/kg topical	Maximal topical dose
Meperidine	1.5 mg/kg IM	Sedative or premedication dose
Morphine	0.2 mg/kg IM	Sedative dose or IM
	0.1 mg/kg IV	Premedication dose
Naloxone	0.005 mg/kg IV *and* IM	Give IM as well as IV, since narcotic effect may outlast IV naloxone effect
Neostigmine	0.07 mg/kg IV	Give in incremental doses following atropine
Pancuronium	*Newborn:*	
	0.05-0.1 mg/kg IV	Initial dose
	1/5 initial dose	Maintenance dose
	Infant:	
	0.12 mg/kg IV	Initial dose
	1/4 initial dose	Maintenance dose
	Child:	
	0.10 mg/kg IV	Initial dose
	1/4 initial dose	Maintenance dose
Pentazocine	1.2 mg/kg IM	Premedication for inpatient
	1.0 mg/kg IM	Premedication for outpatient
Pentobarbital	2-3 mg/kg IM	Sedative or premedication dose
Racemic epinephrine (2.25%)	0.25 to 0.50 ml in 5 ml saline	By aerosol insufflation or IPPB as needed for croup
Sodium bicarbonate	0.3 × wt (kg) × base deficit	Give 1/2 dose and repeat blood gas analysis
Succinylcholine	*Newborn and Infant:*	
	2.0 mg/kg IV	
	3.0 mg/kg IM	
	Child:	
	1.0 mg/kg IV	
Thiopental (2.5%)	3-5 mg/kg IV	Induction dose
	15-25 mg/kg rectal suspension	Rectal premedication dose

than the best estimate should be readily available. We prefer triamcinolone (Kenalog) cream as a lubricant for endotracheal tubes, as it is water-soluble, does not appear to be associated with sensitivity reactions, and may reduce the incidence of post-traumatic subglottic edema.

In the ill, hyporeflexic neonate, tracheal intubation might be safest in the conscious state after inhalation of oxygen for several minutes. In most other patients, a neuromuscular blocker is recommended to facilitate intubation unless contraindicated by factors such as anticipated malignant hyperthermia, presence of a tumor in or about the larynx that can lead to total airway obstruction following loss of muscle tone, or a burned child. Good muscle relaxation permits time for selection of the correct tube size. As the tube is advanced, the fit in the cricoid area may be judged. Either succinylcholine or pancuronium is an excellent drug for the purpose of intubation (see Table 24-8 for doses). Two warnings are in order regarding pancuronium: paralyzing effects may be prolonged in the neonate, and the onset of action is too slow for rapid intubation in the presence of a full stomach.

After neuromuscular blockade, nitrous oxide should be discontinued and halothane decreased below 1.5 per cent as gentle, controlled respiration is begun. Laryngoscopy is then accomplished with the patient's shoulders flat, avoiding overextension of the head, especially in the neonate and infant. The large occiput of the infant head flexes the neck, promoting ready access to the glottis. If resistance to passage of the orotracheal tube is encountered, a smaller tube is used. Nasotracheal intubation is not done without specific reason because of the danger of dislodgement of adenoid tissue into the trachea. Before securing the endotracheal tube, the chest is examined bilaterally for breath sounds, as accidental bronchial intubation easily occurs in pediatric patients. Suctioning of the stomach may follow if decompression is indicated; the catheter is then removed to leave space for an esophageal stethoscope.

MAINTENANCE

Maintenance of body temperature during operation is essential, as previously outlined. Good body contact with a heating mattress must be assured, and if necessary the other techniques mentioned under Monitoring are applied when appropriate.

Two basic inhalation techniques can be used for most operations in children. In the spontaneously breathing patient, halothane delivered with a 50 per cent nitrous oxide-oxygen gas mixture provides a smooth course. Extensive operations in the neonate and infant call for low concentrations of halothane (0.5 to 1.0 per cent) and pancuronium (Table 24-8). This provides muscle relaxation and permits controlled respiration with little depression of the circulatory system. Remember, the newborn is more reactive to nondepolarizing neuromuscular blockers, so that the second and especially third doses must be sharply reduced to avoid prolonged apnea (Table 24-8).

The second technique involves the use of an opioid, nitrous oxide-oxygen, and a nondepolarizing neuromuscular blocker. We have found alphaprodine and pancuronium to be a reliable combination to supplement the inhalants (Table 24-8). This technique results in minimal cardiocirculatory depression and is recommended for the critically ill patient. Others prefer morphine, meperidine, or fentanyl as the opioid of choice (Table 24-8). The nitrous oxide concentration should not exceed 50 per cent in the presence of air entrapment, as occurs in intestinal obstruction. If an intravenous channel has not been established preoperatively, it is started following a ketamine induction, as previously described. (If ketamine is used for induction, alphaprodine should be omitted in the neonate and infant.) Reversibility of the opioid with naloxone and of the neuromuscular blocker with neostigmine make this a useful technique. It is emphasized that naloxone should be given both intravenously and intramuscularly, the dose repeated if necessary along with neostigmine, since both antagonists outlast the effects of the agonists (Table 24-8).

Ketamine is an excellent anesthetic in children for certain operations such as burn debridement and grafting. The circulatory system remains stable with a ketamine-nitrous oxide technique for this kind of operation, and postanesthesia excitement or hallucinations are rarely seen in children under ten years of age. The initial dose is usually 5 to 10 mg per kg intramuscularly *or* 2 to 3 mg per kg intravenously, followed by 1 to 2 mg per kg intravenously as needed. Nitrous oxide is helpful in maintenance of anesthesia.

During operation, meticulous attention must be paid to the ventilatory requirements of the pediatric patient. Especially in thoracic procedures, a shallow, rapid, controlled respiratory pattern is required to provide adequate ventilation and at the same time to keep lung movement from distracting the surgeon. This technique may predispose to progressive atelectasis, necessitating periodic hyperexpansion of the lung and tracheal suctioning if secretions are abundant.

FLUID ADMINISTRATION

Maintenance fluids during operation should consist of a dextrose-containing electrolyte solution such as 5 per cent dextrose in lactated Ringer's solution (10 per cent dextrose and Ringer's in the neonate in view of the tendency toward hypoglycemia), infused at the rate of 5 to 10 ml per kg per hour, depending upon the extent of surgical dissection and estimated fluid loss from exposed viscera.

In general, blood loss should be replaced with whole blood if the loss is greater than 15 per cent of the estimated blood volume (Table 24-2). Small losses are replaced with the dextrose and Ringer's solution mentioned previously. Blood loss is estimated by weighing sponges and collecting suctioned blood into calibrated containers. A minimum of 250 ml of blood must be available preoperatively (even for the small neonate) when loss exceeding 10 per cent of blood volume is expected, since over 100 ml of blood are required to fill the administration set. Rapid transfusion of blood can result in severe metabolic acidosis in the infant, if replacement exceeds 50 per cent of estimated blood volume. Sodium bicarbonate (0.5 to 1.0 mEq per kg) with supplementation if needed should be given during massive transfusions, followed by blood gas analysis. Because blood becomes acidotic and hyperkalemic with the passage of time, the freshest blood available should be used when transfusion in excess of 50 per cent of blood volume is anticipated. Blood should be warmed to body temperature when administered to children, to limit body cooling.

Ten per cent calcium gluconate (0.5 ml/100 ml blood) is given if massive amounts of blood have been transfused, as the small supply of exchangeable calcium in the skeleton of small infants renders them susceptible to hypocalcemia. Plasmanate and albumin are excellent blood substitutes when protein deficiency is suspected (such as in bowel obstruction) and blood loss is marginal.

EMERGENCE

After completion of operation and before the patient is moved to the recovery room, the cardiorespiratory system should be evaluated. Adequacy of respiration is judged by the extent of chest wall expansion, movement of the reservoir bag, breath sounds, peripheral color, and general muscle tone. After extensive operations, blood gas analysis is indicated for more precise assessment. During this period warming of the neonate should be continued to achieve or maintain a minimal body temperature of 36° C. The stomach must be suctioned, when indicated, to prevent limitation of diaphragmatic motion; the nasogastric tube often is left in place for continued decompression postoperatively. Tracheobronchial suctioning is usually not necessary and is only done when there is evidence of secretions.

The trachea should be extubated when the patient is warm and respirations are adequate. Extubation of children, especially neonates and infants, is preferable during light levels of anesthesia. These patients are rarely as deeply anesthetized as one suspects, and extubation during "deep" anesthesia may result in laryngospasm during transport to the recovery room as the anesthesia level lightens. Prior to extubation, 100 per cent oxygen is administered and the tube is gently withdrawn with positive pressure applied to the reservoir bag. Before applying bag and mask to the face, the angles of the mandible should be lifted upward and the chin depressed to open the mouth. This maneuver lifts the tongue forward to clear the posterior pharynx and also causes pain, which stimulates respiration. Oxygen can be provided as needed, but care must be taken to maintain a free airway.

The patient is transported to the recovery room in the lateral position, preferably without an oral airway and with the chest and abdomen clearly in view. Oxygen via bag and mask is used in transporting critically ill patients.

POSTOPERATIVE CARE

Neonates are best cared for postoperatively in an incubator with a head hood, as shown in Figure 24–8, which provides a warm environment and precise control of oxygen concentration. Continuous monitoring of the oxygen level under the hood is recommended. The risks of blindness and possible lung damage in the neonate from oxygen therapy must be balanced against the risks of death or brain damage from hypoxia. The level of Pa_{O_2}

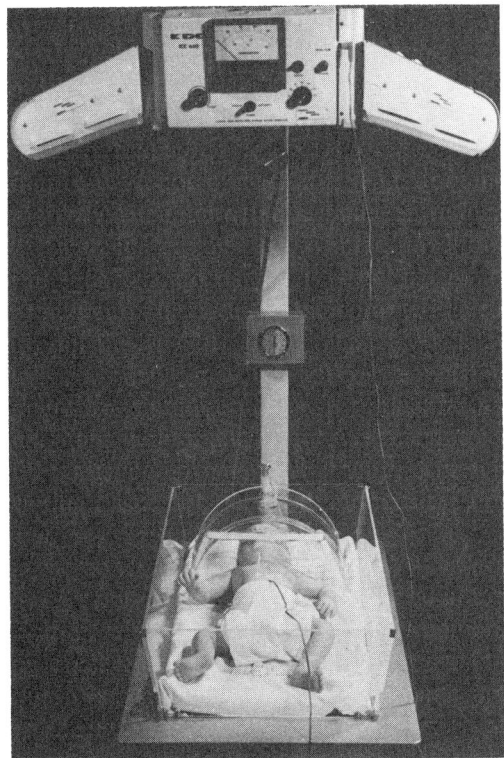

Figure 24-8. Head hood in open incubator for delivery of moist oxygen.

above the normal range, duration of hyperoxia, degree of prematurity, and history of multiple birth are all factors that influence the development of retrolental fibroplasia. We recommend giving supplemental oxygen to the cyanotic infant in respiratory distress, adjusted to maintain Pa_{O_2} between 50 and 70 torr.

Humidification of the oxygen is sufficient in most instances to maintain liquefied secretions. Ultrasonic mist therapy may be indicated to loosen thick, obstructive secretions under the following circumstances: after difficult tracheal intubation; in patients with respiratory infection; after an operation lasting more than three to four hours; in the dehydrated patient; or when signs of croup are noted (see further on).

The early postoperative period is a critical phase for the weak, hyporeflexic newborn infant. Aspiration of gastric contents remains a common cause of death and continuous drainage of stomach contents is therefore desirable.

Constant observation is needed throughout the postoperative phase for early recognition of atelectasis and pneumonia. Respiratory embarrassment readily occurs in the presence of tight abdominal wound closures, with resulting pressure on the diaphragm from below. This occurs postoperatively in diaphragmatic hernia, omphalocele closure, and relief of bowel obstruction.

Periodic orotracheal intubation for tracheal toilet and hyperinflation of the lungs may be necessary. This should be performed with the utmost gentleness, avoiding high airway pressures (Fig. 24–9). Prolonged intubation is undesirable because this bypasses the natural defense mechanisms of the nasopharynx and trachea.

Postintubation laryngeal edema is a complication of pediatric anesthesia that requires special consideration. The incidence of this condition is greatest in the newborn to five-year age group. Use of an appropriate lubricant and the atraumatic insertion of soft, plastic endotracheal tubes that permit a slight airway leak may serve to decrease the incidence of edema. However, if laryngeal swelling occurs, the small diameter of the airway of the infant and child is greatly compromised. One millimeter of edema in the infant's trachea at the cricoid level decreases the lumen by 75 per cent.

The first sign of edema following extubation is a croupy cough beginning within a few minutes to a few hours. Inspiratory stridor and intercostal retraction are warning signs, and tachypnea, tachycardia, and sweating may also be observed. Treatment, instituted at once, consists of administration of oxygen and ultrasonic mist in a head hood or tent. Most croupy coughs disappear with this treatment alone.

Progression of edema is suggested by inability to clear the airway by coughing and by inspiratory stridor with retraction of the costal interspaces and sternum during quiet respiration. Restlessness, pallor, sweating, and cyanosis may follow if hypoxia develops. Dexamethasone given intravenously and racemic epinephrine aerosol are effective in reducing the edema (see Table 24–8 for doses). Secretions distal to the obstruction may have to be removed by tracheal intubation and aspiration. Intubation can be done nasally and the tube left in place for two to three days. If obstruction persists after extubation, a tracheostomy is needed.

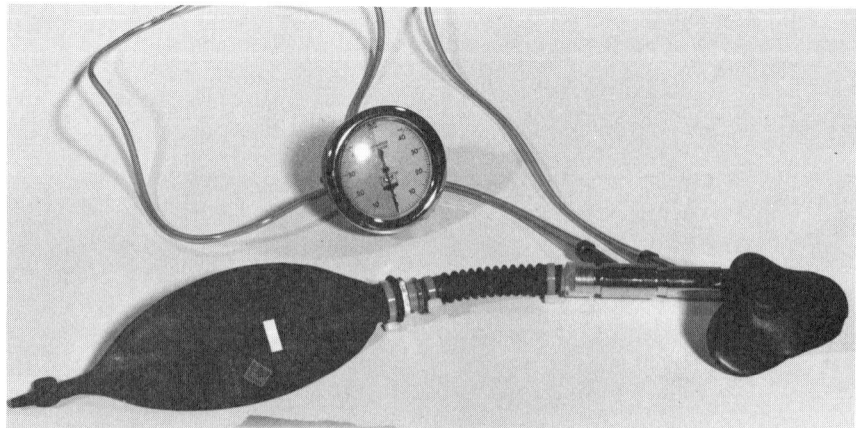

Figure 24–9. Jackson-Rees modification of Ayre's T-piece with pressure gauge in system. For transport of sick neonates. See text.

Should laryngeal edema follow intracranial operation, reintubation should be done immediately. Increased respiratory effort with carbon dioxide retention and venous distention increases intracranial pressure. A tracheostomy may then be required if obstruction persists after 48 to 72 hours of tracheal intubation.

REFERENCES

Avery ME, Fletcher BD: The Lung and Its Disorders in the Newborn Infant. 3rd ed, Philadelphia, WB Saunders Co, 1974.
Bennett EJ, Daughety MJ, Jenkins MT: Fluid requirements for neonatal anesthesia and operation. Anesthesiology 32:343, 1970.
Eckenhoff JE: Some anatomic considerations of the infant larynx influencing endotracheal anesthesia. Anesthesiology 12:301, 1951.
Elliott E, Hanid TK, Arthur LJH, et al: Ketamine anesthesia for medical procedures in children. Arch Dis Child 51:56, 1976.
James LS, Lanman JT: History of oxygen therapy and retrolental fibroplasia. Pediatrics 57 (Suppl): 591, 1976.
Jordan WS, Graves CL, Elwyn RA: New therapy for post-intubation laryngeal edema and tracheitis in children. JAMA 212:585, 1970.
Klaus M, Meyer BP: Oxygen therapy for the newborn. Pediatr Clin North Am 13:731, 1966.
Levin RM: Pediatric Anesthesia Handbook. Flushing, NY, Medical Examination Publishing Co, 1973.
Levin RM, Seleny FL, Streczyn MV: Ketamine-pancuronium-narcotic technique for cardiovascular surgery in infants—a comparative study. Anesth Analg 54:800, 1975.
Mollison PL, Veal N, Cutbush M: Red cell and plasma volume in newborn infants. Arch Dis Child 25:242, 1950.
Nelson NM: Neonatal pulmonary function. Pediatr Clin North Am 13:769, 1966.
Nightingale DA, Richards CC, Glass A: An evaluation of rebreathing in a modified T-piece system during controlled ventilation of anaesthetized children. Br J Anaesth 37:762, 1965.
Nyhan WL: Toxicity of drugs in the neonatal period. J Pediatr 59:1, 1961.
Rackow H, Salanitre E: Modern concepts of pediatric anesthesiology. Anesthesiology 30:208, 1969.
Rita L, Seleny FL, Levin RM: A comparison of pentazocine and morphine for pediatric premedication. Anesth Analg 49:377, 1970.
Schroeder HG, Forbes AR: Massive blood replacement in neonates and children. Br J Anaesth 41:953, 1969.
Silverman WA, Sinclair JC: Temperature regulation in the newborn infant. N Engl J Med 274:92, 1966.
Smith CA, Nelson NM: The Physiology of the Newborn Infant. 4th ed, Springfield, Charles C Thomas Co, 1976.
Smith RM: Anesthesia for Infants and Children. 3rd ed, St Louis, CV Mosby Co, 1968.
Stern L, Lees MH, Leduc J: Environmental temperature, oxygen consumption and catecholamine excretion in newborn infants. Pediatrics 36:367, 1965.
Symposium on Pediatric Anesthesia. Anesthesiology 43:Aug, 1975.
Wilton TNP, Wilson F: Neonatal Anaesthesia. Oxford, Blackwell Scientific Publications, 1965.

Chapter 25

AMBULATORY ANESTHESIA SERVICES

Anesthetics were used originally for the relief of pain in the ambulatory dental patient, and the first surgical patient to receive anesthesia, James Venable, was also afoot. Subsequently, however, administration of anesthetics was almost exclusively restricted to hospitalized patients, although ambulatory anesthesia services have been more available abroad. Over the last decade, largely under the leadership of Dillon and Coakley, a resurgence in outpatient anesthesia has begun. Reed and Ford have fostered the concept of the freestanding ambulatory surgical clinic where surgical patients are treated without need for hospitalization. In addition to an ambulatory anesthesia service, the physician anesthetist has assumed additional roles in the care of ambulatory patients. Anesthesia departments can offer services to ambulatory patients in pain clinics, prenatal clinics, and pulmonary rehabilitation clinics. Each will be discussed in turn.

ANESTHESIA FOR AMBULATORY SURGICAL PATIENTS

AIMS AND ADVANTAGES

Ambulatory surgery offers a reduction in medical costs, release of beds for patients who require hospitalization, protection of patients against risks of unnecessary hospitalization, and avoidance of the disruption of the family unit attendant upon hospitalization.

PATIENT SELECTION

There can be no compromise with patient safety in providing ambulatory anesthesia. Patients of the American Society of Anesthetists' physical status classes 1 or 2 are eligible for operations with an expected duration of less than two hours, and when there is no risk of postoperative bleeding or airway obstruction. The operation should not impede the ability for immediate postsurgical ambulation. Patients must be intelligent and reliable in order to understand the instructions for pre- and postoperative care. Ambulatory surgery is ideal for those leading an active, vigorous life who would like their operations to interfere as little as possible with their daily activity. Patients must be psychologically motivated toward this mode of care.

The surgeon evaluates the patient's preoperative health status and reports it on a form that requires a statement only of pertinent positive and negative findings (Fig. 25-1, top). Nearly all accepted patients are under 40 years of age. Patients with systemic infections or those requiring emergency operations, even if otherwise qualified, may not be accepted in some facilities.

TYPES OF OPERATION

Experience with both freestanding and hospital-associated outpatient facilities shows that about one third of the procedures performed are gynecologic, an equal number general surgical, and the remaining a variety of surgical subspecialty cases. Table 25-1 lists the operations most commonly performed on ambulatory patients.

ORGANIZATION

Outpatient anesthesia services may be provided either by a freestanding clinic or by a hospital-affiliated unit. Ideally, the hospital unit should be administratively separate from the main operating rooms but close by geographically. The freestanding unit is able to deliver health care at a lower cost, not carrying the burden of community service of a general hospital.

Preparation for Anesthesia

Patients will have been screened and given instructions for preanesthetic preparation by the surgeon. A written form is usually used with instructions regarding fasting, dress, and handling of valuables, the need for an escort postoperatively, and the time and place at which to report. Instructions include an estimate of the time of discharge and a notification that hospitalization may be required to insure safety (Fig. 25-1, bottom).

Hemoglobin level, hematocrit reading, and urinalysis are obtained upon arrival at the unit or previously on an outpatient basis. More extensive laboratory evaluation is generally not required. The patient's compliance with instructions is verified and present condition and laboratory tests are checked. A brief physical examination is performed by the anesthetist. An anesthetic technique is chosen that will provide the most rapid return to function consistent with patient safety.

PASSAVANT MEMORIAL HOSPITAL
DEPARTMENT OF ANESTHESIA - OUTPATIENT ANESTHESIA
CHICAGO, ILLINOIS 60611

HOSPITAL COPY

The scheduled surgery is:

Operation _____   Patient's Name _____
Time _____
Date _____   Home Address _____

Anesthesia requested _____

_____ Home Phone No. _____

History for allergy, systemic disease and prior anesthetic problems was negative except for _____

Medications Taken: _____

Medical examination performed on _____ was essentially normal except for _____

Blood Pressure _____   Date of Lab Study _____
Results of:
  Hematology tests _____
  Urine
    Albumin _____
    Sugar _____   _____ M.D.
    Microscopic _____   Referring Surgeon

PATIENT INSTRUCTIONS

BEFORE Surgery Instructions:

1. Report to _____ Passavant Hospital at _____

   (time) _____ on _____ (date), or to Dr. _____

   office at _____ (address).

2. Wear casual clothes and leave dentures, jewelry and valuables at home
3. Eat or drink NOTHING after midnight prior to above. IMPORTANT
4. Be accompanied by an adult who will be able to provide transportation, and to take you home directly after your discharge from the

   Recovery Room area at about _____ AM/PM.

5. Admission to the hospital may be required, subject to the judgment of your attending physicians

AFTER Surgery Instructions:

1. Return home accompanied by an adult. You may be slightly dizzy.
2. Return to see your surgeon when directed.

3. Please call _____ M.D., at telephone number _____
   if you have any questions or problems.

I understand and agree to these instructions.

_____   _____
DATE   SIGNATURE

PATIENT'S COPY

Figure 25–1. Preoperative Form for Ambulatory Surgery.

Table 25-1. OPERATIONS COMMONLY PERFORMED ON AMBULATORY PATIENTS

Diagnostic D and C
Laparoscopy
Inguinal herniorrhaphy*
Myringotomy
Elective abortion*
Excision of skin lesions
Tonsillectomy and adenoidectomy*
Vasectomy
Cystoscopy
Upper extremity procedures
Extraocular muscle resection
Selected oral surgical procedures

*Disagreement exists over the appropriateness of performing these operations on an outpatient basis. A greater need for hospitalization can be anticipated in these groups.

Anesthetic Techniques

Regional anesthesia is often the best choice. Local infiltration, minor peripheral nerve blocks, and some field blocks can be performed by the surgeon. Major regional anesthesia or intravenous regional techniques require an anesthetist. Premedication is usually omitted, although atropine may be given intravenously preceding use of succinylcholine. Drugs with long-lasting effects, such as diazepam, droperidol, or ketamine, are seldom employed for outpatient anesthesia. If general anesthesia is elected, methohexital or thiamylal may be chosen in preference to thiopental because of the probability of earlier recovery. Most agree that nitrous oxide and oxygen are acceptable, supplemented by a short-acting barbiturate or opioid, or by enflurane or halothane. Fentanyl is useful because of its short action; morphine and meperidine are best avoided. Enflurane in low concentrations is cleared from the lung more rapidly than the other volatile anesthetics. Tracheal intubation is employed when necessary, using a tube of smaller size than usual to minimize tracheal irritation. Succinylcholine should be preceded by atropine. Many give 3 mg of d-tubocurarine intravenously prior to succinylcholine to prevent muscle pains postoperatively.

Postoperative Care

Adequate recovery facilities and trained recovery personnel are essential. The ambulatory patient must be more fit when discharged from the recovery room than the inpatient who is returned to a hospital bed. Time for recovery varies with the duration of anesthesia, the drugs used, the extent of the surgical procedure, and the susceptibility of the patient to vertigo, nausea, or postoperative pain. The criteria for estimation of recovery vary. All require stability of vital functions, recovery of orientation, and few residual symptoms of anesthesia or operation. Some have employed psychomotor tests, while most physicians evaluate the patient's ability to ambulate without vertigo. All ask for a responsible adult to take the patient home where recovery can take place in a familiar environment.

Before discharge from the recovery area, the patient is interviewed and examined by the anesthetist. Oral intake is limited to clear liquids until the stomach is settled, and instructions and prescriptions are given for control of pain. The patient is told of possible discomforts from the anesthesia (sore throat or muscle pains) or operation (incisional pain) and provided with a telephone number at which the anesthetist and surgeon can be reached when necessary. A telephone call to the patient the day after operation is suggested to ascertain that recovery is proceeding without complications.

Equipment

An ambulatory facility must be as fully equipped as an operating room. Equipment to monitor blood pressure, heart and breath sounds, and ECG are required. A defibrillator and emergency drugs must be readily available. Anesthesia machines and ancillary equipment must be of the same quality and as well maintained as that used for inpatients.

RESULTS

Safety

Anesthesia is delivered at the same level of safety for both inpatients and outpatients. No deaths occurred in a group of outpatient facilities surveyed by Epstein; at another center there have been no life-threatening complications or deaths in patients given more than 18,000 anesthetics in over four years of operation. Mild complications of short duration occurred in about 45 per cent of patients surveyed: nausea, drowsiness, anorexia, malaise, headache, dizziness, vomiting, and muscle pains. Fewer than 5 per cent had symptoms for more than 24 hours. More than 95 per cent of patients would recommend ambulatory care to their friends and would elect the experience again. Interestingly, the incidence of postoperative infection in herniorrhaphy and of postoperative gastroenteritis in infants operated on as outpatients was less in comparison with inpatients. Care must be taken to avoid a false sense of security because of these early successes. Lack of attention to detail will surely lead to catastrophe.

Economic Savings

Cost savings have averaged about 150 dollars per patient. It is estimated that 20 per cent of the 20 million anesthetics given each year could be given in outpatient facilities. The yearly saving accrued might total 600 million dollars in annual operating costs. Moreover, the hospital beds released could reduce the need for hospital construction at a saving calculated to be about one billion dollars. Indirect cost savings also accrue owing to the reduced incidence of complications that require treatment and the increased ability and productivity of the patient who can return to an occupation or care for a family at an earlier time.

APPRAISAL

Anesthesia care of ambulatory surgical patients can be provided safely and at a significant cost savings. Acceptance by patient and physician is good, so that this kind of care can be expected to expand because of the advantages offered. Attention must be focused continuously on maintenance of high standards of safety when ambulatory care is elected.

PULMONARY REHABILITATION CLINICS

More than 15 million patients in the United States have chronic obstructive pulmonary disease (COPD), while the American Lung Association estimates that 450,000 new patients are seen each year. COPD has become the second highest disease entity requiring social security support as a result of disability.

The patient with COPD may present with any combination of five abnormalities: emphysema, bronchitis, asthma, right heart failure, and left heart failure. The classic "pink puffer" is primarily an emphysematous patient with pulmonary vascular disease, perhaps with some element of chronic left ventricular failure and some bronchospasm. The "blue bloater" is basically the chronic bronchitic with cor pulmonale and right-sided heart failure.

The patient with COPD is chronically ill, with many physical and emotional problems. Exercise tolerance is severely diminished and there is dependence on cardiac reserves for survival. The ability to perform ordinary daily activities is lessened and a state of severe mental depression frequently exists. The physical impairment is irreversible.

The concept of rehabilitation medicine, which focuses on the patient's disability and not on impairment, is useful in approaching these patients. Improvement of disability must be stressed; the degree of impairment must be recognized but not overemphasized. Rehabilitation must stress optimal utilization of remaining lung function, good general medical care, and social, psychological, vocational, and occupational counseling. In this milieu, the anesthetist can apply those skills developed in respiratory therapy, in the operating room, and in intensive care units to assist in rehabilitation.

A program of bronchial hygiene, breathing exercises, oxygen-supported body exercises, chest physiotherapy, and home care training can be used effectively to rehabilitate the patient with COPD and to foster maximal functional performance.

Bronchial hygiene is the keystone of the treatment program. Aerosol therapy is given with one-half normal saline by mask for 15 to 20 minutes with open mouth breathing, utilizing an inspiratory pause and long expiratory times (see Chapter 32). Positive end-expiratory pressure, bronchodilators, and chest physiotherapy are used. In those patients in whom mobilization of secretions is enhanced by chest physiotherapy, members of the family are taught the techniques so that procedures may continue at home. Bronchial hygiene must be coordinated with diaphragmatic breathing; aerosol therapy and IPPB are combined with chest physical therapy. Chest expansion exercises and pursed lip exhalation are taught. Limb exercises condition the peripheral skeletal muscles and reduce oxygen consumption. Breathing and limb exercises are translated into activities of daily living such as walking, stair climbing, and bicycle riding. The patient is taught to clean and maintain the breathing equipment, to keep records of exercise activity, and to monitor sputum production. Periodic re-evaluation and re-education are stressed.

Although this program is best carried out in a rehabilitation setting, it can be delivered to ambulatory patients in any hospital environment by trained respiratory therapists and physiotherapists under the supervision of an anesthesiologist or an internist trained in pulmonary medicine. The results are encouraging. Patients who have been severely debilitated improve markedly and assume additional activities of daily living after a rehabilitation experience. Improvement in pulmonary function is readily documented and is maintained over a period of at least two years if home therapy is continued.

THE PRENATAL ANESTHESIA CLINIC

The anesthetic care of the parturient is discussed elsewhere (Chapter 23). It is important to give prenatal information on anesthesia in a quiet, relaxed atmosphere. Many institutions conduct prenatal classes for the pregnant woman and her spouse, and a few have established prenatal anesthesia clinics to allow for personal evaluation and consultation between patient and anesthetist. A history of prior anesthetic experience is obtained. Examination includes inspection of the sites usually employed for regional anesthesia. An informative discussion is undertaken concerning choice of anesthesia technique and the elements important in its selection. The establishment of a suitable rapport between the obstetric patient and the anesthetist should insure understanding and cooperation between the two.

PAIN CLINICS

Patients suffering chronic pain from both malignant and nonmalignant disease are often neglected in the medical community. Because of training in regional anesthesia, the anesthetist is uniquely equipped to cooperate with other physicians in treating these patients, participating in multidisciplinary clinics that allow full physiologic and psychological evaluation of chronic pain problems. Alternately, the anesthetist may serve as a consultant in a general hospital setting to assist in management of pain amenable to block therapy. In either circumstance, a special knowledge of pain pathways, local anesthetic drugs, and techniques of regional block should assist in the ultimate relief or amelioration of pain. Under any circumstance, it is important that the anesthetist does not serve merely as a technician but functions rather to evaluate the totality of a patient's problems. Only in this way can one discover underlying, serious pathologic processes. Psychological causes of pain occur but should not be accepted until all possible organic causes have been eliminated. A psychologist familiar with the emotional aspects of chronic pain is an essential member of a multidisciplinary pain clinic participating in evaluation and management of pain problems. Behavior modification techniques have been found helpful in rehabilitation of the patient with pain, but require hospitalization. Otherwise, the patient with chronic pain can be evaluated and treated as an outpatient. Even major regional techniques such as the administration of steroids epidurally or intrathecally can be safely managed in the ambulatory patient if adequate recovery facilities are available.

Utilization of neurolytic blocks in the management of pain is best reserved for patients with terminal disease or for treatment of pain in areas in which nerve destruction does not add significantly to disability. Under most circumstances, patients requiring neurolytic blocks are best handled by a group of consultants in a multidisciplinary clinic.

REFERENCES

Bonica JJ (ed): International Symposium on Pain. Advances in Neurology, IV. New York, Raven Press, 1974.
Bonica JJ (ed): First World Congress on Pain. New York, Raven Press, 1976.
Cohen DD, Dillon JB: Anesthesia for Outpatient Surgery. Springfield, Ill, Charles C Thomas, 1970.
Epstein BS: Outpatient anesthesia. *In* Refresher Courses in Anesthesiology, II, 81-96, 1974.
Levy ML, Coakley CS: Survey of "in and out surgery." South Med J 61:995, 1968.
Reed WA, Ford JL: The Surgicenter: An ambulatory surgical facility. Clin Obstet Gynecol 17:217, 1974.
Vandam LD, Eckenhoff JE: The anesthesiologist and therapeutic nerve block: Technician or physician. Anesthesiology 15:89, 1954.

Chapter 26

SPECIAL TECHNIQUES

DELIBERATE HYPOTENSION

Deliberate hypotension reduces bleeding into a wound, thereby providing the surgeon with both better visibility and technical freedom for a more definitive dissection; this is especially important in excision of malignancies. With less bleeding the extent of ligated or cauterized tissue is reduced, the chance of infection is minimized, and wounds heal better; the latter factor is a prime concern of plastic surgeons. In radical dissections, the need for blood replacement is decreased. Attempts at reducing blood loss by deliberate hypotension have been used for over 30 years, first by Gardner who withdrew blood to lower the blood pressure, and subsequently reinfused it. The technique failed because the hypovolemic hypotension and vasoconstriction mimicked shock and the margin of safety was low. Gillies used spinal anesthesia to lower the pressure, but the method was not quite controllable. Around 1950 Enderby and his associates employed ganglionic blockers in conjunction with general anesthesia, the prototype of techniques used today.

During the early 1950s deliberate hypotension was widely and indiscriminately applied with a variety of techniques, for many different operations and on all categories of patients. The basis of the technique was not understood nor were its limitations; thus serious complications resulted and by 1960 few American anesthetists advocated its use. Because of continued favorable experience in a few centers abroad, mainly in England, and because reports appearing in the American literature defined the physiologic and pharmacologic background more clearly, interest has quickened and deliberate hypotension is now commonly practiced.

THEORY

The physiologic basis of the technique is vasodilation, so that tilting the patient with the operative site uppermost allows blood to pool in dependent portions, thereby reducing venous return to the heart and cardiac output. Thus hypotension is most helpful when tilting effectively pools blood, that is, for operations on the head, face, neck, and upper thorax. If blood is not sequestered, venous return and cardiac output cannot be reduced and the technique is ineffective. Thus if a patient is anesthetized and operated upon while supine, bleeding from a cervical operation may be considerable even though systolic blood pressure is at 70 torr. Similarly, if vasodilation is inadequate or the level of anesthesia insufficient to prevent perception of pain, cardiac output cannot be suppressed and conditions will be unsatisfactory.

The principal fear in using deliberate hypotension is the possibility of causing insufficiency of the coronary, cerebral, or renal circulation. As noted in Chapter 27, the circulation to the brain and heart is not adrenergically controlled but responds intrinsically to metabolic demands of the myocardium and to hydrogen ion or baroreceptor alterations in the brain. With deliberate hypotension, the reduction in blood pressure and cardiac output lessens the work of the heart and thus the metabolic demands of the myocardium; a reduction in coronary blood flow is therefore acceptable. In the erect position, because of the height of the brain above heart level, the cerebral circulation is perfused at a mean pressure of from 50 to 55 torr. Consequently, a reduction in arterial pressure to that level in a supine, anesthetized individual breathing high concentrations of oxygen should be of little concern. It should be remembered that perfusion pressure is the resultant of arterial pressure minus resistance to flow across the capillary bed, minus venous pressure. A head-down position provides no protection during hypotension, because both cerebrospinal fluid pressure and cerebrovenous pressure are elevated, thus retarding flow. In the kidney, when the body is tilted head up, perfusion pressure is higher than that at heart level.

These tenets presuppose normovolemia and a normally reactive vasculature. One would not contemplate using the technique in the presence of hypovolemia or if there were symptoms or signs of circulatory insufficiency.

TECHNIQUE

The technique is composed of five components: general anesthesia, body tilt, vasodilation, positive airway pressure, and beta-adrenergic blockade. All are not necessary in every patient.

We have not found any particular regimen of preanesthetic medication better than another, although when dissections are prolonged opioids facilitate maintenance of hypotension because of peripheral circulatory dilation. Anesthesia is usually induced with an intravenous barbiturate followed by nitrous oxide-oxygen and halothane; halothane is an excellent agent because of the myocardial depressant action and facilitation of peripheral blood pooling. Controlled ventilation with at least 50 per cent oxygen via an endotracheal tube is always used to counter the changes in ventilation-perfusion ratios that accompany hypotension and tilting.

The degree of tilt is dependent upon ease of lowering blood pressure and the ability of the surgeon to work with the tilt. In general, tilt is delayed until the patient is prepared, draped, and the surgeon ready to incise; otherwise tilting without the stimulus of pain may lead to excessively low blood pressure. Obviously, the steeper the tilt, the more readily the blood pools. Some anesthetists more or less routinely use a 30-degree tilt; we aim toward 10 to 20 degrees. In many patients, particularly those in the older and less active age groups, the combination of halothane, controlled ventilation, and tilt are sufficient to produce appropriate conditions even in the absence of appreciable hypotension. In the healthy, robust, and physically active, it is necessary to use vasodilators.

Two classes of vasodilators are used. The ganglionic blockers, trimethaphan (Arfonad) and pentolinium (Ansolysen), were commonly used, but recently a vascular smooth muscle relaxant, nitroprusside (Nipride), has achieved popularity. Trimethaphan and nitroprusside both are rapid in onset and of short duration and therefore are given in a continuous infusion; the effect disappears soon after infusion is stopped. Doses of trimethaphan higher than 1 gm are not recommended because the action may persist. A direct vasodilator effect develops, histamine is released and neuromuscular block may appear. The dose of nitroprusside should not exceed 100 mg per hour so that toxic metabolites, cyanide and thiocyanate, are not formed. Pentolinium is given intermittently in intravenous doses from 5 to 15 mg, the effect lasting 45 minutes or so depending upon the level of anesthesia and degree of tilt. One fourth of this amount is repeated if needed. Pupillary dilation and lower than normal blood pressures may outlast the anesthetic; attendants must be cautioned about this. Vasodilators are usually given prior to tilt, allowing for better judgment as to the amount of tilt needed.

With a combination of general anesthesia, tilt, and a vasodilator, blood pressure can be further controlled as dictated by surgical needs by manipulation of airway pressure. Continuous application of end-expiratory pressure, 5 to 20 cm H_2O, further reduces venous return and lowers both cardiac output and blood pressure. Some hold that raised airway pressure increases venous bleeding in a cervical or facial wound, but we do not believe so because blood is returned to the heart via the vertebral venous plexus.

An occasional patient does not respond to any of these measures, especially one who is robust and physically active. Tachycardia sometimes appears, preventing lowering of the cardiac output. Enderby utilizes a beta-adrenergic blocker, propranolol, 0.035 mg per kg intravenously, or practolol, 0.14 mg per kg, to decrease heart rate and the velocity and force of myocardial contraction. Such therapy is used with extreme caution because of potential precipitation of heart failure.

A continuous infusion of an electrolyte and dextrose solution should be given all patients. In the presence of vasodilation, some clinicians give too little fluid. In major dissections, blood loss should be measured and replaced as lost, with either a balanced salt solution or whole blood when indicated.

OPERATIVE CONDITIONS

The purpose of deliberate hypotension is not to create a dry wound but to reduce bleeding to facilitate dissection. All visible vessels must be ligated even though bleeding is not brisk, because bleeding may occur when blood pressure returns to normal. There is no arbitrary level at which blood pressure is best. In the young and healthy, the usual level is 60 to 70 torr, whereas in older individuals satisfactory conditions appear at higher levels. Little is gained by depressing blood pressure more than is necessary. Nor is there an absolute limit to the duration of hypotensive anesthesia. Blood pressure is not kept at a steady level but allowed to fluctuate within reason, depending upon surgical needs. Obviously, operation should proceed with alacrity. Deliberate hypotension has been used successfully in children as young as 5 years and commonly in those in the seventh and eighth decades of life.

MONITORING

Extensive monitoring of the vital signs is not usually indicated, except that blood pressure should be monitored either by an oscillotonometer which permits accurate beat by beat observations at low pressures, or via intra-arterial recording. The electrocardiogram and heart sounds are observed as usual. We have not gained worthwhile information through electroencephalography. In procedures such as radical neck dissection and craniotomy, urinary output should also be monitored.

POSTOPERATIVE CONDITIONS

At the end of the operation, or during operation if hypotension is excessive, the procedures heretofore outlined are reversed. Positive pressure ventilation is discontinued and spontaneous respiration allowed to resume. The table is leveled. Anesthesia is lightened or discontinued. If blood pressure does not return promptly to satisfactory levels, intravenous infusion is quickened and blood volume augmented. Rarely is a vasopressor indicated. Care should be exercised in moving patients from the operating table to the recovery bed and in subsequent transportation, as the circulation may be unstable. In the recovery room monitoring is continued and the nurses are informed of the anesthetic procedure. The head of the bed should be raised only with caution, lest hypotension return. Urine output is checked. The majority of patients enjoy a remarkably smooth and uneventful recovery.

COMPLICATIONS

Unfortunately, there are no controlled studies of sufficient numbers of patients to draw valid conclusions as to the incidence of complications resulting from the use of this technique. The consensus of those most familiar with deliberate hypotension is that complications in such patients are no more frequent, if as frequent as those in similar patients operated on with normotensive levels. To obtain valid data similar risks, the same operations, and comparable age groups should be compared. However, if one fails to discover circulatory insufficiency of a vital organ preoperatively and employs deliberate hypotension, even the closest monitoring may not forewarn of trouble. There is no question that deliberate hypotension is a valuable technique, simplifying some complicated operations, making others possible, and making the results of many superior. However, the technique should not be undertaken by the unwary or the casual clinician, nor by those who have not read the relevant literature.

ANESTHESIA FOR EXTRACORPOREAL CIRCULATION

BACKGROUND

Although sporadic attempts had been made to operate on the heart, cardiac surgery began to expand only in the late 1930s along with pulmonary surgery, when anesthesia could master the problems of the open chest. The first operations were extracardiac: ligation of the patent ductus arteriosus, repair of aortic coarctation, and subclavian–pulmonary artery anastomosis for the pulmonary stenosis of the tetralogy of Fallot. During World War II, a few intrepid surgeons proceeded to remove bits of missiles from the chambers of the beating heart. This experience led to "blind" fracture or dilation of mitral and aortic stenosis. Obviously, for more intricate repair, especially in congenital heart disease, direct vision was necessary. Total body hypothermia in the vicinity of 30°C was then practiced, thus doubling the time of permissible brain ischemia, as the circulation was interrupted to permit work in the interior of the heart. Even this did not allow enough operating time, so cardiopulmonary bypass was introduced. In this procedure venous blood returning to the heart is diverted to an extracorporeal oxygenator and then returned to the aorta. In the presence of a competent aortic valve, brain and heart are thereby perfused with oxygenated blood while the heart chambers are opened and surgical correction of defects is accomplished. This kind of physiologic trespass required solution of many problems, mainly in the effects of prolonged extracorporeal, nonpulsatile blood flow on the formed elements and biochemical constitution of blood. Nonetheless, the totality of the procedure has

Special Techniques

achieved a high degree of perfection as a result of a team approach involving cardiologists, radiologists, surgeons, anesthetists, and several kinds of technicians.

THE PUMP OXYGENATOR

As the name suggests, the oxygenator contains an oxygenating device and an arterial pump. In addition, there is a heat exchanger, two additional pumps for suctioning, a coronary perfusion unit, and other devices (pressure and temperature gauges, flowmeters, injection ports, an oxygen supply, and an anesthesia vaporizer).

Several kinds of oxygenator are available (Figs. 26-1, 26-2). In the bubble type the large surface area needed for gas exchange is provided by bubbling oxygen through a layer of blood; the bubbles are then removed and the residual oxygenated blood is held in a reservoir until returned to the patient via the arterial pump. In the disc or film oxygenator, a thin film of venous blood cascades onto rotating discs or a screen. Since the bubble and disc varieties expose blood directly to the surface material and to the gas stream, a fair degree of trauma to erythrocytes results. A membrane

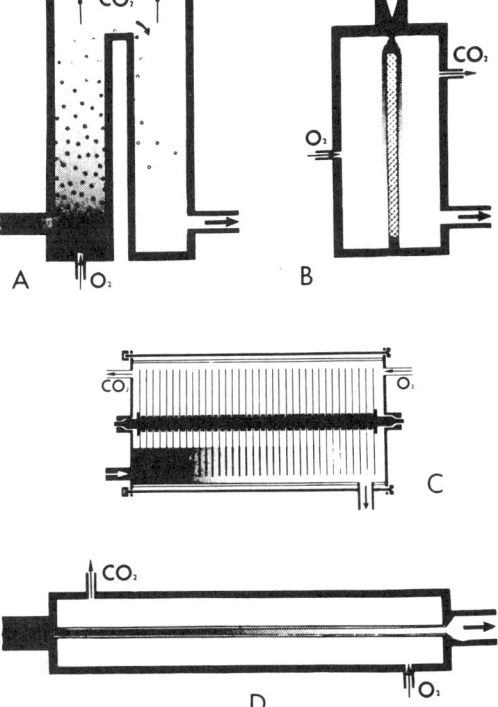

Figure 26-1. Scheme of four basic types of artificial lungs: A, bubble oxygenator; B, stationary film oxygenator; C, rotating disc oxygenator; D, membrane oxygenator. (Reproduced with permission from Norman JC (ed): Cardiac Surgery. 2nd ed, New York, Appleton-Century-Crofts, 1972.)

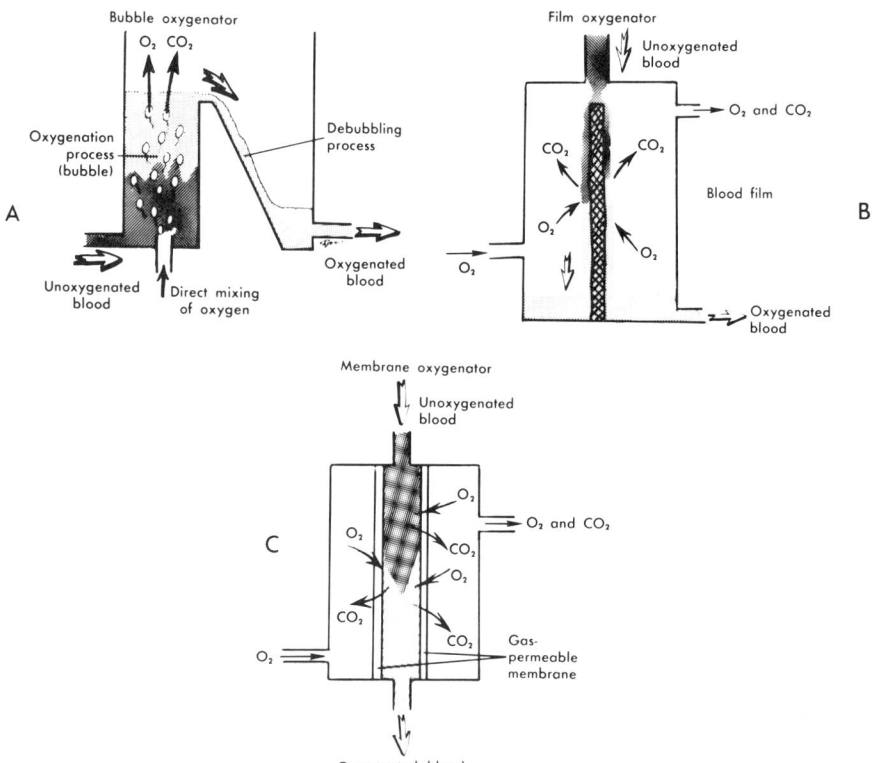

Figure 26-2. Three kinds of oxygenators: *A*, bubble oxygenator; *B*, film-type oxygenator; *C*, membrane oxygenator. (Reproduced with permission from Nosé Y: Manual on Artificial Organs. Vol II. The Oxygenator. St Louis, CV Mosby Co, 1973.)

oxygenator assays to reproduce the biologic situation in the lung, where the gas phase is separated from the film of blood by a membrane that permits diffusion of oxygen and carbon dioxide.

Any oxygenator, some now of the disposable kind, should be capable of oxygenating 5 L of venous blood per minute and removing the necessary amount of carbon dioxide. Flows advocated are based upon body mass—thus 2.4 L per sq m or 60 to 70 ml per kg of body weight. However, as the hypothermia induced lowers metabolism, flows may be lowered to 1.8 L per sq m or 40 to 50 ml per kg. The pumps are of the roller kind, not quite occluding the lines and providing a nonpulsatile flow. The heat exchanger permits control of blood temperature, allowing extracorporeal cooling or warming as required.

The pumps are primed with electrolyte solutions supplemented with albumin, potassium, antibiotics, and the like, each team having its own recipe. Thus a certain degree of hemodilution occurs during bypass circulation, which is well tolerated by patients. Hemodilution may be further augmented by removal of one or two units of the patient's blood, with electrolyte replacement immediately after induction of anesthesia. This affords two units of fresh autologous blood for infusion at the end of the procedure.

HEART DISEASE AMENABLE TO CORRECTION WITH EXTRACORPOREAL CIRCULATION

In the infant and child, for whom anesthesia is quite specialized, all manner of congenital defects are correctable, either very early in life if survival without operation is not possible or later on when operation is better tolerated. Complete transposition of the great vessels, single ventricles or auricles, and major anomalies of venous return or arterial distribution are hardly compatible with survival. Other conditions can await repair: Tetralogy of Fallot and auricular or ventricular septal defects. In all these lesions, hypoxemia, heart failure, and arrhythmias are the major consequences of failure to correct the abnormality.

In adults, acquired heart disease consitutes the main category of operations performed: rheumatic and arteriosclerotic valvular lesions and all the sequelae of coronary arteriosclerosis, such as intractable angina pectoris, old or threatening myocardial infarction, and ventricular aneurysms. Occasionally correction of constrictive pericarditis or removal of a massive pulmonary embolus is accomplished with the aid of extracorporeal circulation. In all, the chief problems are heart pump failure, arrhythmias, and associated pulmonary disease.

PATHOPHYSIOLOGY OF THE DISEASE AND PREOPERATIVE PREPARATION

At one time the mortality in cardiac operations was prohibitively high, but today coronary artery surgery can be done with an overall fatality rate in the vicinity of 1.5 to 2 per cent. This improvement has come as a result of improvement in diagnosis and better preparation for operation. Radiology offers cardiac catheterization, coronary arteriography, and echocardiography. The older therapeutic drugs—digitalis, quinidine, and procainamide—are given with a new understanding of pharmacokinetics, while recent additions such as lidocaine, propranolol, isoproterenol, and dopamine given as supportive measures permit a relatively trouble-free induction of anesthesia. It is a rare cardiac surgical patient who is not given at least ten different drugs preoperatively, some that may interact with anesthetics, as pointed out in Chapter 3. In addition to the available drugs, artificial pacemakers and electric cardioversion and defibrillation help in the management of arrhythmias, while aortic balloon counterpulsation can tide over the failing heart until improved by an operation done with extracorporeal circulation. Even if a catastrophe occurs during induction of anesthesia, the pump oxygenator, rapidly put into use, is at hand to help in resuscitation. Anesthetists must know all these things and understand the nature of the disease according to the test results provided.

Premedication and Choice of Anesthesia

More than in any other kind of patient, the right degree of sedation and analgesia, without depression, is needed in the cardiac patient. The barbiturates, diazepam, and opioids are used, while scopolamine is preferred to atropine because of its amnesic effect and slowing of heart rate. In contrast to the actions of atropine, with scopolamine the relative bradycardia decreases ventricular work and does not counteract the slowing effect of digitalis in auricular fibrillation. A variety of anesthesia techniques is available, according to the preference and experience of the team concerned. In our department the choice lies between the high dose morphine sequence (see Chapter 13) or halothane, both supplemented by nitrous oxide and a neuromuscular blocker. Thiopental, morphine, ketamine, or fentanyl and droperidol may be used for induction, while others elect methoxyflurane or neuroleptanesthesia as the main ingredient of anesthesia. In all the philosophy is the same—to provide the smallest degree of general anesthesia compatible with lack of awareness, minimal circulatory depression or excess of myocardial work, and little arrhythmogenic input. The details of management and their integration into the total scheme of extracorporeal circulation cannot be provided in the context of an introductory text, for they can only be learned by practical experience.

Preparation and Induction of Anesthesia

In Table 26-1 we provide a list of drugs and solutions that must be readied beforehand for use during extracorporeal circulation. Patients are brought to the operating room in the head-up position while breathing oxygen-enriched air, and nitroglycerine is at hand if needed for angina. Oxygen is continued throughout the preliminaries, while the defibrillator is activated as soon as the patient arrives. The pump technician is present and the pump oxygenator readied before induction in case there is a need for early use of extracorporeal assistance to the heart. The anesthesia machine will have been checked, pressure recording devices calibrated, and initial vital signs recorded, including the ECG. All these things plus those that follow require the services of two anesthetists or more. Several units of compatible blood will be at hand.

Various plastic cannulas are placed using local anesthesia beforehand or as anesthesia is induced: a peripheral intravenous infusion with 14-gauge cannula; a radial artery cannula; internal and external jugular lines; a bladder catheter with continual drainage; and a nasal or rectal temperature probe (must be placed before heparinization). The trachea is intubated with the aid of thiopental and succinylcholine, followed by the inhalation agent, attachment of the tracheal tube to a mechanical ventilator, and injection of tubocurarine or pancuronium as required. Basically, anesthesia is induced as for any general anesthetic.

Special Techniques

Table 26–1. Drugs and Solutions for Extracorporeal Circulation

Thiopental, 2.5 per cent
Succinylcholine
Tubocurarine or pancuronium
Atropine
Morphine — if the morphine technique is used.
*Isoproterenol, 2 mg, in 500 ml 5 per cent D/W
Phenylephrine 20 mg in 500 ml 5 per cent D/W
†Heparinized saline, 3000 units in 500 ml 0.9 per cent saline
Lactated Ringer's solution × 2, for peripheral IV and external jugular IV
5 per cent D/W 500 ml, with CVP set, a three-way stopcock, and a length of tubing to connect to internal jugular cannula
Lidocaine, 20 mg per ml (available in prefilled syringes for IV injection)
Sodium bicarbonate, 7.5 per cent (0.89 mEq per ml) (available in prefilled syringes for IV injection)
Heparin, 3 mg/kg body weight and protamine sulfate 4.5 mg/kg body weight, each diluted in 150 ml saline

Drugs Used for Circulatory Complications
*Lidocaine, 1000 mg in 500 ml D_5W (or 2000 mg)
*Levarterenol, 24 mg (3 amp) in 500 ml D_5W (48 μg per ml)
*Epinephrine, 2 mg in 500 ml D_5W (4 μg per ml)
*Dopamine, 800 mg (4 amp) in 500 ml D_5W (1600 μg per ml)

*Minidrip sets are used.
†Plain IV set is used with air excluded from the solution bag and IV set.

An Outline of Extracorporeal Procedure

1. Heparin, 2 to 3 mg per kg of body weight, is given intravenously before venous and aortic cannulation. Activated clotting time is measured repeatedly, held in a range of 300 to 600 seconds.
2. Partial bypass (PBP) is begun, with circulation to the body derived partly from the heart and partly from the oxygenator.
3. Total bypass (TBP) is instituted, when all venous blood is returned to the oxygenator. Ventricular fibrillation is induced electrically and venous infusions and pulmonary ventilation are stopped. Hypothermia to 28 or 30°C is induced. If the aorta is cross-clamped, the duration of occlusion is recorded. The heart may be further cooled (iced) locally and the coronary arteries separately perfused from the pump.
4. While the patient is on TBP, the anesthetist does the following: prepares a blood transfusion set using a microfilter; prepares protamine sulfate (4.5 mg per kg of body weight + 25 mg) for reversal of heparinization; readies isoproterenol for use after TBP; sends blood samples for gas and potassium analysis; and gives morphine, halothane (via a vaporizer attached to the pump), or neuromuscular blocker as required. Since the anesthetist must carefully observe the several monitoring signals, many of the technical things can be done by an assistant.
5. Off TBP and return to PPB: As the surgeon defibrillates the heart, the anesthetist renews pulmonary ventilation by hand to expand atelectatic parts of the lung. The surgeon inserts a left auricular catheter to monitor pressure, and pacemaker wires are applied to the epicardium. Monitoring proceeds and as the heart is warmed, drugs are given to treat arrhythmias or assist myo-

cardial contractility. Protamine is given and both TBP and PBP are concluded when the patient's circulation is deemed adequate. Nitrous oxide is gradually introduced only if the circulation is stable, as it may cause myocardial depression at this time. During and after extracorporeal circulation the complications that can arise are suggested by the pharmacology of the drugs that may be needed (Table 26-1) in relation to adverse changes noted on the monitors.

RETREAT FROM THE OPERATING ROOM AND POSTOPERATIVE CARE

All anesthetics will have been discontinued while respiration is mechanically controlled. Monitoring lines are disconnected from the operating room devices, to be connected to apparatus in the intensive care unit. Arterial pressure can be monitored in transit by allowing the arterial line to pressurize an air column attached to a Tycos blood pressure gauge. Respirations are controlled en route via Ambu bag and oxygen. In the intensive care unit, all monitoring and treatments that prevailed during operation are resumed, and whatever else deemed necessary is instituted.

APPRAISAL

From this brief account one can surmise that the anesthetist is a member of a team that provides a complex array of services during extracorporeal circulation of a pharmacologic, surgical, biochemical, anesthetic, and physical nature. To be at least in mental command of the situation, a considerable degree of knowledge and judgment is to be expected on the part of anesthetists. According to the degree of capability shown, the range of their involvement in the overall procedure can vary from mere giving of the anesthetic, to participation in preparation of the patient for operation, controlling the function of the pump oxygenator, providing all measurements needed, giving ancillary drugs as necessary, and assuming nearly complete responsibility for immediate postoperative care.

ACUPUNCTURE

Traditional Chinese medicine, centuries old, includes the treatment of pain by means of herbal medicines, cupping, exercising, moxibustion (application of heat to the body suface by burning a powder), and acupuncture. In many ways such regimens formed the basis for medical therapy in the United States and abroad until the advent of scientific medicine around the turn of the century. All were based on the humoral theory of disease, that is, a disturbance in the balance between beneficial and noxious influences of endogenous origin. Acupuncture is employed to regulate the flow of humors by the placement of both coarse and fine needles into the stretched skin at one or several of 642 points along 12 imaginary "canals" or medians on the body surface. The needles are usually placed far from the site of pain and the subject helps in their location by reporting on paresthesias, soreness, or discomfort. In recent years, practitioners have twirled the needles or applied mild electric currents to enhance the effect.

In 1958, Chairman Mao Tse-tung of the People's Republic of China decreed that traditional medical therapies should be combined with modern western techniques. While the enthusiasm for acupuncture was modest at first, the proletarian cultural revolution of 1968 hastened its acceptance. Although acupuncture had been in vogue in Europe on a small scale, even introduced to the United States at one time, the procedure was rediscovered in 1971 by a group of American physicians officially invited to observe the methodology of Chinese medicine. This well-meaning group, led by Paul D. White, the eminent cardiologist, subsequently reported on the amazing efficacy of acupuncture both as a method of surgical anesthesia and for the treatment of a variety of ailments, including pain. It is worth noting that the first group of American physicians spent relatively few days in China observing the application of acupuncture by an elite group of Communist physicians to a carefully selected group of patients, with the demonstrations entirely under the surveillance of the government.

As might have been forecast, there was a great rush in this country to use acupuncture in many quarters, both medical and otherwise. More than a few prominent persons thus treated attested to its benefits, legislators clamored for its inclusion in the American system of medicine, and the National Institute of Health was impelled by the Congress to offer support for the scientific study of acupuncture.

As more discerning groups observed the practice and analyzed such data as were available, acupuncture began to approach its leaven. A study group that visited China under the auspices of the American Society of Anesthesiologists came to some important conclusions. Although it had been reported that acupuncture was successful for anesthesia in 90 per cent of operations tried, the "successes" included several grades of acceptance by patients, some requiring local anesthesia in addition to premedication with a barbiturate and meperidine. Proper selection of patients was a necessity, as was considerable indoctrination of patients by both officials and other patients. Surgeons had to be able to operate quickly and gently for otherwise uncomplicated conditions. Probably fewer than 10 or 20 per cent of operations are performed in China with the aid of acupuncture, and at present the Chinese consider the procedure to be experimental with no established scientific basis.

In the United States, acupuncture anesthesia for surgical procedures has not caught on at all, and unpredictable results have been obtained in scattered groups of a few patients undergoing minor operations after lengthy preliminary acupuncture manipulations. Most unbiased observers have concluded that success hinges upon the motivation of the subject, the same reason that hypnosis has occasionally proved successful in the past.

Insofar as nonsurgical applications are concerned, acupuncture appears to be of little value in the treatment of nerve deafness and arthritis, as originally claimed, other than that expected from a placebo effect. In the treatment of chronic pain syndromes it is hardly possible to conduct a double-blind study of efficacy, for the subject perceives some changes as a result of needle placement and manipulation, whether insertions are made at the traditional points or otherwise. Minor degrees of obtundation have been detected both in dentally induced pain and in the experimental production of pain by means of heat. As the experience of pain is an unmanageable combination of sensory (physiologic) and attitudinal (psychological) variables, the two inputs have been measured separately. According to signal detection theory, the subject experiencing some degree of pain relief during acupuncture is merely disinclined to report a stimulus as painful, even though the sensory experience is basically unchanged as at comparable body sites not affected by acupuncture.

Before the effects of acupuncture can be termed mythic, a wide variety of clinical entities should be studied in association with a variety of acupunctural stimuli including voltage, current frequency, wave form, and duration of treatment.

REFERENCES

Deliberate Hypotension

Askrog VF, Pender JW, Eckenhoff JE: Changes in physiological deadspace during deliberate hypotension. Anesthesiology 25:744, 1964.

Eckenhoff JE, Rich JC: Clinical experiences with deliberate hypotension. Anesth Analg 45:21, 1966.

Enderby GEH: A report on mortality and morbidity following 9,107 hypotensive anaesthetics. Br J Anaesth 33:109, 1961.

Enderby GEH (ed): Symposium on Deliberate Hypotension. Postgrad Med J 50:555, 1974.

Epstein HM, Linde HW, Crampton AR, et al: The vertebral venous plexus as a major cerebral outflow tract. Anesthesiology 32:332, 1970.

Fahmy NR, Laver MB: Hemodynamic response to ganglionic blockade with pentolinium during N_2O halothane anesthesia in man. Anesthesiology 44:6, 1976.

Leigh JM, Millar RA (eds): Symposium on Deliberate Hypotension in Anaesthesia. Br J Anaesth 47:743, 1975.

Verner IR: Sodium nitroprusside: Theory and practice. Postgrad Med J 50:576, 1974.

Vesey CJ, Cole PV, Linnell JC, et al: Some metabolic effects of sodium nitroprusside in man. Br Med J 2:140, 1974.

Anesthesia for Extracorporeal Circulation

Laver MB: Anesthesia for open heart surgery: Its contribution to the care of the critically ill. Bull NY Acad Med 51:930, 1975.

Norman JC (ed): Cardiac Surgery, 2nd ed, New York, Appleton-Century-Crofts, 1972.

Nosé Y: Manual on Artificial Organs. Vol II. The Oxygenator. St. Louis, CV Mosby Co, 1973.

Rosky LP, Rodman T: Medical aspects of open-heart surgery. N Engl J Med 274:833 and 886, 1966.

Scheidt S, Wilner G, Mueller H, et al: Intra-aortic balloon counterpulsation in cardiogenic shock. N Engl J. Med 288:979, 1973.

Acupuncture

Bonica JJ: Therapeutic acupuncture in the People's Republic of China. Implications for American medicine. JAMA 228:1544, 1974.

Clark WC: Pain sensitivity and the report of pain: An introduction to sensory decision theory. Anesthesiology 40:272, 1974.

Veith I: Acupuncture therapy—past and present. JAMA 180:476, 1962.

Part F

UNTOWARD SEQUELAE OF ANESTHESIA

Chapter 27

ARTERIAL HYPOTENSION DURING ANESTHESIA

Experienced anesthetists view the significance of blood pressure somewhat differently from most of their medical colleagues, and with good reason. Physicians generally record blood pressure in individuals with normally functioning sympathetic nervous systems, who are conscious, have normal muscle activity, and are breathing room air. The anesthetist commonly supervises the supine, often paralyzed, unconscious patient whose sympathetic nervous activity may be depressed and whose respiration is assisted or controlled by higher than normal concentrations of oxygen. Thus, the two situations are quite different. As recorded peripherally, blood pressure signifies the pressure driving blood through the circulation; considered as an independent observation, pressure means little except at extreme values. Of greater consequence is the resulting tissue perfusion, equally dependent upon sympathetic vasoconstrictor tone.

While many patients manage to maintain a relatively normal blood pressure during anesthesia and operation, it is common to observe a reduction from normal values. Hypotension *per se* is not so important; rather it is the degree and the cause that concern the anesthetist, for one can have adequate perfusion secondary to vasodilation, while at the same low pressure perfusion would be inadequate if vasoconstriction were present. One should learn to appraise the patient's overall condition. The initial reaction to hypotension is often one of alarm—blood pressure should not be so low and energetic treatment must be undertaken! The urge to respond irrationally must be suppressed. Is the skin warm and dry, is the color of blood in the wound satisfactory, and is the pulse full and regular, even though systolic blood pressure may be recorded at 70 torr? If the answers are yes, this hemodynamic situation is obviously different from one at the same level of blood pressure in which the skin is cold and blue, the pulse rapid and thready, and the blood in the wound dark.

We shall discuss some of the common causes of arterial hypotension, as follows: excessive premedication, influence of potent therapeutic drugs given prior to anesthesia, relative or absolute overdose of general anesthetics, circulatory effects of spinal and peridural anesthesia, raised airway pressure, hypovolemia and hemorrhage, surgical manipulation and stimulation, change in position of the patient, and cardiovascular disease. Incompatible transfusion, septic shock, and less common causes of hypotension will also be discussed.

GENERAL CONSIDERATIONS

Blood pressure is the circulatory sign most often recorded during anesthesia, perhaps because the measurement is so relatively simple and traditional. To evaluate the significance of any blood pressure reading, one must consider cardiac output and peripheral vascular reactivity (arteriolar resistance) the principal determinants of blood pressure, and blood volume and peripheral vascular reactivity (venous return) as these contribute to cardiac output. Measurement of these several variables is hardly practical during anesthesia, so their adequacy must be judged indirectly. We shall refer to these judgments throughout this chapter.

Circulation is so regulated to maintain adequate blood flow to the brain and heart, the two most vulnerable vascular beds because of their high metabolic demands. Thus, aspects of the coronary and cerebral circulations are worth noting. The coronary circulation responds to the metabolic demands of the work done by the heart, as determined primarily by mean arterial blood pressure and cardiac output. Coronary vessels are not adrenergically controlled but dilate or constrict in response to oxygen need. Reduction in mean blood pressure decreases cardiac work, and even though accompanied by a lesser volume of coronary blood flow, the requirements of the heart can usually be met. Similarly, with vasodilation, blood pools peripherally, venous return lessens, and cardiac output diminishes. Both can have a salutary effect through lowered cardiac work, unless the decrease in blood pressure precludes adequate coronary blood flow. All these tenets presuppose normally reactive coronary vessels; however, in the presence of coronary arteriosclerosis, the vessels may be unable to respond to myocardial demand. Here blood pressure becomes the principal determinant of coronary flow and a lowering of pressure may be harmful.

The cerebral circulation is likewise essentially without autonomic influence, but flow is regulated by arterial carbon dioxide tension acting through changes in hydrogen ion concentration and also by mean perfusion pressure. In a supine individual mean perfusing arterial blood pressure can fall quite low, to 50 torr, and still be the equivalent of the perfusion pressure in an erect person, assuming an erect mean pressure of 85 torr at the base of the heart and a 35 cm difference in height to the base of the brain. The brain normally extracts only about 25 per cent of the oxygen delivered to it while the heart, a working muscle, removes nearly 80 per cent. The brain, therefore, has considerable oxygen reserves without a need to increase blood flow, while the heart must either increase the volume of coronary blood flow or decrease myocardial oxygen requirements.

CAUSES OF HYPOTENSION

EXCESSIVE PREMEDICATION

The tendency of the opioids to lower arterial blood pressure is well known. Several pharmacologic actions contribute to this, including depression of the vasomotor center, reduction in skeletal muscle tone, depression of respiration, and dilation of peripheral blood vessels owing to a direct action or secondary to release of histamine. Circulatory depression often takes the form of postural hypotension, an intolerance to the upright position. Passive tilt to the 50- or 60-degree head-up position is used experimentally to demonstrate derangement of circulation induced by drugs. The inference then is that the opioids will reduce the ability to compensate for circulatory stress such as hemorrhage, trauma, or change in position. While this can clearly be demonstrated with tilt after administration of morphine or meperidine to the healthy patient, it is of interest that morphine and other opioids in large doses are used as analgetics in poor risk patients for operation, as outlined in Chapter 13. This is not to suggest that the circulatory response to tilt is unimportant or that opioids in the elderly or very ill are not without risk, but rather to point out that advantage is taken of these analgetics under highly controlled conditions in which intra-arterial pressure is monitored continuously and vasopressor drugs and fluids are immediately available. However, opioids administered intravenously during routine anesthesia or postoperatively, before patients recover completely from general anesthesia, may be followed by hypotension. For this reason it is best to reduce the dose of opioid (2.5 mg of morphine or 25 mg of meperidine), to give incremental doses, and to observe the blood pressure response.

Several of the barbituric acid derivatives, secobarbital and pentobarbital, for example, disturb the circulation least when given in 50 to 150 mg doses intravenously or intramuscularly before anesthesia. However, larger doses may depress the circulation at several levels. Similarly, diazepam, now commonly used for premedication, rarely causes hypotension in the usual therapeutic doses. The incidence of complications rises sharply when opioids are combined with either barbiturates or diazepam. Although it is sometimes difficult to judge accurately the amount of premedication that will produce the desired tranquility without reaction, it is safer to err on the side of smaller doses than to seek marked sedation at the risk of arterial hypotension.

INFLUENCE OF POTENT THERAPEUTIC DRUGS USED PRIOR TO ANESTHESIA

Some drugs used in modern therapeutics can affect the course of anesthesia unfavorably, as discussed in Chapter 3. While drugs with this potential do not invariably cause hypotension, it is important to obtain a history of all medications the patient has received. Of chief concern are the adrenal steroids, the antihypertensives, the beta-adrenergic blockers, and the tranquilizers, drugs that may merely potentiate the moderate reduction in blood pressure often seen with general anesthetics. Rarely, a patient may develop profound hypotension during or following anesthesia under these circumstances.

OVERDOSE OF GENERAL ANESTHETICS

Overdose of general anesthetics is a common cause of arterial hypotension. The overdose may be "absolute" or "relative"; in the former case, the amount of drug administered is in excess of that ordinarily tolerated by a normal patient. This may result from a sudden increase in the inspired concentration of an inhalation anesthetic or intravenous injection of a large amount of barbiturate.

Certain additional factors predispose to "absolute" overdose. As the patient's tissues approach saturation, the smaller is the increment of anesthetic required to cause a rise in blood concentration. Overdose, therefore, tends to occur during prolonged anesthesia when large amounts of drug have been absorbed. Overdose with irritant volatile anesthetics occurs more easily if the trachea has been intubated, for the protective action of laryngeal closure is no longer present and pulmonary uptake can be considerable, especially if respiration is assisted or controlled. Overdose also tends to occur at the extremes of age and in the presence of unrecognized hypothermia such as may develop during prolonged thoracic or abdominal operations when appropriate measures to maintain or monitor body temperature have not been taken.

In "relative" overdose the actual amount of drug given is acceptable for the age and weight of the patient but represents, at the time, a larger dose than is tolerable, a sensitivity more apparent than real. In the presence of reduced circulating blood volume the concentration of inhalation anesthetic increases more rapidly. If vasoconstriction in other body areas is present but blood flow to the heart or brain is maintained, depression can result from addition to the blood of ordinarily innocuous amounts of anesthetics. Under either circumstance, a higher concentration of anesthetic is presented to the vital organs than expected from the small amount given.

Though we have referred to hypotension in the context of overdose, we remind the reader that the pharmacologic response to progressive deepening of anesthesia with all general anesthetics entails peripheral vasodilation and reduced myocardial contractility. With halothane, enflurane, and methoxyflurane, for example, the blood pressure response is a good guide to depth of anesthesia, especially when these agents are given without a neuromuscular blocker (see Chapter 16). On the other hand, there are studies that show that the circulatory depressant actions of anesthetics tend to ameliorate with time.

Prevention of arterial hypotension resulting from overdose involves two principles: administering the least amount of anesthetic compatible with adequate surgical conditions, and taking the time to induce anesthesia gradually or to change from one level to another slowly. The surgeon should recognize that the optimal depth of anesthesia is that safest for the patient. A patient may tolerate a given blood concentration of anesthetic provided it develops slowly, whereas the same concentration rapidly produced may cause profound hypotension.

Treatment of overdose with inhalation agents comprises prompt reduction of the inspired anesthetic concentration or elimination of the anesthetic from the circuit and, if necessary, assisted ventilation may be utilized to facilitate lowering the concentration in blood. If the drugs concerned are eliminated in the main by routes other than the lungs, the general supportive measures listed at the end of this chapter are instituted.

VASCULAR ABSORPTION OF LOCAL ANESTHETICS

Rapid absorption of local anesthetics from mucous membranes or other highly vascular tissues may cause marked hypotension (see Chapter 17). Probable causes of lowered blood pressure include depression of the myocardium and the vasomotor centers, as well as dilation of peripheral vessels as a result of direct action. Prior administration of a barbiturate does not protect against these effects and, indeed, may heighten circulatory depression.

Critically ill and elderly patients scheduled for local anesthesia are often unattended during operation; we are aware that deaths have occurred under this circumstance. An anesthetist or another person trained in observing patients and recording blood pressure might well attend all patients, especially those in poor physical condition, in whom extensive use of local anesthesia is planned.

Hypotension can be minimized by reducing the total quantity of anesthetic injected per unit of time. Use of large volumes of concentrated solutions and rapid injection are chiefly responsible for elevation of blood levels to dangerous levels. When topical anesthesia is used, the same principles apply; application is done slowly to avoid rapid vascular absorption. Cocaine limits its own absorption through local vasoconstriction and therefore is less likely to cause hypotension than tetracaine or lidocaine, which are not vasoconstrictors.

Treatment consists of the general supportive measures described at the end of this chapter.

SPINAL AND PERIDURAL ANESTHESIA

The reasons for the fall in blood pressure often observed after spinal and peridural anesthesia have been discussed in Chapters 18 and 19. Briefly, reduction in total peripheral resistance or a decline in cardiac output occurs, the former resulting from paralysis of sympathetic vasoconstrictor fibers to arterioles, the latter a response to pooling of blood in the dilated capacitance vessels with consequent reduction in venous return to the heart. Similar alterations are associated with peridural anesthesia.

A pressor drug such as ephedrine 25 to 50 mg, or phenylephrine 2 to 3 mg, injected intramuscularly three to five minutes prior to administration of anesthesia reduces the incidence of arterial hypotension. Prophylaxis is indicated in the elderly, in whom vascular reactivity may be diminished, and in all patients in whom a decrease in systemic pressure may result in serious impairment of blood flow to the heart and brain, as in patients with hypertension, coronary arterial disease and generalized arteriosclerosis, and those with a history of impaired cerebral blood flow. If, after prophylactic administration of a pressor drug, spinal anesthesia does not result, the rise in systolic arterial pressure resulting from the pressor drug rarely exceeds 40 torr, an elevation that probably occurs spontaneously in all patients from time to time.

Alternative approaches to the prophylactic use of vasopressors should be considered for patients in whom an elevation in blood pressure or cardiac rate is more to be feared. The first is the establishment of a reliable intravenous infusion before performing lumbar puncture. If hypotension appears after intrathecal injection, a previously prepared dilute solution of a vasopressor is infused at a rate approximating the patient's accustomed pressure (phenylephrine 10 mg in 500 ml of 5 per cent dextrose in water). If the fall in blood pressure is precipitous, therapy may be too late. A second alternative is to infuse 500 ml of lactated Ringer's solution rapidly before the lumbar puncture to expand the vascular space and lessen the probability of hypotension.

To prevent a catastrophe that can be associated with a sudden reduction in blood pressure, the anesthetist must recognize that hypotension can develop immediately upon intrathecal injection of the local anesthetic. Repeated measurement of blood pressure is therefore essential until anesthesia stabilizes. Treatment must be prompt. If possible, the legs should be raised to provide autotransfusion. The entire body should not be tilted head down lest a higher level of anesthesia develop. Oxygen supplementation to respiration is begun. A vasopressor is given intravenously and fluids are infused rapidly unless otherwise contraindicated.

RAISED AIRWAY PRESSURE

Positive pressure applied to the airway may lower arterial pressure (Fig. 27-1). Raised airway pressure is transmitted to the large intrathoracic blood vessels and to pulmonary capillaries as well. The higher the mean level of pressure, the lower the blood flow through these vessels, and cardiac output diminishes in proportion to the degree of interference with venous return. As cardiac output and arterial pressure fall, compensatory vasoconstriction in both venous and arterial circulations is initiated via baroreceptor discharge. A normal individual can tolerate reasonable degrees of raised airway pressure through this ability to constrict peripheral vessels, especially those of the venous capacitance system.

This phenomenon is of greater significance in the following situations: in hypovolemia, when the sympathetic nervous system is hypoactive in the physically unfit; following use of ganglionic blocking drugs and general anesthetics, when positive airway pressure is maintained throughout the respiratory cycle; and when the patient is in the head-up position, so that blood is pooled in dependent portions of the body. Other changes occurring during anesthesia can either oppose or enhance the decrease in arterial pressure. These relate to central venous pressure, abdominal muscle tone, and peripheral vasoconstriction (Fig. 27-2). Congested intrathoracic veins collapse less readily in response to external pressure than when venous pressure is normal. Cyclopropane and ether increase central venous pressure, affording a measure of protection, whereas halothane and enflurane decrease central venous pressure. The hypotensive response is muted in the presence of constrictive pericarditis, expanded blood volume, mitral

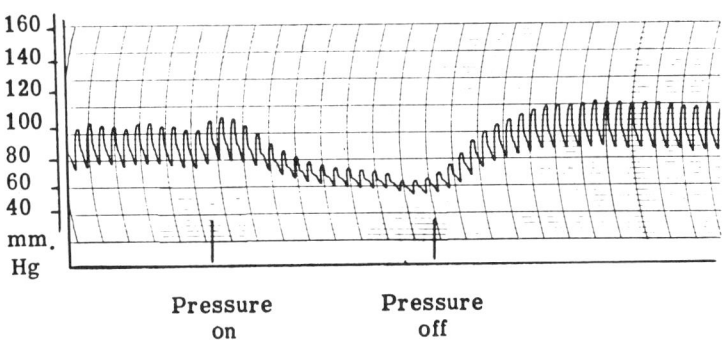

Figure 27-1. Arterial hypotension following the application of 20 cm H_2O pressure to the airway of a patient under general anesthesia.

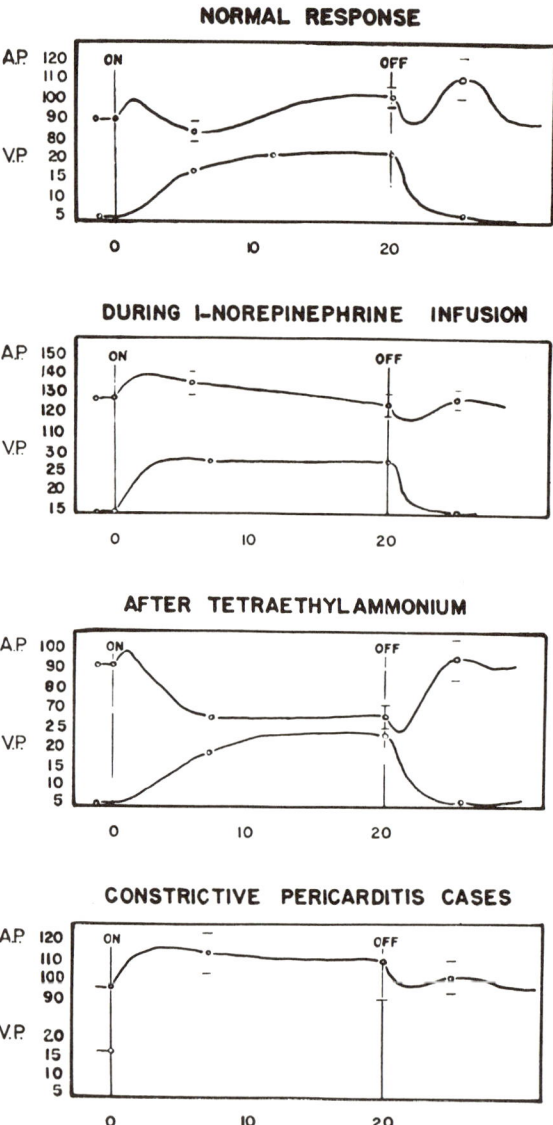

Figure 27–2. Normal arterial pressure response to raised airway pressure, together with alterations in response to the same degree of pressure produced by norepinephrine (normal vasoconstriction), tetraethylammonium (sympathetic blockade), and constrictive pericarditis (raised venous pressure). (Reproduced with permission from Price HL: Proceedings of Conference on the Myoneural Junction, Columbia University and Burroughs Wellcome & Co, 1955.)

stenosis, or congestive heart failure. If abdominal wall tone resists the transmitted intrapulmonic pressure, higher pressures are transmitted to intrathoracic structures. Deep planes of general anesthesia, spinal anesthesia, or neuromuscular blockers afford protection against raised airway pressure through the resulting abdominal muscle relaxation, but the protection is offset by diminished reactive vasoconstriction. If the thorax is open, less pressure is transmitted to the great veins but pressure is still transmitted to the capillaries.

Prevention or treatment of hypotension consists of decreasing the level and duration of pressure applied to the airway. If pulmonary ventilation thereby becomes inadequate, intermittent positive and negative pressure respiration provided by a mechanical ventilator is said to be useful, or a return to spontaneous breathing may be permitted.

HEMORRHAGE

Arterial hypotension follows either loss of whole blood or, in extensive operations, loss of plasma into the tissues. Unfortunately, estimation of the amount of blood lost during operation is faulty. The technique of weighing sponges and subtracting the dry from the wet weight permits a reasonably accurate appraisal of loss, allowing for blood replacement on a sounder basis. This does not, however, take into account "third space loss." Monitoring of central venous pressure is a fair guide to fluid and blood replacement requirements (Chapters 8 and 22), but a high degree of suspicion is important when measured or estimated losses do not account for clinical evidence of hypotension.

Hypotension and tachycardia are often late signs of blood loss in the recumbent healthy patient, except in acute major loss; bradycardia is common, especially in children and in the presence of hypoxia. A pale, moist skin and narrow pulse pressure are suggestive, as are restlessness and ischemic changes on the electrocardiogram. Urinary output is a sensitive guide, particularly so postoperatively when occult bleeding is the basis for progressive hypotension.

Hemodilution takes place slowly so that determination of hemoglobin or hematocrit values is of little immediate value. Determinations of blood volume are not useful unless preoperative measurements are available and bleeding has ceased. Occasionally the presence of blood intraperitoneally can be demonstrated by culdotomy or peritoneal tap.

If considerable blood loss is anticipated, one or more 14- to 16-gauge intravenous catheters is placed so that blood can be administered rapidly, under pressure if necessary. The hazards involved are discussed in Chapter 22.

The necessity of having sufficient whole blood typed, crossmatched, and available prior to elective major operation is obvious. In an emergency, type O universal donor blood of low A or B titer can be used, although a 10-minute saline crossmatch is preferred. On the other hand, considerable hemodilution with lactated Ringer's solution is well tolerated, as witnessed during extracorporeal circulation and in operations on Jehovah's Witnesses who will not accept blood products. One should not overlook the value of blood component therapy or dextran in moderate quantities as plasma expanders.

SURGICAL MANEUVERS

Surgical manipulation in the neck, thorax, or abdomen is a common cause of arterial hypotension, explainable on a mechanical or reflex basis. Venous return to the heart may be obstructed by surgical packs, torsion or compression of large veins by retractors, gallbladder or kidney rests, or by pressure of the gravid uterus or large abdominal tumors upon the inferior vena cava. Rapid release of increased intra-abdominal pressure during drainage of ascites or delivery of a large abdominal tumor may be followed by hypotension as a result of pooling of blood in dilated veins. Rapid decompression of a distended urinary bladder can also cause hypotension.

Hypotension may reflexly follow traction on the gallbladder, bowel, uterus, or mesentery, or stimulation of the parietal peritoneum in the upper abdomen (Fig. 27-3). If the patient is conscious during regional anesthesia, such manipulation may also cause pain, nausea, vomiting, and breath-holding. Reflex hypotension is not limited to stimulation intraperitoneally but may follow manipulation in the chest or stimulation of periosteum or joint cavities. It is presumed that the autonomic nervous system is involved in these reactions, but whether afferent impulses ascend via sympathetic, phrenic, or vagal pathways is not clear. In the upper abdomen the intercostal nerves are believed to carry some of these impulses. As a result of afferent impulses, both inhibition of sympathetic activity and increased vagal tone on the heart have been shown. Atrial contraction contributes to ventricular filling, and vagal-induced reduction in contractility may participate in the diminished stroke volume observed. A puzzling aspect of the hypotension observed during surgical activity is the absence of bradycardia on some occasions and its presence at other times. Atropine given intravenously is useful in its treatment. Peripheral vasodilation may play a role in some instances.

Some evidence suggests that reflexes are more active during the lighter planes of general anesthesia and may be partially or completely blocked in the deeper planes, or inhibited by neuromuscular blockers that interfere with ganglionic transmission (Chapter 14).

Serious hypotension may result when a surgeon removes clamps from

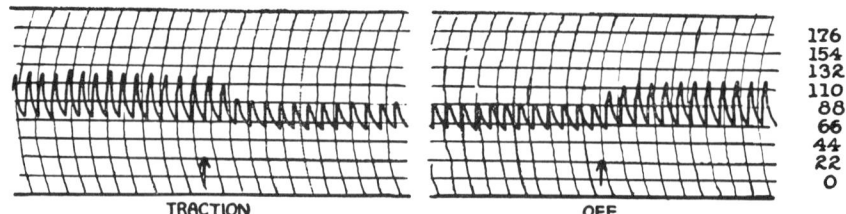

Figure 27-3. Continuous intra-arterial pressure tracing showing abrupt reduction of pulse pressure with traction on the mesentery of the colon of an anesthetized patient. Numbers at right represent torr.

the aorta, or if both aorta and vena cava are occluded simultaneously, obstructing venous return. Hypoxemia, hypotension, and even cardiac arrest have followed total hip replacement owing either to absorption of monomeric methyl methacrylate, a component of the bone cement, or to another as yet undefined cause. More care in preparation of the cement at operation has lessened the incidence of this complication. Carotid sinus stimulation may occur during operations on the neck, resulting in vagal-induced bradycardia and hypotension; local anesthetic infiltration or atropine given intravenously mutes this response.

Gentleness on the part of surgeons and awareness of the consequences of their maneuvers constitute the basis for prevention and treatment of hypotension resulting from surgical manipulation. The anesthetist must be aware of the surgeon's actions at all times and remain in constant communication.

CHANGE IN POSITION OR MOVING THE PATIENT

The circulation of the anesthetized patient is less able to compensate for stress than that of the unanesthetized one, particularly in those critically ill (Fig. 27-4). Change in position to the lateral decubitus may cause a marked reduction in arterial pressure. Positional changes should be accomplished slowly and gently and the blood pressure observed throughout.

Certain operative positions may be poorly tolerated; the lateral decubitus and flexion required for exposure of the kidney or adrenal gland are good examples. Operations performed in the sitting position are often

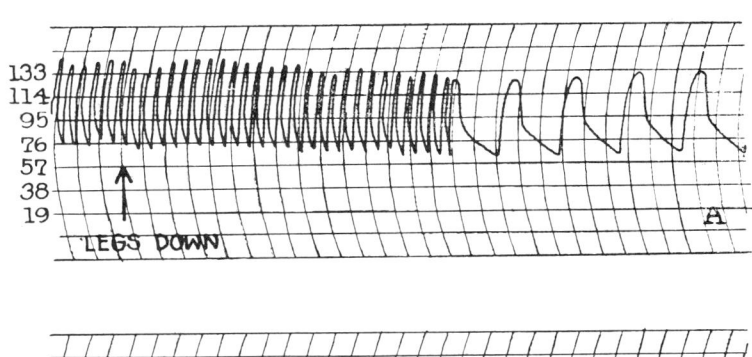

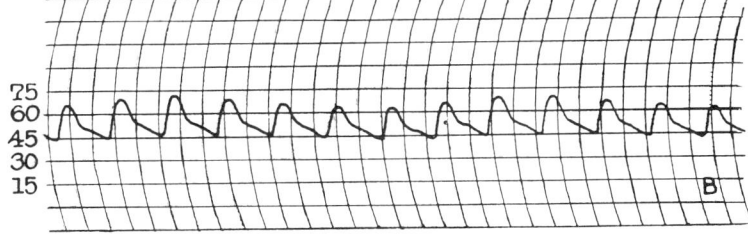

Figure 27-4. Development of postural hypotension after patient who had been in the lithotomy position was placed supine. Time between *A* and *B* in the arterial pressure tracing was two minutes. Numbers represent torr.

complicated by hypotension. Here the legs should be wrapped in Ace bandages beforehand. In patients in poor physical condition it is helpful to test the cardiovascular response to the anticipated position before anesthesia is induced.

CARDIOVASCULAR DISEASE

Myocardial ischemia or infarction during anesthesia may be followed by a profound fall in blood pressure. Diagnosis is usually difficult and rarely established until the ischemia is of several hours' duration. Hypotension may accompany ventricular tachycardia, e.g., in patients with mitral stenosis who are not adequately digitalized. Multifocal ventricular tachycardia commonly noted during cyclopropane anesthesia may compromise diastolic filling of the heart; blood pressure then declines. Nodal rhythm, through alteration of the auricular-ventricular filling pattern, may reduce cardiac output and cause hypotension.

Embolism to any of several vascular beds may lead to hypotension, the cause of which is not readily recognized. Cerebral embolism is a precipitating factor in hypotension as seen during closed mitral valvuloplasty. Usually this involves the brainstem and other neurologic signs are present. Pulmonary embolism from peripheral veins may occur, as may fat embolism from fracture sites, amniotic fluid emboli during delivery, and venous air entrainment during cervical operations or craniotomy. Massive embolism is suspected with the appearance of a pattern of acute cor pulmonale on the electrocardiogram.

Hypovolemia may be present prior to operation. Dehydration, hemorrhage, loss of gastrointestinal fluids, and plasma loss in extensive burns contribute to this state. If hypovolemia is not recognized, dilation of the vascular bed associated with induction of anesthesia is often followed by hypotension. Deficit of both extravascular and intracellular fluid can be a factor in circulatory inadequacy. This is inextricably related to sodium concentration so that both fluid and electrolyte imbalance can be associated with hypotension. Furthermore, the electrolyte environment of the peripheral circulation is a major influence in the response to endogenously secreted catecholamines and adrenal steroids.

Cardiac tamponade may be an unsuspected cause of hypotension. This follows penetrating injury of the heart, or cardiotomy, or may be a complication of anticoagulant therapy.

Heart failure may develop during anesthesia and operation as a result of excessive fluid replacement or in relation to the circulatory complications noted. Failure is relatively easily diagnosed by a rising central venous pressure in the face of a falling arterial pressure, by engorgement of neck veins, and the presence of rales on auscultation of the lungs. Treatment involves digitalization, phlebotomy, and, in resistant cases, cautious intravenous use of isoproterenol or dopamine.

In refractory cardiogenic shock, intra-aortic balloon counterpulsation seems promising in tiding a patient over until blood pressure can be maintained spontaneously.

SEPTIC SHOCK

Septic shock rarely appears for the first time during anesthesia and operation; either it is present preoperatively and operation is attempted in the hope of removing the source of infection, or it develops postoperatively owing to spread of a previously contained infection or contamination of a wound.

Septic shock is commonly caused by *Escherichia coli, Aerobacter aerogenes, Pseudomonas aeruginosa,* clostridia, or *Staphylococcus aureus,* and it is related to the release of endotoxins that potentiate the action of catecholamines, eventually causing major plasma loss in tissues. In the fully developed syndrome, severe hypotension is accompanied by tachycardia, the skin is cold and blanched, and tissue perfusion is inadequate. But early in the course the skin may be hot and dry. Whether endotoxins depress the central nervous system by direct action in addition to depressing the myocardium and the smooth muscle of blood vessels is not known.

Treatment of septic shock varies. In addition to standard supportive therapy, control of fever, and use of antibiotics, vasodilator therapy with concomitant use of large volumes of plasma or balanced salt solution is also instituted. This treatment is predicated upon a significant element of vasoconstriction. Massive steroid therapy has been advised, with repeated doses of 2 gm or more given intravenously; the pharmacologic actions have not been clearly delineated. Presumably, steroids establish a better balance at peripheral vascular sites between catecholamines, steroids, and electrolytes. Since myocardial failure may occur, digitalis is indicated, perhaps isoproterenol or dopamine, and certainly respiratory assistance with oxygen. Central venous pressure is a good guide to therapy but the observation must be correlated with systemic blood pressure, urinary output, and periodic testing with intravenous infusions, as outlined in Chapter 22. Central venous pressure may not be elevated in the presence of left-sided heart failure; hence the suggestion that pulmonary capillary wedge pressure be used as a guide.

INCOMPATIBLE TRANSFUSION

Major blood group incompatibility reactions may be accompanied by hypotension. Indeed, together with generalized cyanosis and oozing at the operative site, unexplained hypotension should suggest the possibility of a hemolytic transfusion reaction (see Chapter 22).

ANAPHYLACTIC REACTION

One kind of allergic reaction to extrinsic antigens involves the presence of circulating antibodies in the serum of the host. Anaphylaxis is an example of this response, which also includes serum sickness, allergy involving the wheal and flare reaction, angioneurotic edema, urticaria, asthma, and certain drug reactions. The reactions observed are frequently referred to as "immediate." This is perhaps the least common cause of hypotension observed by anesthetists, but an anaphylactic reaction with severe hypotension has been reported during spinal anesthesia upon administration of a small amount of dextran (a macromolecular polysaccharide of bacterial origin) and after injection of penicillin. Some degree of protection against anaphylaxis by general anesthetics has been demonstrated, but since there are varying degrees of reaction, it is reasonable to assume that general anesthesia offers protection only against the mild reaction. Treatment consists of administration of oxygen by positive pressure to overcome bronchospasm, administration of epinephrine intramuscularly or by vein, and infusion of aminophylline followed by hydrocortisone. Antihistamines are of little value once the reaction has occurred.

MANAGEMENT OF HYPOTENSION

DIAGNOSIS

The standard means of diagnosing inadequacy of the circulation include measurement of arterial blood pressure, counting the pulse, and estimating the pulse volume as an index of the volume of cardiac ejection or run-off in the peripheral circulation. In healthy young adults a systolic blood pressure of 80 torr may require no treatment, whereas a similar finding in an elderly patient with arteriosclerosis and hypertension constitutes a threat to life. A conscious patient in whom cerebral ischemia develops secondary to a decrease in blood pressure will be restless, anxious, and even disoriented. One can occasionally detect waxing and waning of mental acuity in such patients during alterations in the rate of infusion of a pressor drug. Pallor, cold wet skin, and dilated pupils suggest circulatory inadequacy, as does peripheral cyanosis. The rate of capillary refill upon application of pressure to the skin is sometimes used as an index of the state of the peripheral circulation. Deep sighing respirations or air hunger in a conscious individual suggest a severe degree of shock. Presumably, respiratory stimulation is initiated via carotid sinus pressor receptors. Delayed onset of anesthesia after injection of intravenous anesthetics suggests a sluggish circulation. If an intravenous infusion slows, venoconstriction is suggested as compensating for circulatory inadequacy. Similarly, a reduction in bleeding in the operative field, unusually dark venous blood, and pallor of organs reflect hypotension and compensatory vasoconstriction. Urine output shows a close relationship to the adequacy of renal circulation.

PROPHYLAXIS

Under the several causes of hypotension, preventive measures have been suggested. These include: avoidance of drug overdose in premedication and in local or general anesthesia; gentleness in surgical manipulation; care in movement of the patient; prompt replacement of blood and fluid losses; and circumspect application of pressure to the airway. These and other measures, when coupled with minute-to-minute observation of the patient, go far toward preventing circulatory collapse, which, unfortunately, is not always avoidable. Treatment must be prompt!

GENERAL THERAPEUTIC MEASURES

The aim of treatment should be to augment perfusion of vital organs, which usually does not require a systolic pressure higher than 70 torr so long as other factors impeding oxygen and carbon dioxide transport are not operative. If circumstances permit, elevation of the legs may increase the blood pressure through mobilization of pooled blood, especially after sympathetic blockade. One must also consider relief of pain in the traumatized patient, remembering that use of opioids for pain may produce hypotension. Small doses are safest—such as 2.5 mg morphine given intravenously—and repeated if necessary.

Fluid Therapy

Rapid intravenous administration of any of a variety of solutions may be lifesaving during severe hypotension. The volume of fluid given rather than its composition is vital in the early moments, especially if hypotension is the result of trauma or blood loss. The initial selection, therefore, is based on what is immediately at hand. Physiologic saline, 5 per cent dextrose in water, a balanced salt solution, a plasma expander such as 6 per cent dextran, or plasma or serum albumin are given until whole blood becomes available. Some commercial 5 per cent solutions of plasma protein fractions can worsen hypotension, presumably through a vasodilator action not present in 5 per cent albumin.

Chapters 21 and 22 should be consulted for further details. When possible, and especially in the elderly, critically ill, or injured, therapy should be monitored via measurement of pulmonary wedge pressure, central venous pressure, and urine output.

Oxygen Therapy

Oxygen should be breathed while a diagnosis is being established and continued as therapy. To assure adequacy of ventilation, respiration must be assisted with care to prevent excessive airway pressure. If general anesthetics are administered, they should be discontinued or sharply reduced in concentration. If the patient remains hypotensive at the end of operation, oxygen should be continued postoperatively.

Vasopressor Drugs

These agents are indicated in the therapy of hypotension if the systolic blood pressure has not responded to the measures already outlined or when signs of inadequate perfusion to vital organs persist. The commonly used pressor drugs are sympathomimetic amines that exert a vasoconstrictor action through stimulation of alpha receptors of the sympathetic system, or via increase of myocardial contractile force and heart rate by activation of beta receptors. Vascular responses induced by the two kinds of receptors are as follows: Alpha: constriction of vascular smooth muscle, cutaneous vessels, mucosa, kidney, and splanchnic circulation; beta: positive inotropic activity, stimulation of sinoatrial node, and dilation of blood vessels in skeletal muscle and splanchnic bed.

Selection of the most appropriate pressor drug for therapy of hypotension is not easy. Some drugs have been studied in individuals with normal blood pressures, but few have been completely evaluated in the treatment of hypotension observed under clinical circumstances. As it is in the latter situation that these substances find most use, selection is empiric. Drugs in use today are listed in Table 27-1.

Cardiac Effects. Three cardiac actions are of importance: an effect on the force of ventricular contraction, an effect on the sinoauricular node and conduction system, and production of ventricular irritability. With the following exceptions, the drugs listed increase myocardial contractile force: methoxamine lacks these actions entirely and they are not prominent characteristics of phenylephrine. So far as alteration in sinoatrial nodal activity

Table 27-1. DOSAGES OF PRESSOR DRUGS

	Single Dose (mg)		Continuous IV (mg/500 ml of 5% Glucose in Water)
	IM	IV	
Ephedrine	25–50	10–15	—
Epinephrine	—	—	*
Isoproterenol (Isuprel)	—	—	0.4–0.8
Dopamine	—	—	200‡
Levarterenol (Levophed)	—	—	4 ml†
Mephentermine (Wyamine)	15–30	5–15	35
Metaraminol (Aramine)	2–10	0.5–5.0	20–40
Methamphetamine (Methedrine)	10–20	3–5	—
Methoxamine (Vasoxyl)	10–20	3–5	40
Phenylephrine (Neo-Synephrine)	1–3	0.2–0.4	10–30

*Seldom used as a vasopressor *per se.*
†One ampule contains 4 ml of 0.2% levarterenol bitartrate (0.1% free base).
‡One ampule of Intropin, 5 ml, contains 200 mg dopamine HCl.

is concerned, epinephrine, ephedrine, levarterenol, isoproterenol, and methamphetamine produce tachycardia by direct action. Slowing of the heart after injection of levarterenol, phenylephrine, or methoxamine is reflexly produced by activation of baroreceptors secondary to the rise in pressure, an effect useful in treating supraventricular tachycardia. Ventricular arrhythmias are common after administration of epinephrine, ephedrine, levarterenol, isoproterenol, and methamphetamine and their incidence and severity are enhanced in the presence of hypoxia, hypercarbia, or acidosis. Mephentermine shows relatively little tendency to cause ventricular arrhythmias. Dopamine in low dosage increases myocardial inotropism and blood pressure while acting as a peripheral vasodilator.

Peripheral Vascular Effects. All the drugs listed cause vasoconstriction except isoproterenol and dopamine, and the effect with epinephrine is mitigated by vasodilation in muscle. Constriction is prominent in renal, cutaneous, and splanchnic vessels. A powerful action is exerted upon venules and veins, constricting the large venous reservoir and returning to active circulation blood pooled in this area, important in increasing cardiac output.

Apart from angiotensin, which is not used clinically, levarterenol is the most potent vasoconstrictor but also the shortest acting; it is administered exclusively by intravenous infusion, preferably through a centrally placed catheter. Slough of skin, subcutaneous tissue, and muscle has occurred at the site of superficial intravenous injection. Treatment for extravasation consists of local infiltration with phentolamine. At one time levarterenol was so popular that few patients with serious hypotension escaped its application. Now, treatment is directed more toward the cause and levarterenol is less frequently employed.

Suggested dosages for adults of the commonly used pressor drugs are shown in Table 27-1.

Factors Limiting the Effectiveness of Pressor Drugs. For an optimal pressor effect blood volume must be sufficient to fill the vascular space in its changing capacity. The response of peripheral vessels depends upon a proper balance among endogenous catecholamines, adrenal steroids, sodium and potassium, and hydrogen ion concentration. Imbalance leads to poor reactivity. Either respiratory or metabolic acidosis may counter the action of pressor drugs. Therefore, blood gas measurements should accompany treatment.

Selection of Drug. With coincident hypotension and bradycardia, it seems reasonable to administer a drug that stimulates the sinoauricular node. If hypotension develops during administration of an inhalation anesthetic that sensitizes the myocardium to catecholamines, a pressor drug less likely to cause irritability is indicated. When hypotension exists primarily because of vasodilation, as after spinal anesthesia, a pressor drug with an action primarily on peripheral blood vessels is considered the drug of choice.

REFERENCES

Bland JHL, Laver MB, Lowenstein E: Vasodilator effect of commerical 5 per cent plasma protein fraction solutions. JAMA 224:1721, 1973.

Christy JH: Treatment of gram-negative shock. Am J Med 50:77, 1970.

Due TL, Johnson JM, Wood M, et al: Intraoperative autotransfusion in the management of massive hemorrhage. Am J Surg 130:652, 1975.

Goldberg LI: Dopamine—clinical use of an endogenous catecholamine. N Engl J Med 291:707, 1976.

Jakschik BA, Marshall GR, Kourik JL, et al: Profile of circulatory vasoactive substances in hemorrhagic shock and their pharmacologic manipulation. J Clin Invest 54:842, 1974.

Shoemaker WC, Brown RS: Dilemma of vasopressors and vasodilators in therapy of shock. Surg Gynecol Obstet 132:51, 1971.

Smith LL, Moore FD: Refractory hypotension in man—Is this irreversible shock? Clinical and biochemical observations. N Engl J Med 267:733, 1962.

Smith NT, Corbascio AN: The use and misuse of pressor agents. Anesthesiology 33:58, 1970.

Theye RA, Perry LB, Brzica SM, Jr: Influence of anesthetic agent in response to hemorrhagic hypotension. Anesthesiology 40:32, 1974.

Vandam LD: Drugs for arterial hypotension and shock. In Modell W (ed): Drugs of Choice. St Louis, C V Mosby Co, 1976.

Chapter 28

COMPLICATIONS OF ANESTHESIA

Many complications may arise during the course of anesthesia. These occur because of certain physical or pathologic characteristics of the patient, the drugs or the techniques of anesthetic administration employed, or the supportive measures used. Most of these complications have been discussed in other sections of this text, included under specific agents or techniques. Those discussed here occur with sufficient frequency and serious consequence to warrant emphasis.

ASPIRATION OF GASTRIC CONTENTS

Here and there in this text we have hinted at the serious consequences of aspiration of gastric contents into the lungs, but further emphasis is needed at this point. The possibility of a full stomach exists in any surgical or medical patient; hence the dictum of withholding oral intake of food or drink during the eight to ten hours prior to anesthetization. Obviously aspiration is always a threat in emergency operations, in the presence of pyloric or intestinal obstruction, when diaphragmatic hernia or esophageal diverticula exist, and in those patients with diminished pharyngeal reflexes owing to neurologic or debilitating disease. Above all, the parturient is at highest risk because of the unpredictable time of delivery and the delay in gastric emptying time caused by the processes of labor.

The pulmonary consequences of aspiration relate to both the volume and the character of the material inhaled. Large amounts of fluid will inundate the lungs, while particulate matter may result in obstruction at any level; either will cause varying degrees of asphyxiation. Pathogenic bacteria and colonic bacilli in stagnant secretions or feculent matter will produce infection, but perhaps the most serious consequences result from the relative acidity of gastric secretions. Inhalation of material with a pH less than 2.5 causes an immediate intense bronchoconstriction and destruction of the tracheal mucosa; within hours, a spreading and patchy pneumonitis appears as a fluffiness or "whiteout" on chest x-ray. As a result of obstruction and atelectasis, a major degree of shunting of arteriolar blood occurs, with a widening of the A-a oxygen gradient. Pulmonary edema may develop as a consequence of the chemical insult alone, or secondary to heart failure. Eventually, the full-blown pathogenic picture resembles that of the so-called adult respiratory distress syndrome. The syndrome bears the eponym of Mendelson, who first called attention to the problem in obstetric patients.

As in all complications of anesthesia, prevention is the key. If feasible, before general anesthesia an attempt should be made to empty the stomach via gastric drainage, a method that is hardly effective when solid food is present. Furthermore, upon induction of anesthesia, with relaxation of the pyloric and gastrointestinal sphincters reflux of secretions continues in the presence of intestinal obstruction. Thus, sealing off the trachea at the start of general anesthesia is essential. In cooperative patients while they are still awake the trachea may be intubated with the aid of topical anesthesia, but aspiration may still take place during the process. Otherwise, a rapid induction is done bearing in mind the hazards of drug overdose in these usually ill patients. With the patient's head elevated about 45 degrees and with prior oxygenation, a small dose of induction agent is given intravenously followed by succinylcholine when fasciculations have been eliminated by tubocurarine beforehand. As unconsciousness ensues, an assistant should occlude the esophagus via gentle backward pressure on the cricoid cartilage (Sellick's maneuver). The trachea is intubated as quickly as possible, the cuff on the tube immediately inflated, and induction of general anesthesia begun, although gradually. Gastric drainage is continued throughout and at termination, unless otherwise indicated; extubation is accomplished when pharyngeal reflexes are once again active, with a large tip suction device at hand.

When aspiration occurs or is suspected before the trachea has been sealed, a rapid intubation is again indicated and the trachea suctioned. The pH of the aspirate should be tested by means of litmus paper or one of the commercially prepared papers, even though dilution with alkaline material may already have occurred. Tracheal lavage with saline, 5 ml at a time, followed by suction is advocated even though the inspiration preceding a cough serves to spread the material throughout the lungs. At one time tracheal instillation and parenteral administration of a corticosteroid were practiced in order to diminish the mucosal inflammatory response, but subsequent studies have cast doubt on the efficacy of these measures. Undoubtedly the most effective therapy is that employed for any kind of acute pulmonary insufficiency whether the result of aspiration, drowning, or infection. In all studies the use of PEEP (see Chapter 33) has proved most effective in reversing the pathophysiologic changes. Antibiotics may be given when there is bacterial contamination, and a bronchodilator such as aminophyline used to combat spasm.

MALIGNANT HYPERTHERMIA

The incidence of malignant hyperthermia appearing during anesthesia, first reported in 1922, is judged to be about one in 14,000 with a peak rate of occurrence in the third decade and a preponderance in men. In many cases a distinct familial trait implies a dominant inheritance. Often patients have had congenital muscle or musculoskeletal disorders, some have had hyperthermia upon repeated anesthetization, while others offer no history of previous anesthetic difficulty. Thus it is essential to inquire of patients as to personal or familial complications with anesthesia, particularly unexplained deaths.

No consistent relationship has been found between development of the syndrome and use of specific premedicants. Although halothane is commonly involved, all general anesthetics and techniques have been implicated. In about 65 per cent of reported cases muscle rigidity has appeared upon intravenous injection of succinylcholine for tracheal intubation, aggravated by a second injection, and hardly relieved by a nondepolarizing neuromuscular blocker. Following the onset of rigidity body temperature rises precipitously, as rapidly as 1° C in five minutes. With more insidious onset the earliest signs include warm skin, tachycardia and ventricular arrhythmias, unstable blood pressure, cyanosis and mottling of the skin, profuse sweating, and ultimately cardiac arrest.

At the earliest indication the following procedures are instituted: discontinuance of anesthesia and termination of operation; hyperventilation of the lungs with 100 per cent oxygen to counter the tachypnea that appears concomitant with excess carbon dioxide production; correction of the associated severe lactic acidosis by means of bicarbonate injection; treatment of hyperkalemia with dextrose and insulin; and cooling of the body by whatever means possible (surface cooling, intravenous infusion of iced saline, gastric and rectal lavage, irrigation of the body cavities, and extracorporeal cooling). Cooling is discontinued when the temperature falls below 38° C because of downward drift, but reinstituted if a rise occurs. All these measures require monitoring in the form of the electrocardiogram, temperature probe, bladder catheterization, and placement of arterial and central venous lines to follow the progress of treatment.

Although the biochemical abnormality underlying development of the syndrome has not yet been clearly defined, clues to its origin have come from studies on Poland China pigs that, as a manifestation of an autosomal dominant trait, uniformly develop the fatal syndrome when exposed to halothane. Serum creatine phosphokinase (CPK) levels are elevated beforehand and, after development of the syndrome, *in vitro* studies on muscle slices show both ATP depletion and altered calcium release from the sarcoplasmic reticulum, thus accounting for the muscle rigidity. Drug therapy is based upon these derangements. Lidocaine given for treatment of the cardiac arrhythmias has been shown to worsen the biochemical aberrations, while procainamide, although condemned by some, is considered worthwhile by others. Little benefit has accrued from the use of adrenal steroids or digitalis unless for the treatment of heart failure. Several reports have appeared on beneficial results following injection of dantrolene sodium, a hydantoin derivative still in the investigational phase. The compound has controlled the syndrome in Landrace pigs and both delayed and relaxed muscle rigor in *in vitro* preparations. Since the drug is poorly soluble, a lyophilized preparation is in the making for parenteral use.

Delayed sequelae of malignant hyperthermia include disseminated intravascular coagulation (DIC), acute tubular necrosis of the kidneys (vasoconstrictive nephropathy), inadvertent hypothermia, hyperkalemia, muscle necrosis, and anoxic neurologic damage. Treatment of these entities should be well known to the informed anesthetist. The efficacy of the therapies outlined is still uncertain, and current mortality is judged to be in the 60 to 70 per cent range. Obviously any improvement in these figures lies in prevention, the suspicion that the syndrome may appear, and a vigorous program of action in the earliest phases of development.

NERVE INJURY

Peripheral nerves can be injured during anesthesia through stretch or compression because the anesthetized patient does not perceive pain and lacks protective muscle tone. Among the nerves commonly injured are the several divisions of the brachial plexus and the ulnar, radial, common peroneal, and facial nerves.

The nerves constituting the brachial plexus are held centrally at the transverse processes of the vertebrae and peripherally at the point of entry into the arm. Separation of these points may stretch the nerves with resulting molecular damage, hemorrhage or ischemia, and development of palsy (Fig. 28-1). Lateral flexion of the head to the opposite side with coincident downward displacement of the shoulder places tension on the nerves. Several anatomic fulcrums such as the scalene muscles, the attachment of the pectoralis minor muscle to the coracoid process of the scapula, and the rounded head of the humerus provide additional possibilities for stretch; hyperabduction, extension, and external rotation of the arm stretch the brachial plexus around these fulcrums. A supporting brace improperly applied to the shoulder may act not only as an artificial fulcrum but may compress the brachial plexus against the first rib. A shoulder brace should not be used when the arm is extended on an arm rest. The plexus may also be pinched between the clavicle and first rib.

To avoid brachial plexus injury one must bear the possibility in mind and avoid extremes of position of the head and arm. When palsy develops, a careful neurologic examination should be recorded and measures for restoration of function immediately begun with support of the paralyzed

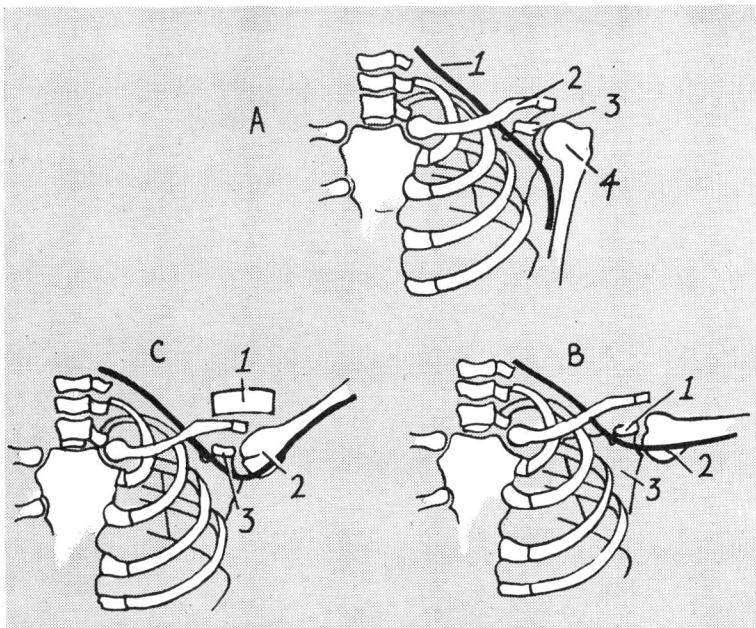

Figure 28-1. Traction on brachial plexus. *A*, Arm at side: *1*, brachial plexus; *2*, clavicle; *3*, coracoid process of scapula; *4*, head of humerus. *B*, Arm at right angle: scapula (*3*) rotates and brachial plexus is stretched beneath the coracoid process (*1*) and around head of humerus (*2*). *C*, Arm hyperextended with shoulder brace (*1*) depressing scapula (*3*). Brachial plexus stretched beneath coracoid process and around head of humerus.

muscles and physiotherapy. In severe injury, restitution of normal function may require as long as six months to a year.

The ulnar, radial, and common peroneal nerves are superficially placed; hence they are easily compressed against bone, stirrups, or the sides of an operating table, or stretched around bony eminences. Certain positions such as lithotomy or the lateral decubitus predispose to injury of these nerves. If paralysis occurs, treatment is the same as that described for brachial plexus injury.

The facial nerve may be injured by overenthusiastic attempts to elevate the jaw via pressure on the rami of the mandible or by tight application of a head strap. Weakness of the muscles about the mouth or eyes is a manifestation of this injury, usually reversible within a week or two. Femoral nerve injury may result from faulty placement of retractors during pelvic operation.

OCULAR INJURY

Careless application of a face mask, the position of the patient on the operating table, anesthetic technique employed, or preparation of the skin for operation on the head and neck may predispose to ocular injury. Open mask techniques for administration of volatile anesthetics are especially prone to cause conjunctivitis or corneal abrasion. Liquid anesthetic or vapor reaching the eye directly may produce corneal ulceration. However, ulceration is more likely to be the result of trauma or drying of the cornea. Large masks pressing on the eyes have resulted in retinal detachment, periorbital edema, and numbness in the distribution of the supraorbital nerve.

The best precaution against corneal injury is to keep the lids closed. One should not elicit the corneal reflex to determine depth of anesthesia. When the eyes are covered by surgical drapes, the lids are best kept closed with tape or adhesive. The same precautions apply when the patient is in the prone position or the head is face down on a cerebellar head rest; the head should be raised periodically to prevent pressure necrosis of the forehead and cheeks. Instillation of sterile mineral oil into the conjunctival sac prevents desiccation of the cornea during deep planes of anesthesia when the lids are partially open.

The eyes should be inspected at the conclusion of anesthesia. If injury is detected, ophthalmologic consultation should be sought. Simple conjunctivitis is best treated by irrigation with a 2.2 per cent solution of boric acid, which is isotonic with lacrimal fluid. Corneal abrasions not only are painful but may progress to inflammation of the uveal tract. If treated early with an antibiotic or one of the sulfonamides, locally instilled, abrasions usually re-epithelialize within 24 hours. During this time the eye is covered with a patch. Atropine is used for mydriasis to prevent formation of synechiae when inflammation is present, and to relieve the pain associated with spasm of the iris and ciliary muscle. Topical local anesthetics for relief of pain should be avoided since they retard corneal epithelial regeneration.

INJURY TO THE LUNGS

EXCESSIVE PRESSURE

Because the gases used in anesthesia are delivered from cylinders and wall outlets at higher than atmospheric pressure, the possibility of damage to the lungs is ever present. Injury can occur not only during anesthesia but whenever inhalation therapy or resuscitation is practiced. The exact limits of pressure that can be safely applied to the lungs have not been defined, and the degree of harm probably differs from patient to patient. It is said that pressure should not exceed 20 to 30 cm of water; however, higher pressures may be required to inflate the lungs after collapse. Whether or not damage occurs depends upon the rapidity of the rise in pressure, the pattern of distribution, and whether the thorax is open at the time. Furthermore, high pressures applied at the nose and mouth are not necessarily transmitted to the alveoli.

Complications of Anesthesia

When high pressure is transmitted to the alveoli, rupture may take place, with hemorrhage and capillary air embolism or dissection into the interstitial tissues (Fig. 28-2). Air in the interstitial tissues of the lungs may collect beneath the pleura, forming blebs and rupturing into the pleural cavity, or it may dissect back via the hilum into the mediastinum (pneumomediastinum). The lungs become distended with air trapped in the interstitium (pulmonary interstitial emphysema), and venous return to the heart may be blocked by collection of air in the mediastinum (air block). Mediastinal emphysema and air block can be recognized by distinctly audible churning sounds synchronous with the heart beat, the so-called mill wheel murmur (Hamman's sign). Air in the mediastinum can dissect downward retroperitoneally or escape into the subcutaneous tissues of the neck or into the pleural cavities when the superior mediastinal pleura ruptures.

Alveolar rupture may occur when there is free transmission of high pressures to the alveoli, as when the trachea is intubated. In the presence of subcutaneous emphysema or otherwise unexplained respiratory distress and hypoxia, pneumothorax, mediastinal and pulmonary interstitial emphysema, and capillary air embolism must be suspected and treated at once if the patient is to survive. In the extreme case there may be little one can do, but the following treatments are suggested.

Pneumothorax. With the patient upright, entry is made into the pleura at the midclavicular line in the second intercostal space anteriorly, with a large gauge needle attached to a 50-ml syringe and a two-way stopcock. Air is aspirated fractionally and underwater drainage instituted. At the same time, pressure is applied to the airway to re-expand the lungs. If tracheal rupture has occurred as a result of trauma or prolonged pressure from a cuffed tracheostomy or tracheal tube, it may be possible to pass a

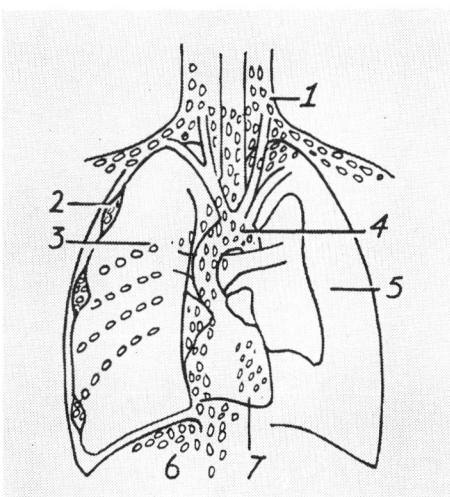

Figure 28-2. Escape of air following rupture of lungs. *1*, Subcutaneous emphysema; *2*, subpleural bleb; *3*, pulmonary interstitial emphysema; *4*, mediastinal emphysema; *5*, pneumothorax; *6*, pneumoperitoneum; and *7*, air embolism to heart.

tracheal tube beyond the site to prevent continued escape of air. A double lumen tube may be useful, near the bifurcation.

Mediastinal and Subcutaneous Emphysema. Superior mediastinotomy may be performed using local anesthesia if the trapped air is under pressure and causing respiratory or circulatory embarrassment; unfortunately, this is not of much value.

Protection against high pressure injury to the lungs can be assured only by careful actions and the obligatory placement of safety valves between the source of pressure and the patient's airway. As a general rule, gas cylinders or wall outlets should be opened and flows adjusted before connection to the patient is made.

AIR EMBOLISM

In addition to positive airway pressure, air embolism may occur as a result of air entrained by negative pressure in the diploic veins during craniotomy, as a complication of cardiopulmonary bypass, thyroidectomy, or intrauterine manipulation. Concurrent administration of nitrous oxide for anesthesia increases the lethality of air embolus by diffusion into the air bubble, enlarging the volume. One hundred per cent oxygen should be substituted immediately.

In suboccipital craniectomy and cervical laminectomy with the patient in the sitting position, prior placement of a catheter in the right ventricle permits immediate withdrawal of trapped air. Air embolism is suspected upon appearance of cardiac arrhythmias or unexplained hypotension. A precordial stethoscope will detect the characteristic bubbling or mill wheel sounds.

When feasible the patient is placed in a steep head-down position with the right side uppermost to prevent tamponade in the outflow tract of the right ventricle. If air is heard within the heart, an attempt can be made to aspirate it by means of ventricular puncture or via the catheter already placed. If heart action stops, cardiac resuscitation as described in Chapter 30 should be undertaken. Closed chest manual systole helps the passage of air emboli lodged in the coronary arteries. Hyperbaric oxygenation has been beneficial in effecting recovery of patients with extensive neurologic damage resulting from massive air embolus occurring during cardiopulmonary bypass. Exposure initially to 6 atm absolute is followed by prolonged decompression, more or less as practiced in other kinds of barotrauma.

MISCELLANEOUS ACCIDENTS

An infinite number of accidents may happen during or following anesthesia. The following is a partial list of complications observed by the authors:

1. A child, left unattended, fell from an operating table, sustaining lacerations of the scalp.

2. A man carelessly positioned in the lateral position for lumbodorsal sympathectomy awoke with pressure contusions of the genitalia.

3. A patient developed marked swelling of the neck resembling parotitis because of manual efforts to elevate the mandible during respiratory obstruction.

4. A young boy about to undergo tonsillectomy struggled during induction, struck his head against the edge of the table, and required sutures for laceration of the scalp.

5. A unit of blood was permitted to extravasate into the tissue of a patient's leg that was out of sight beneath surgical drapes.

6. The hand of an unconscious patient was crushed during elevation of the foot of an operating table.

7. A patient with severe generalized osteoporosis sustained a fracture of the humerus during transfer from operating table to litter.

8. Vigorous tracheal suction with repeated cough at the termination of anesthesia led to rupture of abdominal sutures and wound dehiscence.

9. A bottle containing intravenous fluid fell from its stand, striking the patient's head and causing laceration of the scalp.

REFERENCES

Britt BA, Kalow W: Malignant hyperthermia: A statistical review. Can Anaesth Soc J 17:293, 1970.

Britt BA, Gordon RA, Kalow W (eds): International Symposium on Malignant Hyperthermia. Springfield, Ill, Charles C Thomas, 1972.

Courington FW, Little DM, Jr: The role of posture in anesthesia. In Jenkins MT (ed): Common and Uncommon Problems in Anesthesiology. Clinical Anesthesia 3, Philadelphia, FA Davis, 1968, Chapter 2.

Harrison GG: Control of malignant hyperthermia syndrome by dantrolene. Br J Anaesth 47:66, 1975.

Kalow W, Gordon RA: Malignant hyperthermia: An investigation of five patients. Can Anaesth Soc J 20:431, 1973.

Macklin MT, Macklin CC: Malignant interstitial emphysema of the lungs and mediastinum as an important occult complication in many respiratory diseases and other conditions. Medicine 23:281, 1944.

Ryan JF: Cardiopulmonary bypass in the treatment of malignant hyperthermia. N Engl J Med 290:1121, 1974.

Winter PM, Alvis HJ, Gage AA: Hyperbaric treatment of cerebral air embolus during cardiopulmonary bypass. JAMA 215:1786, 1971.

Chapter 29

ELECTRIC HAZARDS, FIRES, AND EXPLOSIONS

The hazard from the combustion of flammable anesthetics has lessened with the general acceptance of halogenated agents, but the dangers from shock and electrocution have increased because of the widespread use of electric equipment in patient care areas. Monitoring of vital signs, cardiac pacing, electrically operated beds, respirators, and even television sets have increased the potential for electric injury to the patient.

ELECTRIC HAZARDS

When sufficient current flows through tissues, an injury such as a burn or ventricular fibrillation may occur. The kind of injury depends on the magnitude of the current and the tissue affected.

Before an electric injury can occur, current must flow, and for current to flow there must be a complete circuit from the voltage source, through the tissue, and back to the source. Minute electric currents passing through the heart may initiate ventricular fibrillation. If the current flows through a wire or catheter within the heart, as little as 20 μamp (0.00002 amp) can cause fibrillation; about 200 μamp must flow if the current is conducted through the epicardium and 100 mamp if the current flows through the trunk. If a wire stylet or electrode is within the chambers of the heart, as little as 10 mv, or in the case of a saline-filled catheter, 1 v, applied to the proximal end, may be sufficient to electrocute the patient. With good electric contact through moist skin, resistance across the trunk is about 1000 ohms; contact with a 120 v source may easily provide sufficient current for electrocution.

Prevention of electric injury is aimed at eliminating extraneous voltage sources and avoiding connections that result in complete circuits through tissue. Electric energy cannot be completely excluded, as it is used to operate devices essential or useful in patient care. Good practice can, however, elim-

Electric Hazards, Fires, and Explosions 437

inate extraneous sources. Circuits may be completed through wires, conducting liquids such as body fluids or saline, or through "ground." One of the current-carrying wires of hospital (or household) electric systems is at ground potential (there is no voltage difference between it and the earth). The metal conduit that carries these wires and a third, noncurrent-carrying ground wire are also at ground potential, as are the metal cases of many electric devices, water and heating pipes, bed frames, and operating tables. Thus the patient is likely to be grounded and to have one side of an electric circuit completed. To avoid electric injury, a voltage source must not be connected to the patient. Voltages may arise from the hospital electric system or from leakage currents.

What are the potential sources of current leakage and how may they be eliminated (Fig. 29-1)? Improper design or malfunction may cause voltages to be induced in leads from monitoring equipment and virtually any other electric device connected to the patient. Instruments must be so designed that voltage differences do not appear between any pair of patient leads, between any single lead and the case of an instrument, or between these and the ground. Instruments should be ruggedly built so that physical or electric damage or high humidity is unlikely to cause failures that can result in dangerous voltages in patient leads. All instruments should be equipped with three-wire power cords and grounding plugs, as well as grounding terminals by which they may be interconnected with heavy wire. Neither of the two wires bringing electric power to the instrument should be connected to the case. All instruments as well as all electric-conducting objects with which the patient may come into contact should be grounded to a common bus. In anesthetizing locations, the National Fire Protection Association (NFPA) requires that the bus be a highly conductive bare metal bar with terminals for grounding each electric receptacle in the room as well as all metal furniture. The bus must be isolated from all other grounds in the building except at a single common grounding point.

Current flow to a patient through instrument leads can be limited by placing fuses in the leads. Since the smallest fuses available are 1/500 amp (2000 μamp), they offer little protection from electrocution via an intracardiac electrode but are useful with surface electrodes.

BURNS

Burns constitute another electric hazard. Ordinarily if a 60-Hz current of sufficient intensity to cause thermal burns passes through the trunk, fibrillation or sustained myocardial contraction will occur. However, a burn alone may result if the same current passes through an extremity. High frequency current from an electrocautery apparatus is a common cause of burns. The active electrode of the cautery cuts or cauterizes with intense heat because all current flows through a small area. When this current leaves the body through the large ground plate, the current density is small, and significant heating is not produced. If, however, the ground wire is broken or disconnected and the current exits through an ECG electrode, via a conductive face mask, or by contact with a metal table, a burn may result. Current densities higher than 100 mamp/cm^2 can result in skin burns. Large ECG electrodes provide a greater surface area and burns are less likely to result when currents accidentally pass through them. The anesthetist, who is grounded through his conductive shoes, may also be shocked or burned.

CHEMICAL BURNS

Chemical burns resulting from the use of direct current have also occurred. If a few volts are applied to a saline solution, electrolysis occurs with sodium hydroxide formed at the positive pole and chlorine at the anode; the hydroxide thus formed is caustic. In some electrosurgical units a small direct current voltage is applied to the ground plate to detect ground failures; faults occurring in this circuit can also cause electrolysis.

OPTICAL LASERS

Optical lasers have recently come into use as surgical instruments. Their intense, coherent beams of light carry large amounts of energy that focus on small areas of tissue and therefore act as a scalpel that both cuts and effects hemostasis. Papillomas of the larynx, for example, may be vaporized by a carbon dioxide laser beam. This laser operates in the infrared at 10.6 μm. The energy of its beam can obviously cause deep burns and can ignite a rubber endotracheal tube, which must be protected by a reflecting metal tape or foil cover. Laser beams of visible light are transmitted by glass as well as by the ocular lens. Operating room personnel must wear appropriate lenses to protect against stray reflections; patients' eyelids should be taped shut.

MAINTENANCE OF EQUIPMENT

Electric equipment must not only be well designed but properly maintained. Maintenance is ordinarily beyond the ability of physicians and should be delegated to an expert. In small hospitals it is usually not possible to employ a full-time electronic technician or engineer; hence, it may be necessary to rely on the manufacturer or a maintenance firm. Certain faults, however, should be obvious even to the unsophisticated. Equipment with frayed or broken cords, plugs that do not seat firmly in outlets, and damaged instruments should not be used but set aside for repair. If the operator of an instrument receives a shock, use of the instrument for a patient should be avoided.

POWER DISTRIBUTION IN HAZARDOUS AREAS

Isolated power systems are required in anesthetizing locations where flammable agents are used. An isolation transformer eliminates the ground connection of the usual power distribution system. An ungrounded system reduces the danger of electric shock, additionally serving the function of detecting defective electric equipment through the ground indicator system. Personnel and objects in the operating room may be grounded to reduce the electrostatic spark hazard without the danger of shock. A grounded distribution system has one "hot" wire and one wire at ground potential; if contact is made with the hot wire and ground (personnel are grounded through conductive shoes and flooring), current passes through the body (Fig. 29–1). In the ungrounded system the secondary winding of the isolation transformer

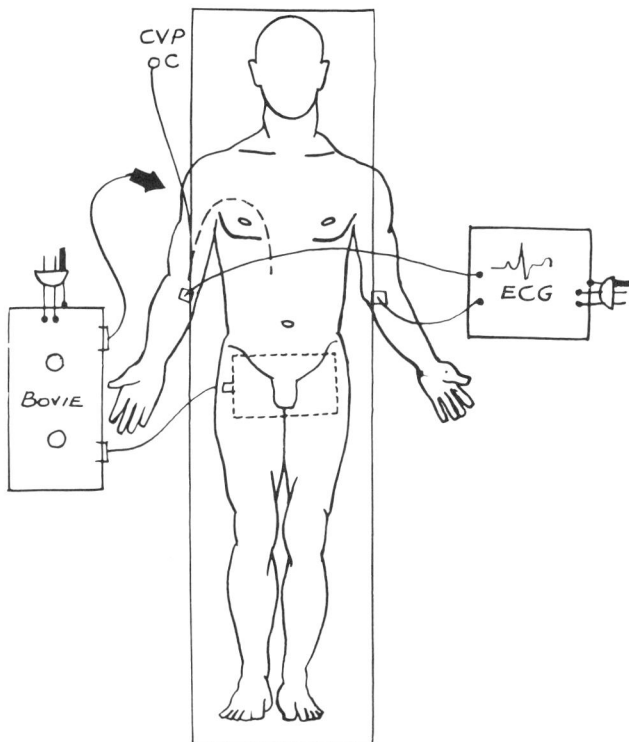

Figure 29–1. Some potential hazards to a patient in the operating room. The patient lies on a conductive mattress on a metal table on a conductive floor. Electrocardiograph electrodes are connected to the arms and the ground plate from an electrocautery is under the buttocks. If a break occurs in the electrocautery grounding line and if the ECG electrodes are grounded or if the patient is grounded at a small area to the table, a burn may result when the cutting current is applied. If the ground to a cardiac monitor is broken, as through faulty connection in the plug, and a fault occurs in the monitor, current could be conducted through one of the arm leads to either the cautery ground or the table and result in electrocution. A central venous pressure catheter could also provide a conducting path to the heart.

does not have a ground connection; for current to pass through the body, both wires supplying power from the transformer must be touched simultaneously, and a grounded person touching either wire alone will not be shocked.

A line isolation monitor (LIM) is incorporated in the isolated system to sound an alarm when a ground has been created on the isolated side, such as when faulty equipment is connected to the power distribution system. The ground warning not only protects personnel but also indicates the need for repair. The warning system relies upon a high-resistance, current-limiting relay, activated when a ground connection occurs on the isolated side. This completes a circuit through the secondary winding of the transformer and the relay activates a warning light and a buzzer (Fig. 29-2). A green light indicates safe conditions, while red warns of a ground in the system.

CODES AND STANDARDS

The applicable codes and standards of the NFPA are prepared by committees representing industry, health care facilities, medical societies, and standards groups. They are continually being analyzed and revised to keep

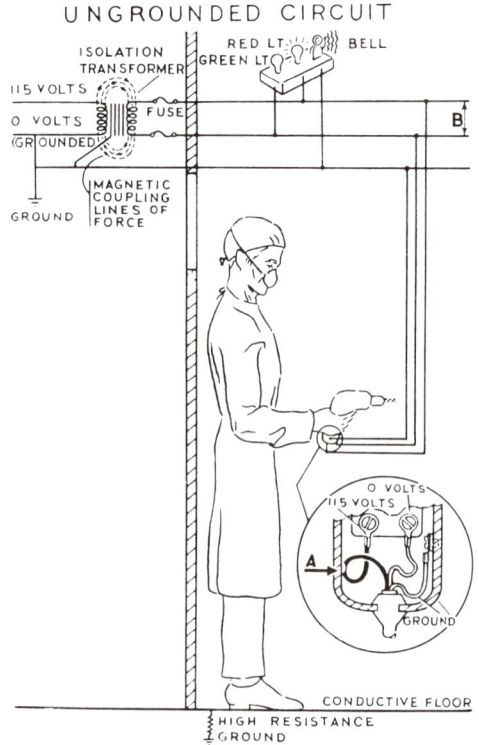

Figure 29-2. The ungrounded circuit and the isolation transformer. Spark or shock occurs only when both live conductors are in circuit. Insulation failure (A) permits a current of 2 milliamperes to flow to ground. The ground contact indicator is activated to warn of the failure. No spark or shock hazard is established. (Reproduced with permission from Walter CW: Anesthesiology 25:505, 1964.)

abreast of advancing technology and to resolve controversy. In many jurisdictions the standards are incorporated into local building codes and therefore are of legal significance. Anesthetists who become involved in the design or administration of facilities must be aware of safety practices and local regulations; technical consultation should be sought when needed.

FIRES AND EXPLOSIONS

In comparison with other hazards of anesthesia, explosions occur so infrequently as to be relatively insignificant. When ether and cyclopropane were in common use, the mortality from explosions was estimated at about one in 1,500,000 patients. The overall death rate attributable to anesthesia is difficult to determine, but probably lies between one in 350 and one in 4000, depending upon the physical condition of the patient. However, the emotional upheaval created by an anesthetic explosion and the resulting publicity cause consternation far out of proportion to the incidence. While widespread use of nonflammable agents in anesthesia has reduced the incidence of explosions, flammable agents continue to be used and ether and acetone are employed to cleanse the skin. So long as flammable vapors are released near the patient, precautions for the prevention of fires and explosions must be taken.

Hepatic or renal complications following halothane, methoxyflurane, or enflurane anesthesia are thought by some to represent contraindications to the use of these drugs. The alternatives are regional anesthesia, balanced drug sequences, or the use of potentially explosive agents. The most useful flammable drugs are cyclopropane and ether. Trichloroethylene, although not flammable at ordinary temperatures, is given primarily as an analgetic or adjuvant to nitrous oxide. Many anesthetists, however, believe that there is no longer any place for flammable agents in anesthesia; that since there are no absolute indications for ether or cyclopropane, adequate alternatives are available and the rare use of these agents does not justify the high cost of installing and maintaining isolated electric circuits and conductive floors.

Fires and explosions are combustive processes differing in speed of reaction and magnitude of forces released. Three elements are necessary for combustion: a combustible substance or fuel, an oxidizing agent, and a source of ignition. For a fire or explosion to occur, the fuel and the oxidizer must be present in appropriate proportions; too little fuel or too little oxidizer will not permit combustion. All flammable anesthetic agents are fuels; oxygen and nitrous oxide are oxidizers, and sparks, flames, or heated surfaces are the common sources of ignition. The lower explosive limits in oxygen (too little fuel) are 2.0 vol per cent for ether and 2.5 vol per cent for cyclopropane. The upper explosive limits (too little oxygen) are above the clinically useful anesthetic concentrations. For all practical purposes any anesthetic given with ether or cyclopropane will be in the flammable range.

A simple method of testing a respired gas mixture for flammability consists of aspirating a gas sample into a 10-ml plastic syringe from the expiratory limb of the anesthesia system. The syringe is taken outside the operating room, the plunger removed, and a lighted match held at the open end. The slightly increased brightness of the flame caused by an oxygen-rich anesthetic mixture should not be confused with the propagated flame resulting from a flammable mixture. When combustion does not result on testing, it is probably safe to use the electrocautery, provided that open cavities such as the chest or abdomen have been flushed out by suctioning to remove anesthetic gases, which are heavier than air.

Measures for prevention of fires and explosions have been suggested by engineers, fire insurance underwriters, manufacturers, and physicians. The most complete set of recommendations is found in the Standard for the Use of Inhalation Anesthetics of the NFPA, revised periodically since it was first promulgated in 1941. We endorse the application of all protective measures that can be adopted within the limits of practicality, unless their adoption involves substitution of a greater hazard.

RECOMMENDED PRECAUTIONS AGAINST EXPLOSIVE HAZARDS

STORAGE OF AGENTS AND CARE OF EQUIPMENT

All gas cylinders, anesthesia machines, and containers of flammable liquids should be stored in well-ventilated areas away from sources of heat. Oxygen and nitrous oxide should be kept apart from combustible substances. Under no circumstances should cylinders be refilled except by the manufacturer. Oil and grease must not be present on equipment, for they may be ignited by oxidizing gases under pressure (Chapter 6).

REMOVAL OF ANESTHETIC VAPORS

Although ventilation or air conditioning of operating rooms and storage places does not completely protect against anesthetic explosions, good ventilation is valuable in minimizing accumulation of an explosive concentration of anesthetic.

SOURCES OF IGNITION

Obvious sources of ignition such as lighted cigarettes or flames are prohibited in operating theaters, corridors, special care units, and storage places. Electric wiring and equipment installed in hazardous anesthetizing locations should conform to the current National Electrical Code of the NFPA and local fire codes and regulations. Among the specifications are:

Electric Hazards, Fires, and Explosions

(1) explosion-proof motors, switches, housings, and outlets; (2) grounded conduits; (3) heavy duty cords with ground wires; (4) distribution of electric current through ungrounded circuits utilizing isolation transformers and ground indicator warning circuits, and (5) conductive flooring, equipment, and footwear.

Static sparks are an important potential source of ignition. These may be generated in many different ways, and hence are the most difficult source of ignition to eliminate. Everyone has had the experience of walking across a heavily piled carpet and discharging a spark upon making contact with another person. A static spark may jump a gap when charged objects of different potential are approximated, but sparking is eliminated if all objects concerned are at the same potential. This condition may be realized by electric interconnection of all objects and persons within the hazardous area. A list of suggested measures follows.

To dissipate any charge, the floor must be conductive to provide a path for static electricity to leak from equipment and personnel. With conductive flooring, an isolated electric system should also be installed to protect personnel from electric shock. Floors must be kept free from dirt and wax, which impair conductivity, and tested at regular intervals for conductivity by the hospital engineering department. Furniture, equipment, and operating tables should make contact with the conductive floor by means of metal or conductive rubber casters or legs.

Wool or nylon blankets are prohibited in locations where flammable anesthetics are in use. Cushions, mattresses, and other interposed objects should be made of conductive materials to connect the patient to the grounded table. Anesthesia machines should not be covered with dust protectors or plastered with adhesive tape because of the danger of static spark during removal. A relative humidity of 50 per cent or higher reduces the danger of static spark, and therefore should be maintained in the operating room.

BEHAVIOR OF PERSONNEL

When connections on anesthesia apparatus are made or broken, both parts should be held in the hands to maintain isoelectric conditions; if this is not done, sparking may occur.

Persons other than the anesthetist should absent themselves from the vicinity of the patient's head and the anesthesia machine, where accumulation of combustible substances is most likely to occur. If contact is necessary between personnel, this is done at a distance from the danger points, initially at the back of the anesthetist's neck.

Equipment and personnel should be moved in a deliberate manner to avoid generation of static electricity. Because tape causes static spark when unrolled and torn, dressings should be prepared away from the operating table.

All personnel in areas in which flammable anesthetics are in use should wear conductive footwear. Shoes should be tested daily to assure optimal conductivity, less than 1,000,000 ohms. Cotton clothing should be worn. Silk, wool, or synthetics may be worn only in intimate contact with the skin and beneath cotton outer garments. Nylon stockings are permissible since they are in close contact with the skin.

REFERENCES

Bruner JMR: Common abuses and failures of electrical equipment. Anesth Analg 51:810, 1972.
Bruner JMR: Hazards of electrical apparatus. Anesthesiology 28:396, 1967.
Graystone P, Towell ME: Electric shock hazard associated with pressure transducers. Anesthesiology 34:79, 1971.
Green HL, Hieb GE, Shatz IJ: Electronic equipment in critical care areas: Status of devices currently in use. Circulation 43:A101, 1971.
Hopps JA: Shock hazards in operating rooms and patient-care areas. Anesthesiology 31:142, 1969.
Leeming MN: Protection of the "electrically" susceptible patient. Anesthesiology 38:370, 1973.
Leeming MN, Ray C Jr, Howland WS: Low voltage direct-current burns. JAMA 214:1681, 1970.
Leonard PF: Characteristics of electrical hazards. Anesth Analg 51:797, 1972.
National Fire Protection Association, 470 Atlantic Avenue, Boston, MA, 02110:
  NFPA 56A Inhalation Anesthetics, 1973.
  NFPA 70 National Electrical Code, 1975.
  NFPA 76B Electricity in Patient Care Areas of Health Care Facilities, 1975.
  NFPA 76C Safe Use of High Frequency Electricity in Health Care Facilities, 1975.
Snow JC, Norton ML, Saluja IS, et al: Fire hazard during CO_2 laser microsurgery of the larynx and trachea. Anesth Analg, 55:146, 1976.

Section 4

ANCILLARY ANESTHESIA CARE

Chapter 30

CARDIOPULMONARY RESUSCITATION

Cardiopulmonary resuscitation extends far back in the history of mankind. Thumping on the chest and mouth-to-mouth breathing were utilized in antiquity, the latter cited in the Bible. However, no concerted attempts at resuscitation were made until the present century, when the prone pressure technique of artificial respiration was widely taught in the United States and other techniques used abroad. During World War II these techniques were re-evaluated, and the advent of operations on the heart brought cardiac resuscitation into focus. In the 1950s thoracotomy and manual compression of the heart, use of resuscitative drugs, and electric defibrillation gained wide acceptance. Mouth-to-mouth breathing was shown to be far more effective for pulmonary ventilation than the manual methods. In the 1960s closed chest manual compression of the heart largely supplanted the open technique.

Respiratory and circulatory resuscitation are treated here as one, for the two are inseparable. When respiration ceases, cardiac arrest soon follows, while circulatory standstill as a primary event is almost coincident with cessation of breathing.

RESPIRATORY RESUSCITATION

Respiratory standstill is easily diagnosed, but not the subtle degrees of ventilatory inadequacy. Both are synonymous with hypoxia and carbon dioxide retention. Cessation of respiration even for brief periods may result in irreversible cerebral damage; hence the need to restore gas exchange as soon as possible. The duration of permissible apnea varies with the adequacy of oxygenation prior to onset and with the metabolic demand. In a denitrogenated, well-oxygenated subject, the safe period of apnea may extend up to five minutes, whereas in hypoxic persons, apnea for 20 to 30 seconds may be fatal.

The causes of respiratory failure may reside in the inhaled atmosphere, the airways and lungs, the oxygen transport system, or the control of respiration. Anesthetists encounter all of these problems in their daily activities.

Inhaled Atmosphere. Decreased oxygen tension in inhaled gas may be the result of lowered oxygen concentration at ambient pressure or reduction in the partial pressure of oxygen at high altitude.

Airway Obstruction or Pulmonary Disease. Obstruction may be caused by tumor, bronchoconstriction, secretions, or solid material; infectious disease such as pneumonia; structural alterations in alveoli, such as occur in severe emphysema; mechanical interference with ventilation, as seen in the fixed chest, paralyzed diaphragm, or flail chest; or impaired diffusion, as is found in pulmonary edema or fibrosis.

Transport System. Interference with blood flow may occur in the lungs, the systemic circulation, or as a result of anemia, or carbon monoxide poisoning.

Control of Respiration. This may be influenced by central nervous system disease; drugs causing central respiratory depression, such as anesthetics and opioids; respiratory acidosis; and trauma to the brain.

An essential criterion of respiratory resuscitation is that the method be immediately available and effective. Mouth-to-mouth breathing has these characteristics.

EXPIRED AIR TECHNIQUES

There is enough oxygen in expired air to assure oxygenation of a victim's blood. Almost all the disadvantages of manual pressure techniques are overcome by positive pressure applied to the airway with expired air via mouth-to-mouth or mouth-to-nose breathing. With either, the resuscitator supports the head and mandible, the adequacy of gas exchange is judged by rise and fall of the chest, and the tidal volume thus estimated. In addition, accumulation of secretions or vomitus and obstruction of the airway can be detected. Little expenditure of energy is required to ventilate the lungs in this manner.

The patient lies supine, the upper airway cleared of obstructing secretions or foreign material. The resuscitator kneels at the side of the patient's head, which is tilted backward maximally with the mandible held forward (Fig. 30–1). This maneuver carries the base of the tongue out of the pharynx and brings oral cavity and oropharynx into line with the larynx and trachea. In mouth-to-mouth breathing the patient's nostrils are closed by the fingers of one hand while the other maintains backward tilt of the head, or leakage of air from the nose is prevented by application of the operator's cheek against the nostrils. The operator's mouth is opened widely and the lips are placed firmly around the patient's open mouth, followed by forceful expiration. The effect is gauged by observing the movement of the chest wall. It may be necessary almost to dislocate the jaw to assure an unobstructed airway, by pulling the mandible forward with the fingers in the mouth or by upward traction at the angles of the jaw. In mouth-to-nose respiration the patient's lips are closed and air is blown into the nose. After inflation of the lungs, the operator removes his or her mouth from the patient's to allow passive expiration. In the mouth-to-nose technique the patient's mouth should be open during expiration because the uvula and soft palate may obstruct escape of air through the nose.

Cardiopulmonary Resuscitation

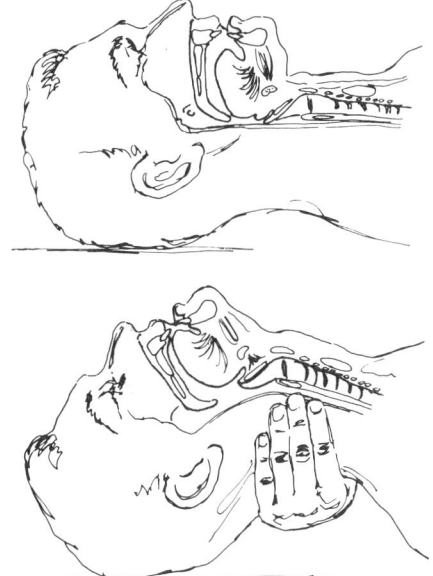

Figure 30-1. Position of the head for mouth-to-mouth breathing. (Reproduced with permission from Gabel RA: Am Fam Physician 7:69, 1973.

A tidal volume of 800 to 1000 ml with a rate of 10 to 12 per minute is sought, to obtain a minute volume of 10 to 12 L in the adult. If the airway is satisfactory, one hand of the operator is placed over the epigastrium to prevent distention of the stomach with air. In the infant or child the operator's mouth is easily placed over both nose and mouth.

Various refinements of the technique have been suggested. These include use of a double oropharyngeal airway; an airway with a one-way valve to avoid return of expired air to the operator's mouth; and a face mask into which the operator blows rather than making direct contact with the patient's mouth. Although an airway may improve ease of expansion of the patient's chest, it has the disadvantage of not being readily available. Placement of a handkerchief over the patient's mouth interferes with gas exchange.

Expired air resuscitation requires no extensive period of training for efficient use. The disadvantages relate principally to contact with the patient's nose or mouth. This is a minor objection, although resuscitation of an apparently drowned or intoxicated individual is not a pleasant prospect. Greater concerns are the possibility of inflation of the patient's stomach with air followed by regurgitation, transmission of infection to the operator, or rupture of the patient's lungs.

BAG AND MASK TECHNIQUE

In expired air techniques, the resuscitator's lungs act as the source of power to expand the patient's lungs. The same result is gained by use of a mask attached to a self-inflating reservoir bag intermittently compressed by hand (Fig. 30-2). Air is the inflating gas, although a source of oxygen can be attached when available. An alternative is the use of an ordinary anesthesia reservoir bag and mask, with gas supplied from a cylinder of compressed air or oxygen. Successful use of these techniques requires a tight mask fit during the compression phase and therefore more training for the civilian. Patency of the airway is maintained by a maximal backward head tilt.

Application of positive pressure at the mouth will not be effective when obstruction is present at the glottic level. Commonly this results from lodgment of a foreign body, rarely from crush injury to the larynx. An attempt should be made to extract the object with the fingers or to dislodge it by pounding the back between the shoulder blades while turning the victim head down. This is more easily done in the infant or child. If an object, a piece of food for example, lodges at the cricoid level, Heimlich recommends embracing the victim from behind and exerting sudden forceful pressure high in the abdomen to dislodge the material. If both measures fail, an airway can be established with a large gauge needle or by an incision, through the cricothyroid membrane. Positive pressure respiration by means of a large syringe or mouth-to-cricothyroid opening is then carried out. We do not advocate attempts to perform tracheotomy in the emergency situation, a difficult procedure even for the expert.

MANUAL METHODS OF RESPIRATION

External compression of the chest is employed in situations in which positive pressure at the airway cannot be applied: severe maxillofacial injury, inaccessibility of the head, or attempted resuscitation in unusual locations, such as treatment of an electrocuted lineman on a telephone pole. At one time the most widely taught method of artificial respiration in the United States was the prone pressure technique. In comparison with other

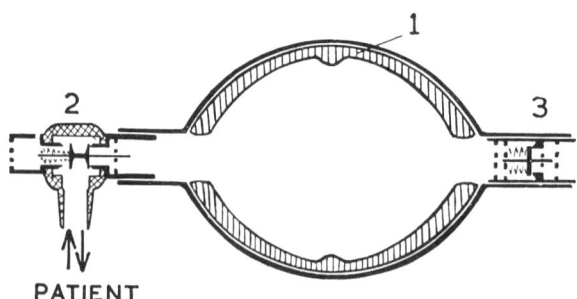

Figure 30-2. Diagram of the Ruben-Ambu resuscitator. *1*, Reservoir bag with sponge rubber lining; *2*, Ruben inflating valve; *3*, one-way valve. (Reproduced with permission from Mushin WW, Rendell-Baker L, Thompson PW, et al: Automatic Ventilation of the Lungs. London, Blackwell Scientific Publications, 1959.)

methods, this is the least effective in moving air and consequently no longer is advocated. Its only advantage is the prone position, which offers a better chance of a clear airway and escape of gastrointestinal contents from the mouth.

Posterior or anterior chest compression may be combined with displacement of the patient's hips or shoulders to expand the thoracic cage. With the patient prone, this is accomplished by elevation of the hips or by lifting the flexed arms over the head. Either maneuver increases chest volume by relieving pressure on the ribs, allowing the abdominal cavity to expand and pulling the diaphragm downward. When the patient is supine, lung volume is increased by hyperextension of the arms. This maneuver increases the anterior-posterior diameter of the chest through traction on the shoulder girdle. A nearly adequate volume of air can be moved with these methods if the trachea is intubated. However, in the usual emergency the resuscitator cannot be certain of a patent airway, and it is difficult to gauge the proper degree of chest compression. Further, these methods are ineffectual when the patient is lying on a mattress that yields to pressure.

CARDIAC RESUSCITATION

Blood flow ceases when the heart stops or the ventricles fibrillate. At normal body temperature the well-oxygenated brain will tolerate ischemia only for about four minutes. Beyond this time, even though blood flow is restored, major and frequently irreversible damage to the brain will have occurred. Should circulatory arrest occur, therefore, the diagnosis must be made at once and a method of moving oxygenated blood to the brain immediately applied. Several factors singly or in combination may precipitate cardiac arrest or ventricular fibrillation: chiefly myocardial depression, heightened irritability, and inadequate coronary blood flow.

Myocardial Depression or Increased Irritability. The common causes are hypoxemia; effects of drugs such as general and local anesthetics, digitalis, quinidine, and procainamide; reflex vagal effects arising from stimulation of the carotid sinus, from pulmonary receptors giving rise to the von Bezold-Jarisch reflex, or attendant upon surgical manipulation of the head, neck, thorax, and upper abdomen; major electrolyte disorders resulting from potassium, sodium, or calcium imbalance — during digitalis therapy, in association with diuresis, following massive transfusion, in uremia, and in intestinal obstruction with vomiting or severe diarrhea; electrocution through use of ungrounded or faulty electric equipment used in diathermy, x-ray, cardiac catheterization, implantation of cardiac pacemakers, or monitoring of physiologic function (ventricular fibrillation may occur in these situations).

Inadequate Coronary Blood Flow. This may involve decreased blood flow to the myocardium or result from increased cardiac work or demands for oxygen that cannot be met. In the former instance, common factors are hypotension from hemorrhage, spinal or peridural anesthesia, overdose of premedicant drugs or local or general anesthetics, traction reflexes, a Stokes-Adams attack, or coronary artery thrombosis. So far as increased demand is concerned, epinephrine, isoproterenol, or aminophylline may cause an increase in cardiac work and a higher oxygen requirement. Cardiac work is increased by elevation of heart rate, heightened myocardial tension and contractile state, as well as impedance to ventricular ejection.

The anesthetist may encounter cardiac arrest during induction of anesthesia, during operation, or in the immediate postoperative period. Arrest is more likely in the elderly or the neonate, in patients with previously diagnosed paroxysmal arrhythmias, in heart block, in digitalis toxicity, following massive hemorrhage, in patients with myocarditis, and during operations on the heart. A treatment plan must be developed that is ready for implementation at a moment's notice.

DIAGNOSIS

The following signs are suggestive or diagnostic of circulatory arrest:
1. Absent radial, carotid, or femoral pulse
2. Inaudible heart sounds
3. Sudden pallor or cyanosis
4. Sudden pupillary dilation
5. Respiratory standstill or apneustic gasps
6. Seizures, convulsions, or loss of consciousness
7. Absence of bleeding and dark blood in the operative field
8. Electrocardiographic evidence of asystole or ventricular fibrillation
9. Electric silence on the electroencephalogram

Most of these signs are unreliable; they may be present during severe hypotension. It must be emphasized that if the blood pressure is not audible, one should not make the error of blaming the apparatus and waste time in trying to readjust it.

EXTERNAL MANUAL CARDIAC SYSTOLE

Before initiating chest compression, a sharp blow is given to the midsternum. This may induce a weak electric current sufficient to start a heart in asystole or terminate certain arrhythmias. The external approach to cardiac arrest involves intermittent application of manual pressure to the sternum just above the xiphoid with the heel of one hand on top of the other and the fingers held straight (Fig. 30-3). The sternum is depressed 4 to 5 cm toward the vertebral column; this may be difficult in the elderly, in whom the chest lacks resiliency. For this to be done effectively the victim must lie on an unyielding surface, either on the floor or on a board placed beneath the chest. Sixty down strokes per minute are necessary to yield a minimally effective cardiac output and blood pressure. In the infant or child, mere compression with the fingers or with the chest held between the fingers is effective. The legs should be raised to increase venous return to the heart. Adequacy of chest compression is judged by reappearance of the peripheral pulses, disappearance of pupillary dilation, and improvement in color.

Cardiopulmonary Resuscitation

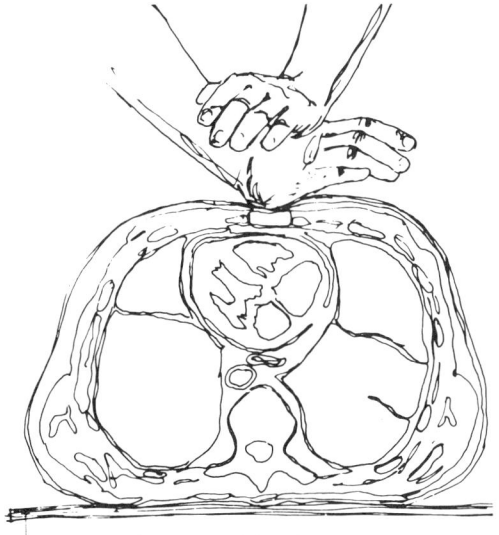

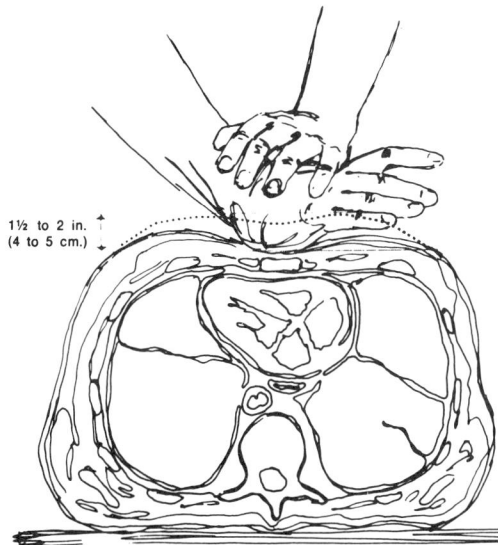

Nonyielding surface to support the spine

1½ to 2 in. (4 to 5 cm.)

Figure 30-3. The heel of the hand is used to depress the chest approximately 4 to 5 cm during closed chest cardiac compression. The patient should lie on a nonyielding surface to support the spine. (Reproduced with permission from Gabel RA: Am Fam Physician 7:69, 1973.)

As manual systole continues the lungs are simultaneously ventilated, for even if sternal pressure results in effective circulation, oxygenation must proceed apace; intermittent sternal pressure alone does not accomplish this. If equipment is not available, mouth-to-mouth or mouth-to-nose ventilation is essential. With bag and mask at hand, 100 per cent oxygen is given by intermittent positive pressure. Tracheal intubation can be carried out after oxygenation has been established, but it is not an essential immediate step. Lung inflation is coordinated with sternal compression: five compressions alternating with one lung inflation are recommended. When only one resuscitator is available, both cardiac and pulmonary resuscitation are carried out by alternating sternal compression and breathing.

The manual method of cardiac resuscitation outlined has met with considerable success; its great value is immediate applicability and avoidance of thoracotomy. Rib fracture, costochondral separation, laceration of the liver or spleen, and fat embolization, all noted occasionally following sternal compression, are a small price to pay if circulation resumes. Mechanical devices manually operated or motor driven have a place in the hospital or an ambulance after hand compression has been instituted, and if recovery is prolonged. A stiff pad at the end of a metal rod is applied rhythmically via pump handle action, as a piston to the precordium.

RECOMMENDED PROCEDURE IN CARDIOPULMONARY RESUSCITATION

In teaching resuscitation, the order of treatment is best remembered by the first four letters of the alphabet: A for airway; B for breathing; C for cardiac compression; and D for definitive therapy. These procedures can be done simultaneously, but require the presence of at least three individuals once initial measures have been instituted. A list of drugs required for resuscitation appears in Table 30-1. Resuscitation may proceed along one of several lines: immediate success; an intervening period of trial with ultimate success; or trial with ultimate failure.

The following steps are taken in resuscitation from cardiac arrest:

1. Establish diagnosis: best signs are apnea, collapse, absence of pulse, pupillary dilation, and absence of heart sounds.
2. Note time. Thump chest sharply two or three times (to counter vagal arrest).
3. Summon help. Sound the alarm for cardiac arrest (hospital alert signal, confirm location).
4. Place support under patient's back, and begin mouth-to-mouth breathing and closed chest compression.
5. With the arrival of others, one physician assumes command; resuscitators are relieved as necessary.
6. Arrival of emergency cart:
    a. Start intravenous infusion by needle or cutdown.
    b. Attach cardiac monitor; prepare defibrillator. If fibrillation is present, shock externally as soon as possible. (DC shock$_1$ 400 watt-seconds in adults, less than 100 watt-seconds in children.)
    c. Inject 44.6 mEq of bicarbonate intravenously, for metabolic acidosis.
    d. For cardiac standstill, primary or after defibrillation, inject epinephrine (0.5 to 1.0 mg or 0.5 to 1.0 ml of a 1:1000 solution) into left ventricle (parasternally, fourth or fifth interspace) (Fig. 30-4).
    e. With appearance of cardiac rhythm, support blood pressure with a vasopressor intravenously (phenylephrine).

Cardiopulmonary Resuscitation

Table 30-1. Drugs for Use in Cardiopulmonary Resuscitation

Drug	Initial Dose	Route	Indication
Epinephrine (Adrenalin)	0.5–1.0 mg	Intravenous or intracardiac	Asystole: To initiate heartbeat Ventricular fibrillation: To improve myocardial tone and induce coarser fibrillation
Sodium bicarbonate	40–50 mEq	Intravenous	Circulatory insufficiency: To correct metabolic acidosis caused by tissue hypoxia
Lidocaine (Xylocaine)	60–80 mg	Intravenous	Ventricular fibrillation: To depress ventricular irritability, facilitating defibrillation
Calcium chloride	1000 mg	Intravenous or intracardiac	Inadequate force of contraction: To increase myocardial contractility
Levarterenol (Levophed)	8 mg in 500 ml	Intravenous drip	Hypotension: To increase myocardial contractility and produce peripheral vasoconstriction
Isoproterenol (Isuprel)	1 mg in 500 ml	Intravenous drip	Bradycardia and inadequate force of contraction: To increase rate and strength of heartbeat
Dopamine (Intropin)	200 mg in 500 ml	Intravenous drip	Hypotension and inadequate force of contraction: To increase myocardial contractility and improve renal blood flow by renal vasodilatation

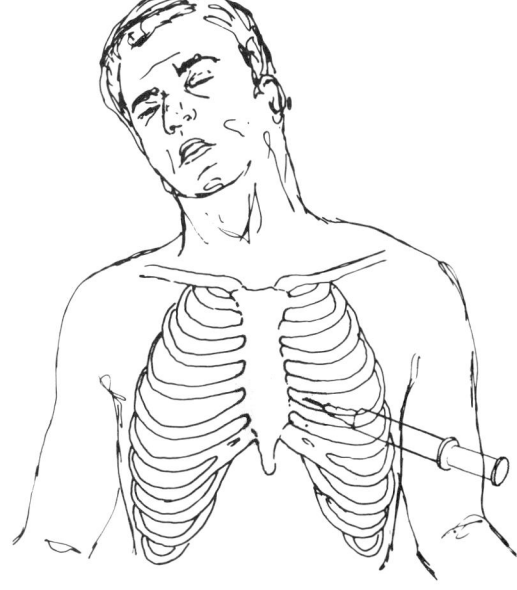

Figure 30-4. Intracardiac injection is made with a 7.5-cm needle through the fourth or fifth interspace, about 5 cm to the left of the midline.

f. At any time, intubate trachea when feasible; give oxygen by intermittent positive pressure. Sample arterial blood for gases and pH; give bicarbonate as necessary. Defibrillate again if needed. Inject lidocaine to control ventricular irritability, isoproterenol by intravenous infusion if blood pressure is not maintained by vasopressors, or calcium gluconate to improve myocardial tone. Administer fluids intravenously to increase blood volume and venous return.
7. Continue with resuscitative efforts so long as there is hope and the patient is salvable. Consider open chest compression under proper circumstances (see following section). The final decision to continue or to desist in resuscitation should rest with the physician in charge.

When signs of good circulation are not immediately evident, the question is how long to persist before opening the thorax. In several situations closed chest compression may be ineffective: the flail or crushed chest, aortic or mitral valvular insufficiency preventing propulsion of blood, pericardial tamponade owing to hemorrhage or effusion, massive myocardial infarction with a toneless ventricle, exsanguinating hemorrhage, and massive pulmonary embolization. It seems reasonable that direct cardiac massage should be more effective in these situations, permitting establishment of the diagnosis at the same time. With the indirect technique the pulse felt peripherally may be merely a shock wave, the mean arterial pressure low, and the central venous pressure high as blood is forced in both directions with compression.

For these reasons we believe there is still a place for thoracotomy and direct compression of the heart and we have experienced success with this when the indirect method failed. But the conditions are sharply defined. Closed chest systole is used to gain time. If not successful within five minutes and if the patient is salvable and circumstances permit management of the open chest, thoracotomy should be done at once. This may be done in the operating room, an emergency room, a recovery room, or an intensive care area, but rarely on the ward.

OPEN CHEST COMPRESSION OF THE HEART

An incision is made in the fourth or fifth left intercostal space, not extending to the sternum lest the internal mammary artery be cut, and not in haste, to avoid lacerating the lung. The pericardium need not be opened at first, but this should be done as soon as possible after first compression of the heart, avoiding injury to the phrenic nerve. A rib spreader is placed because the rib cage cramps the operator's hands. The heart is cradled in the operator's hands, with the ventricles compressed between the thumb and fingers of one hand or the fingers of both hands (Fig. 30–5). Compression is done at the rate of 60 to 80 per minute to insure a sufficient cardiac output. Because of the rapid rate, fatigue occurs rapidly and an alternate operator should be ready to take over.

As in the closed chest technique, adequate venous filling is necessary to supply an adequate stroke volume; all of the ancillary measures ad-

Cardiopulmonary Resuscitation

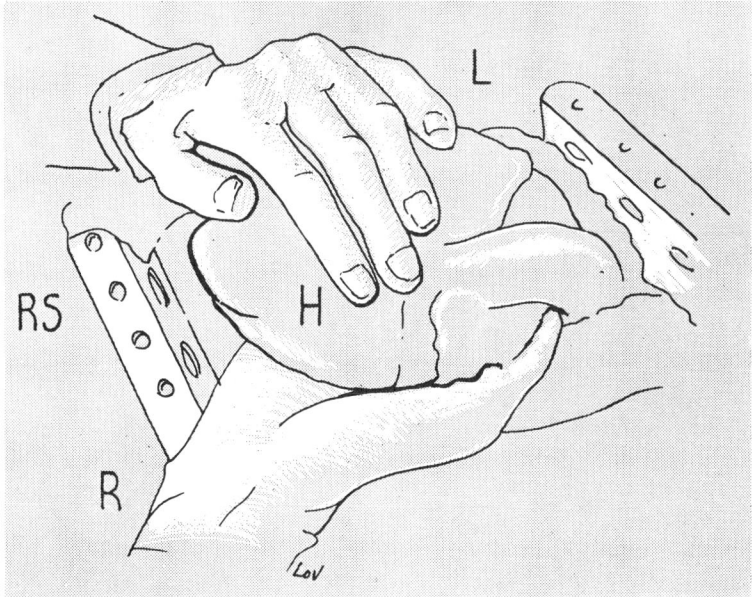

Figure 30-5. Method of performing open chest manual systole. *R*, Right hand; *L*, left hand; *H*, heart; *RS*, rib spreader. (After M. Codding.)

vocated for closed chest resuscitation are applicable when the chest is open. In addition, the aorta can be occluded between the carotid and subclavian arteries to improve coronary blood flow. At the risk of repetition, we again list those signs which suggest that cardiac compression is effective:

1. The heart is full
2. Peripheral pulse becomes palpable
3. Pupils constrict
4. Color of skin, mucous membranes, and blood improves

If the ventricles fibrillate, the first measure is myocardial oxygenation via manual compression. With oxygen ventilating the lungs and circulation through the coronary vessels re-established via compression, the myocardium should lose its dusky color. Defibrillation is then attempted. For internal in contrast to external defibrillation, DC shocks of 30 to 60 watt-seconds are applied by means of disc electrodes at opposite sides of the heart. The larger the mass of the ventricles, the higher the voltage required. Defibrillation is usually followed by asystole, the treatment already outlined. To avoid electrocution, surgeon and anesthetist must avoid contact with the patient as the shocks are applied. When a drug is injected, the aorta is occluded distally to circulate the drug through the coronary system.

PROGNOSIS

Damage to the central nervous system resulting from hypoxia is the determining factor in prognosis when restoration of circulation has been accomplished. If hypoxemia has preceded the cessation of cerebral blood flow associated with cardiac arrest, the capacity of the brain to survive the insult will almost certainly have been reduced below the four-minute figure. There are few measures that can prolong survival time. Hypothermia may be protective, but only if induced immediately and in the right range (30° C). General anesthesia, by reducing cerebral metabolism, may afford slight protection.

Signs presaging recovery include prompt reversal of pupillary dilation, pupillary reaction to light, prompt return of spontaneous respiration, and rapid return of consciousness and orientation. Under these circumstances complete recovery can practically be guaranteed. When there is severe brain damage, decerebrate movements, convulsions, hyperpyrexia, and persistent coma are the manifestations of cell destruction. Continued apnea and hypotension resistant to treatment are ominous, indicative of brainstem damage. Prognosis is guarded, because the longer these conditions persist, the more hopeless the outlook. Serial electroencephalograms offer a means of determining the degree of damage and improvement.

Further anoxia resulting from repeated convulsions should be prevented by the administration of barbiturates or phenytoin. Tracheostomy and assisted or controlled respiration may be necessary. Temperature should be reduced to decrease tissue metabolism and oxygen demand. Cerebral edema and increased intracranial pressure are treated with dexamethasone and osmotic diuretics. Continued surveillance of the patient is necessary until recovery is assured because recurrence of cardiac arrest is not uncommon.

APPRAISAL

Cardiopulmonary resuscitation has saved and will save many lives. It is a dramatic form of therapy which should be thoroughly understood before one is called upon to apply it. Planning is essential. Closed and open chest compression and defibrillation should be practiced in the animal laboratory to develop self-confidence. Personal conviction of the need for prompt diagnosis and immediate action is the key to success.

Heroics in therapy are inappropriate when a favorable outcome cannot be expected. It is poor medical judgment to attempt cardiac resuscitation when the heart has stopped beating in a patient with terminal cancer. Success is less likely if cardiac arrest occurs outside the operating room, although a number of successful resuscitations have been reported under this circumstance. The gamut of resuscitative measures should be attempted outside the operating room only when conditions for success are optimal, that is, when the patient is salvable and individuals who understand the principles of resuscitation are present.

REFERENCES

Bishop R, Weisfeldt ML: Sodium bicarbonate during cardiac arrest. Effect on arterial pH, P_{CO_2} and osmolality. JAMA 235:506, 1976.
Carveth SW, Burnap TK, Bechtel J, et al: Training in advanced life support. JAMA 235:2311, 1976.
Del Guercio LRM, Feins NR, Cohn JD, et al: Comparison of blood flow during external and internal cardiac massage in man. Circulation 31 (Suppl 1):171, 1965.
Gabel RA: Cardiopulmonary resuscitation. Am Fam Physician 7:69, 1973.
Heimlich HJ: A life-saving maneuver to prevent food choking. JAMA 234:398, 1975.
Kouwenhoven WB, Jude JR, Knickerbocker GG: Closed-chest cardiac massage. JAMA 173:1064, 1960.
Lemire JG, Johnson AL: Is cardiac resuscitation worthwhile? A decade of experience. N Engl J Med 286:970, 1972.
Lown B, Neuman J, Amarasingham R, Berkovits BV: Comparison of alternating current with direct current electroshock across the closed chest. Am J Cardiol 10:223, 1962.
National Conference Steering Committee, American Heart Association and National Academy of Sciences–National Research Council: Standards for cardiopulmonary resuscitation (CPR) and emergency cardiac care (ECC). JAMA 277:833, 1974.
Ravin MB, Modell JH (eds): Introduction to Life Support. Boston, Little, Brown, 1973.

Chapter 31

THE IMMEDIATE POSTOPERATIVE PERIOD: RECOVERY AND INTENSIVE CARE

HAZARDS OF THE IMMEDIATE POSTOPERATIVE PERIOD

As an operation draws to a close, there is a tendency for all concerned to "let down." Pressures associated with the surgical procedure are over, and there is an understandable need for those involved to relax; therefore attention is partially diverted from the patient. The senior surgeons often depart from the operating room, leaving the anesthetist without help, although at this time events may occur that threaten the patient's life. Upon emergence from general anesthesia, laryngospasm, retching and vomiting, and excitement may occur, or there may be failure to resume adequate breathing.

An anesthetized patient being moved from the operating table to the litter or bed must be protected against bodily harm. Poorly attended patients have fallen to the floor and been injured. Following abrupt transfer, they have suffered muscle and ligament strain, brachial plexus injury, or dangerous degrees of hypotension. A sufficient number of individuals must assist in the transfer to avoid incidents of this kind. For very heavy patients, roller devices are available to move them onto the litter. Once the patient is moved the sides of the litter or bed must be elevated, a restraining strap put in place, and the patient constantly attended. The unconscious patient is positioned on one side in order to protect the airway.

CIRCULATORY COMPLICATIONS

Hypotension

While the anesthetist is busy disconnecting apparatus from the anesthesia machine, turning off the gas supply, and preparing to move the patient from the operating room, blood pressure or pulse may not be observed for a time, even if monitoring devices are in place. Hypotension may reach serious proportions before being recognized. Chapter 27 lists the causes and treatment of hypotension during and following anesthesia. With a few obvious exceptions these also apply to the postoperative patient, including residual effects of premedication, anesthetics, and neuromuscular blockers, unreplaced blood loss, motion and change of position, cardiac arrhythmias, hypoxia, metabolic acidosis, and electrolyte imbalance.

Hypertension

Although one tends to emphasize the dangers of a decrease in arterial pressure, a certain number of patients will show hypertension. If the rise in pressure is sufficient, a cerebrovascular accident may result, particularly in the arteriosclerotic or hypertensive patient. The more common causes of hypertension are pain, hypercarbia, hypoxia, residual effects of vasopressor drugs, and over-replacement of fluid losses. Treatment is obvious, namely, analgesia, improved alveolar gas exchange, and oxygenation. We have seen marked hypertension after aortic grafts or prolonged abdominal or thoracic operations; the skin appears mottled and cold, and the patient is restless and complains of headache. Whether a rise in pressure represents excessive mobilization of catecholamines is uncertain, but whatever the cause, if dangerously high levels of pressure exist, use of antihypertensive medication is indicated. Trimethaphan or sodium nitroprusside titrated carefully by slow intravenous infusion or fractional administration of chlorpromazine has proved useful under these conditions.

RESPIRATORY PROBLEMS

Hypoxemia

Airway obstruction, laryngospasm, accumulation of secretions, and inadequate gas exchange may be present. Perhaps the most common postoperative respiratory problem today is residual neuromuscular block (Chapter 14). Hypoxemia is a threat. Because of the unreliability of recognition of cyanosis and knowledge that Pa_{O_2} is usually decreased, particularly in the elderly or after major operations, patients are transported to the recovery room with oxygen given via mask and assisted ventilation. Portable oxygen cylinders are easily suspended from litter or bed.

Hypoventilation is commonly observed after anesthesia; tidal volume is reduced after upper abdominal operations, vital capacity and forced expiratory volume are diminished, and cough is restricted by pain. Secretions accumulate and atelectasis develops. Lung compliance is reduced, airway resistance elevated and the work of breathing increased. Abnormal distribution of ventilation and perfusion and shunting cause hypoxemia, which is aggravated when cardiac output is low. Hypoventilation should be searched for and treated promptly. We recommend that oxygen be given to all patients in the recovery room unless the anesthetist states otherwise. Giving oxygen routinely in the absence of orders to the contrary emphasizes our concern with the possibility of postoperative hypoxemia.

This approach also minimizes the diffusion hypoxia that occurs briefly at the termination of nitrous oxide administration. When room air is inhaled, nitrogen diffuses into blood and nitrous oxide into alveoli. Because of higher solubility in blood, the volume of nitrous oxide available for diffusion into the alveoli is greater than the volume of nitrogen entering the circulation. Residual oxygen in the alveoli is therefore diluted and carbon dioxide tension decreased. Provision of a high oxygen concentration for three to four minutes as nitrous oxide is eliminated avoids the hypoxemia. Although diffusion hypoxia is well tolerated by normal individuals, it can summate with other factors in decreasing tissue oxygenation.

In addition to deliberate elevation of $F_{I_{O_2}}$, the tendency today is to reduce the work of breathing and provide better gas exchange through mechanical ventilation for patients who are critically ill. A tracheal tube is often left in place postoperatively and support provided for hours or days, according to the need (see Chapter 33).

Pneumothorax

We have witnessed pneumothorax following brachial plexus or intercostal nerve block, as a result of spontaneous rupture of an emphysematous bleb, during dissection in the neck, or following an operation performed just beneath the diaphragm, such as nephrectomy. Listening to the chest for breath sounds and determination that the trachea is in the midline will usually establish the diagnosis, which is then confirmed by x-ray. Should tension pneumothorax be present, prompt aspiration of the air and institution of underwater drainage are essential.

Restrictive or Obstructive Dressings

Inadequate ventilation may be caused by excessively tight surgical dressings, as after radical mastectomy, and respiratory obstruction may follow application of dressings or plaster jackets about the head and neck.

ASPIRATION OF VOMITUS

This subject is discussed in Chapter 28.

SHIVERING

Shivering has two components, one neurologic and the other relating to temperature control. Pyramidal tract signs are commonly seen as the patient emerges from light planes of general anesthesia, gross clonus sometimes mimicking a convulsion. This can be controlled with methylphenidate given intravenously. Many patients emerge from anesthesia with lowered body temperatures; shivering can be marked, increasing heart rate and work and oxygen consumption, all of which can lead to hypoxemia. Heat loss is engendered by use of semiclosed and open anesthesia systems, by failure to warm infused fluids, by the presence of open body cavities, during deep planes of anesthesia, and in the elderly and cachectic; but the major factor is the air-conditioned operating room. Reduction of body temperature is minimized by maintaining room temperature at least at 21° C.

PAIN

Pain is inevitable after operation, the degree, duration, and effect varying enormously. The very young, the emotionally stable, and the elderly tend to show lesser responses. Superficial operations are accompanied by less pain than following intrathoracic or intra-abdominal procedures or those associated with bladder or anal spasm. Muscle splinting, inadequate ventilation, and diminished cough predisposing to atelectasis are some of the respiratory sequelae of pain, while tachycardia and hypertension are common circulatory reactions.

The patient who is incompletely recovered from general anesthesia is given less than the usual dose of opioid to avoid reanesthetization, hypotension, respiratory obstruction, and hypoventilation. We find that morphine, 5 mg, or meperidine, 50 mg, given intramuscularly, is generally satisfactory for the average adult. It is safer to give a second small dose than administer the larger initially; intravenous administration of a lesser dose results in more immediate relief of pain.

RESTLESSNESS AND EXCITEMENT

Agitation during emergence from general anesthesia may be so severe as to occupy several attendants and require mechanical restraint. A number of factors in addition to pain contribute to the phenomenon. Patients with psychomotor disturbances, those fearful of the findings at operation, or those who confide in the anesthetist that they cannot tolerate pain are likely candidates. Prolonged maintenance of an uncomfortable position or a distended urinary bladder are additional factors. Excitement as a result of hypoxia occurs after thoracic, head and neck, or upper abdominal operations and in the presence of pneumothorax, tracheal collapse, vocal cord paralysis, or respiratory depression from any cause. Arterial hypotension contributes through production of cerebral hypoxia. Scopolamine or the phenothiazines and barbiturates as premedicants are associated with a higher incidence of excitement. However, when these drugs are combined with an opioid, postoperative restlessness is less likely. The role of ketamine in leading to postoperative confusion and hallucination has been discussed in Chapter 13.

Prevention of excitement is apparent from a consideration of the causes. Should agitation develop, however, the following measures are helpful: If the patient has remained in one position on a recovery room bed for a long time, position should be changed. If pain is a factor, an opioid is effective, in small doses by vein if there is delirium, otherwise given intramuscularly. If hypoxemia exists, the underlying causes should be treated if possible while $F_{I_{O_2}}$ is increased. As the anesthetic is eliminated and self-control returns, the patient becomes quiet. Time, therefore, is of the essence, but the experience is upsetting for other patients in the area, for attendants, and for the patient as well.

THE RECOVERY ROOM

A recovery room offers the following advantages: (1) maximal safety for patients; (2) alleviation of the burden of immediate postanesthetic care for the general nursing staff and economy in distribution of nurses; (3) concentration of monitoring and resuscitation equipment; (4) immediate availability of surgeons and anesthetists; (5) opportunity for study of problems associated with the immediate postanesthetic period.

PERSONNEL

Successful operation of a recovery room depends in great measure upon the skill and devotion of the nursing staff. These individuals must be dedicated to their work, for in few other branches of nursing is attention to detail so vital and the need for immediate, intelligent action so necessary. At any moment a patient's condition may worsen. Instant recognition of the change, proper appraisal of its significance, and prompt application of corrective measures are demanded. The luxury of being able to assign a physician to full-time recovery room duty is denied most hospitals, but an anesthetist should be immediately available. In some institutions student nurses obtain their only experience in the care of unconscious patients while on assignment in the recovery room. Under close supervision they learn the problems and management of the unconscious patient: respiratory obstruction, hypotension, emergence excitement, and pain. Orderlies, housekeeping personnel, and respiratory therapists play a major role in the day-to-day operation of the area.

DESIGN AND FACILITIES

Certain features are desirable in the design of a recovery room. Air conditioning is essential and lighting should be uniform and sufficiently bright to permit appraisal of change in color of a patient's skin and mucous membranes. Individual bed lights are helpful for the times when special procedures must be performed. The nurses' station should command a view of all patients, as constant surveillance is essential. The unconscious patient should lie on one side to minimize possibility of aspiration of vomitus, if possible facing the nurses' station to permit observation. During the immediate postanesthetic period, separation of sexes is not essential but care should be taken not to expose patients unnecessarily. Cubicles and curtains can be utilized if an attendant can be assigned to each patient and if the patient can be observed from the central station. At least two telephones are required in the area to be sure that an open line is available in an emergency. A call system permitting nurses to summon additional help is necessary.

An area for assembling, cleaning, and sterilizing equipment and for storing apparatus infrequently used should adjoin the patient area rather than be a part of it; a clinical diagnostic laboratory nearby is a necessity. The recovery room should be adjacent to the operating rooms. If the blood bank is not nearby, a substation is established in the vicinity as well as a storage area for respiratory therapy equipment. It is wise to stock equipment of uniform design so that all understand its use and function. A portable x-ray machine is frequently needed.

Wash basins, adequate electric outlets, bedside tables, work counters, and ceiling suspension of equipment add to the efficiency. The psychological aspects of patient care should not be overlooked. Noise is kept to a minimum; indeed, piped-in music is sometimes provided as a distraction. Conversation about a patient's condition and prognosis should not be audible to the patient.

Oxygen and suction outlets are provided for each patient. Masks capable of providing an $F_{I_{O_2}}$ from 25 to 100 per cent are required. Mechanical ventilation should be at hand or on call from the respiratory therapy service. All kinds and sizes of pharyngeal airways, endotracheal tubes, laryngoscopes, a bronchoscope, and tracheostomy sets are stocked. Few drugs are useful as respiratory stimulants, but bronchodilating agents should be at hand for patients with asthma or bronchoconstriction from other causes; epinephrine, isoproterenol, and aminophylline are used for these conditions.

For hydration and support of the circulation, saline, glucose in water, and one of the plasma expanders such as dextran must be at hand. Several units of type O, Rh negative whole blood are stored in the blood bank for emergency transfusion; these are given until properly crossmatched blood is available. In addition to the usual intravenous sets, provision is made for introducing blood under pressure. Venous cutdown trays, cannulas, and plastic tubing of various sizes are part of resuscitative paraphernalia. To support blood pressure phenylephrine, metaraminol, dopamine, and ephedrine are often used. An electric defibrillating apparatus is a requisite. A cardiac kit with scalpel and thoracic retractors should also be stored. Devices to monitor blood pressure, the electrocardiogram, central venous pressure, and body temperature are at hand. Cooling blankets are essential in the treatment of hyperpyrexia.

Heart failure may occur. Venous tourniquets should be available, as well as facilities for venisection. Digoxin, more rapidly acting drugs of this kind, and antiarrhythmic drugs like quinidine, procainamide, and lidocaine are stored. A recording electrocardiograph is used to permit accurate diagnosis of arrhythmias or myocardial ischemia.

Facilities for management of all types of drainage are needed: gastrointestinal suction apparatus, bladder irrigating sets, underwater chest drainage units, and sump pumps.

Restraining straps, wristlets, armboards, and side rails for beds are needed in the management of restlessness. Opioids, barbiturates, chlorpromazine, and phenytoin are stocked. In case of overdose of opioids, naloxone is a necessity. A locked cabinet for opioids is needed and an accurate record of usage must be kept.

Standard pieces of equipment such as blood pressure cuffs and manometers, stethoscopes, syringes and needles, thermometers, urinary bladder catheters, emesis basins, and urinals and bedpans are always available. A supply of linen and blankets is stocked; a blanket warmer is a useful device and a refrigerator is needed for storage of perishable drugs.

Drugs stocked in the authors' recovery areas are listed in Table 31-1.

Patients with radium implantation for treatment of malignancy are separated from other individuals in the recovery room so that radiation hazards are minimized. Patients with transmissible infections should not be admitted to the recovery room unless isolation techniques are practiced.

RECORDS

An accurate record of the patient's course in the recovery room is kept; one such record is shown in Figure 31-1. Vital signs are recorded. Some anesthetists assign a numerical value to the patient's condition on entry, graded in much the same fashion as the Apgar score for newborns. Criteria include reflex activity, respiration, circulation, state of consciousness, and color. All therapeutic measures are listed in the order administered. Pertinent observations on the patient's appearance and reactions are noted. The record eventually becomes part of the permanent hospital record and is of value to personnel who subsequently assume responsibility for the patient, providing as it does a summary of the early postoperative period. A copy is attached to the anesthetist's copy of the anesthesia chart. A yearly statistical report for the recovery room should include numbers of admissions, length of stay for each patient, mortality, special procedures performed, and unusual problems encountered.

Although complications anticipated in the immediate postoperative period have been listed earlier in this chapter, a few comments on special situations indicate the breadth of problems demanding attention in hospitals providing this kind of care. A neurosurgical patient may develop Cheyne-Stokes respiration, unequal pupils, fixed and dilated pupils, loss of consciousness, and aggravation of hemiparesis as indices of increased in-

Table 31-1. DRUGS KEPT IN THE RECOVERY AREA

Amphetamine	Metaraminol
Atropine sulfate	Methoxamine
Bethanechol chloride	Nalorphine
Calcium chloride	Naloxone
Calcium gluconate	Neostigmine
Chlorpromazine	Nitroglycerin
Cocaine	Opioids
Cortisone	codeine
Dexamethasone	fentanyl
Diazepam	meperidine
Digitoxin	morphine
Digoxin	Oxytocin
Diphenhydramine	Phentolamine
Phenytoin	Phenylephrine
Dopamine	Physostigmine
Doxapram	Phytonadione
Droperidol	Potassium chloride
ϵ-Aminocaproic acid	Procainamide
Edrophonium	Procaine
Ephedrine	Prochlorperazine
Epinephrine	Promethazine
Fibrinogen	Propranolol
Furosemide	Protamine
Glucagon	Quinidine
Glucose, 50 per cent	Secobarbital
Heparin	Sodium bicarbonate
Hydralazine	Sodium iodide
Hydrocortisone	Sodium lactate
Insulin	Sodium nitroprusside
Isoproterenol	Succinylcholine
Lanatoside C	Theophylline ethylenediamine
Levallorphan	Thiopental
Levarterenol	Trimethaphan
Lidocaine	Tripelennamine
Magnesium sulfate	Water for injection, sterile
Mannitol, 25 per cent	

tracranial pressure. Transurethral resection of the prostate may be associated with absorption of a large volume of irrigating fluid through the prostatic bed, resulting in water intoxication, mental confusion, and hypertension. Obstruction of urinary bladder catheters is not uncommon, requiring irrigation. These and other challenging situations require the best in diagnostic acumen and therapy.

GENERAL POLICIES FOR ADMISSION AND RELEASE OF PATIENTS

Admission to and release from the recovery area are the joint responsibility of the services that supervise the recovery area, usually anesthesia, surgery, and nursing, under the overall guidance of the hospital administra-

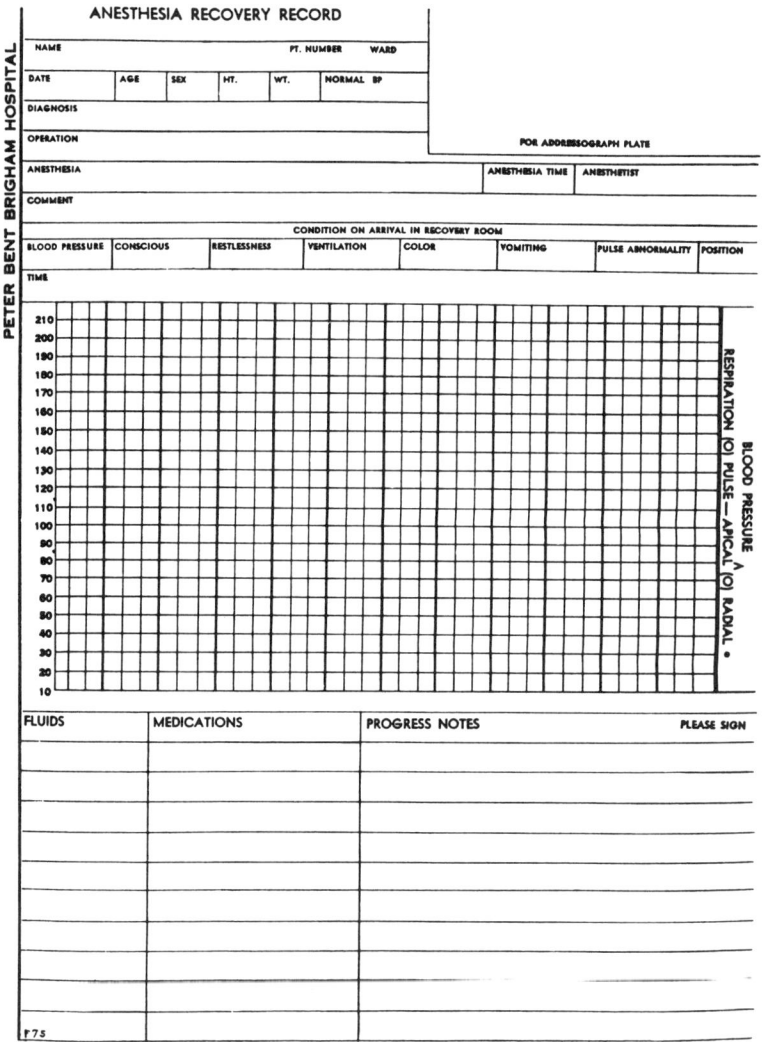

Figure 31-1. An example of an anesthesia recovery record.

tion. This group establishes the rules for conduct in the area: hours of use, admission of visitors, aseptic procedures, hiring of personnel, and charges for services. Only good judgment on the part of the responsible physician and nursing staff can determine when a patient should be discharged from the recovery room. The following criteria are useful: (1) stability of vital signs, (2) control of prior bleeding, (3) sufficient reflexes to prevent aspiration of vomitus, (4) orientation of patient as to time and place, and (5) ability to maintain a safe position in bed, e.g., the optimal position for chest drainage or unobstructed breathing.

Discharge of some patients will depend upon the primary reason for admission; that is, outpatients are kept until they can walk without dizziness or nausea. Patients who have had spinal anesthesia are detained until the level of anesthesia recedes and the blood pressure is stable. Some recovery rooms are open only during the day, others are prepared to keep patients overnight only under exceptional circumstances, while still others retain patients for several days. Ambulatory care surgical units usually maintain their own recovery areas, as do obstetric divisions.

INTENSIVE CARE

When specialized care is needed for days rather than hours, a more versatile unit is necessary, including provision of meals, a waiting area for relatives, a changing area for nurses, sleeping quarters for physicians on call, a clinical laboratory, an x-ray diagnostic unit, and a conference room.

Depending upon the size and function of the hospital, there may be one or several intensive care sections. Individual units have been established for the neonate, the child, patients with suspected or proved myocardial infarction, trauma, burns, and respiratory failure. In a medical intensive care division one finds patients with such varied problems as renal or hepatic failure, gastrointestinal hemorrhage, and neurologic disease, whereas surgical intensive care wards house a wide spectrum of critically ill patients both prior to and following operation. Whether all intensive care areas should be physically adjacent, and whether personnel should rotate among them, is in dispute.

Most of the features and the philosophy of the recovery area pertain to intensive care units, with about 10 per cent of hospital bed capacity devoted to the latter function.

Philosophic and Psychological Problems Posed by Intensive Care

Intensive care can be an effective means of maintaining life as evidenced by reduced mortality, but it is also a costly practice. It is vital, however, that the criteria for instituting care be determined by the implied consent of all involved. Death is no longer defined by absence of spontaneous breathing or heart beat. Thus it is reasonable that selection of patients for prolonged respiratory support should be done with the hope of ultimately providing them with a useful existence. In addition to such criteria as measurement of blood gases and physical findings, considerable judgment and knowledge of the patient's problems are required for selection, and it is by no means certain who should make the final decision for cessation of treatment.

Intensive care medicine is often unnecessarily dehumanizing. Patients with endotracheal intubation or a tracheostomy have difficulty in communicating. They are exposed to the observations and ministerings of many individuals and surrounded by strange and monotonously noisy machinery. Unfortunately, physicians and others occasionally talk carelessly in front of these people. They may be keenly aware of the critical nature of their illness, and death is all around them. They are deprived of such normal experiences as sleep and awareness of night and day, while being constantly suctioned, turned, and punctured with needles.

It is not surprising that such patients frequently develop disorientation, delirium, and psychoses. Thus it is essential that people involved in their care make every effort to add reassurance and psychological support. The experienced nurse serves a vital function in this respect because constant attendance at the bedside provides a calm, friendly, and human approach in this highly charged atmosphere.

REFERENCES

Ali J, Weisel RD, Layug AB, et al: Consequences of postoperative alterations in respiratory mechanics. Am J Surg 128:376, 1974.
Beal JM, Eckenhoff JE (eds): Intensive and Recovery Room Care. New York, The Macmillan Co, 1969.
Becker LD, Paulson BA, Miller RD, et al: Biphasic respiratory depression after fentanyl-droperidol or fentanyl alone used to supplement nitrous oxide anesthesia. Anesthesiology 44:291, 1976.
Gal TJ, Cooperman LH: Hypertension in the immediate postoperative period. Br J Anaesth 47:70, 1975.
Masson AHB, Millar RA: Symposium on the postoperative period. Br J Anaesth 47:89, 1975.
Morris RH, Wilkey BR: The effects of ambient temperature on patient temperature during surgery not involving body cavities. Anesthesiology 32:102, 1970.
Philbin DM, Sullivan SF, Bowman FO, Jr, et al: Postoperative hypoxemia: Contribution of cardiac output. Anesthesiology 32:136, 1970.
Safar P (ed): Public health aspects of critical care medicine and anesthesiology. Clin Anesth 10:3, 1973.

Chapter 32

INHALATION AND CHEST PHYSIOTHERAPY

Thirty years ago the principal concern of hospitals *vis-a-vis* respiratory therapy lay in the maintenance and use of oxygen tents. No attempt was made to define the need for oxygen or to estimate the concentration of oxygen delivered. Most patients breathed concentrations of oxygen far lower than was realized, while measurement of arterial oxygen content, saturation, or tension were confined to the research laboratory.

Gradually more diversified methods of increasing alveolar oxygen tension were developed, with delivery of oxygen by nasal catheter, cannula, mask, or hood. Nevertheless, indications for the use of these devices remained poorly understood, as did the operational aspects of the equipment. Nurses and orderlies were usually assigned to assemble and supervise use of the apparatus. Ultimately the term "oxygen therapy" was coined to define the procedures aimed at increasing the quantity of oxygen breathed by the patient.

Attention next turned to the respiratory tract as a whole. Anesthetists were concerned with pulmonary gas exchange in association with the position of the unconscious patient, the possibilities of airway obstruction, and accumulation of secretions in the respiratory tract. They were consulted when pulmonary complications developed in unanesthetized patients. As a consequence, divisions of oxygen therapy were established in departments of anesthesia.

As knowledge of pulmonary function expanded and the pathologic physiology of respiratory diseases such as pulmonary emphysema, bronchitis, bronchiectasis, and asthma became better understood, the scope of oxygen therapy broadened. Factors other than methods of administering oxygen and maintenance of a patent airway were identified. The value of humidification of inspired gases and of the use of aerosols and bronchodilator drugs was explored. The techniques of intermittent positive pressure breathing (**IPPB**) therapy and chest physical therapy were developed to aid bronchial hygiene and thereby contribute to overall pulmonary care. Under certain circumstances oxygen was given at higher than ambient pressures and in varying concentrations. The aims were to oxygenate blood, to correct hypercarbia, to minimize pulmonary congestion, to diminish the work of breathing, and to decrease the incidence of atelectasis and pneumonia. Arterial puncture and analysis of blood for gases and hydrogen ion concentration became commonplace. This broad approach is now designated respiratory therapy, and its goals are listed in Table 32-1.

OXYGEN THERAPY

The need for oxygen therapy is based upon arterial blood gas measurement and to a lesser extent upon clinical judgment. Unfortunately, tissue hypoxia cannot be measured, although it can be estimated from blood lactate concentrations and Pv_{O_2}. Hypoxia may be present even though Pa_{O_2} is normal. Hypoxemia, a Pa_{O_2} below normal for any age group while breathing room air, increases the work of both ventilation and circulation in compensating for oxygen inadequacy, further worsening the oxygen deficit. If an abnormally low Pa_{O_2} can be raised, ventilatory and myocardial work may decrease while tachycardia, premature ventricular contractions, and dyspnea are eliminated.

Normal values for oxygen and carbon dioxide in atmospheric air, al-

Table 32-1. GOALS OF RESPIRATORY THERAPY

Oxygen:
　　Reverse or prevent tissue hypoxia
　　Treat arterial hypoxemia
　　Decrease work of breathing
　　Decrease myocardial work

Aerosol:
　　Restore and maintain protective mucous secretions
　　　Hydrate desiccated, retained secretions
　　　Promote expectoration
　　　Improve effectiveness of cough

IPPB:
　　Improve distribution of ventilation
　　Re-expand atelectatic alveoli
　　Promote and improve cough
　　Deliver medication

Chest Physiotherapy:
　　Improve distribution of ventilation
　　Mobilize secretions
　　Improve efficiency of ventilation
　　Improve cardiopulmonary work capacity

Table 32-2. NORMAL VALUES FOR OXYGEN AND CARBON DIOXIDE

	Dry Atmosphere	Alveolar Gas	Arterial Blood
P_{O_2} torr	159	105–95	95–70
P_{CO_2} torr	Negligible	42–36	42–36
P_{N_2} torr	601	565	565
Water vapor		47	47
Oxygen content vol per cent			20
CO_2 content vol per cent			48

veolar air, and arterial blood are listed in Table 32-2. Owing to degenerative changes in the lungs occurring with age, the "mean" normal Pa_{O_2} decreases with age (Table 32-3).

INSPIRED OXYGEN CONTENT

Ideally, the concentration of oxygen in inspired air ($F_{I_{O_2}}$) should be that required to maintain a normal alveolar oxygen tension without need for an increase in ventilatory effort; this is usually accomplished with 21 per cent $F_{I_{O_2}}$. Oxygen is appropriately administered via nonrebreathing systems because the expense is little and rebreathing carbon dioxide is easily avoided. However, high concentrations of oxygen add to the threat of accidental combustion. Since one deals with oxygen delivery via nonrebreathing systems, the systems are classified as of high or low flow. A high flow system is defined as one in which gas flow from the apparatus is sufficient to meet total inspiratory requirements. A low flow system is one in which gas flow to the apparatus does not meet total inspiratory demands; thus, room air forms part of the inspired mixture.

Most of the confusion surrounding oxygen therapy results from reference to the technique rather than to the device. Unfortunately, low concentration oxygen techniques have been described in terms of oxygen flow rate through nasal cannulas. Thus "low flow oxygen administration" led many to believe that low flow is synonymous with low concentration. Since it is the oxygen fraction of inspired gas that is important, oxygen flow should be considered only in relation to total gas flow. The concentration of oxygen

Table 32-3. NORMAL ARTERIAL OXYGEN TENSION ACCORDING TO AGE

Age (Years)	Pa_{O_2} Torr
25	95
35	90
45	85
55	80
65	75
75	70

delivered at any flow rate is determined solely by the apparatus and pattern of ventilation.

With a high flow system a large volume of gas provides the total inspired atmosphere, requiring flows of more than 30 L per minute and special devices from which the patient inhales. FI_{O_2} remains constant regardless of change in respiratory pattern. The disadvantages include the extra expense of high gas flows, which can be lessened by the use of equipment that incorporates the Venturi principle (Fig. 32–1 and Table 32–4). Thus, a mask supplied with 5 to 8 L of oxygen per minute can entrain large volumes of room air (50 to 80 L per minute), the mixutre resulting in an FI_{O_2} of 24 to 40 per cent. Escape ports at the perimeter of the mask allow excess gas to vent easily. The flow rate is so high that most patients breathe only that gas in the mask and the relative humidity is close to that of the entrained air. Venti-masks that reliably provide 24, 28, or 35 per cent oxygen concentrations are commercially available.

Face hoods utilizing the Venturi principle incorporated in nebulizers are useful in recovery rooms because patients emerging from general anesthesia do not readily tolerate a mask. Used properly, the hood delivers oxygen concentrations ranging from 40 to 70 per cent. With tracheal tube or tracheostomy in place, a T-piece or Briggs adaptor is attached to deliver the inspired humidified mixture. The reservoir tubing on the exhalation limb tends to eliminate breathing of room air.

Tents and body hoods permitting treatment of the patient in a cooled, oxygen-enriched atmosphere are restricted to pediatric practice. Leaks must be prevented and gas flows sufficient to prevent accumulation of carbon dioxide. Fifteen L of oxygen per minute are required for the first 20 to 30 minutes after the patient is placed in the tent, 10 to 12 L per minute thereafter. Oxygen concentration in a tent rarely reaches 50 per cent and may easily fall to that of room air unless leakage is minimal. However, within a hood oxygen content can approach 90 to 100 per cent. When

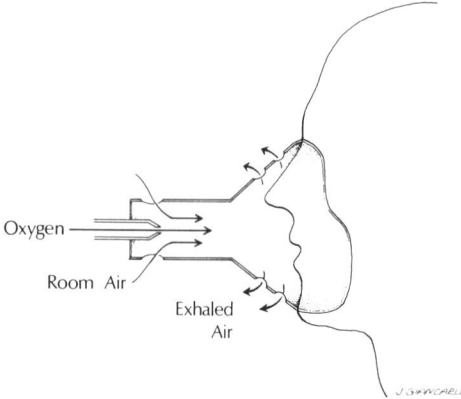

Figure 32–1. A Venturi device providing high total gas flow at fixed FI_{O_2}. Pressurized oxygen is forced through a narrowed orifice. Bernoulli's principle determines the amount of room air "entrained." A Venturi mask is depicted; however, the Venturi mechanism is found in almost all high-flow oxygen delivery systems. (From Suavars, B. A.: Clinical Application of Respiratory Care. Chicago, Year Book Medical Publishers, 1975.)

Table 32-4. LOW FLOW VENTILATORY SYSTEMS

Liter Flow per Minute	Approximate $F_{I_{O_2}}$
Nasal cannula or catheter:	
1	24
2	28
3	32
4	36
5	40
6	44
Plastic mask:	
5	40
6-7	50
7-8	60
Plastic mask with reservoir bag:	
6	60
7	70
8	80
9	90
10	95

either device is used, oxygen concentration should be tested periodically with an analyzer.

The flow system utilizes a reservoir partially or completely filled with 100 per cent oxygen during expiration. On inspiration, the reservoir contents are inhaled along with room air, thus diluting the oxygen with air. The resulting $F_{I_{O_2}}$ depends upon: reservoir size, oxygen flow rate, tidal volume, inspiratory flow rate, and respiratory rate. In low flow systems, $F_{I_{O_2}}$ increases as tidal volume decreases (Fig. 32-2).

Nasal cannulas are a popular means of delivering concentrations of oxygen below 45 per cent. Soft plastic prongs approximately a centimeter in length are placed in the external nares; they are relatively comfortable and well tolerated. The "reservoir" comprises the dead space of the nose, nasopharynx, and oropharynx. Breathing by mouth is inconsequential in the absence of nasal obstruction. Air flowing through the mouth creates a negative pressure as it passes the soft palate, entraining oxygen in the nasopharynx and nose into the oropharynx. Reservoir capacity varies from patient to patient (40 to 80 ml) but is consistent in any one individual. Table 32-5 gives the anticipated $F_{I_{O_2}}$, assuming a normal ventilatory pattern. The smaller the tidal volume, the higher the $F_{I_{O_2}}$ at a given flow rate. Flows exceeding 6 L per minute overload the capacity of the reservoir and increase $F_{I_{O_2}}$ very little.

A plastic mask is used when $F_{I_{O_2}}$ should be above 45 per cent. The added reservoir space of the mask delivers up to 60 per cent inspired oxygen (Table 32-5). The mask fit need not be tight; since room air is drawn in with each breath, several ports are provided for this purpose. So long as the mask approximates the contour of the face, an effective $F_{I_{O_2}}$ is attained.

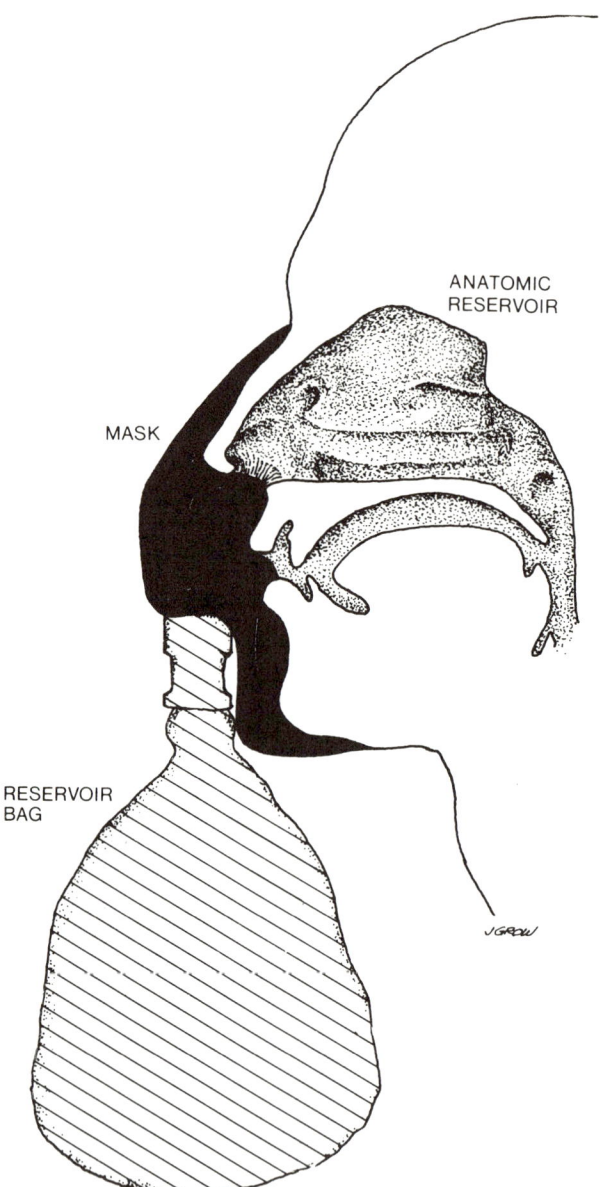

Figure 32–2. Reservoirs in low-flow oxygen therapy. The anatomic reservoir consists of the nose, the nasopharynx, and the oropharynx. This reservoir is estimated to be approximately one third of the anatomic dead space. The appliance reservoir consists of (1) the mask — 100 to 200 ml volume, depending on the appliance; and (2) the reservoir bag — 600 to 1,000 ml of added volume. (From Shapiro, BA: Clinical Application of Blood Gases. Chicago, Year Book Medical Publishers, 1973.)

Table 32-5. APPROXIMATE AIR ENTRAINMENT RATIO

Oxygen Concentration (%)	Air*/100% O_2
24	25/1
28	10/1
34	5/1
40	3/1
60	1/1
70	0.6/1

Examples:
   (a) 40% Venturi device—10 L of O_2 per minute will produce a total gas flow of approximately 40 L per minute.
   (b) 28% Venturi device—4 L of O_2 per minute will produce a total gas flow of approximately 44 L per minute.

*Room air is assumed to be 20.9% oxygen.

A well-fitting plastic mask with reservoir bag is needed for delivery of an FI_{O_2} between 60 and 95 per cent (Table 32-5). Oxygen flows directly into the bag, which should not be allowed to collapse by more than half during inspiration. A one-way valve at the mask provides a nonrebreathing system; without the valve there is some rebreathing, but hardly a significant amount.

HARMFUL EFFECTS OF OXYGEN

Oxygen Toxicity

Much has been written on the toxic effects of high oxygen concentrations. Exposure of mice to high oxygen concentrations for several days is fatal, autopsies revealing a microscopic picture of alveolar hyaline membrane formation, early interstitial fibroblastic changes, and edema. Oxygen causes biochemical abnormalities possibly related to inhibition of enzymes in the tricarboxylic acid cycle, particularly those containing sulfhydryl groups. Inhibition of ciliary action has also been found. However, in humans, major pulmonary changes owing to oxygen inhalation at one atmosphere alone have not been conclusively shown. If oxygen causes pulmonary damage, is this caused by a high Pa_{O_2}? Most observers believe that there is cause for concern only when Pa_{O_2} remains above 100 torr for some time. Hence, in practice, a progressive increase in FI_{O_2} is acceptable so long as Pa_{O_2} remains below 100 torr and after substitute methods such as positive end expiratory pressure (PEEP) fail to raise Pa_{O_2} to safe levels. Oxygen toxicity seems to occur with a combination of high FI_{O_2} and artificial ventilation, but even then only under specific circumstances. While the genesis of oxygen toxicity in man is controversial, appropriate therapy should not be withheld because of fear of the toxic effect of a high FI_{O_2}. A possible clinical alternative may prove to be the use of an extracorporeal membrane oxygenator.

Retrolental Fibroplasia

Prolonged administration of over 40 per cent oxygen to the premature infant is likely to result in retrolental fibroplasia. Apparently spasm of the incompletely developed retinal vessels occurs, followed by perivascular exudation, tissue hyperplasia, scarring, and blindness. The premature neonate, therefore, should not be exposed to atmospheres containing more than 40 per cent oxygen unless Pa_{O_2} is low and a higher FI_{O_2} is required. Development of retrolental fibroplasia is associated with a Pa_{O_2} above 150 torr. As in the adult, a cyanotic infant should not be denied high inspired oxygen concentrations because of fear of complications. Again, PEEP should be given a trial, but at a lower FI_{O_2}.

TREATMENT OF CHRONIC HYPOXIA

Administration of high concentrations of oxygen to patients with chronic hypoxia and carbon dioxide retention may result in confusion and coma. The explanations are several. First, stimulation of carotid and aortic chemoreceptors by a low Pa_{O_2} activates the medullary respiratory and circulatory centers. Sudden correction of chronic hypoxia by inhalation of oxygen removes the stimulus. Second, patients with advanced pulmonary emphysema are deficient in ventilatory exchange of both carbon dioxide and oxygen. The respiratory center becomes relatively insensitive to carbon dioxide and its associated increased hydrogen ion concentration. Under these circumstances, upon inhalation of oxygen the reflex drive to respiration is removed and tidal exchange decreases. Pa_{CO_2} then approaches narcotic levels, leading to confusion and coma. This complication of oxygen inhalation occurs in only a few patients with chronic hypoxia, but when it is present the physician is faced with a dilemma. Untreated, the patient retains consciousness but hypoxic cerebral or cardiac damage may develop. When oxygen is given, hypoxia is corrected but coma ensues. The appropriate treatment therefore is either to increase FI_{O_2} in stepwise fashion over a period of days, as by Venti-mask, or to use IPPB with oxygen. The former avoids abrupt changes in Pa_{O_2} and Pa_{CO_2}, allowing gradual adaptation, and the latter permits control of ventilation.

Oxygen Apnea

A deeply narcotized patient breathing room air may cease to breathe following elevation of FI_{O_2}, a phenomenon termed "oxygen apnea." In part, the explanation is that offered for the appearance of coma in chronic hypoxia. Central depressants reduce the sensitivity of the medullary centers to carbon dioxide and respiration is maintained via hypoxic stimulation of the chemoreceptors. Abrupt correction of hypoxia may result in apnea. This complication appears in patients deeply narcotized with barbiturates and opioids, those with cerebral trauma or edema, and in individuals with hypoxic damage to the respiratory center.

Should oxygen apnea appear, it is convincing indication of the need for treatment, even if artificial ventilation is required.

CARBON DIOXIDE INHALATION

A rise in Pa_{CO_2} increases the depth and rate of respiration unless the respiratory center is depressed by opioids or disease, or the muscles of respiration cannot respond, as in anterior poliomyelitis, or the lungs are diseased, as in emphysema, or the chest wall is stiffened. Carbon dioxide inhalation, once popular in the prevention and treatment of pulmonary atelectasis, has been replaced by positive pressure techniques and other bronchial hygienic regimens. There is still a place for its use, however, perhaps in the treatment of hiccough and to dilate cerebral vessels.

Two methods of administering carbon dioxide are used, one in which carbon dioxide is inhaled by the patient and the other in which it is accumulated by rebreathing. Five or 10 per cent carbon dioxide in 95 or 90 per cent oxygen can be inhaled via bag and mask for two or three minutes; little is accomplished if hyperpnea does not develop in that time. The patient may also be exposed to 100 per cent carbon dioxide by the gravity method, with the delivery tube held three to four inches above the nose or mouth and carbon dioxide allowed to flow over the face. If hyperpnea does not appear within 30 sec, administration is discontinued. A common rebreathing technique involves use of a long plastic tube of wide bore (Schwartz tube) through which the patient breathes via a mouthpiece, a variant of the older technique of rebreathing from a paper bag. Should transient hypoxia be a problem, supplemental oxygen at a low flow, 1 L per minute, is insufflated at the distal end of the tube.

HUMIDIFICATION OF GASES

Adequate humidification and warming of inspired air are necessary for proper functioning of the respiratory mucosa. Normally, inspired air is warmed and humidified as it passes through the nasal and pharyngeal cavities. Secretions produced by the goblet cells and glands of the mucosa contain a mixture of water, polysaccharides, and protein which has a viscosity conducive to optimal function of cilia and protection of epithelial cells. If the nasal passages are bypassed by mouth breathing, tracheal tube, or tracheostomy, or if the moisture content of inspired air is low relative to temperature, water is extracted from the mucous secretions and mucosa. Increased viscosity of secretions and impaired ciliary function follow.

Air saturated with water at body temperature contains 44 mg water per liter of air. Various devices are used in an attempt to saturate the air reaching the trachea with water vapor at body temperature. A bubble jar delivers water in the low range of 6 to 10 mg per liter; hence it is useful only when upper airway humidification mechanisms are intact, as via a nasal catheter, but not through a tracheal tube or tracheostomy.

Inspired air may be raised to body temperature by diversion through a container of heated water. Although the deficit in humidity is eliminated, as the air passes through delivery tubes upon exit from the humidifier temperature decreases, water condenses in the tubing, and once again rewarming and rehumidification are required. To compensate for this, units have been designed to heat air above body temperature. With these systems some water still condenses in the delivery tubing as cooling occurs, and the water must be periodically removed lest it result in air flow obstruction or enter the patient's airway. Systems with heated delivery tubing have been devised to prevent this problem, but if the temperature of inspired gas is raised too vigorously hyperthermia may develop, since the respiratory tract cannot eliminate body heat.

Humidifiers are designed to saturate air with water. Nebulizers suspend tiny water particles in air, directing a rapid flow of gas over an orifice connected to a reservoir, or forcing water onto a metal plate vibrating at ultrasonic frequency. Nebulizers using the capillary jet principle yield particles mostly between 0.1 and 5.0 μ in diameter, and total water delivery ranges between 24 and 35 mg per liter. By adding a heating element to a jet nebulizer, output can be increased to 42 to 50 mg per liter. The ultrasonic nebulizer produces particles between 0.8 and 1.0 μ in diameter. The output from an ultrasonic device need not be warmed, since the supension can easily yield enough molecules to overcome the deficit in humidity arising when inspired air is warmed to body temperature. A particle size from 0.5 to 1.5 μ is effective in avoiding fallout in delivery tubes and the upper airway, allowing deposition of the particles in terminal bronchioles and alveoli. Since by supersaturation the ultrasonic nebulizer can deliver 3 to 6 ml of water per minute into the lungs, water intoxication may result.

The heated water humidifier or ultrasonic nebulizer can be placed in the circuit of a mechanical ventilator without disturbing flow patterns. Capillary jet nebulizers require a share of the total gas flow driving the unit, thus affecting $F_{I_{O_2}}$ and ventilatory volumes.

INTERMITTENT POSITIVE PRESSURE BREATHING (IPPB)

Delivery of gas to the alveoli with minimal respiratory effort can be facilitated by use of a pressure limited ventilator. The ability to inhale and exhale large volumes spontaneously is hindered by airway obstruction, pain, neuromuscular disability, or central nervous system depression. In these instances distribution of air is uneven, resulting in underventilated and collapsed areas of lung. Appropriately administered IPPB can improve distribution of air in two ways. First, delivery of a large volume results in better distribution to underventilated areas, and second, bronchodilation follows raised intraluminal pressures, allowing increased gas flow to bypass mucous plugs in bronchioles. The effects are enhanced by slow, deliberate intake of gas. Cough is improved with the greater volume of air delivered. Many physicians mistakenly consider IPPB only as a means of delivering aerosolized medication to the airway. Although important, this is by no means the greatest asset, for the mechanical benefits of large volume delivery and mechanical bronchodilation are of considerable consequence. Results of treatment, however, depend upon the competence of the technician administering the therapy. IPPB should not be used as the sole means of lowering Pa_{CO_2} or increasing Pa_{O_2} because improvement will only be transient.

Cleaning and sterilization of equipment are essential to prevent cross-infection. High mean positive pressures applied to the airway may impede venous return by increasing intrathoracic pressure. It is important that the respiratory therapy technician recognize signs of circulatory embarrassment and other hazards of positive pressure therapy such as nosocomial infection. The therapist should also be able to recognize the adverse effects of medication delivered by such treatment.

IPPB is commonly used in the therapy of chronic obstructive pulmonary disease. It is only one of a series of measures that should be used, including protection of the airway from irritants, use of bronchodilators, respiratory training and muscle conditioning, adequate hydration, and prevention of infection. IPPB alone is of minimal value. Some believe its use is limited and that it diverts physicians' attention from the total care of patients.

CHEST PHYSIOTHERAPY

Chest physiotherapy has been accepted in Europe for years, but has been slow to be adopted in this country. Through proper instruction and encouragement of the patient, the goal of chest physiotherapy is to improve distribution of ventilation, efficiency of breathing, and elimination of secretions.

Postural drainage in conjunction with chest percussion and vibration is the hallmark of chest physiotherapy. The anesthetist should be conversant with the anatomy of the segmental bronchi so as to be able to give reliable instructions for postural drainage and chest physiotherapy. Chest physiotherapy is helpful in the treatment of segmental atelectasis, drainage of bronchiectasis and lung abscess, and correction of abnormal distribution of ventilation and perfusion. In addition, basic physical therapy techniques aimed at increasing the capacity for exercise in the pulmonary cripple are increasingly applied in the treatment of chronic obstructive lung disease.

INCENTIVE SPIROMETRY

Incentive spirometry encourages the patient to take a voluntary maximal sustained inspiration while inhaling from a spirometer. A light goes on when a preset inspiratory volume is inhaled and remains lit until inspiratory flow ceases. The preset inspiratory volume is increased by increments, the procedure thus providing an incentive for maximal inspiratory effort. Hypocarbia is avoided so long as the rate is limited to 4 or 5 per minute. Physiologic studies on normal subjects show that an intrathoracic subatmospheric pressure of -50 cm of water may be produced by this method, which would allow for all alveoli to open while venous return is transiently increased.

This technique may have a reasonable application in the routine prophylactic stir-up regimen for postoperative patients. In our opinion, little assurance of maximal lung inflation is offered in patients who have a significantly limited vital capacity or in those who are less than cooperative.

DRUGS IN INHALATION THERAPY

The anesthetist takes advantage of the large surface area of the lungs to achieve systemic blood levels of inhalation anesthetics. Similarly, many kinds of medication used in inhalation therapy are delivered by aerosol suspension into the tracheobronchial tree. Commonly used drugs such as bronchodilators are easily absorbed, achieving the degree of bronchodilation that an intravenous dose might otherwise produce. On the other hand, vasoconstrictors and mucolytics exert largely topical actions. Only the more important pharmacologic groupings of drugs administered by aerosol are discussed here.

BETA-ADRENERGIC STIMULATING DRUGS

The substances producing bronchodilation most commonly used in inhalation therapy are the beta-adrenergic stimulants, usually isoproterenol (Isuprel) administered in 1:200 solution. The degree of bronchodilation correlates with systemic blood levels of the drug. Because of systemic absorption, evidences of beta-adrenergic stimulation of the myocardium and peripheral circulation are frequent: tachycardia, palpitation, either hyper- or hypotension, and flushing of the skin. Adverse effects of aerosolized isoproterenol often force discontinuance of treatment and the drug offers no topical vasoconstrictor property. A new class of drug, typified by isoetharine (Bronkosol-2) is claimed to be an active pulmonary beta-receptor stimulant with little effect on cardiac beta receptors.

ALPHA-ADRENERGIC STIMULATING DRUGS

Phenylephrine is often given by aerosol to produce vasoconstriction of the respiratory tract mucosa. More than a few pulmonary diseases may be accompanied by hyperemia and edema of the respiratory mucosa, causing a decrease in bronchiolar lumen and raised airway resistance. Topical application of a vasoconstrictor can reverse many of these changes. Alpha-adrenergic drugs, however, cause hypertension if rapidly absorbed.

RACEMIC EPINEPHRINE

This is a mixture of the levo- and dextroisomers of epinephrine, the levoisomer being the active form. The effect of the combination on cardiovascular receptors is less than that of epinephrine alone because the inactive isomer combines with some of the beta receptors. Both isomers, however, are topical vasoconstrictors. Thus, racemic epinephrine results in a lower incidence of cardiovascular effects while producing effective topical vasoconstriction and bronchodilation.

MUCOLYTICS

When abnormal mucopolysaccharides thicken the sputum, as in cystic fibrosis, certain enzymes may help to break up the long mucopolysaccharide chains, to increase fluidity, and to decrease the viscosity of secretions. An example of such an enzyme is pancreatic dornase (Dornavac). Another compound without enzymatic action, acetylcysteine (Mucomyst), also produces mucolysis while active in the presence of purulent secretions. Acetylcysteine is used as a 10 per cent solution rather than the stronger concentration originally marketed, which was an irritant to the respiratory tract. The compound is not a substitute for hydration and humidification.

DETERGENTS

As a decrease in surfactant is said to occur in some pulmonary diseases, addition of a detergent by aerosol can help to re-expand atelectatic portions of the lung and restore normal alveolar geometry. Although commonly used as vehicles in aerosols and IPPB, there is little evidence to show that detergents are more efficient than normal saline.

ANTIBIOTICS

These drugs are used in aerosol form for treatment of pulmonary infection, but doubt exists that there is any advantage of this route over systemic administration. Antibiotics work best when given systemically, and although there is no decrease in toxicity when the aerosol route is used, certain antibiotics administered by aerosol seem to cause an increased number of sensitivity reactions.

CORTICOSTEROIDS

As potent topical anti-inflammatory agents, these drugs have been used in aerosol therapy to decrease tracheobronchial inflammation. Little steroid is absorbed systemically, and some reports suggest profound improvement in bronchitis following inhalation. There may be some rationale in the use of aerosolized steroids in the treatment of aspiration pneumonitis (see Chapter 28).

REFERENCES

Acute Pulmonary Injury and Repair (the Adult Respiratory Distress Syndrome): The 16th Aspen Lung Conference. Chest 65 and 66 (Suppl):1, 1974.
Allan D (ed): Humidification and mist therapy. Int Anesthesia Clin 8(3):1, 1970.
Clark JM: Toxicity of oxygen. Ann Rev Respir Dis 110:40, 1974.
Egan DF: Fundamentals of Respiratory Therapy. 2nd ed, St. Louis, CV Mosby Co, 1973.
Graff TD, Benson DW: Systemic and pulmonary changes with inhaled humid atmospheres: Clinical application. Anesthesiology 30:199, 1969.
Hayes B, Robinson JS: An assessment of methods of humidification of inspired gas. Br J Anaesth 42:94, 1970.
Hedley-Whyte J: Control of the uptake of oxygen. N Engl J Med 279:1152, 1968.
Kafer ER: Pulmonary oxygen toxicity: A review of the evidence for acute and chronic oxygen toxicity in man. Br J Anaesth 43:687, 1971.
Miller RD, Hepper NGG: The dangers and limitations of IPPB in managing diseases affecting ventilation. In Ingelfinger FJ, Ebert RV, et al (eds): Controversy in Internal Medicine II, Philadelphia, WB Saunders Co, 1974, p 263.
Miller W: Fundamental principles of aerosol therapy. Respir Care 17:295, 1972.
Proceedings of the Conference on the Scientific Basis of Respiratory Therapy. Am Rev Resp Dis 110:1, 1974.
Shapiro BA, Harrison RA, Trout CA: Clinical Application of Respiratory Care. Chicago, Year Book Medical Publishers, 1975.

Chapter 33

RESPIRATION AND RESPIRATORY CARE

Well-functioning lungs are among anesthetists' most important allies during their work in the operating suite and recovery rooms. Therefore we believe that emphasis on the quantitative aspects of gas exchange is of importance not only in reference to the respiratory gases, O_2 and CO_2, but in uptake and elimination of volatile anesthetics. The mechanical properties of the respiratory system are literally felt by the hand of the anesthetist whenever the breathing of an anesthetized patient is controlled or assisted; hence a solid knowledge of respiratory mechanics is essential for good management. Again, because the anesthetist is responsible for maintenance of the patient's fluid balance during operation, understanding of the fluid exchange in the lung and the mechanisms that can derange it cannot be overemphasized.

This chapter is not meant to be a comprehensive text on the physiology of respiration or respiratory failure; coverage of topics is both selective and variable in extent of treatment.

A list of monographs and review articles is given in the references to guide readers to further up-to-date information, and to refer them to original articles in the field of normal and abnormal pulmonary function and the clinical management of failing respiration.

LUNG FUNCTION AND STRUCTURE

The primary function of the lungs is the exchange of the respiratory gases, O_2 and CO_2, between the blood and the atmosphere. The ultimate destination of oxygen is the mitochondria in the tissue cells, where it serves as a proton acceptor in oxidative metabolic pathways and yields "metabolic" water; CO_2 is produced in cells via the various kinds of decarboxylation. Thus the gas exchange between the atmosphere and blood that occurs in the lungs is only one step in the overall transport of O_2 and CO_2 from atmosphere to cells. Intimate functional links between the lungs and the circulatory system are essential, both for the transport of O_2 and CO_2 between the lungs and tissues and for the functioning of the lungs as a gas exchanger.

The structure of the lungs is exquisitely suited to these functions: in an adult man mixed venous blood is exposed to gas within the lungs at an internal surface of 50 to 100 sq m (approximately the size of a tennis court). The gas exchanging membrane consists of about 300 million alveoli with capillary networks in their walls. The membrane separating gas and blood is very thin, on the average about 1 μm, and the diameters of the alveoli also are small, about 150 μm. With this large surface area and the small distances involved, conditions are favorable for efficient diffusional exchange of O_2 and CO_2 between the gas phase and blood.

Gas is transported to the alveoli by mass movement through the conducting airways. The function of the upper airways—nose, mouth, pharynx, and larynx—is to filter out particles of large size, to warm and humidify inspired gas, and to conserve water vapor in expired gas. These conditions are eliminated when the upper airway is bypassed via tracheal intubation or tracheostomy. The lower airways begin at the trachea and its division at the carina, into the two main stem bronchi, with subsequent irregularly dichotomous branching for over 20 generations of division. The diameter of each new generation of tubes decreases; however, the total cross sectional area increases sharply; at the level of the terminal bronchioles it is about 90 times that of the combined main stem bronchi. Thus, the velocity of gas flow decreases markedly toward the periphery.

The airways consist of an epithelial layer with a basal membrane and supporting connective tissue containing cartilage and smooth muscle. The cartilages are U-shaped in the trachea and main stem bronchi and more irregular beyond, disappearing at the level of the bronchioles (about 1 mm in diameter, at the 10th to 11th generations). Maintenance of patency in the small airways depends upon the elastic recoil of the tissues. Smooth muscle is present throughout the tracheobronchial tree down to terminal bronchioles. Upon constriction, as in asthma, airway resistance increases. However, in the normal lung the physiologic role of smooth muscle is not understood. Epithelium is of the pseudostratified columnar type in large airways, the thickness progressively decreasing to a layer of cuboidal cells in terminal bronchioles. Most prominent are the synchronously beating ciliated cells, with mucin-producing goblet cells and serous cells interspersed; large and intermediate bronchi contain glands that penetrate the basal membrane. In chronic bronchitis, the thickness of the glandular layer increases. Ordinarily secretions produced by the epithelial elements form a mucous carpet that is propagated toward the pharynx by the cilia. Because of a functional "blood-bronchial barrier" the liquid component of the mucus is not a simple ultrafiltrate of plasma. One of the consequences of such a barrier is that most antibiotics systemically administered appear in bronchial fluid in appreciably lower concentrations than in plasma. Nutrition of the airways comes from the bronchial circulation, which extends down to the terminal bronchioles. Bronchial veins drain into the pulmonary veins.

Inhaled particles (including bacteria) that bypass the upper airways are deposited on the mucous carpet and removed by continuous motion toward the pharynx. The efficiency of mucociliary clearance mechanisms depends upon the quality of the bronchial secretions, their viscosity, and on the action of cilia. The latter are depressed by irritants such as tobacco smoke or anesthetics. The smallest inhaled particles, less than 3 μm in diameter, upon reaching the alveoli are handled by pulmonary macrophages, presumably derived from blood histiocytes, which engulf and digest particles or microorganisms and clear them via the pulmonary lymphatics and capillary blood vessels.

The airways, from nose to terminal bronchioles, are not endowed with gas-exchanging membranes, thus constituting the anatomic dead space. The respiratory zone, representing some 90 per cent of the lung, begins with the respiratory bronchioles with outpocketings of single alveoli, followed by the alveolar ducts and sacs.

MECHANISMS OF PULMONARY GAS EXCHANGE

These are grouped under three categories: (a) rate of pulmonary ventilation, (b) rate of blood flow through the lung, and (c) diffusional exchange of O_2 and CO_2 between gas and blood. For effective diffusional exchange, it is essential that matching of ventilation with blood perfusion occur throughout the lung. Ideally, the most efficient arrangement would be a perfectly homogeneous distribution of both ventilation and blood flow throughout, and in the first approach to a quantitative evaluation of gas exchange we shall assume this to be the case. However, even in healthy lungs, ideal distribution of ventilation and perfusion does not occur, owing to the effect of gravity on distribution of ventilation and blood flow. In the diseased lung, matching of ventilation and perfusion is further disturbed, with important consequences for gas exchange.

PULMONARY VENTILATION

Distances in the conducting airways are so great that no significant amount of gas can be transported via simple diffusion from atmosphere to alveoli. Thus mass movement of gas, or pulmonary ventilation, is essential for exchange of O_2 and CO_2. In dealing with mechanisms of pulmonary ventilation, we first describe the static volumes of the lungs, then concentrate on the mechanics of respiration, factors that determine bulk movement of gas between the atmosphere and the respiratory zone. Finally, we deal with quantitative aspects of exchange of individual respiratory gases and with the consequent effect on composition of alveolar gas and arterialized blood.

LUNG VOLUMES

Figure 33-1 shows typical values for static volumes in the normal human lung. Of these, tidal volume and vital capacity can be measured with a simple spirometer. Absolute volume of gas present in the lung at functional residual capacity, at residual volume, and at total lung capacity can be measured by gas dilution techniques or with a body plethysmograph.

RESPIRATORY MECHANICS

The tidal volume (V_T) is the volume of gas moved in and out of the lungs in a single breath. At rest, the average V_T is about 500 ml. The product of tidal volume and frequency of breaths per minute is the minute ventilation, usually measured as the expired volume, $\dot{V}_E$, liters per minute. Respiratory rate at rest is about 14 breaths/min; thus a typical resting $\dot{V}_E$ would be 7 L/min.

In order to produce a flow of gas between the atmosphere and the lungs, a pressure difference must exist between the mouth and nose (Pao) and that in alveoli (P_A). In spontaneous breathing, P_A is lowered below atmospheric pressure by the action of inspiratory muscles; during artificial ventilation, the pressure difference (Pao − P_A) is created by applying positive pressure to the airways, or positive pressure ventilation (PPV).

The diaphragm is the essential inspiratory muscle; it is innervated by the phrenic nerves (C3–C5). As the diaphragm contracts, the volume of the chest is increased both by descent of the diaphragm and elevation of the distal margins of the rib cage. The ribs are also elevated by contraction of the

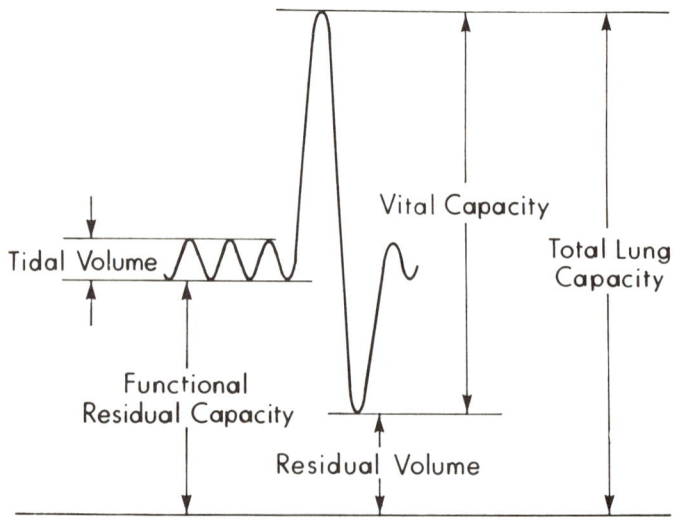

Figure 33-1. Volumes in the lungs.

external intercostal muscles segmentally innervated from the thoracic spinal cord. In forceful inspiration, accessory muscles of inspiration are recruited (shoulder-girdle and neck) to elevate the rib cage.

Expiration is a passive act during quiet breathing caused by elastic recoil of the respiratory system as it returns to resting volume. During the hyperpnea of exercise or in voluntary hyperventilation, expiration becomes active. The important expiratory muscles are those of the abdominal wall which increase intra-abdominal pressure, thrusting the relaxed diaphragm into the chest and exerting traction on the rib cage. The internal intercostals also assist expiration by downward traction. Expiratory muscles are essential for forceful expiration during coughing. In tetraplegic patients, residual sparing of diaphragmatic contraction may be enough to develop adequate inspiratory force during resting ventilation; however, efficient cough is impossible owing to loss of expiratory muscles.

Mechanical Properties of the Respiratory System

Understanding the mechanical or elastic properties of the respiratory system is important for several reasons: First, most of the work of breathing is spent in expanding the chest wall and lungs, not on moving air in and out. Recall that in spontaneous breathing the pressure difference between Pao and P_A required to move air is low, about 1 cm H_2O in quiet breathing. Second, mechanical properties of the lungs determine the distribution of the volume of gas to various parts of the lungs; this, together with the regional perfusion, determines the efficiency of gas exchange and the composition of alveolar gas and arterialized blood. Finally, changes in the mechanical properties of the lung are prominent in most pathologic conditions.

Elastic Properties of the Lungs

The isolated, excised lung changes volume like an elastic balloon; volume increases when the pressure inside increases above that outside, and deflation is spontaneous as a result of elasticity. Static elastic properties of the isolated lung can be described by studying the static pressure-volume relationship. The relevant pressure is the transpulmonary pressure (P_L) or the difference between alveolar pressure (P_A) and the pressure on the surface of the lung. When P_L increases, volume increases, and vice versa. In the excised lung, the surface pressure is the barometric pressure (P_B). To maintain an excised lung at a given volume, P_L must be positive, P_A higher than P_B. With the lung in the chest with no gas flow and the airway open, P_A equals P_B and a positive distending pressure (P_L) results from a subatmospheric negative pleural pressure (P_{pl}) exerted by traction of the chest wall. Figure 33-2 shows a pressure-volume plot of a normal dog lung. Note that the curve during inflation differs from that obtained on deflation, a phenomenon called hysteresis. The slope of the pressure-volume curve at any lung volume is the lung compliance (C_L). Within the range of normal tidal breathing, C_L is about 200 ml/cm H_2O. At high lung volumes, compliance decreases markedly and the lung becomes very stiff.

The elasticity of the lungs is a result of two factors: the presence of a fibrous network in parenchyma, and the effect of surface tension at the gas-liquid interface within the alveoli and small airways. The fibrous network consists of elastin, an extensible protein, and collagen, a rigid material. Elastin probably functions over the whole range of lung volumes, while collagen fibers act as an inextensible net that becomes tense at high lung volumes, not unlike a net around an inflated rubber balloon. Presumably collagen fibers are responsible for the low lung compliance at high lung volumes.

Surface tension is the other and major component of elastic recoil. When the lungs are filled with saline (no gas-liquid interface), lung compliance is greater and the pressure-volume curve shows little hysteresis (Figure 33-2). Considering the very small diameter of alveoli, it is surprising that the contribution of the surface tension to lung elastic recoil is not greater. This is explained by the presence of surfactant, a dipalmitoyl-lecithin bound to a protein, lining the alveoli and terminal airways. Its surface tension is low, about 5 dynes/cm, as compared with plasma surface tension of about 50 dynes/cm and saline of about 70 dynes/cm. In addition to the low surface tension, surfactant exhibits marked hysteresis, that is, the surface tension increases on expansion and decreases on diminution of the surface area. The advantages of surfactant entail increased lung compliance, especially at low volumes.

Surfactant probably also contributes to the inner stability of alveoli. An arrangement of 300,000,000 intercommunicating "bubbles" is very unstable, the smaller bubbles tending to empty into the larger since pressure within a bubble is inversely proportional to its radius. The variable surface

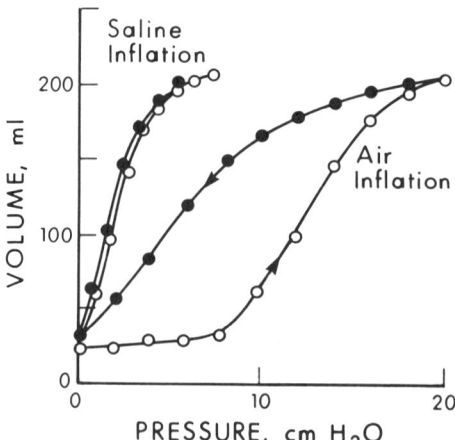

Figure 33-2. Pressure-volume curve of an excised lung showing hysteresis of a gas-filled lung. Open circles, inflation; closed circles, deflation. Note the greater compliance and reduced hysteresis when the lung is filled with saline. (Reproduced with permission from Remington JW (ed): Tissue Elasticity. Bethesda, Md, American Physiological Society, 1957.)

tension of surfactant, decreasing with diminishing radius and increasing with expansion of the alveolus, tends to stabilize the lungs by keeping alveoli open. Another, and perhaps more important mechanism contributing to stability of the alveoli is their interdependence. Any lung region less distended than the surrounding tissue does not collapse because it cannot move independently of contiguous units.

Mechanical (Elastic) Properties of the Chest Wall

The chest wall comprises the rib cage, the diaphragm, and the abdomen. In the chest wall there are passive components with intrinsic elasticity and active components, the respiratory muscles. In the resting state, the chest wall contains a certain volume and resists deformation via compression by expiratory muscles or expansion by inspiratory muscles. Elastic properties of the passive chest wall can be described by the relationship between distending pressure and volume. The distending or transthoracic pressure is the difference between the pressure inside the chest wall (P_{pl}) and the pressure outside (atmospheric pressure). P_{pl} is measured in the esophagus using a balloon-tipped catheter. Figure 33-3 shows a pressure volume plot of the passive chest wall together with that of the lungs, the two contributing to the plot for the total respiratory system. The plot is best described as if it were obtained in a paralyzed subject. Starting from the resting position, known volumes of air would be injected into or removed in steps from sealed airways with the pressures measured statically at the airway opening (Pao) with no gas flow. It can be seen that the compliance of the chest wall over most of the range of the vital capacity is similar to that of the lungs, about 200 ml/cm H_2O; only at very low volumes does the chest wall become stiff. If no deforming force is applied to the system (Pao = 0 in our experiment with a paralyzed subject), the tendency of the lung to collapse is equal and opposite to the tendency of the chest wall to expand, a point

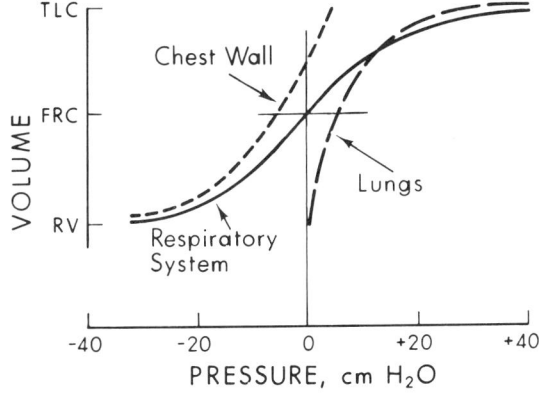

Figure 33-3. Schematic pressure-volume curves of the chest wall, the lungs, and the total respiratory system.

reached at the end of a quiet passive expiration, the functional residual capacity (FRC). It is also apparent in Figure 33-3 that the lung becomes stiff at high volumes while the chest wall becomes very stiff at low volumes.

The total compliance of the respiratory system results from the combined compliance of lungs and chest wall. With the lung within the chest, their elastic resistances, reciprocals of compliances, act in series:

$$\frac{1}{C_L} + \frac{1}{C_{CW}} = \frac{1}{C_{RS}}, \text{ i.e. } \frac{1}{200} + \frac{1}{200} = \frac{1}{100}$$

Thus, the normal compliance (C_{RS}) is 100 ml/cm H_2O.

Intrapleural pressure (P_{pl}) in the relaxed state is subatmospheric, owing to the inward pull of the lungs and outward traction of the chest wall. Upon contraction of inspiratory muscles P_{pl} becomes more negative, and with compression of the chest P_{pl} becomes less negative, reaching positive (higher than atmospheric) values with active compression of the chest by the expiratory muscles. Note that during spontaneous breathing P_{pl} is determined by the elastic properties of the lungs, while with PPV the elastic property of the chest wall governs it.

In the upright position intrapleural pressure is less negative at the base of the lungs than at the apex, with a continuous gradient of pressure presumably owing to the weight of the lungs. Thus, along this gradient in P_{pl}, the lungs are more expanded at the apex than at the bottom and, during tidal breathing, the various parts of the lungs operate along different segments of their pressure-volume curve. With lowering of pleural pressure during inspiration, the lower lung receives more ventilation than the upper; this mechanism is responsible for a gradient of uneven pulmonary ventilation, more ventilation going to the base than to the apex. In the supine position the gradient from apex to base is abolished, and now there is a gradient between the uppermost and lowermost parts of the lung.

Airway Closure

Small airways with no cartilaginous support in their walls depend upon the elastic recoil of the lungs for patency. With low elastic recoil of surrounding tissues the small airways close, mostly in the dependent regions because of the deforming effect of gravity. If perfusion with blood continues in those regions, shunting results. Airway closure occurs in young, healthy individuals only when the lung volume is very low, close to RV; in elderly persons and in those with emphysema, owing to loss of elastic recoil airway closure occurs at higher lung volumes and may exist during tidal beathing. The volume at which closure occurs is called closing volume. The principle of measuring closing volume is as follows:

When inspiration begins at a very low lung volume, near RV, the distribution of inspired gas is such that none initially goes to closed regions; only later, during

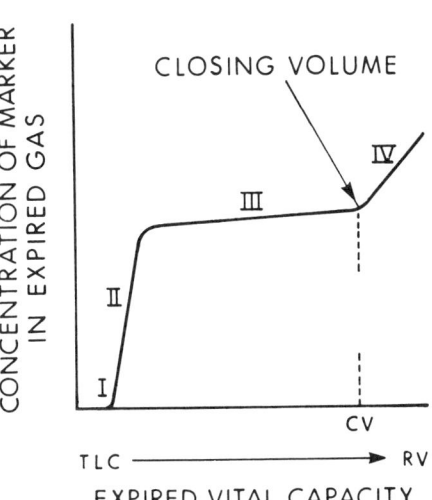

Figure 33-4. Idealized tracing of helium concentration in expired gas during a slow exhalation from total lung capacity (TLC) to residual volume (RV) after the previous breath has been labeled with a bolus of helium. Explanation in the text.

inspiration at a higher lung volume when the closed regions reopen, are they filled with inspired gas. A bolus of a poorly soluble marker gas, such as helium or xenon, is inhaled at the beginning of inspiration starting at RV, followed by inspiration of room air to TLC. Thus, the regions that were closed as the marker gas was being inhaled will contain no marker and will fill with nonmarker gas later during inspiration when opened at a higher lung volume. During subsequent expiration, the concentration of marker gas is measured in exhaled air in the course of a slow expiration from TLC to RV. The concentration of marker gas in exhaled air varies, reflecting the pattern of regional emptying of the lungs. A schematic record is shown in Figure 33-4. Phase I represents gas from the dead space; phase II is a mixture of dead-space gas and alveolar gas; phase III, the "alveolar plateau," represents mixed alveolar gas; and phase IV, with a sudden increase in He concentration, marks the lung volume at which the dependent lung regions, containing a lower He concentration, begin to close and cease to contribute to exhalation. Closing volume is defined as that part of the vital capacity left in the lungs at the turning point between phases III and IV. Closing capacity is the closing volume plus residual volume, RV, usually expressed in per cent of TLC (CC/TLC per cent).

Airway Resistance

A measure of airway resistance is the pressure difference required to produce a given flow of air through the entire system. The driving pressure is Pao − P_A, pressures that can be measured by a body plethysmograph. Physiologically important determinants of airway resistance are the geometry of the airways, including diameter, length, and branching, and the kind of gas flow, whether laminar or turbulent. Recall that resistance increases linearly with the length of a tube, is indirectly proportional to the fourth power of the radius of the tube if flow is laminar, and increases approximately with the fifth power of the radius during turbulent flow. Turbulence is promoted both by high velocity flows and by a large diameter of a tube or its irregularities. In the lungs, laminar flow probably occurs in smaller airways in which air flow is slow; flow is turbulent in the trachea, and in intermediate airways the pattern is probably a mixed one. A typical value for normal airway resistance in the adult is of the order of 1 cm $H_2O/1$ L sec of air flow. In the most severe attack of asthma, resistance can approach values of 50 cm H_2O per L/sec.

About 60 per cent of total airway resistance is contributed by the upper airway, from nose to larynx. Small airways, less than 2 mm in diameter, contribute less than 20 per cent of the total resistance, owing to the large total cross-sectional area of airways that accommodates the flow. The low value for the resistance in small airways creates difficulty in detecting this obstruction. Well-pronounced "small airway disease" can be present without any detectable increase in total airway resistance.

Several factors affect airway resistance; change in lung volume is one. Since the airways form part of the elastic structure, their length and diameter vary with lung volume. At high volumes, above FRC, airway resistance changes little. However, at volumes between FRC and RV resistance increases appreciably with decrease in volume. At volumes close to RV, small airways may close completely and the resistance becomes infinite. Increase in smooth muscle tone and edema of the bronchial mucosa are other factors that influence airway resistance.

Flow Limitation During Expiration

Airways are supported by the elastic recoil of the lung, an important factor in so-called dynamic compression of airways. During forced expiration, the lung is compressed, pleural pressure turns positive, and this in turn is transmitted to both lungs and airways, resulting in airway compression, narrowing, and increased resistance to flow with further expiratory effort. At high lung volumes, close to TLC, the high elastic recoil of the lung preserves the patency of small airways; only the main stem bronchi and trachea are compressed owing to their extraparenchymal location. At progressively lower lung volumes, with decrease in the elastic recoil of the lungs, the compression extends into the more peripheral airways. Thus, maximal expiratory flow is highest close to TLC, progressively decreasing as lung volume diminishes during expiration. In healthy individuals, maximal expiratory flow is about 10 L/sec close to TLC, and about 5 L/sec around FRC. In severe obstructive disease, the maximal expiratory flow rate attainable may be as low as one L/sec, representing the true limits of ventilation. The physiologic limitation imposed on the normal lung during expiration confers an obvious advantage in coughing. With narrowing of the airways, the linear velocity of air flow increases so that the gas exerts a greater shearing force in dislodging mucus or other particles from the bronchial walls.

QUANTITATIVE ANALYSIS OF PULMONARY GAS EXCHANGE

In the first approach, it is useful to state the obvious equalities that apply to gas exchange between lungs and atmosphere:

I. The volume of gas expired per unit of time, $\dot{V}_E$, equals the volume of inspired gas, $\dot{V}_I$, minus O_2 consumed, $\dot{V}O_2$, plus CO_2 produced, $\dot{V}CO_2$:

$$\dot{V}_E = \dot{V}_I - \dot{V}O_2 + \dot{V}CO_2 \tag{1}$$

II. The volume of O_2 consumed equals the volume of O_2 inspired in $\dot{V}_I$, minus the volume of O_2 expired in $\dot{V}_E$:

$$\dot{V}O_2 = \dot{V}_I \cdot F_{IO_2} - \dot{V}_E \cdot F_{EO_2} \tag{2}$$

III. The volume of CO_2 eliminated is equal to the volume of CO_2 in $\dot{V}_E$, minus the volume of CO_2 in $\dot{V}_I$:

$$\dot{V}CO_2 = \dot{V}_E \cdot F_{ECO_2} - \dot{V}_I \cdot F_{ICO_2} \tag{3}$$

When breathing room air or any other CO_2-free gas, the second term on the right side becomes zero, and:

$$\dot{V}CO_2 = \dot{V}_E \cdot F_{ECO_2} \tag{3a}$$

These three equalities implicitly contain all variables necessary in calculations relating to the composition of respiratory gas, as developed further on (gas-exchange ratio, alveolar gas, alveolar equation, and so on).

Note from (1) that $\dot{V}_E$ is not necessarily equal to $\dot{V}_I$; the two volumes will be equal only if $\dot{V}O_2 = \dot{V}CO_2$ (see discussion of respiratory exchange ratio, R).

IV. Nitrogen, an inert gas, is neither consumed nor produced in the body, ie:

$$\dot{V}_{N_2} = 0 = \dot{V}_I \cdot F_{IN_2} - \dot{V}_E \cdot F_{EN_2} \tag{4}$$

Therefore:

$$\dot{V}_I = \dot{V}_E \cdot F_{EN_2}/F_{IN_2}$$

This expression obviates the necessity of measuring of both inspired and expired gas volumes. Fractional concentrations of N_2 can be measured with a nitrogen meter or, if no "foreign" gases (such as anesthetics) are inhaled, N_2 can be derived from measurements of FO_2 and FCO_2, since by definition: $F_{IN_2} = 1 - F_{IO_2} - F_{ICO_2}$, and $F_{EN_2} = 1 - F_{EO_2} - F_{ECO_2}$.

QUANTITIES OF GAS EXCHANGED

The oxygen consumption of a healthy 70-kg individual at rest and at neutral ambient temperature is about 250 ml O_2/min (STPD). The energy equivalent is about 1.2 kcal/min, or about 70 watts. At the same time, about 200 ml of CO_2/min (STPD) are produced. With fever, metabolic rate increases by 10 per cent per 1°C rise in temperature. The volume of O_2 consumed is not necessarily the same as that of CO_2 produced. Recall that, if a mole of carbohydrate is oxidized:

$$C_6H_{12}O_6 + 6\ O_2 \rightarrow 6\ CO_2 + 6\ H_2O + \text{energy};$$
$$CO_2/O_2 = 6/6 = 1$$

Oxidation of a mole of a representative fatty acid would yield:

$$C_{16}H_{32}O_2 + 23\ O_2 \rightarrow 16\ CO_2 + 16\ H_2O + \text{energy};$$
$$CO_2/O_2 = 16/23 = 0.7$$

The ratio $\dot{V}_{CO_2}/\dot{V}_{O_2}$ is called the respiratory exchange ratio (R), its value depending upon the nature of "foodstuff" being oxidized in the body. R is 1.0 for carbohydrate, 0.7 for fat, and 0.8 for protein; the standard value of R on a mixed diet is 0.82. Combining the statements in (1) and (4), one can see that the "nitrogen ratio" ($F_{E_{N_2}}/F_{I_{N_2}}$) is inversely proportional to R.

RESPIRATORY DEAD SPACE AND ALVEOLAR VENTILATION

Not all the gas inhaled reaches the respiratory zone of the lungs. Conducting airways down to the terminal bronchioles are not lined with a gas-exchanging membrane; they represent the anatomic dead space. In addition, in disease some alveoli may be ventilated and devoid of perfusion, contributing to the alveolar dead space, sometimes called parallel dead space. The sum of the anatomic and alveolar dead space is called physiologic dead space, probably a misnomer since alveolar dead space is often the result of pathologic changes.

The volume of the anatomic dead space can be estimated from Radford's empirical formula: anatomic dead space (ml) = body weight (in pounds). About one half the anatomic dead space is located in the upper, extrathoracic airways.

Determination of the physiologic dead space can be explained by means of a model of the respiratory system (Figure 33-5). Visualize the respiratory system as if it consisted of a single conducting tube or dead space, V_D, and an expansible volume in the respiratory zone. Upon inspiration, the first part of a tidal volume, V_T, enters the respiratory zone and instantaneously mixes by diffusion with the gas present, FRC. The first portion of the tidal volume is the effective or alveolar share, V_A. At end inspiration, the latter part of V_T occupies the conducting tube where no blood-gas exchange occurs in the dead space, V_D. During expiration, dead-space gas emerges first and the alveolar component of the tidal volume appears later. Thus, in terms of gas volumes involved:

$$V_T = V_D + V_A, \text{ or } V_A = V_T - V_D$$

What is the composition of the two components of the exhaled volume, V_D and V_A? The dead-space component does not exchange with blood; therefore its composition is the same as that of inspired gas. The alveolar component exchanges with blood, and its composition is a reflection of this. We shall look into its composition

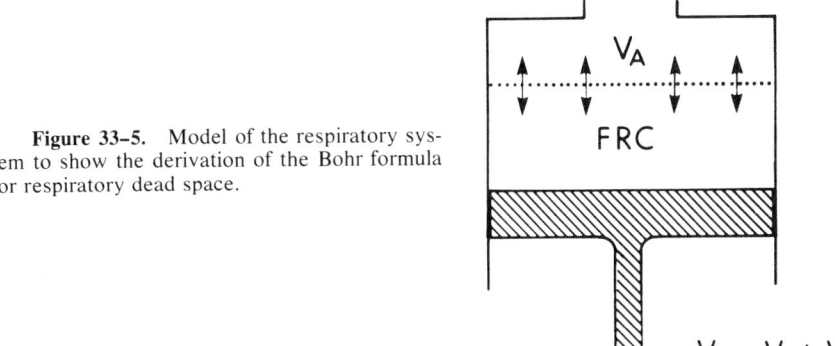

Figure 33-5. Model of the respiratory system to show the derivation of the Bohr formula for respiratory dead space.

later. In terms of quantities of gas that undergo respiratory exchange (O_2, CO_2, or a "foreign" gas, x):

$$V_T FE_x = V_D FI_x + V_A FA_x$$

quantity of gas in mixed expired volume = quantity of gas in dead-space component + quantity of gas in alveolar component

Substitute ($V_T - V_D$) for V_A, and solve for V_D:

$$V_D = V_T \frac{FE_x - FA_x}{FI_x - FA_x}.$$

Since F_x is $P_x/(P_B - P_{H_2O})$:

$$V_D = V_T \frac{PE_x - PA_x}{PI_x - PA_x}$$

This is the Bohr formula employed for determination of physiologic dead space.

The difficulty with the original Bohr formula lies in obtaining a reliable sample of alveolar gas for analysis. The Enghoff modification of the Bohr formula is based upon the assumption that the partial pressure of CO_2 in alveolar gas is the same as that in arterial blood. When room air is inhaled, $PI_{CO_2} = 0$, and the equation for dead space is simplified:

$$V_D = V_T \frac{Pa_{CO_2} - PE_{CO_2}}{Pa_{CO_2}}$$

Thus, physiologic dead space, sometimes expressed as the wasted fraction of ventilation, V_D/V_T, can be simply measured by collecting mixed expired gas and measuring the partial pressure in this and in a sample of arterial blood. In normal individuals, V_D/V_T is about 0.3, so that approximately 30 per cent of ventilation is "wasted" on dead-space ventilation.

The effective or alveolar ventilation, $\dot{V}_A$, is the total minute ventilation, $\dot{V}_E$, less wasted dead space ventilation, $\dot{V}_D$:

$$\dot{V}_A = \dot{V}_E - \dot{V}_D$$

To maintain a given $\dot{V}_A$ with increase in physiologic dead space, it is obvious that the total ventilation, $\dot{V}_E$, has to increase. A large increase in V_D/V_T, for example, to 0.8, as sometimes is seen in patients with acute respiratory insufficiency, can require very high total ventilations, over 20 L/min for adequate gas exchange.

Alveolar ventilation can be simply determined by measuring total ventilation, $\dot{V}_E$, and subtracting the wasted part (dead space times respiratory frequency). Another way of determining $\dot{V}_A$ is as follows: since $\dot{V}CO_2$ equals $\dot{V}_E \cdot F_{ECO_2}$, it also equals $\dot{V}_A \cdot F_{ACO_2}$. Thus, $\dot{V}_A = \dot{V}CO_2/F_{ACO_2}$. $\dot{V}CO_2$ can be measured in mixed expired gas ($\dot{V}_A \times F_{ECO_2}$) and F_{ACO_2} derived from $P_{ACO_2} = P_{aCO_2}$, as measured in a sample of arterial blood: $F_{ACO_2} = P_{aCO_2}/(P_B - P_{H_2O})$.
Thus

$$\dot{V}_A = \frac{\dot{V}_{CO_2}}{Pa_{CO_2}} (P_B - P_{H_2O})$$

or, since

$$\dot{V}_{CO_2} = R \cdot \dot{V}_{O_2},$$

$$\dot{V}_A = \frac{\dot{V}_{O_2}}{Pa_{CO_2}} R (P_B - P_{H_2O})$$

ALVEOLAR GAS

One can visualize alveolar gas as a compartment interposed between atmospheric air and capillary blood in the lungs. Oxygen is continuously removed and CO_2 added as blood flows, while O_2 is supplied to alveolar gas and CO_2 removed by the cyclic process of alveolar ventilation ($\dot{V}_A$). By means of $\dot{V}_A$, alveolar gas tends to approach the composition of inspired gas, while through perfusion ($\dot{Q}$) it tends to approach the gas composition of mixed venous blood, the latter being determined by the influence of cardiac output, O_2 consumption, and CO_2 production. The stead state composition of alveolar gas is determined by the contribution of $\dot{V}_A$ and $\dot{Q}$. The higher the $\dot{V}_A/\dot{Q}$ ratio, the more alveolar gas approaches inspired gas in composition; the lower the ratio, the more alveolar gas resembles the gas composition of mixed venous blood. In summary, the composition of alveolar gas is determined by (1) the rate of alveolar ventilation ($\dot{V}_A$); (2) the rate of pulmonary perfusion with mixed venous blood ($\dot{Q}$); and (3) the composition of inspired gas.

Pulmonary ventilation is so regulated that a healthy human breathing air at sea level maintains effective alveolar ventilation, thus keeping P_{ACO_2} at 40 torr; P_{AO_2} is close to 100 torr, the other constituents of the alveolar gas being water vapor, 47 torr at 37°C, and N_2, adding up to P_B. Note that once the value of P_{ACO_2} has been "chosen" by the regulatory mechanisms of pulmonary ventilation, it follows from the gas exchange ratio ($\dot{V}CO_2/\dot{V}O_2$)

that PA_{O_2} is also determined for any given composition of inspired gas. This is stated by the simplified alveolar equation:

$$PA_{O_2} = PI_{O_2} - PA_{CO_2}/R$$

The term PI_{O_2} can also be stated as $FI_{O_2} \cdot (P_B - P_{H_2O})$. If $R = 1$, the equation simplifies to $PA_{O_2} = PI_{O_2} - PA_{CO_2}$.

Note that the PA_{O_2} is directly related to the concentration of O_2 in inspired gas (FI_{O_2}) and to barometric pressure (P_B). PA_{O_2} is less than the inspired O_2 tension in proportion to PA_{CO_2} as O_2 is removed from and CO_2 delivered to the alveolar gas. The ratio of the two processes is the respiratory ratio R. PA_{CO_2}, in turn, is determined by regulation of $\dot{V}_A$.

PULMONARY VENTILATION AND METABOLIC RATE

Earlier we showed that:

$$\dot{V}_A = \frac{\dot{V}_{O_2}}{PA_{CO_2}} R (P_B - 47)$$

By rearrangement, to solve for PA_{CO_2}:

$$PA_{CO_2} = \frac{\dot{V}_{O_2}}{\dot{V}_A} R (P_B - 47)$$

Two important implications emerge from this relationship: (1) With varying $\dot{V}_{O_2}$, as during fever or muscular activity, in order to maintain a constant PA_{CO_2}, and thus a constant composition of alveolar gas, $\dot{V}_A$ must vary in precise proportion to increase in metabolic rate. For the usual values of P_B, R, and PA_{CO_2},

$$\dot{V}_A (L/min, STPD) = \frac{\dot{V}_{O_2} (L/min, STPD)}{40 \text{ torr}} \cdot 0.82 \cdot 713 \text{ torr} = 15 \cdot \dot{V}_{O_2}$$

Thus, for each liter of O_2 consumed, 15 L of $\dot{V}_A$ must be provided to maintain PA_{CO} at 40 torr. (2) At a given metabolic rate ($\dot{V}_{O_2}$), PA_{CO_2} is reciprocally related to effective pulmonary ventilation ($\dot{V}_A$). Thus doubling $\dot{V}_A$ will, at a given $\dot{V}_{O_2}$ halve PA_{CO_2} and, conversely, halving V_A will double PA_{CO_2}. This relationship is the basis for the important role the respiratory system plays in short-term adaptation to disturbances in acid balance. As CO_2 is an acid ($CO_2 + H_2O \rightleftarrows H_2CO_3$), lowering of P_{CO_2} by increasing $\dot{V}_A$ at a given $\dot{V}_{O_2}$ will remove H^+ from the body fluids to compensate for metabolic acidosis. Conversely, a decrease in $\dot{V}_A$ at a given $\dot{V}_{O_2}$ will increase P_{CO_2} in alveolar gas and body fluids, thus effectively adding H^+ to compensate for metabolic alkalosis. This is referred to as respiratory compensation for metabolic disturbances in acid-base balance.

If the lung were a perfect and homogeneous gas exchanger, Pa_{CO_2} and Pa_{O_2} in the systemic circulation would be the same as in alveolar gas. However, this is not true because of two factors: (1) presence of physiologic right-to-left shunts — bronchial veins drain into the pulmonary veins while some thebesian veins in the myocardium drain into the left heart; (2) the distribution of $\dot{V}_A$ and $\dot{Q}$ to various parts of the lungs is not uniform, producing $\dot{V}_A/\dot{Q}$ inhomogeneity reflected in the composition of alveolar gas and of the pulmonary end-capillary blood. We shall point out later how $\dot{V}_A/\dot{Q}$ inhomogeneity produces differences between mixed alveolar gas and arterialized blood.

PULMONARY CIRCULATION

The lung accommodates the cardiac output (CO); nevertheless, perfusion pressure is low. The mean pulmonary artery pressure (PAP) is normally about 15 torr, or 25/8 torr systolic/diastolic. The pressure in pulmonary veins is nearly the same as that in the left atrium, about 8 torr, in reference to atmospheric pressure. The pulmonary wedge pressure (PWP) is obtained by occluding blood flow to an arterial branch; this measures the pressure in the pulmonary capillaries and small veins, usually indistinguishable from left atrial pressure. Thus, the pressure drop across the pulmonary vascular bed is only about 7 torr, more than ten times than the pressure gradient across the systemic circulation. Typical values for pulmonary vascular resistance (PVR) in the resting state (CO = 5 L/min), defined as the ratio of perfusion pressure to flow, would be $(15 - 7)$ torr over 5 L/min, or 1.6 units, as compared with the systemic vascular resistance of $(95 - 5)/5 = 18$ units. However, because of the special structure and mechanical behavior of the pulmonary vessels, PVR as defined does not provide meaningful insight into pressure-flow relationships as a means of evaluating pulmonary hemodynamics, both in respect to the whole lung and especially in respect to regional perfusion.

The pulmonary arteries, like the veins, are thin-walled and therefore both distensible and collapsible. Pulmonary arterioles possess an incomplete layer of smooth muscle. The capillaries form a mesh within the alveolar walls, occupying most of the alveolar surface, and their walls are collapsible. Lymphatics begin as capillaries in the bronchovascular spaces in the vicinity of respiratory bronchioles; alveolar septa contain no lymphatics.

The shape and caliber of the pulmonary vessels vary with transmural pressure, that is, the difference between the pressure inside and that outside. Being both distensible and collapsible, the vessels remain open only with positive transmural pressure, or when the pressure within the vessel is higher than in the perivascular space.

In relation to perivascular pressure, the pulmonary vessels can be divided into (a) "alveolar" vessels (capillaries, small arterioles, and venules) with perivascular pressures equal to the gaseous pressure in the alveoli, which in spontaneous breathing is close to barometric pressure; and (b) "extra-alveolar" vessels (arteries and veins) that are "tethered" to the lung parenchyma, their perivascular pressures usually similar to pleural pressure. Like the pleural pressure, the perivascular pressure around the extra-alveolar vessels is determined by elastic recoil of the lungs. Thus, in the erect position, the perivascular pressure of extra-alveolar vessels is more negative or subatmospheric at the apices than at the base.

Changes in lung volume exert differing effects on the two kinds of vessel: increase in lung volume, either total or regional, increases the "pull" on the walls of the tethered vessels, increases their diameters, and decreases resistance. On the other hand, the alveolar vessels will be stretched and their cross-sectional area decreased by stretching the alveolar walls at high lung volumes. With decrease in lung volume, the perivascular pressure of the extra-alveolar vessels becomes less subatmospheric, transmural pressure is less, and resistance increases. Thus, lung volume is one determinant of the variable pulmonary vascular resistance.

Another determinant is perfusion pressure. As the pulmonary vessels are distensible, increase in perfusion pressure increases their diameters. Since the vessels are also collapsible, increase in perfusion pressure recruits additional vessels, thus increasing the total cross-sectional area of the perfused vessels and decreasing the calculated PVR.

Although probably of little clinical significance, the neurogenic and humoral control of pulmonary vessels is under continuing investigation. Hypoxia is important in producing active constriction of the pulmonary resistive vessels. Hypoxia in both alveolar gas and systemic blood produces vasoconstriction and an increase in PAP. Hypoxemic influences on pulmonary vasoconstriction are augmented by both low pH and elevated Pa_{CO_2}. The mechanism of vasoconstriction probably entails a direct action on vascular smooth muscle. Presumably the usefulness of this mechanism is to divert blood from hypoventilated parts of the lung with a low $P_{A_{O_2}}$, thus tending to match ventilation and perfusion. In chronic hypoxemia, however, the generalized pulmonary vasoconstriction results in pulmonary hypertension and cor pulmonale.

REGIONAL DISTRIBUTION OF PULMONARY BLOOD FLOW

As the pulmonary circulation is a low pressure system, the hydrostatic pressure differences caused by gravity in the lung are large enough to modify effective arterial inflow pressure. Local perfusing pressure in various parts of the lungs is determined by the pressure in the main pulmonary artery (PAP) and the hydrostatic pressure difference away from the hilum. Figure 33-6 is a schematic representation of the effective pressure heads available for perfusion in the vertical lung. Pressures within the vessels decrease with height above the heart and increase below. At the apex, PAP may not be sufficient to raise the blood; thus effective perfusion pressure will be less than the pressure in alveolar gas (equal to barometric pressure). As a result, the alveolar vessels collapse and flow ceases (Fig. 33-6, zone 1 of West). In the normal lung with spontaneous breathing, a zone of no flow probably does not exist; however, if PAP is lowered as in hemorrhage or hypotension, or if the pressure in alveolar gas is raised as in PPV, there will be a pronounced zone 1—unperfused and ventilated—of alveolar dead

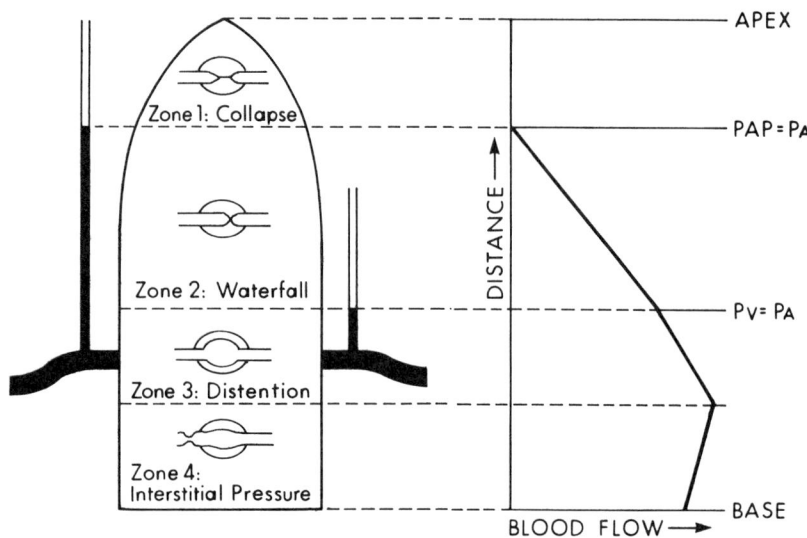

Figure 33-6. Schematic representation of the four zones of the lung in which different hemodynamic conditions govern blood flow. For discussion, see text. PAP, mean pulmonary arterial pressure; P_A, pressure in the alveolar gas; P_V, pulmonary venous pressure. (Redrawn with permission from Hughes JMB, Glazier JB, Maloney JE, and West JB: Resp. Physiol 4:58, 1968.)

space. In lower parts of the lung (zone 2) the effective inflow pressure is higher because the height above the heart is less; effective inflow pressure will be higher than alveolar pressure. Pulmonary venous pressure, however, is still lower than alveolar pressure; blood flow is determined by the difference between effective inflow pressure and alveolar pressure. The change in venous pressure—unless it exceeds alveolar pressure—will have no effect on local blood flow (waterfall effect). Further down the lung, venous pressure will be higher than that in the alveoli (zone 3) and blood flow will be governed by the difference between effective inflow pressure—PAP now increased by the hydrostatic effect—and venous pressure. Since in zone 3 the pressure within the alveolar vessels must lie between that of arterial inflow and venous outflows, it will be higher than the pressure in the alveoli; the alveolar vessels will be distended and their resistance to flow will be low. Thus there is a gradient in local perfusion, with less blood flow at the apex and progressively increasing flow toward the base of the erect lung.

We have described the perfusion gradient produced by gravity in relation to variations in regional resistance of alveolar vessels. However, the true picture is more complicated, owing to the contribution of extra-alveolar vessels to local resistance to flow. As noted, the pressure about the extra-alveolar vessels is influenced by lung recoil, thus depending upon lung volume. In poorly inflated lung regions, as at the base, the perivascular pressure around extra-alveolar vessels can approach positive collapsing values. Transmural distending pressure is low, local resistance to flow increases, and when the lung is upright blood flow is reduced, presumably the result of this mechanism (zone 4).

In the supine position, the apex-to-base gradient in perfusion is abolished and a gradient between the uppermost and lowermost parts of the lung prevails. The gradient is less pronounced as the distance between the frontal and dorsal regions lessens.

FLUID EXCHANGE IN THE LUNGS

As in other vascular beds, fluid exchange across the pulmonary capillaries is governed by Starling's law. Net filtration ($\dot{n}$) is proportional to the difference between the filtering and reabsorbing forces. The force producing filtration is the difference between the hydrostatic pressure within the pulmonary microvasculature (P_c) and the hydrostatic pressure in pulmonary interstitial fluid (P_{isf}). The reabsorptive force is the difference between oncotic pressure in plasma (π_c) and that in interstitial fluid (π_{isf}):

$$\dot{n} = K\,[(P_c - P_{isf}) - (\pi_c - \pi_{isf})]$$

where K is the permeability coefficient of the capillary membrane.

In the pulmonary capillaries not all the pressures involved in the Starling equilibrium are known. The colloid-osmotic pressure of plasma protein is about 25 torr; oncotic pressure in the interstitial fluid, as estimated from protein concentration in the lung lymph, is about 19 torr. This would give a net colloid osmotic pressure of about 6 torr for fluid reabsorption. Hydrostatic pressure within the capillaries must lie between that of the pulmonary arterioles and that of the left atrium; owing to the effect of gravity on arterial inflow pressure, the pressure in the arterioles, and thus in capillaries, is not uniform throughout, varying between 7 and 12 torr from the apex to the base of the lung, with an average of about 10 torr. The hydrostatic pressure in pulmonary interstitial fluid is not known with certainty. At present there are two schools of thought concerning its magnitude: one holds that P_{isf} is slightly positive in reference to atmospheric pressure (about 4 torr), while the other maintains that the pressure is distinctly subatmospheric (−2 to −4 torr). According to the first assumption, the net balance of Starling forces in the capillaries would be (10−4) − (25−19) = 0, and the lung should be "dry." In the second case, the balance would be [10 − (−4) − (25 − 19)] = +8 torr of net filtering pressure, suggesting an appreciable continuous filtration of fluid to be carried away by lymph. Indeed, recent observations indicate that there is continuous lymph outflow from the lungs of experimental animals, presumably also applying to human lungs. Fluid formed by filtration in the alveolar capillaries moves along the interstitial spaces of the alveolar septa where lymphatics are lacking toward the perivascular and peribronchial spaces, thence absorbed into lymph capillaries. Lymph flows toward the hilum as a result of rhythmic contraction of smooth muscle in lymphatic vessels; the unidirectional propulsion of the lymph results from the presence of funnel-shaped valves.

Pulmonary Edema

Interstitial fluid accumulates in the lungs when the rate of formation exceeds the transporting capacity of the lymphatic system. The latter can increase its capacity about 10 times. From the preceding considerations, it is apparent that an increase in intracapillary hydrostatic pressure, a decrease in plasma colloid pressure, and increased permeability of the capillary membrane will induce accumulation of fluid if the capacity for lymphatic drainage is exceeded.

Lowering of plasma oncotic pressure alone is hardly ever severe enough to cause pulmonary edema; in patients with nephrosis there may be anasarca and ascites but not pulmonary edema, in the absence of left ventricular failure. Lymphatic obstruction, such as a tumor, may cause localized edema. The commonest causes of pulmonary edema, however, are an increase in intracapillary pressure (high pressure pulmonary edema), as in left ventricular failure or fluid overload, and leaky capillaries (low pressure pulmonary edema), as in septicemia, acute post-traumatic pulmonary insufficiency, or after inhalation of noxious gases. Traditionally hypoxemia has been considered one of the causes of increased permeability of pulmonary capillaries, but there are no data to support this belief. Measurement of pulmonary wedge pressure is essential for differentiating the two kinds of edema.

Excess fluid accummulates first in perivascular and peribronchial spaces, where it interferes with local perfusion and ventilation. Wheezing in cardiac asthma is produced by compression of small airways by edema fluid. Further accumulation of fluid propagates toward alveolar septa, lowering lung compliance and thickening the gas-exchanging membrane. During this interstitial stage of pulmonary edema, interference with gas exchange is not pronounced at rest since for both O_2 and CO_2 the diffusing capacity appreciably exceeds the need for gas exchange in an otherwise normal lung. Only in the final stages of fluid accumulation are the alveoli filled and the typical rales, frothy sputum, and hypoxemia observed.

TRANSPORT OF O_2 AND CO_2 BETWEEN LUNGS AND TISSUES

The next step in gas exchange, between alveolar gas and pulmonary capillary blood, is a matter of simple diffusion as molecules of O_2 and CO_2 move in the gas phase through the gas-exchanging membrane and blood.

The transfer rate of a gas by passive diffusion ($\dot{V}$, ml of gas per minute) in lungs is directly proportional to the area available for diffusion

(A), and to the difference in partial pressures in the gas phase (PA) and capillary blood (P_c), while inversely proportional to the distance over which the diffusion occurs (d). This is Fick's law of diffusion:

$$\dot{V}_{gas} = D \frac{A}{d}(P_A - P_c)$$

The diffusion coefficient (D) is characteristic for each gas. The heavier the gas molecule, the slower the movement, and the more soluble the gas in tissue water, the more rapid the diffusion. Carbon dioxide is somewhat heavier than O_2 but much more soluble in tissues, and the diffusion coefficient for CO_2 is about 20 times higher than that for O_2.

In the lungs, area and distance cannot be evaluated separately, so they are considered together and measured as the diffusing capacity for a given gas, D_L. Thus, the diffusing capacity for O_2 is:

$$D_{L_{O_2}} = \dot{V}_{O_2} / (P_{A_{O_2}} - P\bar{c}_{O_2})$$

where $P\bar{c}_{O_2}$ is the mean partial pressure of O_2 in pulmonary capillary blood; the latter is not easily determined, so instead of measuring $D_{L_{O_2}}$, carbon monoxide is employed as a marker gas. This offers the advantage that, with the very low concentration of CO inhaled—a fraction of 1 per cent—and the avid binding of CO to hemoglobin, $P\bar{c}_{CO}$ is negligibly small. Thus, $D_{L_{CO}} = \dot{V}_{CO}/P_{A_{CO}}$. The normal value for $D_{L_{CO}}$ is 25 to 40 ml/min/torr of driving pressure.

During exercise the diffusing capacity increases two to three times, owing to recruitment of alveolar vessels. In pulmonary fibrosis, diffusing capacity is decreased and values as low as 5 to 10 ml/min/torr are found in ambulatory patients. The reduction in D_L is produced by decrease in the area available for diffusion; increased thickness of the membrane is probably a minor factor and the apparent diffusion barrier observed in diseased lungs results mainly from abnormalities of $\dot{V}/\dot{Q}$.

TRANSPORT OF O_2 IN BLOOD

After crossing the alveolar capillary membrane, O_2 is carried in blood in two forms: in physical solution, and in reversible combination with hemoglobin. The quantity present in solution is determined by the solubility coefficient and partial pressure (Henry's law). The solubility of O_2 in blood is very low, 0.003 ml O_2/100 ml blood per torr, at 37°C. With the usual Pa_{O_2} about 100 torr, only 0.3 ml of O_2 is present in physical solution in 100 ml of arterial blood, 0.3 vol per cent.

Oxygen combines with hemoglobin (Hb) reversibly to form oxyhemoglobin (HbO_2). At full saturation, each gram of Hb binds 1.36 ml O_2 and the oxygen capacity is the maximum that can be carried by available hemoglobin. With the usual Hb concentration of 15 gm per 100 ml, the normal O_2 capacity is 20 ml/100 ml blood. The O_2 content, or O_2 concentration (C_{O_2}) in blood is the sum of the dissolved O_2 and that bound to Hb. Oxygen saturation of hemoglobin (S_{O_2}) is the ratio of O_2 combined with Hb over O_2 capacity, expressed in per cent. Oxygen transport is the product of oxygen content in arterial blood and the cardiac output: $Ca_{O_2} \times CO$.

Saturation of Hb with O_2 is primarily determined by the Pa_{O_2}. The relationship between So_2 and Pa_{O_2} is complex and best described and analyzed in graphic form such as the oxygen dissociation curve (Fig. 33–7). The peculiar shape of this curve offers certain physiologic advantages. A flat top prevents wide fluctuations in Sa_{O_2} with changes of Po_2 normally prevailing in alveolar gas. The steep part is advantageous in unloading O_2 in tissues: a large decrease in So_2 is produced by a relatively small drop in Po_2. The location of the dissociation curve is also of importance in loading and unloading Hb as it is affected by temperature, pH, and Pco_2 (Bohr effect), and by the concentration of 2,3-diphosphoglycerate (2,3-DPG) in erythrocytes. By convention, the position of the dissociation curve is defined by the Po_2 value that produces 50 per cent saturation (P_{50}). The P_{50} of normal human Hb is 26 to 27 torr at 37°C, pH 7.40, Pco_2 40 torr, and a normal concentration of 2,3-DPG. P_{50} increases with shift to the right of the curve, or decreased affinity of Hb for O_2; with shift to the left, or increased affinity, P_{50} is lowered. With decreased affinity of Hb for O_2, unloading of O_2 in tissues is facilitated. A shift to the right is produced by increase in temperature, decrease in pH, increase in Pco_2, and increase in 2,3-DPG; opposite changes shift the curve to the left. The increase in affinity of Hb for O_2 produced by the leftward shift impedes unloading of O_2 in tissues; a lower tissue Po_2 must prevail for unloading of a given O_2 from blood.

Among other factors the pH within erythrocytes is important in determining the concentration of 2,3-DPG: acidosis reduces and alkalosis increases 2,3-DPG levels. The shift of the curve instantaneously produced by the Bohr effect is counterbalanced by changes in 2,3-DPG, although on a much slower time scale—a matter of hours. Therefore, acidosis initially causes a rightward shift; however, after several days the curve shifts back, in spite of persisting acidosis, owing to lowering of 2,3-DPG. Sudden cor-

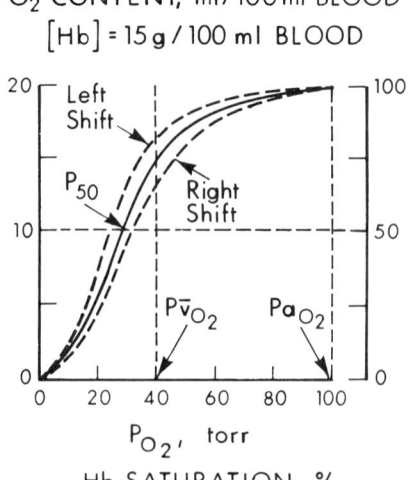

Figure 33–7. Dissociation curve of O_2 in blood. Pa_{O_2} and Pv_{O_2} are the usual normal values in arterial and mixed venous blood. Note how shifts in the dissociation curve affect the saturation (and O_2 content) in the range of Pv_{O_2}.

rection of acidosis leads to a shift to the left until the level of 2,3-DPG readjusts to the new acid-base balance.

The amount of O_2 transported to tissues is the product of Ca_{O_2} and CO. Ca_{O_2} depends upon the concentration of Hb and its saturation, the latter in turn a function of Pa_{O_2} and of the position of the Hb dissociation curve. Thus, all these variables—CO, Hb concentration, Pa_{O_2}, and the position of the dissociation curve—affect the efficiency of oxygen transport to tissues. Hypoxia can result from disturbance of any or a combination of these variables.

TRANSPORT OF CO_2

CO_2 is produced in tissues and then diffuses into capillary blood, where it is present both in physical solution and chemically bound. The solubility coefficient of CO_2 in blood is 0.03 mM/L/torr P_{CO_2}. Thus, in mixed venous blood with the usual P_{CO_2} of 46 torr, about 1.38 mM of CO_2 is physically dissolved; in arterial blood, with the usual Pa_{CO_2} of 40 torr, 1.2 mM/L of CO_2 is dissolved. Chemical binding occurs in two ways: (a) via hydration of CO_2 to H_2CO_3 and subsequent involvement in the complex process of buffering; (b) through direct reaction with NH_2 groups of proteins, to form carbamino compounds: $CO_2 + R-NH_2 \rightleftharpoons R-NHCOOH$, fairly strong acids (pK < 6). Hemoglobin plays a primary role in transporting CO_2 in blood, both by providing most of the buffering of the carbonic acid formed by hydration of CO_2 and by forming the carbamino compound carboxyhemoglobin. In plasma, hydration of CO_2 to H_2CO_3 is a slow process; however, within erythrocytes the process is accelerated by the enzyme carbonic anhydrase. Thus, most of the H_2CO_3 and subsequent buffering and formation of HCO_3^- is provided by erythrocytes. HCO_3^- subsequently diffuses into plasma, and Cl^- diffuses into erythrocytes to maintain electric equilibrium. The reduction of HbO_2 that occurs simultaneously with loading of blood with CO_2 increases the capacity of Hb to form the carbamino compound carboxyhemoglobin, also making the molecule of Hb a weaker acid. Both factors increase the capacity of reduced Hb to bind CO_2 (the Haldane effect). In the lungs, these processes are reversed and as Hb is oxygenated to HbO_2, CO_2 is released both from carboxy Hb and bicarbonate.

The relationship between P_{CO_2} and total content of CO_2 in blood is described by the CO_2 dissociation curve (Fig. 33–8). Unlike the dissociation curve for O_2, within the range of P_{CO_2} values present in mixed venous and arterial blood the relationship is almost linear.

MATCHING OF VENTILATION AND PERFUSION IN LUNGS

We have stated that the composition of alveolar gas is determined by the ratio of effective pulmonary ventilation to rate of perfusion with mixed

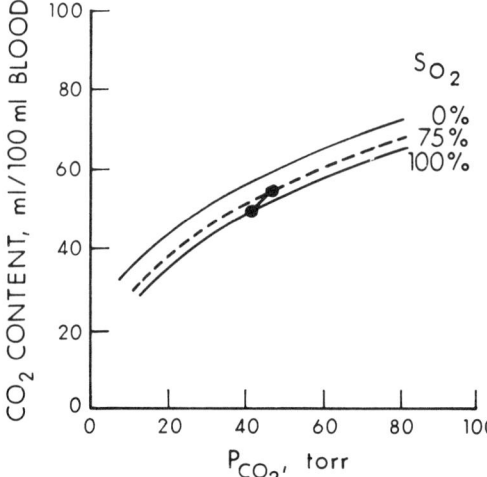

Figure 33-8. CO_2 dissociation curves for whole blood at 0.75, and 100 per cent oxyhemoglobin saturation (S_{O_2}). The Haldane effect between arterial and mixed venous blood is shown by the heavy straight line.

venous blood—$\dot{V}_A/\dot{Q}$—the composition of mixed venous blood and of inspired gas being additional factors. The composition of alveolar gas and of the blood leaving each alveolus is determined by the local $\dot{V}/\dot{Q}$. In a normal person at rest, the lungs receive about 4 L/min of $\dot{V}_A$ and 5 L/min of blood or cardiac output ($\dot{Q}$). Thus, the overall value of $\dot{V}_A/\dot{Q}$ for the whole system is 4/5 or 0.8. If this $\dot{V}/\dot{Q}$ prevailed everywhere, that is, if ventilation and perfusion were distributed equally to all parts of the lungs, the composition of alveolar gas and of blood leaving pulmonary capillaries would be the same in all gas-exchanging units. On the other hand, if there were units in which $\dot{V}/\dot{Q}$ was high (> 0.8), the composition of local alveolar gas would approach that of inspired gas, a low $P_{A_{CO_2}}$ and high $P_{A_{O_2}}$. In ventilated alveoli with no perfusion, $\dot{V}/\dot{Q} = \infty$, thus constituting alveolar dead space. Units with low $\dot{V}/\dot{Q}$ (< 0.8) would contain alveolar gas with a composition approaching that of mixed venous blood, or a high $P_{A_{CO_2}}$ and low $P_{A_{O_2}}$. Perfused alveoli with no ventilation are characterized by $\dot{V}/\dot{Q} = 0$, constituting an intrapulmonary shunt or venous admixture.

In a normal, upright person with more ventilation and perfusion at the base of the lung, the gradient from apex to base is more pronounced for perfusion than for ventilation; therefore $\dot{V}/\dot{Q}$ ratios are high at the apex, about 3, and low at the base, about 0.6, with a continuum of $\dot{V}/\dot{Q}$ values along the gradient. The presence of regions with low and high $\dot{V}/\dot{Q}$ carries important consequences for efficiency of gas exchange. A simplified presentation of this intriguing problem follows. Readers interested in a more rigorous treatment are referred to West's monograph on $\dot{V}/\dot{Q}$, or to Farhi's text.

Assuming that blood leaving each alveolus is in equilibrium with $P_{A_{CO_2}}$ and $P_{A_{O_2}}$ within the alveolus, then blood coming from alveoli with low $\dot{V}/\dot{Q}$ will have an abnormally high P_{CO_2} and an abnormally low P_{O_2}, while blood coming from alveoli with high $\dot{V}/\dot{Q}$ will have an abnormally low P_{CO_2} and a high Po_2. When contingents of blood from various regions with differing $\dot{V}/\dot{Q}$ values are mixed, the *content* of O_2 and CO_2 in arterialized blood will be the weighted average of the *content* of the two gases. The resulting *partial pressures* of the two gases in mixed arterialized blood will depend on their dissociation curves. For CO_2, the dissociation curve is almost a straight line over the range of Pco_2 between 25 and 50 torr (Fig. 33-8). Thus, a change in Pco_2 is simply proportional to change in CO_2 content. If, for instance, equal volumes of blood, one with a Pa_{CO_2} of 30 and the other of 50 torr, were mixed, the resulting Pco_2 would be 40. On the other hand, the dissociation curve of O_2 is nonlinear (Fig. 33-7). If equal volumes of blood with a Po_2 of 50 torr, So_2 83 per cent, and 120 torr, Sa_{O_2} 99 per cent, were mixed, the resulting Sa_{O_2} is $(83 + 99)/2 = 91$, corresponding to a Po_2 of only 63 torr. The O_2 dissociation curve is flat in the range of Po_2 values over 80 torr; therefore, when breathing room air, the moderate increase in Pa_{O_2} in blood coming from regions with high $\dot{V}/\dot{Q}$ cannot compensate for the low saturation of the blood coming from regions of low $\dot{V}/\dot{Q}$. Upon inhalation of air, hypoxemia is an inevitable consequence of maldistribution of ventilation and perfusion with low $\dot{V}/\dot{Q}$ values. If inspired gas is enriched with O_2, hypoxemia can be relieved, since with a fairly high $F_{I_{O_2}}$ even poorly ventilated alveoli will fill with gas containing $P_{A_{O_2}}$ high enough to saturate the circulating blood.

The presence of low $\dot{V}/\dot{Q}$ regions also affects elimination of CO_2. A tendency to hypercapnia in mixed arterialized blood results from admixture of blood from underventilated and overperfused regions with a low $\dot{V}/\dot{Q}$. However, the increased Pa_{CO_2} drives respiration, and hypercapnia can be averted if the total ventilation is increased. Owing to the linearity of the CO_2 dissociation curve, it is possible to further lower the content of CO_2 in already well-ventilated areas; however, this is at the cost of a large increase in the work of breathing.

High $\dot{V}/\dot{Q}$ regions do not cause hypoxemia; they merely increase the wasted fraction of ventilation, requiring a higher total ventilation ($\dot{V}_E$) to maintain a given $\dot{V}_A$. This, together with the increase in ventilation required to forestall the hypercapnia resulting from low $\dot{V}/\dot{Q}$ regions, eventually leads to respiratory failure and CO_2 retention, when the limits of total resting ventilation are reached.

Abnormality in matching $\dot{V}$ and $\dot{Q}$ is the most common cause of hypoxemia in patients with chronic lung disease. Maldistribution is produced by regional differences in compliance and resistance to air flow, by vascular obstruction as occurs in pulmonary embolization, and by other factors. Other common causes of hypoxemia involve alveolar hypoventilation and intrapulmonary shunting. Alveolar hypoventilation is synonymous with hypercapnia, causing hypoxemia when room air is inhaled. Hypoventilation can occur in skeletal, muscular, neuromuscular, or CNS disorders, including curarization and administration of CNS depressants, or in pulmonary disease when an increase in V_D/V_T is so high that adequate $\dot{V}_A$ is not achieved by the attainable total ventilation.

True intrapulmonary shunt, when mixed venous blood is not exposed to gas on passage through the lungs, is probably not the most important cause of hypoxemia in patients with acute respiratory failure; true venous admixture does occur with atelectasis and lung collapse. Rather, it is the $\dot{V}/\dot{Q}$ abnormality with extremely low values of $\dot{V}/\dot{Q}$ that underlies most of what is commonly called "shunt" in patients with acute respiratory distress. The magnitude of the true shunt, that is, the fraction of pulmonary blood flow completely bypassing alveolar gas, can best be evaluated after prolonged inhalation of 100 per cent O_2, to abolish the contribution of low $\dot{V}/\dot{Q}$ to hypoxemia. If a sample of mixed venous blood is then taken, the magnitude of shunt can be evaluated quantitatively; however, this is seldom justifiable in acutely ill patients because of the risk of accelerating development of atelectases in diseased lungs, caused by absence of N_2 in alveolar gas upon inhalation of 100 per cent O_2.

REGULATION OF PULMONARY VENTILATION

The "respiratory pump," unlike the heart, has no intrinsic rhythmicity, but is operated by skeletal muscles that do not contract unless stimulated through appropriate somatic innervation. The rhythmic stimuli are generated in the respiratory centers, a network of oscillator neurons located in the pons and medulla. An intact efferent pathway from centers down to respiratory muscles is essential for spontaneous breathing.

Smooth operation of the rhythmic contraction and relaxation of respiratory muscles is achieved through various modulating reflexes, the receptors being located in the lungs and chest wall. The afferent limb of reflexes originating in the lungs reaches the respiratory centers via the vagi (Hering-Breuer inflation reflex, deflation reflex). In man the function of most of these reflexes is poorly understood. The intercostal muscles and the diaphragm are equipped with muscle spindles that sense the tension in muscle fibers. This reflex control of muscle tone is integrated at the spinal level and helps to stabilize contraction in the face of variable mechanical loads, as in changing resistance or compliance.

What is the nature of the information reaching the respiratory centers that influences rate and depth of breathing? First, many physiologic functions unrelated to the needs of steady state gas exchange require that the normal breathing pattern be interrupted or modified. Some of these functions are voluntary: breath-holding, voluntary hyperventilation, straining, speech, or playing a wind instrument. Others are reflex in nature: sneezing, swallowing, vomiting, and hiccoughing. These inputs originating in various parts of the CNS merely interfere with the primary function of respiratory regulation, which is to provide gas exchange. The important input in this respect comes to respiratory centers through chemoreflexes that detect the concentration of respiratory gases in blood and other body fluids. Chemoreception for respiration customarily has been linked with the composition of arterial blood. This seems logical, since the blood is a natural link between the lungs—the effector—and the respiratory center—the regulator. The effect of O_2 on respiration is indeed brought about by chemical stimuli originating in arterial blood, in the peripheral carotid chemoreceptors. On the other hand, the respiratory drive owing to CO_2 and to accompanying changes in pH is not simply explained by chemical stimuli in blood. The acidity of cerebral fluids detected by central medullary chemoreceptors appears to be the important stimulus.

The remarkable sensitivity of respiration to CO_2 can be demonstrated by inhalation of various CO_2 mixtures. An increase in Pa_{CO_2} of 1 torr produces an increase in $\dot{V}_E$ of 2 to 3 L/min. If a reduction of Pa_{CO_2} is induced, as by means of artificial hyperventilation, ventilation may be completely suppressed temporarily; posthyperventilation apnea may be pronounced in anesthetized patients. The ventilatory response to CO_2 is reduced by CNS depressants—anesthetics, opioids, and sedatives. Also the state of wakefulness influences the respiratory response to CO_2; during sleep it is reduced.

Ondine's curse is a syndrome observed in patients after operations involving the brain stem and higher segments of the cervical cord or during bulbar poliomyelitis. The patients have long periods of apnea; however, while awake they breathe on command. A similar phenomenon occurs with an overdose of opioids. Marked insensitivity to CO_2 seems to be the underlying disturbance. Recently it has been suggested that a related disturbance is responsible for some crib deaths in infants.

The respiratory drive derived from CO_2 is mainly detected by the central medullary chemoreceptors. These receptors are exposed to cerebrospinal fluid (CSF), thus detecting the acidity of this fluid. CSF is separated from blood by the blood-brain barrier. Molecular CO_2, being lipid soluble, crosses the blood-brain barrier freely, while HCO_3^- is presumably regulated by active transport between blood and CSF, the functional blood-brain barrier. The pH in CSF that results from a given CSF $[HCO_3^-]$ and P_{CO_2} sets the level of resting pulmonary ventilation. In metabolic acidosis, therefore, lowered CSF $[HCO_3^-]$ results in hyperventilation, thus lowering Pa_{CO_2}. In metabolic alkalosis, an increase in CSF $[HCO_3^-]$ lowers ventilation, thus producing the compensatory CO_2 retention found in arterial blood. The extent of respiratory compensation for metabolic acid-base disturbances as observed in arterial blood results in changes in Pa_{CO_2} of approximately 1 torr for each mM per liter of base excess or base deficit. Thus, the physiologically normal Pa_{CO_2} in a patient with a base excess of +10 mM/L is regulated close to 50 torr, and with a base deficit of −10 mM/L, Pa_{CO_2} is normally set close to 30 torr. In patients with chronic lung disease and CO_2 retention, the buildup of $[HCO_3^-]$ in CSF is appreciable, probably one of the contributing factors to the notorious insensitivity of these patients to increases in Pa_{CO_2}. It follows from the Henderson-Hasselbalch equation that the higher the CSF $[HCO_3^-]$, the smaller the change in pH resulting from a given increase in P_{CO_2} in CSF.

The effect of O_2 on respiration can be studied by inhaling abnormal concentrations of O_2. At sea level, the effect on $\dot{V}_E$ of decreasing $F_{I_{O_2}}$ is surprisingly small: no appreciable change in breathing is seen until about one half of the O_2 concentration in air is reached, and even at $F_{I_{O_2}}$ values less than 8 per cent there is a large variation in sensitivity among individuals. However, this is not a fair appraisal of the isolated effect of O_2 on respiration; as soon as respiratory rate increases, P_{CO_2} decreases, thus reducing the total respiratory drive. Still, if Pa_{CO_2} is maintained constant while inhaled O_2 is lowered (isocapnic hypoxia), the effect on ventilation is not dramatic until Pa_{O_2} values around 60 torr are reached. Thus, the bodily mechanisms for detecting O_2 lack are not very sensitive.

Hypoxemia combined with hypercapnia increases ventilation more than the mere additive effect of both stimuli. This is referred to as interaction of the respiratory drives of O_2 and CO_2, but the site of interaction is not known.

Chemoreceptors detecting lack of O_2 are located in the bifurcation of the carotid arteries, the carotid bodies, and at the aortic arch or aortic chemoreceptors. The stimulus is a fall in Pa_{O_2}, not in O_2 content. Thus, anemia or poisoning with carbon monoxide does not stimulate respiration. Afferent impulses from peripheral chemoreceptors reach the respiratory centers through the glossopharyngeal nerve from the carotid bodies, and via the vagus nerves from the aortic bodies. Thus the anoxic drive for respiration is of a reflex nature; the direct effect of anoxia on respiratory centers is purely depressive.

Patients with chronic obstructive pulmonary disease and CO_2 retention as a result of a virtually abolished sensitivity to CO_2 depend upon the coexisting hypoxemia for respiratory drive. If given high concentrations of oxygen to relieve hypoxemia while breathing spontaneously, they lose the only effective respiratory drive and may die from CO_2 narcosis.

Surprisingly enough, recent observations indicate that individuals who are hypoxemic from birth, such as people living at high altitudes or patients with cyanotic congenital heart disease, have very low O_2 respiratory drives. It is not clear whether this phenomenon derives from the chemoreceptors *per se* or from the CNS.

RESPIRATORY FAILURE

Respiratory failure occurs when gas exchange is inadequate for metabolic needs; consequently, arterial blood gases are deranged, and this is manifested as hypoxemia alone or hypoxemia with hypercapnia.

Because the normal values for Pa_{CO_2} and Pa_{O_2} have a certain range, depending upon age, tension of O_2 in inhaled gas, acid-base balance, and other factors, it is not easy to quantify exactly the derangements in arterial blood gases that define respiratory failure. Most workers consider as indicators of respiratory failure a Pa_{O_2} lower than 60 torr at sea level while breathing room air at rest, with no abnormal intracardiac right-to-left shunt, and a Pa_{CO_2} of 50 torr or higher. However, Pa_{O_2} decreases with age and is of course affected by $F_{I_{O_2}}$. Most clinicians consider a Pa_{O_2} of 70 torr when breathing O_2 via face mask to be an indication of significant hypoxemia; those who measure alveolar-arterial gradients in P_{O_2} during inhalation of 100 per cent O_2 consider an A-a gradient of more than 450 torr an indication of failure. Pa_{CO_2} varies with the respiratory compensation for metabolic acid-base imbalance: a Pa_{CO_2} of 50 torr in a patient with metabolic alkalosis and a base excess of +12 mM/L of several days' duration is a normal physiologic response, while a Pa_{CO_2} of 40 torr in a patient in metabolic acidosis with a base deficit of −10 mM/L would indeed indicate relative hypercapnia.

Hypercapnia has only one cause—alveolar hypoventilation. Hypoxemia can result from hypoventilation while breathing air, a low $F_{I_{O_2}}$, high altitude, $\dot{V}/\dot{Q}$ abnormalities, intrapulmonary shunt, and as a result of decrease in the lung diffusing capacity. A combination of these factors may also be the cause.

An attempt at a clinical classification of respiratory failure is given in Table 33–1. The problems posed in management of the various kinds of respiratory failure differ, as do the underlying pathophysiologic mechanisms. With failure of the respiratory pump the principal problem is hypoventilation, usually combined with inability to protect airways and to clear bronchial secretions. Pathologic changes in the lungs can develop secondarily: aspiration, infection, atelectasis, or barotrauma as a result of mechanical ventilation. The task is to assure adequate artificial ventilation, to protect the airways, and to provide general supportive therapy including pulmonary toilet.

In failure of the gas-exchanger, the initial and important problem is hypoxemia caused by $\dot{V}/\dot{Q}$ abnormalities and pulmonary shunts. Initially, PA_{CO_2} is normal or low owing to the hypoxic drive; secondarily, with increase in V_D/V_T as a result of pulmonary pathology and with increase in alveolar dead space, hypoventilation and CO_2 retention may set in. The most common clinical entity in this category is the so-called adult respiratory distress syndrome (ARDS) seen after trauma, burns, aspiration,

Table 33–1. CLINICAL CLASSIFICATION OF RESPIRATORY FAILURE

I. Acute Respiratory Failure with Previously Normal Lungs:
  (a) Without initial pulmonary pathology
    (Failure of the "respiratory pump")
    Examples: myasthenia, botulism muscular paralysis, drug overdose
  (b) With pulmonary pathology
    (Failure of the "gas-exchanger")
    Examples: severe pneumonia, post-traumatic pulmonary insufficiency
II. Acute Failure Superimposed on Chronic Lung Disease:
  (a) Without pre-existing CO_2 retention
    Example: bronchopneumonia in chronic pulmonary fibrosis
  (b) With chronic CO_2 retention
    Example: bronchopneumonia in COPD

shock, immune reactions to transfusions of blood, gram-negative septicemia, viral infection, and after prolonged inhalation of high concentrations of O_2, among other conditions. The clinical manifestations are breathlessness with patchy pulmonary infiltrates that can culminate in the white lungs seen on chest x-ray, severe hypoxemia, initially with a normal or low P_{CO_2}, and subsequent hypercapnia. The pathologic changes in the lung are not specific. Interstitial infiltrates, microemboli, and alveolitis, sometimes with formation of hyaline membranes, are seen. The main pathophysiologic disturbance is a severe reduction in lung compliance or stiff lung, owing to the infiltrates and increase in lung water. FRC is low, leading to closing of lung units and shunt, and there is a severe $\dot{V}/\dot{Q}$ mismatch that contributes to hypoxemia and a large alveolar dead space, the latter eventually leading to hypercapnia. The main therapeutic problems entail treatment of hypoxemia and controlled, mechanical ventilation when CO_2 elimination is inadequate.

Although it is the chest physician who sees most of the acute complications of chronic pulmonary disease, postoperative pulmonary complications are well within the anesthetist's domain. Here, the problem is usually severe hypoxemia, especially in patients who are already hypoxemic with chronic pulmonary fibrosis. Adequate O_2 administration is mandatory. The situation differs in patients with chronic obstructive disease with CO_2 retention and hypoxemia. Here the derangement lies in the chemical regulation of respiration, with depressed sensitivity to CO_2 and dependence on hypoxic respiratory drive, together with abnormal pulmonary mechanics (increased lung compliance and airway obstruction). These patients usually have values both for Pa_{CO_2} and Pa_{O_2} between 50 and 60 torr and Sa_{O_2} is about 80 per cent. Artificial ventilation must be avoided if possible because of subsequent difficulties in weaning. Controlled oxygen therapy (see Chapter 32) with moderately increased O_2 concentrations (24 to 30 per cent) aims at relieving hypoxia by gaining somewhat on Sa_{O_2} without abolishing the hypoxemic respiratory drive.

DIAGNOSIS OF RESPIRATORY INSUFFICIENCY

In the first approach, the presence of conditions predisposing to respiratory insufficiency must be recognized: drug overdose, aspiration, neuromuscular dysfunction, trauma, or presence of chronic lung disease. Clinical indicators of hypoxemia and hypercapnia are sought: breathlessness with tachypnea and mental derangement are common signs of impending respiratory failure. Hypoxemia may be present without cyanosis; nevertheless, cyanosis should be looked for in the mucosa of the mouth, so-called central cyanosis. When present, central cyanosis indicates severe hypoxemia with a Pa_{O_2} usually less than 40 torr. CO_2 retention produces few and variable clinical signs. Prominent is restlessness, followed by depression and coma. The periphery is warm and sweaty, and the pulse bounds with a rise in blood pressure owing to sympathetic stimulation. On the whole, clinical impressions of respiratory failure are unreliable and should be confirmed by measurement of arterial blood gases.

THE ROLE OF ANESTHETISTS IN RESPIRATORY CARE

In their work in the operating room, anesthetists support respiration and circulation of anesthetized patients, therefore the care of more prolonged respiratory problems is a natural extension and application of their knowledge and skills.

Because of the complexity of care for patients in acute respiratory failure, the team approach provides the best solution, involving anesthetist, surgeon, internist, pediatrician, neurologist, and microbiologist. Nursing of these patients is difficult and requires special skills, notably related to the complex monitoring equipment in use. Pulmonary physiotherapy is an essential component of intensive care (see Chapter 32). As the equipment used in respiratory care is complex, its proper use calls for the collaboration of well-trained respiratory therapists. All these activities require collaboration and continuous communication among the specialists mentioned and are best organized in the setting of an intensive care unit. An efficient laboratory working around the clock is essential for measurement of arterial blood gases.

PRINCIPLES OF RESPIRATORY SUPPORT IN ACUTE PULMONARY INSUFFICIENCY

For hypercapnia, there is only one treatment: adequate ventilation. If the patient is unable to do this spontaneously, mechanical ventilatory support is provided.

Treatment of hypoxemia relies upon three principal measures: (a) enrichment of inspired gas with O_2, (b) careful fluid management both to prevent and to treat pulmonary edema, and (c) mechanical measures to prevent and remedy the causes of intrapulmonary venous admixture. The latter is achieved by artificially operating the lungs at large volumes through application of positive pressure to the airways to prevent and treat atelectasis. Prolonged use of extracorporeal membrane oxygenation (ECMO) for treatment of intractable hypoxemia is currently being evaluated.

TRACHEAL INTUBATION AND TRACHEOSTOMY

The indications for tracheal intubation in patients in respiratory failure are summarized in Table 33–2. Techniques of tracheal intubation are described in Chapter 15. Nasotracheal tubes, as compared with oral ones, are better tolerated by awake patients, are more securely anchored, and enter the larynx at an angle that applies less pressure to the posterior wall. On the other hand, the size of the tube is limited by the diameter of the nasal passages, posing problems in suctioning and adding appreciable resistance during spontaneous breathing.

Tubes with flaccid low pressure cuffs are used for prolonged tracheal

Table 33-2. INDICATIONS FOR ENDOTRACHEAL INTUBATION

I. Maintenance and protection of airways (patency, prevent aspiration)
II. Application of positive pressure to airways
   1. Intermittent positive pressure ventilation (IPPV)
   2. Continuous positive airway pressure (CPAP)
      (a) spontaneous breathing with CPAP (continuous positive pressure breathing, CPPB)
      (b) positive end-expiratory pressure (PEEP) in combination with IPPV
III. Pulmonary toilet

intubation because they adapt over a large tracheal surface, thus better stabilizing the tube. Moreover, low pressure cuffs provide a satisfactory seal while still pliable, whereas a rubber or latex tube with a rigid cuff inflates to a spherical shape; contact with the tracheal mucosa is therefore over a narrow ring. When adequately inflated to seal the airway the stiff cuff is unyielding and rigid, applying unnecessary force to the tracheal wall.

The decision to perform tracheostomy in patients needing prolonged tracheal intubation is usually postponed unless it is obvious that the need for control of the airways may extend over weeks. Translaryngeal intubation is maintained for two or more weeks by some clinicians. However, intubation via tracheostomy is better tolerated by awake patients, and tracheostomy tubes with soft cuffs are used. With respect to avoiding the damage of prolonged tracheal intubation, the only advantage of tracheostomy over translaryngeal intubation is the consideration of laryngeal trauma, for the trachea incurs damage with both. Tracheostomy is not without risk, however, and the wound acts as a portal of entry for infection. Moreover, partial resection of the tracheal cartilage must be performed as part of the procedure. Chondromalacia is a possible complication, and fatal hemorrhage resulting from erosion of the innominate artery by a tracheostomy tube has occurred.

Once an endotracheal tube is placed, regardless of kind, a sterile technique is employed in manipulating the tube and in clearing secretions. When the tube is removed, certain complications should be anticipated: after prolonged intubation laryngeal reflexes are obtunded and there is a high risk of aspiration. Further complications of prolonged intubation are edema and ulceration of the larynx with the translaryngeal tube, and damage to the tracheal wall with both translaryngeal intubation and tracheostomy that can result in tracheoesophageal fistula or tracheal stenosis.

VENTILATORY SUPPORT

Factors are complex that lead to and ultimately precipitate respiratory failure to the extent that mechanical respiratory support is needed. To mention a few: mechanical derangements of the respiratory system, in turn increasing the work of breathing; alterations in distribution of flow of gas and blood and efficiency of gas exchange; variable metabolic needs in ill patients; the state of consciousness; and the still poorly understood failure of chemical regulation of respiration. It is, therefore, impossible to quantify all possible derangements that ultimately call for ventilatory support. Instead, one relies upon predictive indicators of need that are established empirically as guidelines (Table 33-3).

Mechanical ventilators produce intermittent expansion of the lungs by application of positive pressure to the airways (IPPV) or by creating subatmospheric pressure around the chest wall. The prototype of such negative-pressure ventilators is the tank ventilator or iron lung; cuirass ventilators are also occasionally used. The latter consist of a plastic shell that covers the anterior aspect of the thorax and abdomen, while subatmospheric pressure is intermittently applied beneath the shell. Nowadays, practically all patients who need mechanical ventilation are treated with IPPV.

There are two basic designs of positive pressure ventilators: those in which a preset volume of gas is delivered, and those in which gas flow ceases when the pressure reaches a preset level. With the latter, variations in compliance or resistance of the respiratory system can result in large variations in tidal volumes delivered. Ventilators are also classified according to the capacity to control or assist respiration. With respiratory assist, the patient's inspiratory efforts initiate delivery of a tidal volume. Thus the patient's respiratory center regulates the rate of minute ventilation and Pa_{CO_2}. With controlled ventilation, the rate of delivery of the chosen tidal volumes is determined by the setting on the machine. The expiratory phase in IPPV is passive, thus utilizing the elastic recoil of the patient's respiratory system. It is beyond the scope of this text to enter into details of design or operation of the ventilators available.

Table 33-3. INDICES OF NEED FOR VENTILATORY SUPPORT

	Normal Range	Ventilatory Support Indicated
I. Indices of the mechanical properties of the respiratory system and of the respiratory muscles		
Vital capacity (ml/kg of body weight)*	65-75	<15
FEV_1 (ml/kg of body weight)*	50-60	<10
Inspiratory force (cm H_2O)	75-100	<25
II. Indices of adequacy of $\dot{V}_A$ and of oxygenation		
Resting respiratory rate (breath/min)	12-20	>35
Pa_{CO_2}, torr	35-45†‡	>55‡
V_D/V_T	0.25-0.40	>0.60
Pa_{O_2}, torr: breathing air	75-95	<60 torr‡
O_2 mask	variable	<70
FI_{O_2} 1.0	>600	<200

*In very obese patients, use "ideal" weight.
†See page 511 for modifying influence of metabolic acid-base imbalance.
‡Applies to acute elevation of P_{CO_2}, not to patients with chronic CO_2 retention.
(Modified from Pontoppidan H, Geffin B, Lowenstein E: Acute Respiratory Failure in the Adult. Boston, Little Brown and Co, 1973.)

MANAGEMENT OF RESPIRATORY SUPPORT

In patients with stiff lungs, large tidal volumes are used—10 ml/kg of body weight, more than twice the normal spontaneous V_T. This provides a continuous "sighing" to prevent or treat the hypoxemia presumably caused by closure of lung units in association with high elastic recoil of diseased lungs. The rate of ventilation is set at 10 to 14 breaths per minute; lower frequencies are poorly tolerated. However, in patients with chronic obstructive lung disease in whom lung compliance is increased, large tidal volumes and a high minute ventilation are avoided. With airway obstruction and highly compliant lungs, very high FRC values can be produced and peak inspiratory volumes beyond the patient's spontaneous TLC can result, causing difficulty in weaning and resumption of spontaneous breathing. Tidal volumes of more than 600 ml are seldom used in these patients.

Depending on the need of $\dot{V}_E$ to achieve adequate $\dot{V}_A$, adjustments are made: if the setting of the machine results in hyperventilation, additional dead space is added to the circuit; if more ventilation is needed to maintain adequate CO_2 elimination, frequency is increased. FI_{O_2} is initially set high and subsequently adjusted to provide adequate oxygenation. These adjustments are evaluated by serial blood gas determinations. Humidification of the inspired gas is provided (see Chapter 32).

For controlled ventilation, synchronization of the patient's breathing efforts with the machine is desirable. Sedation is usually necessary. In agitated hypoxic patients, especially in those with abnormally high respiratory drives as in pulmonary embolus, hyperammonemia, or head trauma with CNS acidosis, neuromuscular blockade and sedation are sometimes necessary.

While on mechanical ventilation close monitoring of the patient is essential, especially blood pressure, serial determinations of arterial blood gases, and evaluation of the effective compliance of the respiratory system. Effective compliance is the tidal volume delivered divided by peak inspiratory pressure registered by the ventilator, influenced both by compliance and resistance to flow in the system. Obstruction of airways or decreased compliance is thus detected, as in pneumothorax or voluntary use of expiratory muscles opposing the respirator. Expired volumes are continuously monitored by a spirometer included in the respiratory circuit, and alarm systems signal failure of delivery of the preset tidal volumes.

Treatment of hypoxemia requires careful selection of FI_{O_2} to achieve adequate oxygenation. Pulmonary edema is forestalled by careful regulation of fluid balance. Bedside measurement of pressures in the pulmonary circulation with the flow-directed catheter is useful in differentiating between low pressure and high pressure edema. Selective use of diuretics in combination with colloids can produce dramatic reductions in the pulmonary shunt.

The purpose of positive end-expiratory pressure (PEEP) is to counterbalance the high elastic recoil of stiff lungs and to prevent the lungs from reaching very low volumes at expiration, where closing occurs. Some ventilators offer built-in valves to provide PEEP, but PEEP can also be improvised by submerging the end of the expiratory line under water, the depth determining end-expiratory pressure. In treatment of pulmonary edema, PEEP improves gas exchange. The mechanism is thought to entail improvement of distribution of ventilation and blood flow rather than reduction of accumulated fluid. There are no simple rules for recommending any specific level of PEEP. Each patient has to be "titrated" to achieve the desired effect of improved oxygenation while avoiding potentially toxic $F_{I_{O_2}}$ values. Increments of 5 cm H_2O PEEP are usually tried and levels up to 15 to 20 cm H_2O are routinely used. Recently very high levels of PEEP, approaching 60 cm H_2O, have been found useful and tolerable.

Continuous positive pressure can also be applied to the airways of spontaneously breathing patients (CPAP or CPPB). CPPB can be devised by submerging the expiratory line of a T-piece under water and providing a flow of inspired gas high enough to maintain positive pressure during the entire breathing cycle, including inspiration. This is facilitated by incorporating a reservoir bag at the inspiratory line. CPPB is useful in combating hypoxemia in some patients who do not require mechanical ventilation for CO_2 elimination.

The two main complications of positive airway pressure, with either IPPV or PEEP, are depression of cardiac output owing to an increase in mean intrathoracic pressure and pulmonary barotrauma.

If depression of cardiac output occurs, it is manifest as systemic hypotension and decreased urinary output. Thus with use of PEEP, a decrease in cardiac output can reduce oxygen transport to tissues in spite of improved arterial oxygenation. Hemodynamic consequences of increased intrathoracic pressure resulting from IPPV and PEEP are complex and are now under investigation. Prevention and treatment of hypovolemia are essential hemodynamic adjustments needed to maintain adequate venous return in the face of increased intrathoracic pressure.

Pulmonary barotrauma results from disruption of lung tissue as occurs when a bulla is ruptured, or more commonly from local disruption of lung parenchyma, with gas entering the pulmonary interstitium and propagating along bronchovascular bundles (pulmonary interstitial emphysema), thus compressing small airways and vessels (see Chapter 28). Through these interstitial channels the gas can reach the mediastinum (pneumomediastinum) and subcutaneous tissues of the neck (subcutaneous emphysema), or enter the retroperitoneal space. If any of the visceral coverings are disrupted, pneumothorax, pneumopericardium, or pneumoperitoneum results. Gas under positive pressure can also enter disrupted pulmonary vessels and cause air embolization.

Accumulation of secretions in the respiratory tract should be avoided. Obstruction of airways by mucus leads to maldistribution of ventilation and patchy or massive atelectases. Stagnant secretions, especially in atelectasis, provide a nidus for infection. Humidification of inspired gases, adequate fluid balance, and chest physiotherapy help to move the secretions toward the large airways.

Weaning from the Ventilator

Indicators for weaning from the ventilator are the reverse of those that suggest the need for mechanical respiratory support (Table 33–3). In principle, mechanical indices such as vital capacity and inspiratory pressure should predict that the patient will be able to provide adequate ventilation, and indices characterizing the performance of the lung, such as arterial blood gases, V_D/V_T, and shunt should be satisfactory according to empirically established rules.

A T-piece is attached to the endotracheal tube and humidified O_2 or air enriched with O_2 is inhaled. Attempts to wean may begin while the patient is still on PEEP; a CPPB circuit is then used in trials of spontaneous breathing. Sedation is avoided and weaning is best carried out during the day when sufficient personnel are present. The patient is closely observed for tachypnea, tachycardia, increase in blood pressure, arrhythmias, or general distress. If spontaneous breathing is tolerated, arterial blood gases are checked to evaluate the efficiency of gas exchange. Periods of spontaneous breathing may be short, 10 to 15 min, alternating with controlled ventilation, especially after long periods of mechanical ventilation. Progressively, as tolerated, spontaneous breathing is prolonged.

Recently, intermittent mandatory ventilation (IMV) has been used in the process of weaning from mechanical ventilation. Here, as opposed to the previously described technique of alternation between spontaneous breathing with a T-piece and periods on ventilatory support, the process is continuous and gradual. In principle, the endotracheal tube is attached to a T-piece and a ventilator delivers tidal volumes at a preset rate, while the patient can inhale spontaneously through the inspiratory line. This allows gradual progression from complete ventilatory control by the respirator to a situation in which the patient provides more and more of the ventilation spontaneously. All the while the frequency of tidal volumes delivered by the machine is gradually lowered until weaning is complete. IMV can easily be combined with CPAP. In some patients with difficult weaning problems, IMV has been helpful.

REFERENCES

Bendixen HH, Egbert LD, Hedley-Whyte J, et al: Respiratory Care. St Louis, CV Mosby Co, 1965.
Bushnell, SS: Respiratory Intensive Care Nursing. Boston, Little, Brown and Co, 1973.
Farhi LE: Ventilation-perfusion relationship and its role in alveolar gas exchange. *In* Caro CG (ed): Advances in Respiratory Physiology. Baltimore, Williams & Wilkins Co, 1966, 148–197.
Fenn WO, Rahn H: Handbook of Physiology. Section 3, Respiration, vols I and II. Washington, DC, American Physiological Society, 1964.
Murray JF: The Normal Lung. The Basis for Diagnosis and Treatment of Pulmonary Disease. Philadelphia, WB Saunders Co, 1976.
Mushin WW, Rendell-Baker L, Thompson PW, et al: Automatic Ventilation of the Lungs. Philadelphia, FA Davis Co, 1969.
Nunn JF: Applied Respiratory Physiology, with Special Reference to Anaesthesia. London, Butterworth, 1969.

Pontoppidan H, Geffin B, Lowenstein E: Acute Respiratory Failure in the Adult. Boston, Little Brown and Co, 1973.
Shoemaker WC (ed): The Lung in the Critically Ill Patient. Baltimore, Williams & Wilkins Co, 1976.
Skillman JJ: Intensive Care. Boston, Little, Brown and Co, 1975.
Staub NC: Pulmonary edema. Physiol Rev 54:678, 1974.
Sykes MK, McNicol MW, Campbell EJM: Respiratory Failure. 2nd ed, Oxford, Blackwell Scientific Publications, 1976.
West JB: Ventilation/Blood Flow and Gas Exchange. 2nd ed, Oxford, Blackwell Scientific Publications, 1970.
West JB: Respiratory Physiology—the Essentials. Baltimore, Williams & Wilkins Co, 1974.

APPENDIX I

COMMON ABBREVIATIONS

a – arterial blood
A – alveolar gas
ACD – acid citrate dextrose
Ach – acetylcholine
ACTH – adrenocorticotropic hormone
ADH – antidiuretic hormone
AR – assisted respiration
ATN – acute tubular necrosis
ATP – adenosine triphosphate
B – barometric
c – capillary blood
C – concentration of gas in blood phase
CGA – Compressed Gas Association
cm – centimeter
CO – cardiac output
CPAP – continuous positive airway pressure
CPK – creatine phosphokinase
CPPB – continuous positive pressure breathing
CPPV – continuous positive pressure ventilation
CR – controlled respiration
CRF – corticotropin-releasing factor
CSF – cerebrospinal fluid
CVP – central venous pressure
D – dead-space gas
D – diffusing capacity
DIC – disseminated intravascular coagulation
E – expired gas
EACA – epsilon-aminocaproic acid
ECG – electrocardiogram
EEG – electroencephalogram
EO – ethylene oxide
ER – endoplasmic reticulum
ERV – expiratory reserve volume
f – respiratory frequency
F – fractional concentration in dry gas phase
FRC – functional residual capacity
GFR – glomerular filtration rate
gm – gram
HB$_s$Ag – hepatitis B surface antigen
Hz – hertz
I – inspired gas
IC – inspiratory capacity
IPPB – intermittent positive pressure breathing
IPPV – intermittent positive pressure ventilation
IRDS – idiopathic respiratory distress syndrome
IRV – inspiratory reserve volume
kg – kilogram
kcal – kilocalorie
L – liter
LP – lumbar puncture
MAC – minimum alveolar concentration
mamp – milliampere
MAO – monoamine oxidase
mEq – milliequivalent
mg – milligram
ml – milliliter
mm – millimeter
mOsm – milliosmole
mv – millivolt
NE – norepinephrine
NFPA – National Fire Protection Association
opioid – a narcotic, either synthetic or opium-related
P – gas pressure
P̄ – mean gas pressure
PAH – para-aminohippurate
PEEP – positive end-expiratory pressure
ppm – parts per million
PPV – positive pressure ventilation
psi – pounds per square inch
PTF – post-tetanic facilitation
PVR – peripheral vascular resistance
PWP – pulmonary wedge pressure
Q – volume of blood
Q̇ – volume of blood/unit time
R – respiratory exchange ratio
REM – rapid eye movement
RIHSA – radioactive iodinated human serum albumin
RPF – renal plasma flow
RV – residual volume
S – per cent saturation of hemoglobin
STPD – 0°C, 760 torr, dry
T – tidal gas
TBT – tracheobronchial toilet
TLC – total lung capacity
torr – mm Hg
μamp – microampere
μm – micrometer
v – venous blood
V – gas volume
V̇ – gas volume/unit time
VC – vital capacity

APPENDIX II

NUMERICAL EQUIVALENTS

Volume

1 liter = 1.057 qt	1 cu ft = 0.028 cu m
= 61 cu in	1 qt = 0.946 L
1 cu m = 35.26 cu ft	= 946 ml
1 ml = 0.0338 oz	1 US fluid oz = 29.57 ml
= 16.231 minims	1 minim = 0.0616 ml

Mass or Weight

1 kg = 2.205 lb	1 lb (AV) = 0.453 kg
1 gm = 0.035 oz	1 oz (AV) = 28 gm
= 15.45 grains	1 grain = 0.0647 gm
1 mg = 0.015 grain	= 64.7 mg

Force

1 dyne = 2.24×10^{-6} lb weight*	1 lb weight = 453.59 gm weight
= 1.01×10^{-3} gm weight	= 4.44×10^{5} dynes
= 0.015 grain weight	= 4.44 newtons
1 newton = 10^5 dynes = 0.224 lb weight	
= 101 gm weight	
= 1573 grain weight	
1 gm weight = 980.665 dynes	
1 kg weight = 9.80×10^5 dynes	
= 9.8 newtons	

*All weights based on acceleration due to gravity of 9.8 meters/sec^2

Pressure

1 mm Hg = 0.019 lb/sq in
          = 1.35 gm/sq cm
          = 13.5 kg/sq m
          = 1333.22 dynes/sq cm
          = 133.32 newtons/sq m
         1 lb/sq in (psi) = 51.715 mm Hg
                          = 70.307 gm/sq cm
                          = 6.8×10^4 dynes/sq cm
                          = 6.8×10^3 newtons/sq m
                          = 703.07 kg/sq m

Work or Energy

1 joule = 0.239 cal (gm)	1 calorie = 4.18 joules
= 2.39×10^{-4} cal (kg)	1 BTU = 1054.8 joules
= 9.48×10^{-4} BTU	
= 2.77×10^{-7} kw-hr	1 kw-hr = 3.6×10^6 joules
= 1 watt-sec	1 watt-sec = 1 joule
= 0.62×10^{19} electron volts	1 electron volt = 1.6×10^{-19} joules
1 curie = 3.7×10^{10} disintegration/sec	
1 rad (radiation absorbed dose) = 1×10^{-2} joule/kg	
1 roentgen = 2.57×10^{-4} coulomb/kg	

Power

1 watt = 0.056 BTU/min	1 BTU/min = 17.58 watts
= 0.00131 horse power	1 horse power = 745.7 watts
= 0.00134 horse power (electric)	1 horse power (electric) = 746 watts
= 0.737 ft-lb/sec	1 ft-lb/sec = 1.35 watts
= 1 × 10^7 ergs/sec	1 gm-cm/sec = 9.8 × 10^{-5} watts
= 0.239 cal/sec	1 erg/sec = 1 × 10^{-7} watts
	1 cal/sec = 4.18 watts

Temperature

Temperature Fahrenheit = 9/5 × C + 32
Temperature centigrade = 5/9 (F − 32)
Temperature Kelvin = 273.15 + C

INDEX

Note: Page numbers in *italics* refer to illustrations.
Page numbers followed by (t) refer to tables.

Abdomen, surgery in, and hypotension, 418
Abdominal muscle, tone of, raised airway pressure and, 415
Abdominal wall, intercostal block and, 291
Abducens nerve, paralysis of, lumbar puncture and, 275
Abortions, trace anesthetics in operating room and, 147
Abscess, lung, chest physiotherapy in, 481
Accidents, miscellaneous, 434–435
  to patient, recording of, 57
Accommodation, of nerve and muscle membrane, 196
ACD, 332
Acetylcholine
  in muscle relaxation, 146
  in neuromuscular block, 197
    reversal of, 213
  local anesthetics and, 244
Acetylcysteine, in inhalation therapy, 483
Acid, 324
  barbituric, derivatives of. See *Barbiturates*.
  carbonic, 324
Acid-base balance, 309–329
  and neuromuscular blockers, 208
  metabolic disturbances in, respiratory compensation for, 499, 511
Acid citrate dextrose, 332
Acidemia, 324
Acidosis, 324, 325–329
  and 2,3-diphosphoglycerate, 506
  and intravenous barbiturates, 177
  fetal, 357
  in newborn, 361
  in pregnancy, 348
  metabolic, 327
    in dehydrated infant, 372
    in newborn, 366
    respiratory compensation for, 499
  respiratory, acute, 326

Acidosis (*Continued*)
  respiratory, arterial blood carbon dioxide in, 97
    chronic, 327
    cyclopropane and, 152
Action potential, of nerve and muscle membrane, 196
Acupuncture, 406–408
Acute tubular necrosis, hemolysis and, 333
  postoperative, 20
Addiction, drug, 34
ADH, in extracellular fluid tonicity, 316
  secretion of, 321
Adhesive arachnoiditis, spinal anesthesia and, 275
Adhesive tape, and static electricity, 443
Adrenals, drugs affecting, 31
Adrenocorticoids, increased levels of, 322
Adult respiratory distress syndrome, 513
Age, patient, and anesthetic overdose, 412
  and minimum alveolar concentration of halothane, *122*, 123
  anesthesia record of, 104
Air, inspired, 488
  humidification of, 479
Air block, 433
Air embolism, 434
  excessive lung pressure and, 433, *433*
  monitoring of, 94
Airway
  anatomy of, *222*, 486
  closure of, 492
  dynamic compression of, 494
  foreign body in, 450
  insertion of. See *Tracheal intubation*.
  obstruction of, and respiratory failure, 448
    in anesthesia induction, in child, 378
    in laryngeal edema, 386
    in newborn, 364
    in positive pressure respiration, 450
    ketamine and, 188
  of newborn, clearing of, 360

525

Airway (*Continued*)
  pharyngeal, in respiratory obstruction, 127, *128*
  pressure at, 100
    complications of, 519
    positive, continuous, in respiratory distress syndrome of newborn, 362
    in resuscitation, 450
    raised, and hypotension, 415–417, *415, 416*
  problems with, in inhalation anesthesia, 126–130
  resistance of, 493
Albumin, in intravascular volume expansion, 331
Alcohol(s), as cutaneous antiseptics, 80
  effects of, 32
  in sterilization, 83
Aldosterone, increased levels of, 322
Alkalemia, 324
Alkalosis, 324, 325–329
  and 2,3-diphosphoglycerate, 506
  metabolic, 328
    respiratory compensation for, 499
  respiratory, 328
Allen's test, 93
Allergy, to analgetics, 43
  to blood transfusion, 334
  to local anesthetics, 258
N-Allylnormorphine, as analgetic, 43
Alpha-adrenergic stimulating drugs, in inhalation therapy, 483
Alveolar anesthetic tension, 119, *119*
  factors affecting, 117–118, 117(t)
  inspired tension and, 118–120, *119*
  of nitrous oxide, 150, *151*
Alveolar gas, 498–499
  and pulmonary blood, diffusion of carbon dioxide and oxygen between, 504
  composition of, 507
  inhalation anesthetics in, 116, 170
    partial pressure of. See *Alveolar anesthetic tension.*
Alveolar hypoventilation, 509
  and hypercapnia, 513
Alveolar ventilation. See *Ventilation, alveolar.*
Alveolus(i). See also *Alveolar anesthetic tension,* and *Alveolar gas.*
  development of, 364
  excessive pressure on, 432
  in gas exchange, 486
Ambulatory anesthesia services, 388–395
Ambulatory patient
  anesthesia for, 5, 388–395
    equipment for, 392
    preparation for, 389, *390*
    results of, 392
    techniques for, 391
  surgery for, anesthesia in, 5, 388–393
    patient selection for, 388, 391(t)
    types of, 389, 391(t)

Amethocaine. See *Tetracaine.*
Amides, 248–250, 252(t)
Ammonium compounds, quaternary, in sterilization, 83
Amnesia, in ether anesthesia, 232
Amphetamine, anesthesia and, 35
Analgesia
  diethyl ether and, 154, 232
  inhalation anesthetics and, 147
Analgetics
  allergy to, 43
  anesthesia record of, 105
  and respiration, 41, *42*
  preoperative, 40
  undesirable effects of, 41
Anaphylaxis, and hypotension, 421–422
  blood transfusion and, 334
Anectine. See *Succinylcholine.*
Anemia, in children, 370, *370,* 371(t)
  of pregnancy, physiologic, 347
Anemometer, Wright, 96
Anesthesia
  ancillary care, 445–521
  and operation, 113–444
  as speciality, development of, 2
  asepsis in, 78–86
    technique for, 79–80
  authorization for, by patient, 55
  barbiturate. See *Barbiturates.*
  caudal. See *Caudal anesthesia.*
  choice of, 16–21
  complications of, 427–435
  consultation before. See *Preanesthetic consultation.*
  depth of, and blood pressure, 238
    anesthesia record of, 106
  dissociative. See *Dissociative anesthesia.*
  emergence from, restlessness and excitement during, 463
  endotracheal, Ayre's T-piece in, 166
  epidural. See *Peridural anesthesia.*
  equipment for. See *Equipment.*
  ether. See also *Diethyl ether.*
    and analgesia, 154, 232
    Guedel's signs and stages of, 232–236, *233*
  for ambulatory patient. See *Ambulatory patient.*
  for extracorporeal circulation, 400–406
  general, for ambulatory patients, 391
    for delivery, 353
    overdose of, and hypotension, 412–413
  Gillespie's signs and stages of, 231, *233*
  induction of, anesthesia record of, 104
    in children, 377, *378*
    in extracorporeal circulation, 404
    with intravenous barbiturates, 180
  intravenous. See *Intravenous anesthesia.*
  maintenance of, with intravenous barbiturates, 181
  obstetric, 5, 346–363. See also *Delivery,* and *Labor.*

Index

Anesthesia (*Continued*)
  obstetric, caudal, 286
    peridural, 278
    regional, *350*, 351–353
  pediatric. See *Pediatric anesthesia.*
  peridural. See *Peridural anesthesia.*
  preliminary considerations in, 9–48
  premedication for. See *Premedication.*
  preparation for, 36–48
    minimizing legal risk in, 55
  presurgical, 237
  record of. See *Anesthesia record.*
  regional. See *Regional anesthesia.*
  research in, 5–6
  risk of, 13–16
  sacral. See *Sacral anesthesia.*
  special services in, 4–5
  special techniques in, 396–408
  specialities of, 346–408
  spinal. See *Spinal anesthesia.*
  steroid, 190
  subarachnoid, in labor, 352
  surgical, 234–236
  technique for, aseptic precautions in, 79–80
  topical, 251–255
  untoward sequelae of, 409–444
  Woodbridge's components of, 238–*239*
Anesthesia machines, 59, *60*
  checklist for, 76
  fail-safe devices for, *60*, 63, *64*
  hazards of, 75–76
  in pediatric anesthesia, 373
  pressure within, 100
  storage of, 442
  use of mechanical ventilators of, 73–75, *74*
Anesthesia record, 47, 101–111, *102*–*103*
  charting of, 105–106
  early use of, 101
  face of, 104–105
  in malpractice claims, 101
  in minimizing legal risk, 57
  in recovery room, 466, *468*
  information from, 103–108
  reverse of, 106–108
Anesthesiologist, 2–3. See also *Anesthetist.*
  functions of, 3–4
Anesthesiology, realm of, 1–8
  teaching of, 6
Anesthetic. See also *Anesthesia,* and names of specific anesthetics.
  alveolar tension of. See *Alveolar anesthetic tension.*
  anesthetic record of, 105
  arterial concentration of, 240
  clinical assessment of, 236–240, *237*
  early use of, 1
  gaseous, 149–153
  in subarachnoid space, action and fate of, 260–261

Anesthetic (*Continued*)
  in subarachnoid space, injection of, 284
  inhalation. See *Inhalation anesthetic.*
  intravenous, blood levels of, 136
  local. See *Local anesthetic.*
  overdose of. See *Overdose, anesthetic.*
  peridural, 282, 282(t)
    action of, site of, 279–280
    injection of, 283
  rectal, blood levels of, 136
  response to, evaluation of, 231–241
  spinal. See *Spinal anesthetic.*
  trace in operating room, 72, 100, 172
    and abortions and congenital anomalies, 147
    removal of, 442
  volatile, 153–160
    vaporization of, 171
Anesthetist
  approach to pregnant patient, 355–356
  in postoperative period, 460
  in recovery room, responsibility of, 57
  in respiratory care, role of, 515–520
  in transmission of disease, 78
  nurse, 2–3
    responsibility of, 54–55
  personal hygiene and behavior of, 78–79
  physician, 2–3
    functions of, 3–4
  relationship to surgeon, 6–8
  role of, in respiratory care, 515–520
Angiotensin II, and extracellular fluid volume, 316, *316*
Anhidrosis, in paravertebral lumbar block, 306
  in stellate ganglion block, 304
Anion(s), extracellular, 313, *314*
Anion gap, 313
Ankle, nerve block of, 302, *303*
Ansolysen, in deliberate hypotension, 398
Antacid, in delivery, 356
Antiarrhythmics, 28, 255
Antibiotics, 31–32
  and neuromuscular blockers, 208
  in inhalation therapy, 483
Antibody, and hemolysis, 334
Anticholinergics, preoperative, 44–45
Anticholinesterases, 213
Anticoagulants, 30, 332
  and hypoprothrombinemia, 337
Antidepressants, anesthesia and, 33
Antidiuresis, anesthesia and, 146
Antidiuretic hormone, in extracellular fluid tonicity, 316
  secretion of, 321
Antigen, hepatitis type B surface, 335
Antihemophiliac globulin, 336
Antihistamines, in allergic reactions to blood transfusion, 334
Antihypertensives, 29
  and hypotension, 412

Antilirium, in postoperative reaction to scopolamine, 44
Anti-Parkinson therapy, 34
Antiseptics, cutaneous, 80
Anuria, hemolysis and, 333
Apgar score, 360, 360(t)
Apnea, 447
 oxygen, 478
 succinylcholine and, 206
AR. See *Respiration, assisted.*
ARDS, 513
Arachnoiditis, adhesive, spinal anesthesia and, 275
Aramine, in hypotension, 424, 424(t)
Arfonad, in deliberate hypotension, 398
 in hypertension, 461
Arrhythmias, cardiac
 air embolism and, 434
 cyclopropane and, 153
 detection of, 90
 halothane and, 156
 in cardiac arrest, 452
 management of, in cardiac surgery, 403
 treatment of, 28
 trichloroethylene and, 158
 ventricular, vasopressors and, 425
Arterial blood. See *Blood, arterial.*
Arterial pressure. See *Blood pressure.*
Arterial pump, 401
Arteriosclerosis, coronary, blood pressure in, 410
Artery, coronary, surgery on, 403
 ulnar, evaluation of, 93
Arthritis, anesthesia in, 19
Asepsis, in anesthesia, 78-86
 technique for, 79-80
Asphyxia, and neonatal depression, 359
Aspiration
 meconium, 361
 of gastric contents, 427-428
  after tracheal extubation, 230
  in labor, 349
  in newborn, 385
  prevention of, 130
   during tracheal intubation, 225
Asthma, bronchial
 anticholinergics in, 45
 diethyl ether in, 154
 halothane in, 157
 in chronic obstructive pulmonary disease, 393
Atelectasis
 analgetics and, 41
 anesthesia and, 19
 chest physiotherapy in, 481
 postoperative, in child, 385
ATN, hemolysis and, 333
 postoperative, 20
Atrial pressure, left, monitoring of, 91
Atropine
 in reversal of neuromuscular block, 213

Atropine (*Continued*)
 preoperative, 44, 129
  in ambulatory patients, 391
  in child, 372
Autoclave, in sterilization, 81
Axillary block of brachial plexus, 293-294, *294*
Ayre's T-piece, 166-167, *167*
 in pediatric anesthesia, 374, *374, 386*
Azotemia, methoxyflurane and, 147

Bacteria, cutaneous antiseptics and, 80
 transmission of by blood, 335
Bag, reservoir. See *Reservoir bag.*
Bag and mask technique, of respiratory resuscitation, 449-450, *450*
Baralyme, as carbon dioxide absorber, 70
Barbiturates, 33, 174-183
 alcohol and, 33
 and hypotension, 411
 anesthesia and, 33
 biotransformation of, 177
 in labor, 349
 in preventing adverse effects of local anesthetics, 257
 injection of, intra-arterial, 182
  extravascular, 181
 intravenous, anesthesia induction with, 180
  anesthesia maintenance with, 181
  anesthesia management with, 180
  anesthetic action of, 178
  central nervous system effects of, 179
  circulatory effects of, 178-179
  clinical use of, 179-181
  complications of, 181-183
  controllability of, 174
  distribution of, 175
  fate in the body, 175
  respiratory effects of, 178
  selection of patients for, 179
  theoretic considerations in, 174-178
 preoperative, 38
 solutions of, alkalinity of, 177
Barbituric acid, derivatives of. See *Barbiturates.*
Barotrauma, pulmonary, positive airway pressure and, 519
Base, 324
Belladonna alkaloids, preoperative, 44
 with ketamine, 188
 pupil response to, 235
Benzalkonium, tincture of, as cutaneous antiseptic, 80
Benzodiazepines, anesthesia and, 33
 preoperative, 40
Beta-adrenergic block, and hypotension, 412
 in deliberate hypotension, 398
Beta-adrenergic stimulating drugs, in inhalation therapy, 482

Index 529

Bicarbonate, 324
  extracellular, 313, *314*
  in acute respiratory acidosis, 326
  in malignant hyperthermia, 429
  in regulation of pulmonary ventilation, 511
  plasma, in newborn, 366
Bile, excretion of neuromuscular blockers in, 206
Biotransformation, of barbiturates, 177
  of drugs, 24–25
    enzymes in, 25, *26–27*
  of inhalation anesthetics, 141
Birth. See *Delivery*.
Bishydroxycoumarin, in thromboembolic disease, 30
Bladder, urinary, anesthesia and, record of, 108
  catheterization of, 97
Bleeding
  and cardiac failure, 452
  and hypotension, 417
  measurement of, 94
  reduction of, deliberate hypotension and, 396
Blind nasotracheal intubation, 226
Block, air, 433
  nerve. See *Nerve block*.
Blood
  arterial, carbon dioxide in, monitoring of, 97
    removal of, 142
  concentration of anesthetic in, 240
  inhalation anesthetics in, 116
    tension of, 119, *119*
  oxygen in, 131
    monitoring of, 96–97
    tension of, 472, 473(t)
  capillary, fetal, 359
  carbon dioxide in, content of, 508
    transport of, 507
  coagulation of, anesthesia and, 30
  concentration of local anesthetics in, 255
  crossmatching of, 334, 417
  flow of. See *Circulation*.
  in dehydration, 319
  intravascular volume of, maintenance of, 331–332
  intravenous administration of, 341–344, *343, 344*
  intravenous anesthetic in, level of, 136
  isotonic saline as substitute for, 323
  loss of, 330
    and cardiac failure, 452
    and hypotension, 417
    measurement of, 94
    reduction of, deliberate hypotension and, 396
  oxygen in, content of, 508
    maintenance of, 332
    transport of, 505–507

Blood (*Continued*)
  pH of, 324
  pulmonary, alveolar gas and, diffusion of carbon dioxide and oxygen between, 504
  transfusion of, and overload of circulation, 338–340
    in child, 383
    incompatible, and hypotension, 421
    insertion of catheter for, 342–344, *343, 344*
    minimizing legal risk in, 57
    reactions to, 333
    transmission of disease by, 334
  venous, inhalation anesthetics in, 117
    during inhalation anesthesia, 131
  volume of, 330
    extracellular fluid volume and, 310–311
    in children, 368, *368*
    in pregnancy, 347
    monitoring of, 90, 94
  volume expanders of, 331–332
  volume replacement of, 94
    rapid, 339
  whole, therapy with, 332–336
Blood component therapy, 330–345, 333(t)
Blood gases, analysis of, 325, 326(t), 327(t)
  fetal, 359
Blood pressure. See also *Hypertension*, and *Hypotension*.
  anesthesia and, 18
  anesthesia record of, 106
  depth of anesthesia and, 238
  during anesthesia, 409–426
    measurement of, 47
  gallamine and, 204
  halothane and, 155, 413
  in newborn and child, 366, 367(t)
  measurement of, direct, 93–94
    during anesthesia, 47
    indirect, 88–89
    Riva-Rocci method of, 88, 101
  monitoring of, in pediatric anesthesia, 377
  pancuronium and, 204
  significance of, 410
  tubocurarine and, 203
Blood pressure cuff, 88
Blood-bronchial barrier, 486
Bohr formula, for respiratory dead space, 497, *497*
Boiling point, of inhalation anesthetics, 137–138, 139(t)
Bowel
  distention of, nitrous oxide and, 150
  effect of analgetics on, 42
  inhalation anesthesia and, 131
  spinal anesthesia and, 262
  traction on, and hypotension, 418
Brachial plexus
  anatomy of, 293
  block of, 292

Brachial plexus (*Continued*)
  block of, axillary, 293–294, *294*
    interscalene, 295
    supraclavicular, 295–296, *295*
  injury to, 430, *431*
Bradycardia, blood loss and, 417
  cyclopropane and, 152
  during anesthesia, anticholinergics in, 44
Brain
  anesthetics and, 125
  circulation of, 411
    inhalation anesthetics and, 143
  damage to, in circulatory failure, 458
  inhalation anesthetics and, 115
Breath sounds, in tracheal intubation, 227
Breathing. See also *Respiration*.
  continuous positive pressure, 519
  intermittent positive pressure, 480–481
  in respiratory insufficiency, 19
Breathing circuit, losses of gas from, 170
Brevital, 174, *175*
Bronchial circulation, 486
Bronchial hygiene, in chronic obstructive pulmonary disease, 394
Bronchial intubation, 227, 229
Bronchiectasis, chest physiotherapy in, 481
Bronchitis, anesthesia in, 18
  anticholinergics in, 45
  in chronic obstructive pulmonary disease, 393
Bronchodilation
  diethyl ether and, 154
  halothane and, 157
  inhalation therapy for, 482
  intermittent positive pressure breathing and, 481
Bronchopneumonia, anesthesia and, 19
Bronchospasm, anesthesia in, 18
  tubocurarine and, 203
Bronchus(i), 486
  intubation of, 227, 229
Bronkosol-2, in inhalation therapy, 482
Bubble oxygenator, 401, *401*, *402*
Buffer system, 324
Bupivacaine, 249, 253(t)
  in cesarean section, 355
  in stellate ganglion block, 305
Burns, chemical, 438
  electric, 437–438
Butterfly needle, 341
Butyrophenones, in neuroleptanesthesia, 183
Bypass
  cardiopulmonary, air embolism in, 434
  in cardiac surgery, 400
  in extracorporeal circulation, partial, 405
    total, 405

Calcium
  anesthetics and, 125
  binding of, local anesthetics and, 244

Calcium (*Continued*)
  extracellular, 313, *314*
    abnormalities of, 313, 315(t)
  Calcium chloride, in cardiopulmonary resuscitation, 455(t)
    in heart failure, 340
  Calcium gluconate, in child, 383
    in heart failure, 340
  Cannula, nasal, for oxygen therapy, 475, 475(t)
    radial artery, in direct measurement of blood pressure, 93
  Capillary blood, fetal, 359
  Carbocaine, 249, 252(t)
    in caudal anesthesia, 286
  Carbon dioxide
    absorption of, chemical, 69–71
      in inhalation anesthesia, 162, 163(t)
    and ventilation, 142, *142*
    arterial blood, monitoring of, 97
    removal of, 142
    combining power of, 328
    compressed, 62, 63(t)
    diffusion of, between alveolar gas and pulmonary blood, 504
    in blood, content of, 508
      transport of, 507
    in regulation of pulmonary ventilation, 511
    inhalation of, 479
    production of, 495
    pulmonary exchange of, quantitative analysis of, 495
    respiratory response to, analgetics and, 41, *42*
      premedication and, *39*
    retention of, 478
      anesthesia in, 18
      in respiratory failure, 447, 513
    transport of, between lung and tissues, 485, 504–510
      in blood, 507
    values for, 472, 473(t)
  Carbon dioxide absorbers, 69–71
  Carbon dioxide dissociation curve, 507, *508*
  Carbon dioxide ventilation diagram, 142, *142*
  Carbon dioxide ventilatory response curve, 142, *142*
  Carbonic acid, 324
  Carboxyhemoglobin, 507
  Carcinoma, of lung, anesthesia in, 20
    of pancreas, celiac block in, 306
  Cardiac. See also *Heart*.
  Cardiac arrest, causes of, 451
    Innovar and, 186
  Cardiac glycosides, 28
  Cardiac output, 410
    and oxygen transport in blood, 506
    cyclopropane and, 152
    depression of, positive airway pressure and, 519

Cardiac output (*Continued*)
  enflurane and, 159
  in deliberate hypotension, 397
  in newborn, 366, 367(t)
  in pregnancy, 347
  monitoring of, 92–93
  raised airway pressure and, 415
  spinal anesthesia and, 261
Cardiac resuscitation, 451–454
Cardiac tamponade, and hypotension, 420
Cardiopulmonary bypass, air embolism in, 434
  in cardiac surgery, 400
Cardiopulmonary resuscitation, 5, 447–459
  procedure for, 454–457, *455*, 455(t)
Cardiopulmonary system, in child, preoperative assessment of, 371
Cardiotachometer, 90
Cardiovascular drugs, 28–30
Cardiovascular system
  disease of, and hypotension, 420
  in dehydration, 318
  local anesthetics and, 255
  neuroleptanesthesia and, 185
Cartilage, in airway, 486
Catecholamines, acidosis and, 325
  antiarrhythmics and, 28
  antihypertensives and, 29
Catheter
  for continuous spinal anesthesia, 271
  for intravenous fluid therapy, 341
  for peridural anesthesia, 283
  insertion of, for blood transfusion, 342–344, *343, 344*
  intravenous, in pediatric anesthesia, 378
  tracheal, anesthesia record of, 104
Catheterization, urinary bladder, 97
Cations, extracellular, 313, *314*
Cauda equina syndrome, spinal anesthesia and, 275
Caudal anesthesia, 278–287
  in labor, 351
    continuous, 352
  techniques and complications of, 285–286, *286*
Celiac plexus, block of, 306
Central nervous system
  anesthetics and, 133, *134*
    record of, 106
  diethyl ether and, 154
  hypoxia and, 458
  intravenous barbiturates and, 179
  local anesthetics and, 255
  neuroleptanesthesia and, 184
  preanesthetic evaluation of, 98
Central nervous system, active agents, 32–34
Central venous pressure, in dehydration, 319
  monitoring of, 90–91, *92*
  and rapid fluid replacement, 339

Cerebral circulation, 411
  inhalation anesthetics and, 143
Cerebral ischemia, hypotension and, 422
Cerebral palsy, diazepam in, 191
Cerebral vessels, dilatation of, carbon dioxide inhalation in, 479
Cerebrospinal fluid, in lumbar puncture, 104, 269
  in regulation of pulmonary ventilation, 511
  spinal anesthetic in, 261
Cerebrovascular accident, postoperative, 461
Cerebrovascular dilatation, carbon dioxide inhalation in, 479
Cervical laminectomy, air embolism in, 434
Cervical nerves, 289
Cervical plexus, block of, 289–290, *290*
Cervix, dilatation of, during labor, 354, *354*
Cesarean section, 354–355
Chart, anesthesia. See *Anesthesia record*.
  hospital, notes on, 108
Chemical(s), and muscle membrane, 196
  in carbon dioxide absorption, 69–71
Chemical burns, 438
Chemical endarteritis, intra-arterial barbiturate injection and, 182
Chemical sterilization, 82–83
Chest
  external compression of, in cardiac resuscitation, 452, *453*
    in respiratory resuscitation, 450
  movement of, in tracheal intubation, 227
  wall of, mechanical (elastic) properties of, 491, *491*
  spasm of, in tracheal intubation, 229
Chest physiotherapy, 471–484, 481
Child(ren). See also *Pediatric anesthesia*.
  anemia in, 370, *370*, 371(t)
  anesthesia induction in, 377, *378*
  blood volume in, 368, *368*
  body temperature of, control of, *367–368*, 376–378
    monitoring of, 376, 378
    postoperative, 384
  circulatory system of, 366–367, 367(t)
  fluid administration in, 378, *379*, 383–384
  fluid balance and metabolism in, 368–369, *368*
  fluid requirements in, 368, 369(t)
  hemoglobin in, 370, 371(t)
  hydration of, 371–372
  hyperthermia in, 368
  inhalation anesthesia in, 372
  ketamine in, 189, 382
    in anesthesia induction, 377
  monitoring of, 376–377
  postoperative care of, 384–387
  preoperative evaluation and preparation of, 370–373
    psychological considerations in, 370
  preoperative feeding of, 372–373, 373(t)

Child(ren) (*Continued*)
  respiratory system of, 364–366, 365(t)
  tracheal intubation in, 379–382
    postoperative, 386, *386*
Chloral hydrate, 39
Chloride, extracellular, 313, *314*
Chlorine, in sterilization, 82
Chloroform, early use of, 1, 16, 65
Chloroprocaine, 247
  in cesarean section, 355
Chlorpromazine, 183, 187
  anesthesia and, 33
  in hypertension, 461
Cholecystostomy, intercostal block for, 291
Cholinesterase, and succinylcholine, 206
  in reversal of neuromuscular block, 213
Chronic obstructive pulmonary disease, intermittent positive pressure breathing in, 481
  treatment of, 393
Cidex, in sterilization, 84
Cinchocaine, 248
Circle absorber, 59, *60*
Circle technique, for inhalation anesthesia, 169
Circulation
  abnormalities of, and choice of anesthesia, 18
  and respiratory failure, 448
  anesthesia and, 143
  bronchial, 486
  cerebral, 411
  complications of, postoperative 460–461
  coronary, 410
    inadequate, and circulatory failure, 451
  depression of, excessive premedication and, 411
    treatment of, 257
  diazepam and, 190
  diethyl ether and, 154
  extracorporeal, anesthesia for, 400–406
    drugs for, 404, 405(t)
    procedure for, 405
  failure of, 236
    diagnosis of, 452
    hemolysis and, 333
    prognosis in, 458
  halothane and, 156
  in pregnancy, 347–348
  inhalation anesthetics and, 143–145
  insufficiency of, in deliberate hypotension, 397
  intravenous barbiturates and, 178–179
  local anesthetics and, 255
  monitoring of, 87–95
  morphine and, 41
    intravenous, 191
  peridural anesthesia and, 281
  pulmonary, 500–504
    regional distribution of, 501–503, *502*

Circulation (*Continued*)
  spinal anesthesia and, 261
  volume overload of, 338–340
Circulatory failure, 236
  diagnosis of, 452
  hemolysis and, 333
  prognosis in, 458
Circulatory insufficiency, in deliberate hypotension, 397
Circulatory system, anesthesia and, record of, 107
  of child, 366–367, 367(t)
Cirrhosis, anesthesia in, 19
Citanest, 249
Cleft palate, repair of, Ayre's T-piece in, 166
Clinic, pain, 395
  pulmonary rehabilitation, 393–394
Closed systems, for inhalation anesthesia, 168–169
Closing volume, 492, *493*
Closure, airway, 492
Clotting, anesthesia and, 30
Clotting factors, deficiencies of, fresh frozen plasma in, 338
  maintenance of, 336–338
CNS. See *Central nervous system.*
CO. See *Cardiac output.*
Coagulation, anesthesia and, 30
Coagulation factors, deficiencies of, fresh frozen plasma in, 338
  maintenance of, 336–338
Coagulopathy, blood transfusion and, 336
  consumption, 337
  disseminated intravascular, 337
Cocaine, 245
  and hypotension, 414
  early use of, 16, 292
Codeine, preoperative, 40
Collagen, in lung, 490
Colloids, bacterial contamination of, 335
  in dehydration, 319
Colon, mesentery of, traction on, and hypotension, 418, *418*
Colostomy, loop, intercostal block for, 291
Coma, oxygen in chronic hypoxia and, 478
Combustion hazards, minimizing legal risk in, 56
Competitive agents, action of, 199–201
Compliance, lung, 100, 490, 492
  of respiratory system, 492
  with mechanical ventilation, 518
Compressed gases. See *Gases, compressed.*
Compression, external chest, in cardiac resuscitation, 452, *453*
  in respiratory resuscitation, 450
  of airway, dynamic, 494
Concentration effect, in uptake of inhalation anesthetics, 120
Conjunctivitis, 432

Index 533

Connector, for tracheal tubes, 219, *219*
Consciousness, loss of, 232
   peridural anesthesia and, 284
Consumption coagulopathy, 337
Continuous positive airway pressure, in respiratory distress syndrome of newborn, 362
Continuous positive pressure breathing, 519
Convulsions, diethyl ether and, 154
   local anesthetics and, 257
   peridural anesthesia and, 284
Coombs test, in blood crossmatching, 334
COPD, intermittent positive pressure breathing in, 481
   treatment of, 393
Copper Kettle vaporizer, *60*, 66, *67*
Cornea, injury to, 432
Coronary arteriosclerosis, blood pressure in, 410
Coronary artery, surgery on, 403
Coronary circulation, 410
   inadequate, and circulatory failure, 451
   inhalation anesthetics and, 143
Corticosteroids. See *Steroids*.
Cortisol, anesthesia and, 31
Cough
   expiratory muscles in, 489
   in postintubation laryngeal edema, 386
   in tracheal intubation, 129, 225, 227
      prolonged, 229
   intravenous barbiturates and, 182
   topical anesthesia and, 251
CPAP, in respiratory distress syndrome of newborn, 362
CPD, 332
CPPB, 519
CR. See *Respiration, controlled*.
Craniectomy, air embolism in, 434
Crossmatching, of blood, 334, 417
Crystalloids, bacterial contamination of, 335
   in intravascular volume expansion, 331
Cuff, blood pressure, 88
   for tracheal tubes, 219, 516
Cuirass ventilator, 517
Culdoscopy, caudal anesthesia in, 284
Curare, 4
   early use of, 2
CVA, postoperative, 461
CVP, in dehydration, 319
   monitoring of, 90–91, *92*
   and rapid fluid replacement, 339
Cyanosis
   central, 514
   in hypotension, 422
   in inadequate arterial blood oxygenation, 96
   intravenous barbiturates and, 183
   tracheal extubation in, 228
Cyanotic congenital heart disease, preoperative medication in, 373

Cyclopropane, 152–153
   and electroencephalogram, 133, *135*
   and explosions, 441
   and neuromuscular block, 209
   compressed, 62, 63(t)
   pupil response to, 235
Cylinders, for compressed gases, 59, *60, 61*, 442
Cystic fibrosis, inhalation therapy in, 483
Cytochrome P-450, in drug metabolism, 25

Dalmane, preoperative, 40
Dantrolene sodium, in malignant hyperthermia, 430
Dead space, respiratory, 496–500, *497*
Death, maternal, anesthesia and, 346
   patient, anesthesia and, 14, 109
   reports of, 109–110
Decamethonium, 197
   uptake and distribution of, 204
Decelerations, periodic, in fetal heart rate, 357, *358*
Defibrillation, in cardiopulmonary resuscitation, 454
Dehydration, fluid therapy in, 317–320
   in infant, 371, 372(t)
Delirium
   after ketamine anesthesia, 189
   in ether anesthesia, 232
   in water intoxication, 322
   postoperative, 464
Delivery
   aspiration of gastric contents during, 427
   cesarean section, 354–355
   forceps, anesthesia and, 354
   general anesthesia for, 353
   monitoring during, 356
   trauma during, and neonatal depression, 359
Delta factor, 339
Demerol. See *Meperidine*.
Dentures, removal of, before anesthesia, 12
   before tracheal intubation, 221
Depletion syndrome, 318
Depolarization, and muscle twitch response, 199, *200*
   of end plate, 197
   of nerve membrane, 243, *244*
Depolarizing agents, action of, 197–199
Depression, neonatal, 359
   treatment of, anesthesia and, 33
Desensitization, of nerve and muscle membrane, 197
Detergents, in inhalation therapy, 483
Dexamethasone, in postintubation laryngeal edema, 386
Dextran, and anaphylaxis, 422
Dextran-70, in intravascular volume expansion, 331

Dextrose, in malignant hyperthermia, 429
Diabetes, treatment of, 30
Dialysis, in kidney disease, 20
Diaphragm, in respiration, 488
  paralysis of, brachial plexus block and, 293
  spinal anesthesia and, 262
Diaphragmatic hernia, and aspiration of gastric contents, 427
Diazepam
  and hypotension, 411
  anesthesia and, 33
  in convulsions, 257
  in labor, 351
  in neuroleptanesthesia, 187
  in preventing adverse effects of local anesthetics, 257
  intravenous, 190–191, *191*
  preoperative, 39
    and minimum alveolar concentration, 123
    in child, 373
Dibucaine, 248
DIC, 337
Dichloracetylene, 158
Dicumarol, in thromboembolic disease, 30
Diethyl ether, 153–155. See also *Ether anesthesia.*
  and analgesia, 154, 232
  and electroencephalogram, 135, *137*
  and explosions, 441
  and neuromuscular block, 209
  early use of, 1, 16, 65, 153
Diffusion, Fick's law of, 505
  of oxygen and carbon dioxide, between alveolar gas and, pulmonary blood, 504
Diffusion hypoxia, postoperative, 462
Digit(s), nerve block of, 299–300, *299*
Digitalis
  and cardiac arrest, 452
  anesthesia and, 28
  anticholinergics and, 45
  diuretics and, 29
  in malignant hyperthermia, 430
  in septic shock, 421
Digoxin, in heart failure, 340
Dihydromorphinone, preoperative, 41
Dilaudid, preoperative, 41
Dimethyltubocurarine, 199
2,3-Diphosphoglycerate, 332
  and oxygen dissociation curve, 506
Directional valves, in inhalation anesthesia systems, 163, 163(t)
Disc oxygenator, 401, *401*
Disseminated intravascular coagulopathy, 337
Dissociation curve, carbon dioxide, 507, *508*
  oxygen, 506, *506*
Dissociative anesthesia, 187–189
  clinical management of, 188–189
  contraindications to, 189

Dissociative anesthesia (*Continued*)
  indications for, 189
  postoperative course of, 189
Distress, respiratory, in infant, 371
  syndrome of, adult, 513
  of newborn, 362
Diuresis, after hemolysis, 334
  maintenance of, 323
Diuretics, 29
  in heart failure, 340
Diverticula, esophageal, and aspiration of gastric contents, 427
Dopamine, in cardiopulmonary resuscitation, 455(t)
  in heart failure, 340
  in hypotension, 424, 424(t)
Doppler flowmeter, monitoring of blood pressure by, 89
Doppler transducer, in diagnosing air embolism, 95
Dornase, pancreatic, in inhalation therapy, 483
Dornavac, in inhalation therapy, 483
2,3-DPG, 332
  and oxygen dissociation curve, 506
Dressings, restrictive or obstructive, and respiratory obstruction, 462
Droperidol, pharmacologic actions of, 184
Drug(s). See also names of specific drugs.
  absorption of, in intestines, 23
  and concurrent therapy, 28–35
  and endocrine organs, 30–31
  and neuromuscular blockers, 208
  anesthesia and, 3
  biotransformation of, 24–25
  excretion of, 25–28
  for cardiopulmonary resuscitation, 455(t)
  for extracorporeal circulation, 404, 405(t)
  history of, on anesthesia record, 104
  in cardiopulmonary resuscitation, 455(t)
  in inhalation therapy, 482–484
  in pediatric anesthesia, 380(t)–381(t)
  in recovery room, 467(t)
  interactions of, 22–35
  maternal, and neonatal depression, 359
  metabolism of, in newborn, 369
  pharmacokinetics of, 22, *22*
  psychoactive, 33
  therapeutic, and hypotension, 412
  transfer of, across placenta, 359
  uptake of, 23–24
Duranest, 250, 253(t)
  in stellate ganglion block, 305
Dyes, in carbon dioxide absorbers, 69
Dystrophy, muscular, anesthesia in, 19

Ear, lumbar puncture and, 275
Ear oximeter, in measuring arterial blood oxygenation, 97

Index

ECG, monitoring of, 90
  in pediatric anesthesia, 377
ECMO, in hypoxemia, 515
Edema
  laryngeal, after tracheal extubation, 229
    after tracheal intubation, in child, 386
  pulmonary, 504
    aspiration and, 428
    excess saline administration and, 322
    positive end expiratory pressure in, 519
  tracheal, after tracheal extubation, 229
Edrophonium, in reversal of neuromuscular block, 213
EEG, anesthesia and, 133-135, *134-137*
  in evaluating central nervous system function, 98
  monitoring by, 240
Elastin, in lung, 490
Elbow, nerve block at, 296-298, *297*
Electric burns, 437-438
Electric equipment, maintenance of, 438
Electric shock, 439
  in assessing neuromuscular block, 211
  in cardiopulmonary resuscitation, 454
Electricity
  and injury, 436, *439*
  and muscle membrane, 196
  codes and standards for, 440-441
  hazards of, 436-444
    minimizing legal risk in, 56
  power distribution of, in hazardous areas, 439-440, *439, 440*
  static, 443
Electrocardiogram, monitoring of, 90
  in pediatric anesthesia, 377
Electrocution, 436
Electroencephalogram, anesthesia and, 133-135, *134-137*
  in evaluating central nervous system function, 98
  monitoring by, 240
Electrolytes, administration of, excess, hazards of, 320-323
Electrophoresis, serum, 23
Embolism
  air, 434
    excessive lung pressure and, 433, *433*
    monitoring of, 94
    and hypotension, 420
Emergency surgery, 13, 15
  aspiration of gastric contents during, 427
Emphysema
  anesthesia in, 18
  in chronic obstructive pulmonary disease, 393
  mediastinal and subcutaneous, *433,* 434
  pulmonary interstitial, 519
Endarteritis, chemical, intra-arterial barbiturate injection and, 182
Endocrine disease, and choice of anesthesia, 20
Endocrine organs, drugs and, 30-31

Endotracheal anesthesia, Ayre's T-piece in, 166
Endotracheal intubation. See *Tracheal intubation.*
End-plate potential, of nerve and muscle membrane, 197
Endotracheal tubes. See *Tubes, tracheal.*
Enflurane, 17, 159
  and blood pressure, 413
  and electroencephalogram, 135, *136*
  and myocardial contractility, 159, 160(t)
  and neuromuscular block, 209, *210*
  for ambulatory patients, 391
  for delivery, 353
  vaporizer for, 67
Enzyme(s), in biotransformation of drugs, 25, *26-27*
Enzyme induction, 25, *26-27*
  microsomal, and hepatic necrosis, 149
EO, in sterilization, 83
Ephedrine, in circulatory depression, 257
  in hypotension, 414, 424, 424(t)
Epidural anesthesia. See *Peridural anesthesia.*
Epiglottis, in tracheal intubation, 221
Epinephrine
  and duration of spinal anesthesia, 263, 280
  and peridural anesthetics, 280
  in cardiopulmonary resuscitation, 454, 455(t)
  in caudal anesthesia, 286
  in hypotension, 424, 424(t)
  in postintubation laryngeal edema, 386
  in preventing adverse effects of local anesthetics, 256
  in stellate ganglion block, 305
  racemic, in inhalation therapy, 483
Equipment, 59-77
  cleaning of, 84-85
  electric, maintenance of, 438
  explosive, care of, 442
  for ambulatory patient, 392
  for intravenous blood administration, 341, *343*
  for pediatric anesthesia, 373-376, *374, 375*
  for peridural anesthesia, 281
  for spinal anesthesia, 266-267, *267*
  for tracheal intubation, 216-220, *217, 218(t), 219, 221*
    in child, 375, *375,* 376(t)
  mechanical limitations of, in regulation gas flow, 172
  recovery room, 465
  sterilization of, 81-84
Equivalents, numerical, 523
Erythrocytes, pH of, and 2,3-diphosphoglycerate, 506
Escape valve, and gas flow rate, 172
  for anesthesia machines, 72
Esophageal intubation, 228

Esophagus, diverticula of, and aspiration of gastric contents, 427
  in temperature measurement, 99
Ester compounds, 245–248, 252(t)
Ethanol, extracellular, 312
Ether. See *Diethyl ether.*
Ether anesthesia. See also *Diethyl ether.*
  and analgesia, 154, 232
  Guedel's signs and stages of, 232–236, *233*
Ethrane. See *Enflurane.*
Ethylene oxide, in sterilization, 83
Etidocaine, 250, 253(t)
  in stellate ganglion block, 305
Eugenols, 192
Evipal, 174, *175*
Excitement, postoperative, 463
Expert witnesses, in malpractice claims, 52
Expiration, 489
  flow limitation during, 494
  muscles of, 489
Expired air techniques, of respiratory resuscitation, 448–449, *449*
Expired gases, rebreathing of, 162–163, 163(t)
Explosions, 436–444
  hazards of, precautions against, 442–444
Explosive equipment, care of, 442
Extracorporeal circulation, anesthesia for, 400–406
  drugs for, 404, 405(t)
  procedure for, 405
Extracorporeal membrane oxygenation, in hypoxemia, 515
Extraocular muscles, succinylcholine and, 202
Extremity, lower, anatomy of, 300
  nerve blocks of, 300–302
  upper, nerve blocks of, 292–300
Extubation, tracheal, 228
  complications of, 229–230
  in child, 384
Eye(s)
  in central nervous system depression, 98
  in stages of ether anesthesia, 232, *233*
  injury to, 431–432
  lumbar puncture and, 275
  protection of, from ultraviolet light, 79
Eyelid, ptosis of, stellate ganglion block and, 304
Eyelid reflex, 232

Face mask, 71
  fit of, 126
  in anesthesia induction, in child, 377, *378*
  in bag and mask resuscitation, 450
  in oxygen therapy, 475, 475(t)
  in pediatric anesthesia, 374, *375*
  temperature of, in open drop method, 165
Facial nerves, injury to, 431
Factor V, 336

Factor VIII, 336
Fail-safe devices, for anesthesia machines, 60, 63, *64*
Fasciculation, 198
  abdominal, succinylcholine and, 203
  post-tetanic, 212
Feeding, preoperative, anesthesia record of, 104
  of child, 372–373, 373(t)
Femoral nerve, block of, 300
Fentanyl, 184, *184*
  and alveolar ventilation, 41, *42*
  in ambulatory patients, 391
  in labor, 350
  pharmacologic actions of, 184
Fetus
  effect of thiopental on, 355
  lung of, 364
    maturity of, 362
  monitoring of, 356–359
    heart rate of, 356, *358*
Fibrillation, ventricular, causes of, 451
Fibrinolysis, blood transfusion and, 337
Fick's law of diffusion, 505
Film oxygenator, 401, *401*, *402*
Fingers, nerve block of, 299, *299*
Fires, 436–444
  sources of, 442–443
Fistula, tracheoesophageal, tracheal intubation and, 516
Flammability, of anesthetics, 441
  of inhalation anesthetics, 140
Flaxedil, 199
  biliary excretion of, 206
  side effects of, 204
Floor, conductive, in operating room, 443
Flowmeter, Doppler, measurement of blood pressure by, 89
  for anesthesia machines, 60, 64
Fluid(s)
  administration of, excess, hazards of, 320–323
    in deliberate hypotension, 398
    in pediatric anesthesia, 378, *379*, 383–384
  balance of, in child, 368–369, *368*
  body, compartments for, 309–313
    chemical structure of, 313, *314*
    volume of, 311(t)
  cerebrospinal, in lumbar puncture, 104, 269
    in regulation of pulmonary ventilation, 511
    spinal anesthetic in, 261
  exchange of, in lung, 503–504
  extracellular, tonicity of, physiologic control of, 316, *316*
    volume of, 311(t)
      and blood volume, 310–311
      and intracellular fluid volume, 311–313
      physiologic control of, 316, *316*

Fluid(s) (*Continued*)
  interstitial, 309
    accumulation of, 504
    transfer to intravascular space, 331
  intracellular, volume of, and extracellular fluid volume, 311-313
  intravascular, 309
  intravenous, 309-329, 341-344
  loss of, preoperative, 317
  parenteral, composition of, 319(t)
  replacement of, 4, 94
    anesthesia record of, 105
    rapid, central venous pressure monitoring and, 339
    urine output in measuring, 98
  requirements of, in children, 368, 369(t)
Fluid therapy
  in dehydration, 317-320
  in hypotension, 423
  intravenous, 317-320
    technique for, 341-344
  routine parenteral, in elective surgery, 317
Fluoride, and nephrotoxicity, 147
Fluoromar, 17, 157-158
  and neuromuscular block, 209
  pupil response to, 235
Fluotec vaporizer, 68, *68*
Fluothane. See *Halothane*.
Flurazepam, preoperative, 40
Fluroxene, 17, 157-158
  and neuromuscular block, 209
  pupil response to, 235
Forane, 17, 160
  and neuromuscular block, 209
Forceps delivery, anesthesia and, 354
Foreign body, in airway, 450
Functional residual capacity, in pregnancy, 347
Furosemide, and diuresis, 334
  maintenance of, 323
  in heart failure, 340

Gallamine, 199
  biliary excretion of, 206
  side effects of, 204
Gallbladder, traction on, and hypotension, 418
Gangrene, intra-arterial barbiturate injection and, 182
Gap, anion, 313
Gas(es)
  alveolar. See *Alveolar gas*.
  anesthetic, waste, 72, 100, 172
    and abortions and congenital anomalies, 147
    removal of, 442
  blood, analysis of, 325, 326(t), 327(t)
    fetal, 359

Gas(es) (*Continued*)
  compressed, 59-63
    conducting tubes for, 71
    cylinders for, 59, *60, 61*, 442
    for mechanical ventilator, 74
    properties of, 62, 63(t)
    specifications for use of, 61
  concentration of, 116
  dilution or washout of, 171
    pulmonary exchange of, mechanisms of, 487-494
    quantitative analysis of, 495-496
  expired, rebreathing of, 162-163, 163(t)
  flow of, in anesthesia systems, 170-173
    mechanical limitations of, 172
  humidification of, 479-480
  inspired, oxygen content of, 473-477
  liquefied, 62
  losses of, from breathing circuit, 170
Gas scavenger systems, for anesthesia machines, 72, *73*
Gas sterilization, 83-84
Gaseous anesthetics, 149-153
Gastric contents, aspiration of. See *Aspiration, of gastric contents*.
Gastrointestinal tract
  anesthesia and, record of, 107
  circulation to, inhalation anesthetics and, 144
  fluid losses from, 317
  in pregnancy, 349
Gastrostomy, intercostal block for, 291
General anesthesia, for ambulatory patient, 391
  for delivery, 353
  overdose of, and hypotension, 412-413
Germicides, liquid, 82
GFR, inhalation anesthetics and, 144, 146
Gillespie's signs and stages of anesthesia, 231, *233*
Glaucoma, anticholinergics in, 45
Globulin, antihemophiliac, 336
Glomerular filtration rate, inhalation anesthetics and, 144, 146
Glucocorticoids, increased levels of, 322
Glucose
  extracellular, 312
  in alcohol intoxication, 33
  in diabetes, 31
  in pediatric anesthesia, 369
Glycopyrrolate, preoperative, 45
Glycosides, cardiac, 28
Granuloma, of vocal cords, after tracheal extubation, 229
Guedels' signs and stages of ether anesthesia, 232-236, *233*

Haldane effect, 507, *508*
Halogen(s), in sterilization, 82

Halogenated hydrocarbons, 129
Halothane, 16, 155–157
  and blood pressure, 155, 413
  and cerebral circulation, 143
  and heart rate, 155, *156*
  and hepatic disease, 148
  and hypotension, 238
  and malignant hyperthermia, 429
  and myocardial contractility, 155, *156*, 160(t)
  and neuromuscular block, 209, *210*
  for delivery, 353
  in anesthesia induction, in child, 377
  in cesarean section, 355
  in deliberate hypotension, 397
  minimimum alveolar concentration of, patient age and, *122*, 123
  monitoring of, 100
  solubility of, in rubber, 140(t), 155
  vaporizer for, 67, *68*
Hamman's sign, 433
Hand, nerve block of, 299–300, *299*
Harelip, repair of, Ayre's T-piece in, 166
Head, lifting of, in assessing neuromuscular block, 213
  position of, for tracheal intubation, 223, *223*
Headache, anesthesia record of, 106
  lumbar puncture and, 273, 274(t)
Hearing, lumbar puncture and, 275
Heart
  arrhythmias of. See *Arrhythmias, cardiac.*
  alcohol and, 32
  anticholinergics and, 44
  circulation of, 410
    inadequate, and circulatory failure, 451
    inhalation anesthetics and, 143
  cyclopropane and, 152
  diazepam and, 191
  diethyl ether and, 154
  disease of, anesthesia in, 18
    cyanotic congenital, preoperative medication in, 373
    extracorporeal circulation in, 403
    preanesthetic assessment of, 12
  electric currents through, 436
  external manual compression of, 452–454, *453*
  inhalation anesthetics and, 144, *145*
  intravenous barbiturates and, 178
  levodopa and, 34
  local anesthetics and, 255
  morphine and, 41
  open chest manual compression of, 456–457, *457*
  output of. See *Cardiac output.*
  peridural anesthesia and, 281
  resuscitation of, 451–454
    external chest compression in, 452, *453*

Heart (*Continued*)
  succinylcholine and, 202
  surgery on, 400
    analgetics in, 41
    and cardiac arrest, 452
  vasopressors and, 424
Heart failure
  blood transfusion and, 349
  cardiac resuscitation in, 451
  during anesthesia, 420
  in chronic obstructive pulmonary disease, 393
  inotropic drugs in, 340
Heart rate
  cyclopropane and, 152
  fetal, monitoring of, 356, *358*
  halothane and, 155, *156*
  in newborn, 366, 367(t)
  monitoring of, 87–88, *88*
  pancuronium and, 204
Heat sterilization, 81–82
Hematocrit, in blood loss, 331
  in dehydration, 319
Hemochromatosis, anesthesia in, 19
Hemodialysis, in kidney disease, 20
Hemodilution, and hypotension, 417
  in extracorporeal circulation, 402
Hemoglobin
  in blood loss, 331
  in carbon dioxide transport, 507
  in child, 370, 371(t)
  in dehydration, 319
  in packed red blood cells, 335
  in urine, 333
  oxygen-carrying capacity of, 332, 505
Hemolysis, blood administration and, 333
Hemorrhage, and cardiac arrest, 452
  and hypotension, 417
  reduction of, deliberate hypotension and, 396
Henderson-Hasselbalch equation, 23, 324
Heparin, in disseminated intravascular coagulopathy, 337
  in thromboembolic disease, 30
Hepatic. See *Liver.*
Hepatitis
  anesthesia in, 19
  halothane and, 148
  transmission of, by anesthetist, 78
    by blood, 334
Hepatitis type B surface antigen, 335
Hepatotoxicity, inhalation anesthetics and, 148
Hernia, diaphragmatic, and aspiration of gastric contents, 427
Hexachlorophene, in sterilization, 83
Hexobarbital, 174, *175*
Hiccough, carbon dioxide inhalation in, 479
High flow oxygen therapy, 473, *474*

Hip, replacement of, and hypotension, 419
Histamine, release of tubocurarine and, 203
Hoarseness, after tracheal extubation, 299
Hood, head, incubators with, 384, *385*
  oxygen, 474
Horner's syndrome, brachial plexus block and, 293
  stellate ganglion block and, 304
Hospital chart. See also *Anesthesia record.*
  notes on, 108
Humidification, of gases, 479–480
Humidifiers, 480
Hyaline membrane disease, 362
Hydration, of child, 371, 372
  of infant, 371, 372(t)
Hydrocarbons, halogenated, 129
Hydrocortisone, 31
Hydrolysis, of local anesthetics, 256
Hydroxyzine, in labor, 351
  preoperative, 40
Hypercapnia, 509
  alveolar hypoventilation and, 513
  treatment of, 515
Hypercarbia, 325
Hyperesthesia, anesthesia record of, 107
Hyperkalemia, dehydration and, 320
Hyperpnea, for blind nasotracheal intubation, 226
  in carbon dioxide inhalation, 479
Hyperosmolarity, 312
Hypertension
  cyclopropane and, 152
  gallamine and, 204
  pancuronium and, 204
  postoperative, 461
  psychoactive drugs and, 33
  treatment of, 29, 461
    and hypotension, 412
Hyperthermia, 99
  and general anesthetic overdose, 412
  in child, 368
  malignant, 429–430
Hyperthyroidism, anesthesia and, 30
Hyperventilation, 325
  in pregnancy, 347
Hypnotics, preoperative, 37
Hypocarbia, 325
Hypochloremia, in respiratory acidosis, 327
Hypoesthesia, anesthesia record of, 107
Hypoglycemia, anesthesia and, 31
Hypokalemia, dehydration and, 320
  in metabolic alkalosis, 328
Hypo-osmolarity, 312
Hypoprothrombinemia, 337
Hypotension
  air embolism and, 434
  anaphylaxis and, 421–422
  cardiovascular disease and, 420
  causes of, 411–422

Hypotension (*Continued*)
  deliberate, 396–400
    complications of, 400
    technique for, 397–399
  depressed cardiac output and, 519
  depth of anesthesia and, 238
  diagnosis of, 422
  during anesthesia, 409–426
  excessive premedication and, 411–412
  general anesthetic overdose and, 412–413
  halothane and, 238
  hemorrhage and, 417
  in dehydration, 320
  incompatible transfusion and, 421
  isotonic saline in, 323
  management of, 422–425
  maternal, regional anesthesia and, 352
  morphine and, 41
  moving of patient and, 419–420, *419*
  peridural anesthesia and, 281, 284, 414–415
  postoperative, 460
  prevention of, vasopressors in, 414
  psychoactive drugs and, 33
  raised airway pressure and, 415–417, *415, 416*
  septic shock and, 421
  spinal anesthesia and, 261, 272, 414–415
  supine position in pregnancy and, 348
  surgical maneuvers and, 418–419, *418*
  tubocurarine and, 203
  vascular absorption of local anesthetics and, 413–414
  vasopressors in, 414, 424–425, 424(t)
  volume overload of circulation and, 339
Hypothermia, 99
  and minimum alveolar concentration, 123
  for cardiac surgery, 400
Hypothyroidism, treatment of, 30
Hypoventilation, 325
  alveolar, 509
    and hypercapnia, 513
  postoperative, 461
Hypovolemia, and hypotension, 420
  raised airway pressure in, 415
Hypovolemic shock, whole blood in, 332
Hypoxemia
  abnormal ventilation-perfusion matching in, 509
  and pulmonary vessels, 501
  in respiratory failure, 512
  nitrous oxide and, 151
  postoperative, 461
  treatment of, 515
Hypoxia
  and central nervous system, 458
  and pulmonary vessels, 501
  cerebral, local anesthetics and, 257
  chronic, treatment of, 478–479
  diffusion, postoperative, 462

Hypoxia (*Continued*)
in respiratory failure, 447
nitrous oxide and, 121
Hysteresis, 489, *490*

IMV, 520
Incubator, with head hood, 384, *385*
Inderal, anesthesia and, 28
  in deliberate hypotension, 398
  in thyrotoxicosis, 30
Infant. See also *Child(ren)*, and *Newborn*.
  anemia of, 370, *370,* 371(t)
  dehydration in, 371, 372(t)
  larynx of, 379
  preoperative evaluation of, 370-373
Infarction, myocardial, and hypotension, 420
Infection
  lumbar puncture and, 275
  of larynx or trachea, after tracheal extubation, 229
  pulmonary, aspiration and, 427
  respiratory, in child, 370
  transmission of, by anesthetist, 78
    prevention of, 79
  virulent, sterilization in, 85
Inferior laryngeal nerve, paralysis of, brachial plexus block, and, 293
Inflatable cuffs, for tracheal tubes, 219, 516
Infusion, intravenous, operative, 47
Inhalation anesthesia, 115-173
  airway and respiratory problems in, 126-130
  and analgesia, 147
  carbon dioxide absorption in, 162, 163(t)
  emergence from, 131-132
  fundamentals of, 115-132
  in child, 382
  induction of, 125-126
    speed of, 120
  intravenous barbiturates with, 180
  maintenance of, 130-131
  open drop method for, 165-166, *166*
  open or nonrebreathing systems for, 164-165, *164*
  semiclosed systems for, 168
  semiopen systems for, 165-168
  techniques of, 162-173, 163(t)
Inhalation anesthetics, 133-161
  alveolar tension of. See *Alveolar anesthetic tension*.
  and circulation, 143-145
  and myocardial contractility, 144, *145,* 413
  and neuromuscular blockers, 209, *210*
  and respiration, 141-147
  biotransformation of, 141
  boiling point of, 137-138, 139(t)
  characteristics of, 135-137
  flammability of, 140

Inhalation anesthetics (*Continued*)
  in alveolar gas, 116, 170
    partial pressure of. See *Alveolar anesthetic tension*.
  in arterial blood, 116
    tension of, 119, *119*
  in labor, 351
  in venous blood, 117
  inspired tension of, and alveolar tension of, 118-120, *119*
  mechanism of action of, 123-125
    neurophysiologic and biochemical mechanisms of, 125
  overdose of, and hypotension, 412
  partition coefficient of, 118, 118(t)
  pharmacologic characteristics of, 140-141
  physical and chemical properties of, 124, 137-140, 139(t)
  potency of, 121, 121(t), 140-141
  reactivity and stability of, 138-139
  solubility of, 118, 118(t),
    in rubber, 138, 140(t)
  toxicity of, 147-149
  uptake and distribution of, 115-121, *116*
    physical consequences of, 120-121
Inhalation therapy, 471-484
  drugs in, 482-484
  equipment for, sterilization of, 81-84
Injections, aseptic precautions in, 80
  of barbiturates, extravascular, 181
  intra-arterial, 182
Innovar, 184
  anesthesia induction with, 185
Inotropic drugs, in heart failure, 340
Inspiration, 488
Inspired air, 488
  humidification of, 479
Inspired anesthetic tension, alveolar anesthetic tension and, 118-120, *119*
Inspired tension of inhalation anesthetics, and alveolar anesthetic tension, 118-120, *119*
Insufficiency, acute pulmonary respiratory support in, 515
  respiratory, and choice of anesthesia, 18-19
    diagnosis of, 514
Insufflation, 164
Insulin, in diabetes, 30
  in malignant hyperthermia, 429
Intensive care, 460-470
  psychological problems in, 469
Intercostal muscles, in anesthesia, 235
  spinal anesthesia and, 262
Intercostal nerves, block of, 291
Intermittent mandatory ventilation, 520
Intermittent positive pressure breathing, 480-481
  in respiratory insufficiency, 19
Intermittent positive pressure ventilation, 517

Index

Interscalene brachial plexus block, 295
Intestines, absorption of drugs in, 23
  obstruction of, and aspiration of gastric contents, 427
  tracheal extubation in, 228
Intoxication, water, 321
Intra-abdominal pressure, and spinal anesthetic, 265–266
Intracranial pressure
  anesthesia in, 18
  decreased, lumbar puncture and, 273
  increased, inhalation anesthetics and, 143
  intravenous barbiturates in, 179
Intragastric pressure, succinylcholine and, 203
Intraocular pressure, succinylcholine and, 202
Intrapleural pressure, 492
Intravascular volume, maintenance of, 330–332
Intravenous anesthesia, 174–241
  local, 250–251
  regional, 306–307
  technique for, 307
Intravenous anesthetic, blood levels of, 136
  elimination of, 137
Intravenous barbiturates. See *Barbiturates, intravenous.*
Intravenous fluids, 309–329, 341–344
Intravenous therapy, aseptic precautions in, 80
  supportive, 309–345
Intubation
  bronchial, 227, 229
  endotracheal. See *Tracheal intubation.*
  esophageal, 228
  nasotracheal. See also *Tracheal intubation.*
    blind, 226
    in child, 382
  orotracheal. See also *Tracheal intubation.*
    in conscious patient, 225
    postoperative, in child, 386, *386*
  tracheal. See *Tracheal intubation.*
  translaryngeal, 516
Iodine, in sterilization, 82
Iodophors, as cutaneous antiseptics, 80
  in sterilization, 82
Ionization, of drugs, 23
IPPB, 480–481
  in respiratory insufficiency, 19
IPPV, 517
Ischemia, cerebral, hypotension and, 422
  myocardial, and hypotension, 420
  peripheral artery cannulation and, 93
Isoetharine, in inhalation therapy, 482
Isoflurane, 17, 160
  and neuromuscular block, 209
Isoproterenol
  in cardiopulmonary resuscitation, 455(t)

Isoproterenol (*Continued*)
  in heart failure, 340
  in hypotension, 424, 424(t)
  in inhalation therapy, 482
Isuprel. See *Isoproterenol.*

Jaws, malformation of, tracheal intubation in, 225

Kanamycin, anesthesia and, 31
Ketamine, 187, *187*
  in anesthesia induction, in child, 377
  in pediatric anesthesia, 382
Kidney
  anesthesia and, record of, 108
  circulation of, inhalation anesthetics and, 144
  disease of, and choice of anesthesia, 19–20
  excretion of antibiotics by, 32
  excretion of barbiturates by, 38
  excretion of neuromuscular blockers by, 205
  function of, monitoring, 97–98
  in drug excretion, 25
  in water conservation, 317
  inhalation anesthetics and, 146
    toxic effects of, 147–148
  protection of, isotonic saline and, 323
  transplantation of, dialysis before, 20
Korotkoff sounds, detection of, 89
Kyphoscoliosis, anesthesia in, 19

Labor
  cardiac output during, 348
  effect of anesthesia on, 354, *354*
  first stage of, pharmacologic agents in, 349–351
  nerve block, in, 349, *350*
  pain pathways in, 349
  pain relief in, 349–353
Lambert-Eaton syndrome, neuromuscular blockers in, 207
Laminectomy, cervical, air embolism in, 434
Largon, as analgetic, 40
Laryngeal nerve, inferior, paralysis of, brachial plexus block and, 293
Laryngoscope, 216
  in pediatric anesthesia, 375
Laryngospasm
  anticholinergics in, 45
  during tracheal intubation, 225
  after tracheal extubation, 229
  in inhalation anesthesia, 129
  intravenous barbiturates and, 182
  thiopental and, 178

Larynx
 edema of, after tracheal extubation, 229
  after tracheal intubation, in child, 386
 in infant and adult, 379
 infection of, after tracheal extubation, 229
 topical anesthesia of, 251
 tumors displacing, tracheal intubation in, 225
Lasers, optical, 438
Lateral femoral cutaneous nerve, block of, 301
Law suits, malpractice. See *Malpractice claims.*
Left atrial pressure, monitoring of, 91
Left ventricular function, monitoring of, 91
Leg, surgery on, nerve blocks for, 300
Legal risk, how to minimize, 55-57
Leukocytes, allergic reaction to, 336
Levarterenol, in cardiopulmonary resuscitation, 455(t)
 in hypotension, 424, 424(t)
Levodopa, in Parkinson's disease, 34
Levophed, in cardiopulmonary resuscitation, 455(t)
 in hypotension, 424, 424(t)
Levoprome, as analgetic, 43
Lidocaine, 248, 253(t)
 and hypotension, 414
 antiarrhythmic action of, 255
 in cardiopulmonary resuscitation, 455(t)
 in caudal anesthesia, 286
 in cervical plexus block, 289
 in cesarean section, 355
 in malignant hyperthermia, 429
 intravenous use of, 251
 serial injection of, 283
Light, ultraviolet, to prevent transmission of infection, 79
LIM, 440, *440*
Line isolation monitor, 440, *440*
Lipid solubility, of anesthetics, 124
 of drugs, 23
Litigation, malpractice. See *Malpractice claims.*
Liver
 alcohol and, 33
 anesthesia and, record of, 107
 biopsy of, intercostal block for, 291
 biotransformation of drugs by, 24
 circulation to, inhalation anesthetics and, 144
 disease of, and choice of anesthesia, 19
  and cholinesterase, 207
  and hypoprothrombinemia, 337
 excretion of antibiotics by, 32
 excretion of barbiturates by, 38
 in diabetes, 31
 necrosis of, halothane and, 148
  microsomal enzyme induction and, 149
 neoplasms of, anesthesia in, 19
 toxic effects of inhalation anesthetics on, 148-149

Local anesthetics, 242-259
 action of, 243-245, *244*
 adverse effects of, 255-258
 concentration of, for spinal anesthesia, 264-265
 intravenous use of, 250-251
 long-acting, 250
 transfer of, across placenta, 249, 353
 use of, 254(t)
 vascular absorption of, and hypotension, 413-414
Low flow oxygen therapy, 473, 475(t), *476*
Lower extremity, anatomy of, 300
 nerve blocks of, 300-302
LSD, anesthesia and, 35
Lubricants, for tracheal tubes, 220, 380
Lumbar epidural anesthesia, in labor, 351
Lumbar paravertebral block, 305-306
 in labor, 351
 technique for, 305
Lumbar puncture
 and headache, 273, 274(t)
 record of, 106
 anesthesia record of, 104
 for spinal anesthesia, 268-271, *270*
 sequelae of, 273-275, *273*
 traumatic, 275
Lumbar sympathetic ganglia, 305
Lung
 abscess of, chest physiotherapy in, 481
 and tissues, transport of carbon dioxide and oxygen between, 485, 504-510
 aspiration of gastric contents into. See *Aspiration, of gastric contents.*
 carcinoma of, anesthesia in, 20
 circulation of, 500-504
  regional distribution of, 501-503, *502*
 compliance of, 100, 490, 492
 development of, 364
 diffusion of carbon dioxide and oxygen in, 504
 disease of, and respiratory failure, 448
  chronic, hypoxemia in, 509
  chronic obstructive, intermittent positive pressure breathing in, 481
   treatment of, 393
  in inhalation anesthesia, 127
 edema in. See *Edema, pulmonary.*
 elastic properties of, 489, *490, 491*
 fetal, 364
  maturity of, 362
 fluid exchange in, 503-504
 function of, 485-487
  anesthesia and, 18
  preanesthetic assessment of, 12
  in infant, 371
 gas exchange in, mechanisms of, 487-494
  quantitative analysis of, 495-496
 infection of, aspiration and, 427
 injury to, 432-434
 rupture of, 433, *433*
 structure of, 485-487

Index

Lung (*Continued*)
  ventilation of, 487
    and metabolic rate, 499
    regulation of, 510–512
  ventilation-perfusion matching in, 487, 507–510
  volumes in, 488, *488*
  and pulmonary vessels, 501
Lymph, in lungs, 503
Lysergic acid diethylamide, anesthesia and, 35

MAC, 121–123, 121(t), 123(t), 140
  of halothane, patient age and, *122*, 123
Magill attachment, 167–168, *169*
  in pediatric anesthesia, 374, *375*
Magnesium, extracellular, 313, *314*
  abnormalities of, 313, 315(t)
Malignancy, terminal, local anesthetics in, 250
Malignant hyperthermia, 429–430
Malpractice, proof of, 52
Malpractice claims, 51
  anesthesia chart in, 101
  causes of, 53–54, *55*
  character of, 51–53
Mannitol, and diuresis, 334
  maintenance of, 323
  extracellular, 312
Manometer, aneroid, in measuring anesthesia machine pressure, 100
Marcaine, 249, 253(t)
  in cesarean section, 355
  in stellate ganglion block, 305
Marijuana, anesthesia and, 35
Mask, face. See *Face mask*.
Meal, preoperative, anesthesia record of, 104
  of child, 372–373, 373(t)
Mechanical ventilators, use of, on anesthesia machines, 73–75, *74*
Meconium, aspiration of, 361
Median nerve, block of, at elbow, 296, *297*
  at wrist, 298, *299*
Medical students, responsibility of, 54–55
Medicolegal considerations, 51–58
Megacolon, celiac block in, 306
Membrane(s)
  biologic, anesthetics and, 124
  muscle, 196
  nerve, 196
    local anesthetics and, 243, *244*
  tympanic, in temperature measurement, 99
Membrane expansion theory, of local anesthetics, 244
Membrane oxygenator, 401, *401*, *402*
Membrane potential, of nerve and muscle, 196

Mendelson, syndrome of, 428
Mental response, 238, *239*
  anesthesia record of, 107
Meperidine, 183
  and hypotension, 411
  for postoperative pain, 463
  in cardiac surgery, 42
  in labor, 350
  preoperative, 41
    in child, 372
Mephentermine, in hypotension, 424, 424(t)
Mepivacaine, 249, 252(t)
  in caudal anesthesia, 286
Meprobamate, anesthesia and, 33
Meralgia paresthetica, 301
Mescaline, anesthesia and, 35
Mestinon, in reversal of neuromuscular block, 213
Metabolic acidosis. See *Acidosis, metabolic*.
Metabolic alkalosis, 328
  respiratory compensation for, 499
Metabolism
  and disturbances in acid-base balance, respiratory compensation for, 499, 511
  in child, 368–369
  of inhalation anesthetics, 141
  of neuromuscular blockers, 205
  rate of, pulmonary ventilation and, 499
Metaraminol, in hypotension, 424, 424(t)
Methamphetamine, in hypotension, 424, 424(t)
Methedrine, in hypotension, 424, 424(t)
Methemoglobinemia, prilocaine and, 249
Methohexital, 174, *175*
Methotrimeprazine, as analgesic, 43
Methoxamine, in hypotension, 424, 424(t)
Methoxyflurane, 17, 157
  and myocardial contractility, 157, 160(t)
  and nephrotoxicity, 147
  and neuromuscular block, 209
  biotransformation of, 141
  in cesarean section, 355
  in labor, 351
  solubility of, in rubber, 140(t), 157
  vaporization of, 171
  vaporizer for, 7
Methyldopa, in hypertension, 29
Methylphenidate, in postoperative shivering, 463
Metubine, 199
Microsomal enzyme induction, and hepatic necrosis, 149
Microsomes, 25
Minimum alveolar concentration, 121–123, 121(t), 123(t), 140
  of halothane, patient age and, *122*, 123
Minute ventilation, 488
Minute volume, monitoring of, 95–96
Mitochondria, anesthetics and, 124
MAO inhibitors, anesthesia and, 34
Monitor, line isolation, 440, *440*

Monitoring, 4, 87-100
  during delivery, 356, *358*
  fetal, 356-359
  in deliberate hypotension, 399
  miscellaneous devices for, 99-100
  of air embolism, 94
  of arterial blood carbon dioxide, 97
  of arterial blood oxygenation, 96-97
  of blood pressure, in pediatric anesthesia, 377
  of blood volume, 90, 94
  of body temperature, 98-99
    in pediatric anesthesia, 376
  of cardiac output, 92-93
  of central venous pressure, 90-91, *92*
    and rapid fluid replacement, 339
  of child, 376-377
  of circulation, 87-95
  of electrocardiogram, 90
    in pediatric anesthesia, 377
  of electroencephalogram, 240
  of heart rate, 87-88, *88*
    fetal, 356, *358*
  of minute volume, 95-96
  of patient, on mechanical ventilation, 518
  of pulmonary wedge pressure, 91-92
    and rapid fluid volume replacement, 339
  of renal function, 97-98
  of respiration, 95-97
Monoamine oxidase inhibitors, anesthesia and, 34
Mood elevators, anesthesia and, 33
Morphine
  and circulation, 41
  and hypotension, 411
  for postoperative pain, 463
  intravenous, 191-192
    postoperative management of, 192
  preoperative, 40
    in child, 372
  pupil response to, 235
Morphine sulfate, in labor, 350
Mortality, maternal, anesthesia and, 346
  patient, anesthesia and, 14, 109
  reports of, 109-110
Motor response, 238, *239*
  block of in peridural anesthesia, 281
  spinal anesthesia and, 261
  disturbances of, anesthesia record of, 107
Mouth-to-mouth respiration, 448, *449*
Mouth-to-nose respiration, 448
Mucolytics, in inhalation therapy, 483
Mycomyst, in inhalation therapy, 483
Mucus, secretion of, in inhalation anesthesia, 129
Muscle(s)
  abdominal, tone of, raised airway pressure and, 415
  circulation to, inhalation anesthetics and, 144

Muscle(s) (*Continued*)
  expiratory, 489
  extraocular, succinylcholine and, 202
  hyperactivity of, enflurane and, 159
  intercostal, in anesthesia, 235
    spinal anesthesia and, 262
  membrane, 196
  pain of, succinylcholine and, 203
  relaxation of, diethyl ether and, 154
    inhalation anesthetics and, 131, 146
    intravenous barbiturates and, 179
    spinal anesthesia and, 261
  respiratory, 510
  rigidity of, in malignant hyperthermia, 429
  smooth, in airway, 486
  sternocleidomastoid, in stellate ganglion block, 303
  sternomastoid, in cervical plexus block, 290, *290*
  tone of, anesthesia and, 235
    suppression of, 195
  twitch response of, depolarization and, 199, *200*
    in assessing neuromuscular block, 211, *212*
  neuromuscular block and, 200, *201*, *202*
Muscular dystrophy, anesthesia in, 19
Musculoskeletal system, neuroleptanesthesia and, 185
Myasthenia gravis, anesthesia in, 19
  neuromuscular blockers in, 207
Myelitis, transverse, spinal anesthesia and, 275
Myocardial contractility
  acidosis and, 325
  enflurane and, 159, 160(t)
  halothane and, 155, *156*, 160(t)
  inhalation anesthetics and, 144, *145*, 413
  methoxyflurane and, 157, 160(t)
  vasopressors and, 424
Myocardial depression, and circulatory arrest, 451
Myocardial infarction, and hypotension, 420
Myocardial ischemia, and hypotension, 420
Myocardial oxygen consumption, 143
Myotonia congenita, neuromuscular blockers in, 207
Myotonia dystrophica, neuromuscular blockers in, 207

Nalline, as analgesic, 43
Naloxone, after morphine anesthesia, 192
  in pediatric anesthesia, 382
  in resuscitation of newborn, 361
Narcotics. See *Opioids*.
Nasal cannula, for oxygen therapy, 475, 475(t)
Nasotracheal intubation. See also *Tracheal intubation*.

Nasotracheal intubation (*Continued*)
  blind, 226
  in child, 382
Nasotracheal tubes, lubricants for, 220
Nausea, anesthesia record of, 107
  spinal anesthesia and, 272
Nebulizers, 480
Neck, surgery in, and hypotension, 418
Necrosis
  acute tubular, hemolysis and, 333
    postoperative, 20
  hepatic, halothane and, 148
    microsomal enzyme induction and, 149
Needle, butterfly, 341
  scalp vein, 341
Nembutal. See *Pentobarbital*.
Neomycin, anesthesia and, 31
Neoplasms, liver, anesthesia in, 19
Neostigmine, anticholinergics and, 44
  in reversal of neuromuscular block, 213
Neo-Synephrine. See *Phenylephrine*.
Nephrectomy, dialysis before, 20
Nephrotoxicity, inhalation anesthetics and, 147
Nerve(s)
  abducens, paralysis of, lumbar puncture and, 275
  cervical, 289
  differential blockade of, 245
  facial, injury to, 431
  femoral, block of, 300
  inferior laryngeal, paralysis of, brachial plexus block and, 293
  injury to, 430–431
  intercostal, block of, 291
  lateral femoral cutaneous, block of, 301
  median, block of, at elbow, 296, *297*
    at wrist, 298, *299*
  membrane of, 196
    local anesthetics and, 243, *244*
  obturator, block of, 301
  peroneal, block of, 301
    injury to, 431
  phrenic, paralysis of, brachial plexus block and, 293
  pudendal, block of, in labor, 353
  radial, block of, at elbow, 297, *297*
    at wrist, 298, *299*
    injury to, 431
  sciatic, block of, 301
  spinal, anatomy of, 288, *289*
  thoracic, block of, 291
  tibial, block of, 302, *303*
  ulnar. See *Ulnar nerve*.
Nerve block. See also *Regional anesthesia*.
  aseptic preparation for, 80–81
  at elbow, 296–298, *297*
  at wrist, 298–299, *299*
  in labor, 349, *350*
  in popliteal space, 301
  of ankle, 302, *303*

Nerve block (*Continued*)
  of hand and digits, 299–300, *299*
  of lower extremity, 300–302
  paravertebral, 289–292
  regional, 288–308
  sympathetic, 302–306
Nerve fibers, differential block of, 280
Nervous system, central. See *Central nervous system*.
Nesacaine, 247
  in cesarean section, 355
Neuroleptanesthesia, 183–187
  clinical use of, 185–186
  pharmacologic actions of, 184–185
  postoperative course of, 186
Neuroleptics. See *Neuroleptanesthesia*.
Neurologic complications, of peridural anesthesia, 284
  of spinal anesthesia, 276
Neurologic disease, spinal anesthesia and, 276
Neuromuscular block
  and muscle twitch response, 200, *201*, *202*
  depth of, assessment of, 210–213, *212*
  factors influencing, 207–209
  phase I, 198
  phase II, 198–199
  residual, postoperative, 461
  reversal of, 213–214
Neuromuscular blockers, 195–215
  action of, factors influencing, 207–209
    rapid onset of, 206
    sites of, 198(t)
  clinical use of, 210–214
  distribution of, 204–206
  elimination of, 205
  in tracheal intubation, 224
    in child, 381
  inhalation anesthetics and, 209, *210*
  intravenous barbiturates with, 181
  metabolism of, 205
  plasma protein binding of, 205
  uptake of, 204–206
  with neuroleptics, 186
Neuromuscular junction, monitoring of, 98
Neuromuscular pharmacology, 195–197
Neuromuscular physiology, 195–197
Neuroplegia, 183
Newborn
  Apgar score of, 360, 360(t)
  blood pressure in, 366, 367(t)
  circulatory system of, 366
  depression of, 359
  evaluation and care of, 359–362
  heart rate in, 366, 367(t)
  postoperative care of, 384, *385*
  respiratory distress syndrome of, 362
  respiratory system of, 364, 365(t)
  temperature control in, 367
Nipride, in deliberate hypotension, 398

Nitrogen, pulmonary exchange of, 495
Nitroprusside, in deliberate hypotension, 398
Nitrous oxide, 149–151
 alveolar tension of, 150, *151*
 and diffusion hypoxia, 462
 and electroencephalogram, 135, *137*
 and hypoxia, 121
 compressed, 62, 63(t)
 early use of, 16, 59, 149
 escape valves for, 72
 in anesthesia induction, in child, 377
 in cesarean section, 355
 in labor, 351
 in neuroleptanesthesia, 183
 in pediatric anesthesia, 382
 intravenous barbiturates with, 181
 monitoring of, 100
 uptake of, 120
Nonrebreathing system, for inhalation anesthesia, 164–165, *164*
 for oxygen, 473
Novocain. See *Procaine.*
Numbness, spinal anesthesia and, 276
Numerical equivalents, 523
Nupercaine, 248
Nurse anesthetist, 2–3
 responsibility of, 154–155
Nursing staff, in recovery room, 464

Obesity, and spinal anesthetic, 265–266
 anesthesia in, 18
 monitoring of blood pressure in, 89
Obstetric anesthesia, 5, 346–363. See also *Delivery,* and *Labor.*
 caudal, 286
 peridural, 278
 regional, *350,* 351–353
Obstruction
 airway. See *Airway, obstruction of.*
 intestinal, and aspiration of gastric contents, 427
  tracheal extubation in, 228
 of tracheal tubes, 229
 respiratory, correction of, 127, *128*
  in inhalation anesthesia, 127
  restrictive or obstructive dressings and, 462
 superior vena cava, and increased central venous pressure, 90
Obturator nerve, block of, 301
Oil, solutions of local anesthetics in, 250
Ointments, anesthetic, 251
Oliguria, anesthesia and, 146
Omnopon, preoperative, 41
Ondine's curse, 511
Open drop method, for inhalation anesthesia, 165–166, *166*
Open or nonrebreathing systems, for inhalation anesthesia, 164–165, *164*

Operating room
 asepsis in, 78
 care of patient in, 79
 conductive floor in, 443
 electric hazards, fires, and explosions in, 436–444
 immediate preanesthetic care in, 46
 minimizing legal risk in, 56
 trace anesthetics in, 100, 172
  and abortions and congenital malformations, 147
  removal of, 442
 transport of patient to, 37, 46
Operating table, moving of patient from, 460
Operation. See *Surgery.*
Opioids
 and addiction, 34
 and hypotension, 411, 423
 in labor, 349
 in neuroleptanesthesia, 183
 in pediatric anesthesia, 382
 in postoperative restlessness and excitement, 464
 preoperative, 40–44
  and minimum alveolar concentration, 123
  vs. preoperative barbiturates, 39
  with barbiturate anesthesia, 180
Opioid antagonist, preoperative, 43
Opium, alkaloids of, preoperative, 40
Optical lasers, 438
Organophosphorous compounds, and cholinesterase, 207
Orotracheal intubation. See also *Tracheal intubation.*
 in conscious patient, 225
 postoperative, in child, 386, *386*
Oscillotonometer, 89
Osmolality, 312
Osmolarity, 312
Outpatient. See *Ambulatory patient.*
Overdose
 anesthetic, and hypotension, 412–413
  in labor, 353
  patient age and, 412
  prevention of, 240
  with anesthesia machine, 75
 premedication, and depressed respiration, 126
Overpressure, 126
Oximeter, in measuring arterial blood oxygenation, 97
Oxybarbiturates, 174
 biotransformation of, 177
Oxygen
 administration of, after nitrous oxide, 151
 and retrolental fibroplasia, 385, 478
 compressed, 62, 63(t)
 consumption of, 495
  anesthesia and, 18
  in newborn, 367
  myocardial, 143

Index

Oxygen (*Continued*)
  diffusion of, between alveolar gas and pulmonary blood, 504
  for tracheal extubation, 228
  harmful effects of, 477–478
  in blood, arterial, 131
    monitoring of, 96–97
    tension of, 472, 473(t)
    content of, 508
      maintenance of, 332
    transport of, 505–507
  in cerebral circulation, 411
  in chronic hypoxia, 478
  in hypotension, 423
  in inspired gas, 473–477
  in malignant hyperthermia, 429
  in newborn, 384
    consumption of, 367
  in packed red blood cells, 335
  in regulation of respiration, 511
  in respiratory failure, 447
  inadequate delivery of, from anesthesia machine, 75
  metabolic demand for, 170
  nonrebreathing system for, 473
  postoperative, 461
  pulmonary exchange of, quantitative analysis of, 495
  saturation of hemoglobin with, 332, 505
  toxicity of, 477
  transport of, between lung and tissues, 485, 504–510
    in blood, 505–507
  values for, 472, 473(t)
Oxygen apnea, 478
Oxygen dissociation curve, 506, *506*
Oxygen hoods, 474
Oxygen tents, 474
Oxygen therapy, 472–479
  early use of, 471
  high flow, 473, *474*
  low flow, 473, 475(t), *476*
Oxygenator, pump, 401–403, *401*, *402*
Oxyhemoglobin, 505
Oxytocin challenge test, 357

Pain
  acupuncture in, 406
  clinic for, 395
  local anesthetics for, 243
  muscle, succinylcholine and, 203
  pathways of, in labor, 349
  postoperative, 463
  relief of, in hypotension, 423
    in labor, 349–353
  tourniquet, brachial plexus block and, 296
  treatment of, 5, 44
Palate, cleft, repair of, Ayre's T-piece in, 166

Palsy. See also *Paralysis*.
  cerebral, diazepam in, 191
Pancreas, carcinoma of, celiac block in, 306
  circulation to, inhalation anesthetics and, 144
Pancreatitis, celiac block in, 306
Pancuronium, 199
  in tracheal intubation, in child, 381
  metabolism of, 205
  side effects of, 204
Pantocaine. See *Tetracaine*.
Pantopon, preoperative, 41
PAP, 500, *502*
Paracervical block, in labor, 352
Paralysis
  abducens nerve, lumbar puncture and, 275
  brachial plexus, 430
  diaphragmatic, brachial plexus block and, 293
  inferior laryngeal nerve, brachial plexus block and, 293
  phrenic nerve, brachial plexus block and, 293
  respiratory, antibiotics and, 31
  spinal anesthesia and, 276
  vocal cord, after tracheal extubation, 230
    brachial plexus block and, 293
Paraplegia, muscle spasm of, local anesthetics in, 250
Paravertebral lumbar block, 305–306
  in labor, 351
  technique for, 305
Paravertebral somatic nerve block, 292
Paresthesias
  brachial plexus block and, 296
  paravertebral somatic nerve block and, 292
  peridural anesthesia and, 283
  spinal anesthesia and, 269
Parkinson's disease, treatment of, 34
Partial bypass, in extracorporeal circulation, 405
Partial pressure, of inhalation anesthetic. See *Alveolar anesthetic tension*.
Patient
  age of, and anesthetic overdose, 412
    and minimum alveolar concentration of halothane, *122*, 123
  anesthetic record of, 104
  accident to, recording of, 57
  admission to and release from recovery room, 467–469
  ambulatory. See *Ambulatory patient*.
  and choice of anesthesia, 17–20
  and malpractice claims, 53
  anesthesia record of, 104
  authorization for anesthesia by, 55
  body habitus of, and choice of anesthesia, 18
  and choice of premedication, 37

Patient (*Continued*)
  care of, in operating room, 79
    negligence in, 52
  conscious, orotracheal intubation in, 225
  death of, anesthesia and, 14, 109
    reports of, 109–110
  emotional status of, and choice of anesthesia, 17
  monitoring of, 4, 87–100
  movement of, after surgery, 131
    and hypotension, 419–420, *419*
    from operating table, 460
    to operating room, 37, 46
  physical status of, and anesthetic risk, 13–16
    anesthesia record of, 104
    classification of, 14
  position of, and spinal anesthetic, 266
    and tracheal intubation, 227
    for caudal anesthesia, 285
    for peridural anesthesia, 282
    for spinal anesthesia, 266
  pregnant, approach of anesthetist to, 355–356
  preoperative anxiety of, 37
  preparation of, for anesthesia, 13
  rapport with physician, lack of, 53
  selection of, for ambulatory surgery, 388, 391(t)
    for intravenous barbiturates, 179
  tilting of, in deliberate hypotension, 396
Pavulon. See *Pancuronium.*
PBP, in extracorporeal circulation, 405
Pediatric anesthesia, 5, 364–387
  Ayre's T-piece in, 166
  drugs used in, 380(t)–381(t)
  emergence from, 384
  equipment for, 373–376, *374, 375*
  fluid administration in, 378, *379*, 383–384
  induction of, 377–379, *378*
  ketamine in, 189, 382
  maintenance of, 382–383
  management of, 377–384
PEEP, in aspiration of gastric contents, 428
  in mechanical ventilation, 518
  in oxygen inhalation, 477
Penicillin, and anaphylaxis, 422
Pentazocine, as analgetic, 43
  preoperative, in child, 373
Penthrane. See *Methoxyflurane.*
Pentobarbital
  and hypotension, 411
  and local anesthetics, 257
  preoperative, 38
    in child, 373
    vs. preanesthetic consultation, 36, 37(t)
Pentolinium, in deliberate hypotension, 398
Percaine, 248
Percutaneous procedures, aseptic preparation for, 80–81

Perfusion, ventilation and, in lungs, 487, 507–510
Perfusion pressure, 501, *502*
Pericardial tamponade, and increased central venous pressure, 90
Pericarditis, constrictive, raised airway pressure in, 415, *416*
Peridural anesthesia, 278–287
  and hypotension, 281, 284, 414–415
  anesthesia record of, 104
  equipment for, 281
  in labor, 351
  level of, anesthesia record of, 106
  management and sequelae of, 284
  physiologic effects of, 281
  results of, 279–280
  serial, 283
  single dose, 282
  spread, onset, and duration of, 280
  technical aspects of, 281–284
Peridural anesthetics, 282, 282(t)
  action of, site of, 279–280
  injection of, 283
Peridural space, anatomy of, 278–279
  negative pressure in, 279
  vascularity of, 280
Perinatology, 346–363
Perivascular pressure, and pulmonary vessels, 500
Peroneal nerve, block of, 301
  injury to, 431
pH, 324
Pharmacologic principles, 22–35
Pharyngeal airway, in respiratory obstruction, 127, *128*
Pharynx, suctioning of, 130
  topical anesthesia of, 251
Phenergan, 183
  preoperative, 40
Phenobarbital, in enzyme induction, 25, *26–27*
Phenol, in stellate ganglion block, 305
  in sterilization, 82
Phenothiazines, anesthesia and, 33
Phenylephrine
  and hypotension, 414
  in cardiopulmonary resuscitation, 454, 455(t)
  in circulatory depression, 257
  in hypotension, 424, 424(t)
  in inhalation therapy, 483
Pheochromocytoma, anesthesia in, 20
Phosphorus, inorganic, serum, 313
Phrenic nerve, paralysis of, brachial plexus block and, 293
Physical examination, by anesthetist, 12
Physician, rapport of patient with, lack of, 53
  resident, responsibility of, 54–55
Physician anesthetist, 2–3
  functions of, 3–4

Index

Physiologic anemia, of infant, 370, *370*, 371
  of pregnancy, 347
Physiologic dead space, 496, *497*
Physostigmine, in postoperative reaction to scopolamine, 44
Placenta
  transfer of drugs across, 359
  transfer of local anesthetics across, 249, 353
  transfer of neuromuscular blockers across, 206
  transfer of thiopental across, 355
Plasma, cryoprecipitated, 338
  fresh frozen, 338
  volume of, restoration of, after blood loss, 331
Plasma protein(s), in intravascular volume expansion, 331
Plasma protein binding, of barbiturates, 177
  of drugs, 23
  of neuromuscular blockers, 205
Plasmapheresis, 338
Platelet(s), reduced, and coagulopathy, 337
Platelet concentrates, 337–338
Pneumoencephalography, nitrous oxide in, 150
Pneumomediastinum, 433, 519
Pneumonia, aspiration and, 428
  postoperative, in child, 385
Pneumotachograph, 95
Pneumothorax, 433, *433*
  brachial plexus block and, 297
  nitrous oxide and, 150, *151*
  postoperative, 462
  stellate ganglion block and, 304
  tension, monitoring of blood pressure in, 90
Poliomyelitis, anesthesia in, 19
Polyuria, methoxyflurane and, 147
Pontocaine. See *Tetracaine.*
Popliteal space, nerve block in, 301
Position of patient. See *Patient, position of.*
Positive end expiratory pressure, in aspiration of gastric contents, 428
  in mechanical ventilation, 518
  in oxygen inhalation, 477
Postoperative period
  care during, 460–470
    for ambulatory surgical patient, 391
    in minimizing legal risk, 57
    of child, 384–387
  hazards of, 460–464
  in deliberate hypotension, 399
Post-tetanic fasciculation, 212
Potassium
  diuretics and, 29
  extracellular, 313, *314*
    abnormalities of, 313, 315(t)
  in dehydration, 320
  neuromuscular blockers and, 207
  serum levels of, in kidney disease, 20

Practolol, in deliberate hypotension, 398
Preanesthetic considerations, essential, 49–111
Preanesthetic consultation, 11–21
  and choice of premedication, 36
  guidelines for, 11–13
  in minimizing legal risk, 55
  in pregnancy, 356, 394
  notes from, 15–16
  vs. premedication, 36, 37(t)
  with children, 370
Pregnancy, physiologic changes in, 347–349
  preanesthetic consultation in, 356, 394
Pregnanediones, 190, *190*
Pregnant patient, approach of anesthetist to, 355–356
Preload function, 339
Premedication, 36–48. See also names of specific drugs.
  anesthesia record of, 104
  and respiratory response to carbon dioxide, *39*
  choice of, 36
  excessive, and hypotension, 411–412
  for extracorporeal circulation, 404
  for spinal anesthesia, 268
  in ambulatory patients, 391
  in child, 372–373
  overdose of, and depressed respiration, 126
  vs. preanesthetic consultation, 36, 37(t)
Preservatives, accumulation of, in vaporizers, 69
Pressure
  airway. See *Airway, pressure at.*
  arterial. See *Blood pressure.*
  blood. See *Blood pressure.*
  central venous, in dehydration, 319
    monitoring of, 90–91, *92*
    and rapid fluid replacement, 339
  intra-abdominal, and spinal anesthetic, 265–266
  intracranial. See *Intracranial pressure.*
  intragastric, succinylcholine and, 203
  intraocular, succinylcholine and, 202
  intrapleural, 492
  left atrial, monitoring of, 91
  lung, excessive, 432
    and air embolism, 433, *433*
  partial, of inhalation anesthetics, in alveolar gas. See *Alveolar anesthetic tension.*
  perfusion, 501, *502*
  perivascular, and pulmonary vessels, 500
  pulmonary artery, 500, *502*
  pulmonary venous, 500, *502*
  pulmonary wedge, 500
    monitoring of, 91–92
    and rapid fluid replacement, 339
  transpulmonary, 489
  transthoracic, 491

Pressure (*Continued*)
  vapor, of inhalation anesthetics, 137–138, *138*
  of volatile anesthetics, and temperature, 65, *66*
  within anesthesia machine, 100
Pressure-reducing valves, for anesthesia machines, *60*, 63–64, *64*
Prilocaine, 249
Proaccelerin, 336
Procainamide, in cardiac arrhythmias, 28
  in malignant hyperthermia, 430
Procaine, 247, 252(t)
  antiarrhythmic action of, 255
  early use of, 16
  for continuous spinal anesthesia, 271
  in caudal anesthesia, 286
  in cervical plexus block, 289
  in intra-arterial barbiturate injection, 182
  intravenous use of, 251
Promazine, as analgesic, 40
Promethazine, 183
  preoperative, 40
Propanidid, intravenous, 192–193
Propiomazine, as analgesic, 40
Propranediol carbamates, anesthesia and, 33
Propranolol, anesthesia and, 28
  in deliberate hypotension, 398
  in thyrotoxicosis, 30
Prostigmine, anticholinergics and, 44
  in reversal of neuromuscular block, 213
Protein, anesthetics and, 124
  extravascular, transfer of to intravascular space, 331
Prothrombin, in blood transfusions, 337
Pseudocholinesterase, abnormal activity of, and neuromuscular blockers, 207
  and succinylcholine, 206
Psychoactive drugs, 33
Psychological causes of pain, 395
Psychological problems, in intensive care, 469
PTF, 212
Ptosis, of eyelid, stellate ganglion block and, 304
Pudendal nerve, block of, in labor, 353
Pulmonary artery pressure, 500, *502*
Pulmonary barotrauma, positive airway pressure and, 519
Pulmonary circulation, 500–504
  regional distribution of, 501–503, *502*
Pulmonary insufficiency, acute, respiratory support in, 515
Pulmonary rehabilitation clinics, 393–394
Pulmonary vascular resistance, 500
Pulmonary venous pressure, 500, *502*
Pulmonary wedge pressure, 500
  monitoring of, 91–92
  and rapid fluid replacement, 339
Pulse, anesthesia record of, 106
  monitoring of, 87

Pump, arterial, 401
Pump oxygenator, 401–403, *401, 402*
Punch card system, for anesthesia records, 108
Pupils, in cardiopulmonary resuscitation, 458
  in stages of anesthesia, 232, *233*
PVR, 500
Pyloric stenosis, metabolic acidosis of, 372
Pyridostigmine, in reversal of neuromuscular block, 213

Quaternary ammonium compounds, in sterilization, 83
Quelicin. See *Succinylcholine.*
Quinidine, in cardiac arrhythmias, 28

Rachi-resistance, 272
Radial artery cannula, in direct measurement of blood pressure, 93
Radial nerve, block of, at elbow, 297, *297*
  at wrist, 298, *299*
  injury to, 431
RDS of newborn, 362
Receptors, of nerve and muscle membrane, 197
Record, anesthesia. See *Anesthesia record.*
  recovery room, 466–467, *468*
  use of, for statistical purposes, 108–109
Recovery room, 464–469
  admission and release of patients, 467–469
  care in, 460–470
  design and facilities of, 464–466
  after deliberate hypotension, 399
  for ambulatory patient, 391
  drugs in, 467(t)
  personnel in, 464
  record of, 466–467, *468*
  responsibility of anesthetist in, 57
Rectal anesthetic, blood levels of, 136
Red blood cells, leukocyte-deficient, 336
  packed, 335–336
  reconstituted frozen, 336
Reflex, eyelid, 232
  vomiting, 234
Reflex response, 238, *239*
Regional anesthesia, 5, 242–308
  for ambulatory patients, 391
  for cesarean section, 354
  in labor, *350*
  in pain, 395
  intravenous, 306–307
    technique for, 307
  obstetric, *350*, 351–353
Regional nerve block, 288–308
Rehabilitation, in chronic obstructive pulmonary disease, 393
  in chronic pain, 395

Index   551

Relaxation, muscle. See *Muscle, relaxation of.*
Renal. See also *Kidney.*
Renal plasma flow, inhalation anesthetics and, 144
Renin, and extracellular fluid volume, 316, *316*
Reserpine, in hypertension, 29
  in thyrotoxicosis, 30
Reservoir bag, 162, 163(t)
  compression of, in assisted respiration, 75
  for anesthesia machines, 60, 64–65
  in bag and mask resuscitation, 450
  in oxygen therapy, 475, *476*
Resident physician, responsibility of, 54–55
Resistance, airway, 493
  in tracheal intubation, 229
Respiration, 485–521
  abnormal patterns of, in inhalation anesthesia, 127
  anesthesia and, 4
  anesthesia record of, 106
  assisted, anesthesia record of, 105
    by compression of reservoir bag, 75
    mechanical ventilator on anesthesia machine for, 73
  carbon dioxide and, analgetics and, 41, *42*
    premedication and, *39*
  controlled, and respiratory failure, 448
    anesthesia record of, 105
  cyclopropane and, 152
  depressed, analgetics and, 41, *42*
    in inhalation anesthesia, 126
    opioids and, 349
    premedication overdosage and, 126
  diethyl ether and, 154
  exercises for, in chronic obstructive pulmonary disease, 394
  failure of, 236, 512–514, 513(t)
    acute, intrapulmonary shunt in, 510
    causes of, 447
    tracheal intubation in, 515–516, 516(t)
  frequency of, monitoring of, 95–96
  halothane and, 157
  in metabolic disturbances in acid-base balance, 499, 511
  in pregnancy, 347
  in stages of anesthesia, 232, *233*
  increased resistance to, in tracheal intubation, 229
  inhalation anesthetics and, 141–147
  intravenous barbiturates and, 178
  intravenous morphine and, 191
  ketamine and, 188
  local anesthetics and, 255
  mechanics of, 488–494
  monitoring of, 95–97
  mouth-to-mouth, 448, *449*
  mouth-to-nose, 448
  neuroleptanesthesia and, 184

Respiration (*Continued*)
  obstruction of, correction of, 127, *128*
    in inhalation anesthesia, 127
    restrictive or obstructive dressings and, 462
  positive pressure, in resuscitation, 450
  postoperative, in child, 384
  premedication and, 38, *39*
  problems with, anesthesia record of, 107
    in inhalation anesthesia, 126–130
    postoperative, 461–462
  regulation of, oxygen in, 511
  spinal anesthesia and, 262, 272
  support of, in acute pulmonary insufficiency, 515
    management of, 518–519
Respiratory acidosis. See *Acidosis, respiratory.*
Respiratory alkalosis, 328
Respiratory care, 485–521
  role of anesthetist in, 515–520
Respiratory dead space, 496–500, *497*
Respiratory distress, in infant, 371
Respiratory distress syndrome, adult, 513
  of newborn, 362
Respiratory exchange ratio, 496
Respiratory insufficiency, and choice of anesthesia, 18–19
  diagnosis of, 514
Respiratory muscles, 510
Respiratory paralysis, antibiotics and, 31
Respiratory resuscitation, 447–451
  bag and mask technique of, 449–450, *450*
  expired air techniques of, 448–449, *449*
  manual methods of, 450–451
Respiratory system
  compliance of, 492
    with mechanical ventilation, 518
  mechanical properties of, 489
  of child, 364–366, 365(t)
Respiratory therapy, 471, 472(t)
Respiratory tract, anesthesia and, record of, 107
  infection of, in child, 370
Response assessment, 238, 239(t). See also *Motor response,* and *Sensory response.*
Restlessness, postoperative, 463
Resuscitation
  cardiac, 451–454
    external chest compression in, 452, *453*
  cardiopulmonary, 5, 447–459
    procedure for, 454–457, *455*, 455(t)
  of newborn, 359
  respiratory, 447–451
    bag and mask technique of, 449–450, *450*
    expired air techniques of, 448–449, *449*
    manual methods of, 450–451
Resuscitator, Ruben-Ambu, *450*
Retching, in inhalation anesthesia, 130

Retrolental fibroplasia, oxygen and, 385, 478
Ringer's solution, in intravascular volume expansion, 331
  in prevention of hypotension, 414
Riva-Rocci method of measuring blood pressure, 88, 101
Robinul, preoperative, 45
Rotameters, for anesthesia machines, *60, 64*
RPF, inhalation anesthetics and, 144
Rubber, solubility of halothane in, 140(t), 155
  solubility of inhalation anesthetics in, 138, 140(t)
  solubility of methoxyflurane in, 140(t), 157
Ruben-Ambu resuscitator, *450*

Sacral anesthesia. See *Caudal anesthesia.*
Sacral approach, for spinal anesthesia, 269
Sacral canal, anatomy of, 284
Sacrum, anatomy of, 284
Saline
  administration of, excess, 321(t), 322
  in intravascular volume expansion, 331
  isotonic, 319
    administration of, excess, 322
    indications for, 323
Saliva, secretion of, in inhalation anesthesia, 129
Salt. See *Saline,* and *Sodium.*
Scalp vein needle, 341
Scavenger systems, for anesthesia machines, *72, 73*
Sciatic nerve, block of, 301
Scopolamine, in cardiac surgery, 404
  preoperative, 44
Secobarbital, and hypotension, 411
  and local anesthetics, 257
  preoperative, 38
Second gas effect, in uptake of inhalation anesthetics, 120
Secretions, bronchial, mucociliary clearance of, 487
  mucous and salivary, in inhalation anesthesia, 129
  respiratory tract, in mechanical ventilation, 519
Sedatives, 33
  preoperative, 37–40
    nonbarbiturate, 39
Seizures, enflurane and, 159
Sellick's maneuver, 428
Semiclosed systems, for inhalation anesthesia, 168
Semiopen systems, for inhalation anesthesia, 165–168
Sensory response, 238, *239*
  block of, peridural anesthesia and, 280
    spinal anesthesia and, 261
  disturbance of, anesthesia record of, 106
  intravenous barbiturates and, 178

Septic shock, and hypotension, 421
Shivering, postoperative, 462
Shock
  electric, 439
  in assessing neuromuscular block, 211
  in cardiopulmonary resuscitation, 454
  hypovolemic, whole blood in, 332
  septic, and hypotension, 421
Shunt, intrapulmonary, 510
Sierra nonrebreathing valve, 374, *375*
Sighing mechanism, depression of, 142
Sight, lumbar puncture and, 275
Sinoauricular node, vasopressors and, 424
Skin
  circulation to, inhalation anesthetics and, 144
  in cyanosis, 96
  preparation of, for lumbar puncture, 269
    for nerve blocks, 80
    for peridural anesthesia, 282
    for venipuncture, 342
  temperature of, in paravertebral lumbar block, 306
  in stellate ganglion block, 304
Sleep, sedatives and, 37
Slip joint, for tracheal tubes, 219, *219*
Soda lime, as carbon dioxide absorber, 69
  reaction of trichloroethylene with, 158
Sodium, extracellular, 312, *314*
  in extracellular fluid tonicity, 316, *316*
  in water intoxication, 322
Sodium bicarbonate, in acidosis in newborn, 361
  in cardiopulmonary resuscitation, 454, 455(t)
  in dehydration, 319
Sodium nitroprusside, in hypertension, 461
Somatic nerve, paravertebral, block of, 292
Sparine, as analgetic, 40
Spinal anesthesia, 260–277
  and hypotension, 261, 272, 414–415
  anesthesia record of, 104
  choice of, 267–268
  continuous, 271
  delayed sequelae of, 273–276
  equipment for, 266–267, *267*
  factors influencing, 262–266
  in labor, 352
  level of, anesthesia record of, 106
  lumbar puncture for, 268–271, *270*
  management of, 271–273
  physiologic effects of, 261–262
  preparation for, 268
  sterilization for, 266–267
Spinal anesthetic
  dosage of, 263, *264,* 264(t)
  duration of action of, 262–263
  injection of, 268–271, *270*
    sequelae of, 275–276
    serial, 263
  intra-abdominal pressure and obesity and, 265–266

Spinal anesthetic (*Continued*)
  patient position and, 266
  solution of, specific gravity of, 265
Spinal column, curvature of, and spinal anesthesia, 265, *265*
Spinal nerve, anatomy of, 288, *289*
Spirometer, in measuring tidal volume, 95, *96*
  incentive, 482
Splanchnic circulation, inhalation anesthetics and, 144
Starling's law, 503
Static electricity, 443
Stellate ganglion
  anatomy of, 302
  block of, 302
    complications of, 304
    technique for, 303, *304*
Stenosis, pyloric, metabolic acidosis of, 372
  tracheal, tracheal intubation and, 516
Sterilization
  chemical, 82-83
  for peridural anesthesia, 281
  for spinal anesthesia, 266-267
  gas, 83-84
  heat, 81-82
  in pediatric anesthesia, 376
  of equipment for anesthesia and inhalation therapy, 81-84
Sternocleidomastoid muscle, in stellate ganglion block, 303
Sternomastoid muscle, in cervical plexus block, 290, *290*
Sternum, compression of, in cardiac resuscitation, 452
Steroid(s)
  and hypotension, 412
  anesthesia and, 31
  in inhalation therapy, 484
  in malignant hyperthermia, 430
  in septic shock, 421
Steroid anesthesia, 190
Stethoscope, in operating room, 47, 87, *88*
  in pediatric anesthesia, 377
Stimulus assessment, 238
Stimulus-response assessment, 237-240
Stomach, absorption of drugs in, 23
  contents of, aspiration of. See *Aspiration, of gastric contents.*
  drainage of, prior to anesthesia, 428
Streptomycin, anesthesia and, 31
Subarachnoid anesthesia, in labor, 352
Subarachnoid space, action and fate of anesthetics in, 260-261
  injection of anesthetics in, 284
Sublimazine. See *Fentanyl.*
Succinylcholine, 197
  action of, 198, *200*
    rapid onset of, 206
  in ambulatory patients, 391
  in cesarean section, 355

Succinylcholine (*Continued*)
  in convulsions, 257
  in tracheal intubation, 224
    in child, 381
  side effects of, 202-203
Superior vena cava obstruction, and increased central venous pressure, 90
Supine hypotensive syndrome, 348
Supraclavicular brachial plexus block, 295-296, *295*
Surfactant, in lung, 490
Surgeon, relationship to anesthetist, 6-8
Surgery
  abdominal, and hypotension, 418
  and changes in gas flow, 172
  anesthesia and, 113-144
  cardiac, 400
    analgetics in, 41
  and cardiac arrest, 452
  consent for, on anesthesia record, 104
  coronary artery, 403
  elective, routine parenteral fluid therapy in, 317
  emergency, 13, 15
    aspiration of gastric contents during, 427
  for ambulatory patients, anesthesia in, 5, 388-393
    patient selection for, 388, 391(t)
    types of, 389, 391(t)
  in deliberate hypotension, 399
  maneuvers in, and hypotension, 418-419, *418*
  neck, and hypotension, 418
  on leg, nerve blocks for, 300
Surgical anesthesia, 234-236
Surital, 174, *175*
Sympathetic nerve block, 302-306
Synapse, anesthetics and, 125
Systemic diseases, and neuromuscular blockers, 207
Systemic reactions, to local anesthetics, 255-257
Systole, open chest manual, 456-457, *457*
  external manual cardiac, 452-454, *453*

Tachycardia
  anticholinergics in, 45
  blood loss and, 417
  gallamine and, 204
  vasopressors and, 425
  ventricular, and hypotension, 420
Tachypnea, 127
  inhalation anesthetics and, 141
Talwin, as analgetic, 43
  preoperative, in child, 373
Tamponade, cardiac, and hypotension, 420
  pericardial, and increased central venous pressure, 90
Tape, adhesive, and static electricity, 443
Taylor approach, for spinal anesthesia, 269

TBP, in extracorporeal circulation, 405
Teeth, in tracheal intubation, 221
Temperature
  and newborn, 360
  and vaporization of volatile gases, 65, 66
  body. See also *Hyperthermia* and *Hypothermia*.
    and neuromuscular blockers, 208
    and postoperative shivering, 462
    monitoring of, 98–99
    in child, control of, 367–368
      monitoring of, 376
      postoperative, 384
  of face mask, in open drop method, 165
  of inspired air, 480
  skin, in paravertebral lumbar block, 306
    in stellate ganglion block, 304
Tensilon, in reversal of neuromuscular block, 213
Tension, alveolar anesthetic. See *Alveolar anesthetic tension*.
  arterial blood anesthetic, 119, *119*
Tension pneumothorax, monitoring of blood pressure in, 90
Tent, oxygen, 474
Test, Allen's, 93
  Coombs, in blood crossmatching, 334
  oxytocin challenge, 357
Tetanic fade, 212
Tetanus, diazepam in, 191
  in assessing neuromuscular block, 211, *212*
Tetracaine, 247, 252(t)
  and duration of spinal anesthesia, 262
  and hypotension, 414
  dosage of, for spinal anesthesia, 263, *264*, 264(t)
  for continuous spinal anesthesia, 271
  in cesarean section, 355
  in stellate ganglion block, 305
Thermistor, in monitoring cardiac output, 92
  in temperature monitoring, 99
Thermocouple, in temperature monitoring, 99
Thermometers, in pediatric anesthesia, 377
  in temperature monitoring, 99
Thiamylal, 174, *175*
Thiazides, anesthesia and, 29
Thigh, surgery on, nerve blocks for, 300
Thiobarbiturates, 174
  biotransformation of, 177
Thiopental, 16, 174, *175*
  and laryngospasm, 178
  and local anesthetics, 257
  distribution of, 176, *176*
  for delivery, 353
  in cesarean section, 355
  preoperative, in child, 373
Thoracic nerves, block of, 291
Thoracotomy, 456
Thorax, surgery in, and hypotension, 418

Throat, sore, following tracheal extubation, 229
Thrombocytopenia, blood transfusion and, 337
  platelet transfusion in, 337
Thromboembolic disease, treatment of, 30
Thrombophlebitis, plastic catheter for fluid therapy and, 341
Thromboplastins, in coagulopathy, 337
Thrombosis, arterial, intra-arterial barbiturate injection and, 182
Thymol, accumulation of, in vaporizers, 69
Thyroid, drugs affecting, 30
Thyroid storm, 30
Thyroidectomy, air embolism in, 434
Thyrotoxicosis, anesthesia in, 20
  anticholinergics in, 45
  treatment of, 30
Tibial nerve, block of, 302, *303*
Tidal volume, 488
  in assessing neuromuscular block, 213
  monitoring of, 95–96, *96*
Tissue(s), carbon dioxide transport to, from lung, 485, 504–510
  destruction of, local anesthetics and, 257–258
  inhalation anesthetics in, 116
To-and-fro technique, for inhalation anesthesia, 168
Toe, nerve block of, 302
Tolerance, to barbiturates, 177
Topical anesthesia, 251–255
Tourniquet, for intravenous regional anesthesia, 306
Tourniquet pain, brachial plexus block and, 296
Total bypass, in extracorporeal circulation, 405
T-piece, Ayre's, 166–167, *167*
  in pediatric anesthesia, 374, *374, 386*
Trachea, 486
  collapse of, after tracheal extubation, 229
  edema or infection of, after tracheal extubation, 229
  mucous membrane of, ulceration of, after tracheal extubation, 229
  topical anesthesia of, 255
  tumors displacing, tracheal intubation in, 225
Tracheal catheter, anesthesia record of, 104
Tracheal extubation, 228
  complications of, 229–230
  in child, 384
Tracheal intubation, 174–241, 216–230
  anesthesia record of, 104
  care after, 227–228
  complications of, 228–230
  cough in, 129, 225, 227
  equipment for, 216–220, *217*, 218(t), *219, 221*
  in child, 375, *375*, 376(t)

Index

Tracheal intubation (*Continued*)
  for delivery, 353
  in ambulatory patients, 391
  in child, 379–382
  in preventing aspiration of gastric contents, 428
  in respiratory failure, 515–516, 516(t)
  intravenous barbiturates with, 179
  laryngeal edema after, in child, 386
  neuroleptanesthesia for, 186
  neuromuscular blockers in, 224
  sequelae of, anesthesia record of, 107
  succinylcholine in, 210
  techniques of, 220–227
  topical anesthesia for, 251
  with curved blade, 224
  with straight blade, 223, *223*
Tracheal stenosis, tracheal intubation and, 516
Tracheal tug, 236
Tracheoesophageal fistula, tracheal intubation and, 516
Tracheostomy, in respiratory failure, 515–516
Train-of-four, in assessing neuromuscular block, 211, *212*
Tranquilizers, 33
  after ketamine anesthesia, 189
  and hypotension, 412
  in labor, 349
  preoperative, 39
Transfusion, blood. See *Blood, transfusion of.*
Translaryngeal intubation, 516
Transmural pressure, and pulmonary vessels, 500
Transpulmonary pressure, 489
Transthoracic pressure, 491
Trauma, during tracheal intubation, 229
Trichloroethylene, 158
  in carbon dioxide absorption systems, 71
  solubility of, in rubber, 140(t), 158
Tricyclic antidepressants, anesthesia and, 33
Triflupromazine, as analgetic, 40
Trilene, 158
  in carbon dioxide absorption systems, 71
  solubility of, in rubber, 140(t), 158
Trimethaphan, in deliberate hypotension, 398
  in hypertension, 461
Trimethylene. See *Cyclopropane.*
Tube(s)
  conducting, for compressed gases, 71
  nasotracheal, 226, 515
  tracheal, 216–219, *217*, 218(t)
    connectors for, 219, *219*
    dislodgment of, 229
    in pediatric anesthesia, 375, *375*, 376(t)
    inflatable cuffs for, 219, 516
    lubricants for, 220, 380
    obstruction of, 229

Tuberculosis, sterilization in, 85
Tubocurarine, 199
  action of, 199, *201, 202*
  biliary excretion of, 206
  plasma protein binding of, 205
  side effects of, 203–204
Tubules, renal, in drug excretion, 25
  necrosis of, acute, hemolysis and, 333
  postoperative, 20
Tumors, displacing trachea or larynx, tracheal intubation in, 225
Twitch response of muscle, depolarization and, 199, *200*
  in assessing neuromuscular block, 211, *212*
  neuromuscular block and, 200, *201, 202*
Tympanic membrane, in temperature measurement, 99

Ulceration, of tracheal mucous membranes, after tracheal extubation, 229
  of vocal cords, after tracheal extubation, 229
Ulnar artery, evaluation of, 93
Ulnar nerve
  block of, at elbow, 298
    at wrist, 298, *299*
  injury to, 431
  stimulation of, in assessing neuromuscular block, 211
Ultraviolet light, to prevent transmission of infection, 79
Upper extremity, nerve blocks of, 292–300
Urea, extracellular, 312
Urinary bladder, anesthesia and, record of, 107
  catheterization of, 97
Urinary tract, spinal anesthesia and, 262
Urine
  hemoglobin in, 333
  output of, blood loss and, 417
    depressed cardiac output and, 519
    in dehydration, 318
    in measuring fluid replacement, 98
  measurement of, 97
  volume of, decrease in, anesthesia and, 146
Urticaria, blood transfusion and, 334
Uterus, contractions of, monitoring of, 356, *358*
  traction on, and hypotension, 418

Valve(s)
  directional, in inhalation anesthesia systems, 163, 163(t)
  escape, and gas flow rate, 172
  for anesthesia machines, 72
  for carbon dioxide absorbers, 69

Valve(s) (*Continued*)
  gas scavenger, for anesthesia machines, 72, 73
  pressure-reducing, for anesthesia machines, 60, 63–64, 64
  Sierra nonrebreathing, 374, 375
  waste gas scavenger, 72, 73
Valium. See *Diazepam*.
Vapor pressure, of inhalation anesthetics, 137–138, 138
  of volatile anesthetics, and temperature, 65, 66
Vaporization, of volatile anesthetics, 171
  of volatile liquids, 65–66, 138
Vaporizers, 65–69, 67, 68
  agent-specific, 68, 68
  and concentration of anesthetic, 171
  Copper Kettle, 60, 66, 67
  Fluotec, 68, 68
Vascularity, of peridural space, 280
Vasoconstriction
  blood loss and, 331
  cocaine and, 246
  inhalation therapy for, 482
  raised airway pressure and, 415
  renal, halothane and, 144
  spinal anesthesia and, 262
  vasopressors and, 425
Vasodilation
  cerebral, carbon dioxide inhalation in, 479
  inhalation anesthetics and, 143
  cutaneous, inhalation anesthetics and, 144
  in deliberate hypotension, 396
  inhalation anesthetics and, 413
  isotonic saline in, 323
Vasopressors
  in cardiopulmonary resuscitation, 454
  in circulatory depression, 257
  in hypotension, 414, 424, 424(t)
    prevention of, 414
  in spinal anesthesia, 269, 272
Vasoxyl, in hypotension, 424, 424(t)
Vena cava, superior, obstruction of, and increased central venous pressure, 90
Venipuncture, 342, 344
Venous blood, concentration of inhalation anesthetics in, 117
  during inhalation anesthesia, 131
Ventilation
  alveolar, analgetics and, 41, 42
  determination of, 498
  in newborn and adult, 365, 365(t)
  monitoring of, 95, 97
  and perfusion, in lungs, 487, 507–510
  carbon dioxide and, 142, 142
  controlled, 4, 518
  in deliberate hypotension, 397
  enflurane and, 159
  intermittent mandatory, 520
  intermittent positive pressure, 517
  mechanical, 517

Ventilation (*Continued*)
  minute, 488
  pulmonary, 487
    and metabolic rate, 499
    regulation of, 510–512
  respiratory, 496–500
  support of, 516–517, 517(t)
Ventilation diagram, carbon dioxide, 142, 142
Ventilator(s)
  compressed gases for, 74
  mechanical, monitoring of patient on, 518
  use of, on anesthesia machines, 73–75, 74
  types of, 517
  weaning from, 520
Ventilatory response curve, carbon dioxide, 142, 142
Ventricular fibrillation, causes of, 451
Ventricular tachycardia, and hypotension, 420
Venturi device, for high flow oxygen therapy, 474, 474, 477(t)
Vesprin, analgetic, 40
Vessels
  construction of. See *Vasoconstriction*.
  dilation of. See *Vasodilation*.
  peripheral, vasopressors and, 425
  pulmonary, 500
Visceral function, disturbances of, anesthesia record of, 107
Vision, lumbar puncture and, 275
Vistaril, in labor, 351
  preoperative, 40
Vocal cords
  paralysis of, after tracheal extubation, 230
    brachial plexus block and, 293
  ulceration and granuloma of, after tracheal extubation, 229
Volatile anesthetics, 153–160
  vaporization of, 171
Volatile liquids, boiling point of, 137, 139(t)
  vapor pressure of, 137, 138
  vaporization of, 65–66, 138
Vomiting
  analgetics and, 42
  anesthesia record of, 107
  in inhalation anesthesia, 130
  intravenous barbiturates and, 182
  local anesthetics and, 258
  postoperative, prevention of, 40
  spinal anesthesia and, 272
Vomiting reflex, 234
Vomitus, aspiration of. See *Aspiration, of gastric contents*.

Wall, abdominal, intercostal block and, 291
  chest, mechanical (elastic) properties of, 491, 491
  spasm of, in tracheal intubation, 229

Waste gas scavenger systems, for anesthesia machines, 72, *73*
Water
 administration of, excess, 321–322, 321(t)
 conservation of, 317
 in inspired air, 480
 intoxication with, 321
 total body, 310
Weight, of patient, anesthesia record of, 104
Wescodyne, in sterilization, 84
Woodbridge's components of anesthesia, 238, *239*

Wright anemometer, *96*
Wrist, nerve block at, 298–299, *299*
Wyamine, in hypotension, 424, 424(t)

Xylocaine. See *Lidocaine*.

Y-piece, in endotracheal anesthesia, 167

Zephiran, as cutaneous antiseptic, 80